INTERNAL
MEDICINE
CLERKSHIP GUIDE

INTERNAL
MEDICINE
CLERKSHIP GUIDE

THIRD EDITION

Douglas S. Paauw, MD, FACP

Professor
Division of General Internal Medicine
Director, Medicine Student Program
Rathman Family Foundation Endowed Chair for Patient-Centered
  Clinical Education
Department of Medicine
University of Washington School of Medicine
Seattle, Washington

Mary B. Migeon, MD

Associate Professor
Division of General Internal Medicine
Department of Medicine
University of Washington School of Medicine
Seattle, Washington

Lisanne R. Burkholder, MD, MPH, FACP

Associate Professor
School of Rural Health
University of Melbourne
Specialist Consultant in General Medicine
Goulburn Valley Health
Shepparton, Australia

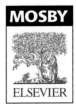

MOSBY

ELSEVIER

MOSBY
ELSEVIER

1600 John F. Kennedy Blvd.
Ste 1800
Philadelphia, PA 19103–2899

INTERNAL MEDICINE CLERKSHIP GUIDE   ISBN: 978-0-323-04558-2
Copyright © 2008, 2003, 1999 by Mosby, Inc., an affiliate of Elsevier Inc.

Notice

Knowledge and best practice in this field are constantly changing. As new research and experience broaden our knowledge, changes in practice, treatment and drug therapy may become necessary or appropriate. Readers are advised to check the most current information provided (i) on procedures featured or (ii) by the manufacturer of each product to be administered, to verify the recommended dose or formula, the method and duration of administration, and contraindications. It is the responsibility of the practitioner, relying on their own experience and knowledge of the patient, to make diagnoses, to determine dosages and the best treatment for each individual patient, and to take all appropriate safety precautions. To the fullest extent of the law, neither the Publisher nor the Authors assume any liability for any injury and/or damage to persons or property arising out or related to any use of the material contained in this book.

The Publisher

Library of Congress Cataloging-in-Publication Data
Internal medicine clerkship guide / [edited by] Douglas S. Paauw, Mary B. Migeon, Lisanne R. Burkholder. – 3rd ed.
   p.; cm.
  Includes bibliographical references and index.
  ISBN-13: 978-0-323-04558-2
  ISBN-10: 0-323-04558-8
  1. Internal medicine. 2. Clinical clerkship. I. Paauw, Douglas S. (Douglas Stephen), 1958- II. Migeon, Mary B. III. Burkholder, Lisanne R.
  [DNLM: 1. Clinical Clerkship. 2. Internal Medicine. WB 115 I6065 2008]
RC46.G896 2008
616–dc22
                                            2007006395

Acquisitions Editor: James Merritt
Developmental Editor: Nicole DiCicco
Publishing Services Manager: Linda Van Pelt
Project Manager: Francisco Morales
Design Direction: Louis Forgione

> ### Working together to grow libraries in developing countries
> www.elsevier.com | www.bookaid.org | www.sabre.org
>
> ELSEVIER   BOOK AID International   Sabre Foundation

Printed in USA
Last digit is the print number: 9 8 7 6 5 4 3 2 1

To Kathy and Carly
Glen and Kristen
Jacques, Sophie and Jonathan
In memory of Bruce Gilliland, invaluable mentor and teacher
In memory of George Aagaard

Contributors Listing

Bradley D. Anawalt, MD
Associate Professor
Department of Medicine
University of Washington School of Medicine
Associate Chief of Medicine
VA Puget Sound
Seattle, Washington

Amy Baernstein, MD
Assistant Professor
Division of General Internal Medicine
Department of Medicine
University of Washington School of Medicine
Seattle, Washington

Ernie-Paul Barrette, MD, FACP
General Internal Medicine
Belle Greve 317
Metrohealth Medical Center
Cleveland, Ohio

Lisanne R. Burkholder, MD, MPH, FACP
Associate Professor
School of Rural Health
University of Melbourne
Specialist Consultant in General Medicine
Goulburn Valley Health
Shepparton, Australia

Andrea Akita Chun, MD
Internal Medicine
Group Health Cooperative
Poulsbo, Washington

Sarah L. Clever, MD
Assistant Professor
Department of Medicine
Johns Hopkins School of Medicine
Baltimore, Maryland

Dawn E. DeWitt, MD, MSc, FACP, FRACP
Professor
Head, School of Rural Health
Dean, Rural Clinical School
University of Melbourne
Melbourne, Australia

Anne Eacker, MD
Assistant Professor
Division of General Internal Medicine
Department of Medicine
University of Washington School of Medicine
Seattle, Washington

Keith D. Eaton, MD, PhD
Assistant Professor
Division of Medical Oncology
University of Washington School of Medicine
Seattle, Washington

Timothy C. Evans, MD, PhD, FACP
Associate Professor
Medicine and of Medical Education and Biomedical Informatics
Medical Director
MEDEX Northwest University of Washington School of Medicine
Seattle, Washington

Kelly Fryer-Edwards, PhD
Assistant Professor
Department of Medical History & Ethics
University of Washington School of Medicine
Seattle, Washington

Gregory C. Gardner, MD
Professor, Rheumatology
Adjunct Professor, Orthopaedic Surgery and
    Rehabilitation Medicine
University of Washington School of Medicine
Seattle, Washington

Barak Gaster, MD
Associate Professor
Division of General Internal Medicine
Department of Medicine
University of Washington School of Medicine
Seattle, Washington

Karna Gendo, MD
Hospitalist/Allergist
Group Health Permanente
Redmond, Washington

Deborah L. Greenberg, MD
Associate Professor
Division of General Internal Medicine
Department of Medicine
University of Washington School of Medicine
Seattle, Washington

Melissa M. Hagman, MD
Assistant Professor
Division of General Internal Medicine
Department of Medicine
University of Washington School of Medicine
Seattle, Washington

Matthew F. Hollon, MD, MPH
Assistant Professor
Division of General Internal Medicine
Department of Medicine
University of Washington School of Medicine
Seattle, Washington

Robert R. Kempainen, MD
Assistant Professor
Pulmonary and Critical Care Medicine
Department of Medicine
University of Minnesota
Minneapolis, Minnesota

Lindsey S. Klaff, MD
Acting Instructor
Harborview Medical Center
Division of General Internal Medicine
Department of Medicine
University of Washington School of Medicine
Seattle, Washington

Christopher Knight, MD
Assistant Professor
Division of General Internal Medicine
Department of Medicine
University of Washington School of Medicine
Seattle, Washington

Eric E. Kraus, MD
Associate Professor
Department of Neurology
University of Washington School of Medicine
Seattle, Washington

Mary B. Laya, MD, MPH
Associate Professor
Division of General Internal Medicine
Department of Medicine
University of Washington School of Medicine
Seattle, Washington

Abhijit P. Limaye, MD
Associate Professor
Division of Laboratory Medicine and Medicine
Department of Medicine
University of Washington School of Medicine
Seattle, Washington

Mary B. Migeon, MD
Associate Professor
Division of General Internal Medicine
Department of Medicine
University of Washington School of Medicine
Seattle, Washington

George Novan, MD
Clinical Professor
Department of Medicine
University of Washington School of Medicine
Seattle, Washington
Clerkship Coordinator
Internal Medicine Residency Spokane
Spokane, Washington

Kim O'Connor, MD
Assistant Professor
Division of General Internal Medicine
Department of Medicine
University of Washington School of Medicine
Seattle, Washington

Douglas S. Paauw, MD, FACP
Professor
Division of General Internal Medicine
Director, Medicine Student Program
Rathman Family Foundation Endowed Chair for Patient-Centered
   Clinical Education
Department of Medicine
University of Washington School of Medicine
Seattle, Washington

Genevieve L. Pagalilauan, MD
Assistant Professor
Division of General Internal Medicine
Department of Medicine
University of Washington School of Medicine
Seattle, Washington

Linda E. Pinsky, MD
Associate Professor
Division of General Internal Medicine
Department of Medicine, Director of Residency Ambulatory Education
University of Washington School of Medicine
Seattle, Washington

Heidi S. Powell, MD
Associate Professor
Division of General Internal Medicine
Department of Medicine
University of Washington School of Medicine
Seattle, Washington

Caroline S. Rhoads, MD
Associate Professor
Division of General Internal Medicine
Department of Medicine
University of Washington School of Medicine
Seattle, Washington

Henry Rosen, MD
Professor and Associate Chair
Department of Medicine
University of Washington School of Medicine
Seattle, Washington

Alexander D. Schafir, MD
Clinical Assistant Professor
Oregon Health Sciences University
Providence St. Vincent Medical Center
Portland, Oregon

Anneliese M. Schleyer, MD, MHA
Medical Director of Inpatient Hospitalist Service
Harborview Medical Center
Assistant Professor
Division of General Internal Medicine
Department of Medicine
University of Washington School of Medicine
Seattle, Washington

John V. L. Sheffield, MD
Professor
Division of General Internal Medicine
Department of Medicine
University of Washington School of Medicine
Seattle, Washington

C. Scott Smith, MD, FACP
Professor
Department of Medicine
Adjunct Associate Professor
Medical Education and Biomedical Informatics
University of Washington School of Medicine
Seattle, Washington

Siang Yong Soh, MBBS
Medical Intern
Goulburn Valley Health
Shepparton, Australia

Thomas O. Staiger, MD
Associate Professor
Division of General Internal Medicine
Department of Medicine
University of Washington School of Medicine
Seattle, Washington

Karen Stout, MD
Assistant Professor
Division of Cardiology
Department of Medicine
Department of Pediatrics
Director, Adult Congenital Heart Disease Program
University of Washington School of Medicine
Seattle, Washington

Eliza L. Sutton, MD, FACP
Assistant Professor
Division of General Internal Medicine
Women's Health Care Center
Department of Medicine
University of Washington School of Medicine
Seattle, Washington

Jeffrey I. Wallace, MD, MPH
Associate Professor and Director
Clinical Geriatrics
University of Colorado Health Sciences Center
Denver, Colorado

Acknowledgments

We would like to thank our authors for their timely and excellent efforts, D.C. Dugdale and Dawn DeWitt for sage advice about the world of publishing, and Michael Richardson for enthusiastic and generous sharing of his extensive radiologic website resources. We also appreciate the indispensable support of the Division of General Medicine at the University of Washington Medical Center. Finally, we would like to thank our students, who inspire us with their enthusiasm and whose thoughtful feedback helped shape this book.

Preface

Guide to Internal Medicine
Third Edition

This Guide aims to accompany and aid third-year medical students in that all-important transition from book-learning to the real-world practice of medicine. We present core concepts in Internal Medicine in a purposefully brief format to allow cover-to-cover reading during the Medicine Clerkship. Our goal is to help the third-year clerk build a solid foundation of knowledge on which future detailed reading and study may be layered. Although targeted for third-year students, as the Guide has evolved we have received positive feedback about its utility for learners and educators in other fields including those in Physician Assistant, Nursing, Nurse Practitioner, Family Practice, and Internal Medicine residency training programs.

The Guide is divided into three sections covering basic skills, common symptoms, and common conditions. The text is structured around basic questions frequently asked of students to keep the learner engaged and to keep the learning practical. *Key points* in each chapter help learners focus on core concepts. *Practice cases* apply new learning to real clinical scenarios. *Learning objectives* accompany answers to each case-based problem and emphasize common Internal Medicine problems. A *multiple-choice exam* at the end of the Guide tests your mastery of the material and prepares learners for clinical and board exams.

We sincerely hope this Guide helps students enjoy the process of learning and mastering basic concepts and skills in Internal Medicine.

Abbreviation Terms

A1C	glycosylated hemoglobin
ABG	arterial blood gas
ABI	ankle-brachial index
ACEI	angiotensin-converting enzyme inhibitor
ACIP	Advisory Committee on Immunization Practice
ACTH	adrenocorticotropic hormone
AFB	acid-fast bacillus
AFP	alpha-fetoprotein
AIDS	acquired immune deficiency syndrome
AIN	acute interstitial nephritis
ALL	acute lymphocytic leukemia
ALT	alanine aminotransaminase (same as SGPT)
ANA	antinuclear antibody
Anti LKM1	antibody to liver, kidney microsome type 1
APAS	antiphospholipid antibody
AR	aortic regurgitation
ARF	acute renal failure
AS	aortic stenosis
ASCUS	atypical cells of undetermined significance
ASIS	anterior superior iliac spine
AST	aspartate aminotransaminase (same as SGOT)
ATN	acute tubular necrosis
AUA	American Urology Association
AVNRT	AV node reentrant tachycardia
AZT	zidovudine (azidothymidine)
BCC	basal cell carcinoma
β-HCG	beta human chorionic gonadotropin
BMI	body mass index
BP	blood pressure
BPH	benign prostatic hyperplasia
BPV	benign positional vertigo
BUN	blood urea nitrogen
BV	bacterial vaginosis
CABG	coronary artery bypass graft

CAD	coronary artery disease
cANCA	cytoplasmic antineutrophil cytoplasmic antibody
CBC	complete blood count
CCU	cardiac care unit
CDC	Centers for Disease Control
CEA	carcinoembryonic antigen
CFS	chronic fatigue syndrome
CHF	congestive heart failure
CIE	counterimmunoelectrophoresis
CK	creatine kinase
CLL	chronic lymphocytic leukemia
CML	chronic myelogenous leukemia
CMV	cytomegalovirus
CNS	central nervous system
COPD	chronic obstructive pulmonary disease
CP	creatine phosphokinase
CPAP	continuous positive airway pressure
CPK	creatine phosphokinase
CPR	cardiopulmonary resuscitation
CR	complete remission
CRH	corticotropin-releasing hormone
CSF	cerebrospinal fluid
CT	computed tomography
CV	cardiovascular
CXR	chest x-ray
d4T	stavudine
DCCT	Diabetes Control and Complications Trial
DDAVP	1-deamino(8-D-arginine) vasopressin
ddC	zalcitabine
ddI	didanosine
DGI	disseminated gonococcal infection
DHT	dihydrotestosterone
DIC	disseminated intravascular coagulation
DKA	diabetic ketoacidosis
DLCO	diffusing lung capacity to carbon monoxide
DM	diabetes mellitus (type 1 or 2)
DMARD	disease modifying antirheumatic drug
DNR	do not resuscitate
DUB	dysfunctional uterine bleeding
DVT	deep venous thrombosis
Dx	diagnosis

DXA	dual electron x-ray scan absorptiometry, bone density test
EBV	Epstein-Barr virus
ED	emergency department
EEG	electroencephalogram
EF	ejection fraction
EGD	esophagogastroduodenoscopy
EMG	electromyogram
EOMI	extraocular movements intact
ERCP	endoscopic retrograde cholangiopancreatogram
ERT	estrogen replacement therapy
ESR	erythrocyte sedimentation rate
ETT	exercise tolerance test exercise treadmill test
FAP	familial adenomatous polyposis
FMP	first menstrual period
FNA	fine needle aspiration
FSH	follicle stimulating hormone
FTA-ABS	fluorescent treponemal antibody absorption (test)
GE	gastroesophageal reflux
GERD	gastroesophageal reflux disease
GGT	serum gamma-glutamyltransferase
GI	gastrointestinal
GYN	gynecologic gynecology
H&P	history and physical
HAART	highly active antiretroviral therapy
HBsAg	hepatitis B surface antigen
HBV	hepatitis B virus
HCM	hypertrophic cardiomyopathy
HcT	hematocrit
HCV	hepatitis C virus
HDV	hepatitis D virus
HEENT	head, eyes, ears, nose, and throat
HEV	hepatitis E virus
HF	hot flash
HGSIL	high grade squamous intraepithelial lesion
HHNC	hyperglycemic hyperosmolar nonketotic (diabetic) coma
HIT	heparin-induced thrombocytopenia
HITT	HIT-associated thrombosis
HIV	human immunodeficiency virus

HMG CoA	3-hydroxy-3-methylglutaryl coenzyme A
HNPCC	hereditary nonpolyposis colorectal cancer
HPI	history of present illness
HPV	human papillomavirus
HRT	hormone replacement therapy
HSCT	hematopoietic stem cell transplantation
HSP	Henoch-Schönlein purpura
HSV	herpes simplex virus
HTLV	human T-cell leukemia/lymphoma virus
IBD	inflammatory bowel disease
IBS	irritable bowel syndrome
ICU	intensive care unit
ID/CC	identification and chief complaint
IDU	injection drug user
IL-RA	interleukin/receptor agonist
INH	isoniazid
INR	international normalized ratio, a standardized prothrombin time
ITP	immune thrombocytopenic purpura
IVDU	intravenous drug user
IVIG	intravenous immunoglobulin
JVP	jugular venous pressure
KOH	potassium hydroxide
KS	Kaposi's sarcoma
LCR	ligase chain reaction
LDH	lactate dehydrogenase
LE	leukocyte esterase
LEEP	loop electrical excision procedure
LFTs	liver function tests
LGSIL	low grade squamous intraepithelial lesion
LH	luteinizing hormone
LHRH	luteinizing hormone-releasing factor
LLQ	left lower quadrant
LMW	low molecular weight
LMWH	low-molecular-weight heparin
LOC	level of consciousness
LP	lumbar puncture
LV	left ventricle
LVF	left ventricular failure
LVH	left ventricular hypertrophy
MAC	*Mycobacterium avium* complex
MCA	middle cerebral artery

MCP	metacarpophalangeal
MCV	mean corpuscular volume
MEN-2	multiple endocrine neoplasia syndrome
MI	myocardial infarction
MMR	measles, mumps, rubella
MP	micronized progesterone
MPAN	microscopic polyarteritis nodosa
MR	mitral regurgitation
MRI	magnetic resonance imaging
MSH	melanocyte-stimulating hormone
MSLT	multiple sleep latency test
MTP	metatarsophalangeal
MVA	motor vehicle accident
Na	sodium
NCEP	National Cholesterol Education Program
NG	nasogastric
NHL	non-Hodgkin's lymphoma
NIPPV	noninvasive positive pressure ventilation
NNRTI	non-nucleoside reverse transcriptase inhibitors
NOF	National Osteoporosis Foundation
NPH	no previous history
NPO	nothing by mouth
NPV	negative predictive value
NRTI	nucleoside reverse transcriptase inhibitors
NSAID	nonsteroidal anti-inflammatory drug
NSCLC	non-small cell lung cancer
OCP	oral contraceptive pill
OSA	obstructive sleep apnea
PA (view)	posteroanterior
PAC	premature atrial contractions
PAN	polyarteritis nodosa
PANCA	perinuclear antineutrophil cytoplasmic antibody
PCOS	polycystic ovary syndrome
PCP	*Pneumocystis carinii* pneumonia
PCR	polymerase chain reaction
PE	pulmonary embolus
PEEP	positive end expiratory pressure
PERRLA	pupils equal, round, reactive to light and accommodation
PET	positron emission tomography
PHN	postherpetic neuralgia
PI	protease inhibitors

PID	pelvic inflammatory disease
PLMD	periodic leg movement disorder
PMH	past medical history
PMI	point of maximal impulse (of the heart against the chest wall)
PMN	polymorphonuclear neutrophil (leukocytes)
PMR	polymyalgia rheumatica
PN	peripheral neuropathy
PND	postnasal drip or paroxysmal nocturnal dyspnea
PPD	packs per day (cigarettes)
PPI	proton pump inhibitor
PPV	positive predictive value
PSA	prostate-specific antigen
PSC	primary sclerosing cholangitis
PSG	polysomnogram
PT	prothrombin time
PTA	prior to admission
PTH	parathyroid hormone
PTT	partial thromboplastin time
PTU	propylthiouracil
PUD	peptic ulcer disease
PVC	premature ventricular contractions
PVD	peripheral vascular disease
PVR	postvoid residual
RA	radionuclide angiography rheumatoid arthritis
RAS	reticular activating system
RBC	red blood cells
RF	rheumatoid factor
RLQ	right lower quadrant
RLS	restless leg syndrome
RNA	ribonucleic acid
ROM	range of motion
ROS	review of systems
RPR	rapid plasma reagin
RR	respiratory rate
RUQ	right upper quadrant
SAAG	serum-ascites albumin gradient
SAH	subarachnoid hemorrhage
SBE	subacute bacterial endocarditis
SBP	spontaneous bacterial peritonitis
SCLC	small cell lung cancer

SERMs	selective estrogen receptor modulators
SGOT	serum glutamic-oxaloacetic transaminase (same as AST)
SGPT	serum glutamic-pyruvic transaminase (same as ALT)
SIADH	syndrome of antidiuretic hormone secretion
SLE	systemic lupus erythematosus
SMBG	self-monitoring blood glucose
SPEP	serum protein electrophoresis
SS-A	Sjögren's syndrome antigen A
SS-B	Sjögren's syndrome antigen B
SSRI	selective serotonin reuptake inhibitor
SVT	supraventricular tachycardia
T	temperature
TA	temporal arteritis
TB	tuberculosis
TC	total cholesterol
TCA	tricyclic antidepressant
TEE	transesophageal echocardiography
TG	triglycerides
TIA	transient ischemic attack
TIBC	total iron-binding capacity
TIPS	transjugular intrahepatic portosystemic shunt
TLC	total lung capacity
TMP-SMX	trimethoprim-sulfamethoxazole
tPA	tissue plasminogen activator
TSH	thyroid-stimulating hormone
TTE	transthoracic echocardiography
TURP	transurethral resection of the prostate
U/A	urinalysis
UBT	urea breath test
UPEP	urinary protein electrophoresis
URI	upper respiratory infection
US	ultrasound
UTI	urinary tract infection
VDRL	Venereal Disease Research Laboratory (a test for syphilis)
VS	vital signs
VT	ventricular tachycardia
vWd	von Willebrand's disease
WBC	white blood cell/count
WOB	work of breathing

Table of Contents

Section 3

Patients Presenting with a Known Condition 219

Introduction to the Medicine Clerkship

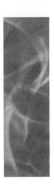

Secrets to Being a Successful Medical Student

1

JOHN V. L. SHEFFIELD

Medicine is not a trade to be learned but a profession to be entered. It is an ever-widening field that requires continued study and prolonged experience in close contact with the sick. All that the medical school can hope to do is to supply the foundations on which to build.
— *Francis W. Peabody, 1927*

 ## WHAT CAN I DO TO BE SUCCESSFUL IN THE INTERNAL MEDICINE CLERKSHIP?

Within the lecture hall, success is often defined by grades. As you enter the clinical years, performance evaluations remain important, but you also must define personal goals and definitions of success that are broader than pass/fail. In the medicine clerkship, you may hope to learn how to provide excellent patient care, develop your history-taking and physical examination skills, improve your presentations, acquire time management skills, and become a careful diagnostician. In addition to building these important clinical skills, a vital measure of success is the degree to which you build a foundation of professionalism in your work habits, behavioral attributes, and values as a caretaker and colleague. In this introductory chapter, the suggestions made are based on extensive experience working with students, and it is hoped that they will help you excel in the clerkship and enjoy the experience.

Be Enthusiastic

Your energy level, desire to learn, and spirit will motivate your residents and attendings to teach and involve you in patient care. With enthusiasm, a student with an average knowledge base provides exceptional care and is a vital team member. Without enthusiasm, a brilliant student appears disinterested and is a less effective team member and physician.

Know Your Patients

An excellent student has complete and timely command of a patient's history, physical exam, and lab test results; strives to understand basic pathophysiologic principles underlying patient conditions; is aware of diagnostic and therapeutic options available; and seeks to understand the personal and social factors that may influence the patient's response to therapy.

Care About Your Patients

Assume personal responsibility for the quality of care your patients receive. Monitor their progress closely, and spend time at the bedside to answer questions and discuss matters other than symptoms. Although team hierarchy gives residents and attendings precedence, your patients will view you as their primary physician if you establish a caring rapport.

Communicate with Precision

Your chart notes and oral presentations are your opportunity to show your fund of knowledge, problem-solving skill, and ability to think clearly. Legible and precise order writing is essential to good patient care. Careful explanation of the treatment plan to nursing staff ensures that your intended plan is followed.

Distinguish Between Major and Minor Problems

As important as being able to identify all of your patient's problems is the ability to put major and minor problems in perspective. At first, it is natural to consider all problems important, but time constraints make it essential that you prioritize when presenting cases and planning your workday. Attend to all of your patient's issues, but keep a steady focus on the big picture, and you will be able to budget time more efficiently and manage patients more effectively.

Acknowledge Your Knowledge Deficits and Seek Guidance when Necessary

At the beginning of the clerkship, you are not expected to know much about taking care of patients. When you encounter uncertainty, take note of it, and do not try to hide it from others. Seek guidance from house staff, nurses, attendings, patients, therapists, and reading. Don't judge yourself harshly. Instead, get excited to learn something new. Your patients will benefit greatly from your honesty about what you don't know.

Develop Sound Reading Habits to use Throughout Your Career

It is impossible to know everything, but it's a good idea to avoid being ignorant about the same thing twice. Each day, keep a list of things you don't understand and read about them later. You may be amazed by how much you retain when the material you read is relevant to your patients.

Behave Professionally

You are expected to approach patients with empathy and respect their individual dignity and confidentiality. Strive to be cooperative, patient, and attentive at all times, even with difficult individuals. It is a privilege to care for fellow human beings. When in doubt, treat others as you would have them treat you or your family.

Be a Team Player

Medical care is provided by professionals from multiple disciplines who share the common goal of serving the patient. To contribute, you must understand the special role of nurses, therapists, and pharmacists and use them appropriately. Strong team spirit can motivate you to provide excellent care despite fatigue and stress. Earn respect by being respectful.

Be Proactive About Follow-up

Whether you are on the wards or in the clinic, follow up on all patient lab test results, tests, or questions that arise in the care of the patient. Check on patients by phone call after they have left the hospital. Phone follow-up also is important for clinic patients. Talk to your attending or resident you are working with in the clinic before calling the patients.

Work Well with Nurses

Nurses spend their entire day at patients' bedsides and can provide valuable insight into patient progress. Experienced nurses know a lot about patient assessment and ways to provide comfort. Some students find this intimidating and end up treating nurses unpleasantly. It is far preferable to acknowledge nursing expertise openly and try to learn from the suggestions made.

Strike a Healthy Balance Between Medicine and Personal Life

Sleep, exercise, good food, and leisure activities with family and friends are vital to your soul. To sustain your energy and focus at the hospital, you must attend to your personal happiness. A healthy balance in your life can help you cope with the anxiety of adapting to your new role and responsibilities and to accept this challenge eagerly. If all goes well on the rotation, you will glimpse the profound satisfaction available to individuals who care for the sick and gain insight into the kind of physician you want to become.

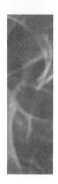

2

Day-to-Day Inpatient Skills

JOHN V. L. SHEFFIELD

What are a Student's Responsibilities on a Ward Team?

On the inpatient wards, your primary responsibility is being the team's "expert" on all your patients; you perform the admission history and physical exam, and you actively participate in all aspects of their care. In addition to knowing everything about your patients (and always having patient data readily available), you should write all but emergent orders (cosigned by house staff or attending), represent and speak for your team wherever your patients are discussed, complete daily chart notes in timely fashion, perform procedures with appropriate supervision, and contribute to all diagnostic and treatment planning. You also may be asked to research aspects of your patients' cases and teach the team during rounds. In addition, you should pay attention on rounds to learn from all patients on the team, and you should be ready and willing to help care for any patient as necessary. Finally, students can be an important source of energy, enthusiasm, curiosity, and fresh humanitarian spirit for their teams. This energy is often crucial to team morale.

Do I Need to Pre-round?

Yes. The workday officially begins with work rounds, at which time the team sets a plan for the day for each patient. Before work rounds, you should pre-round, which consists of reviewing chart notes (for new consult recommendations and acute events overnight) and vital signs, speaking to the patient briefly, doing a directed physical exam, and checking lab results. Allow 10–15 minutes per patient, and be ready to start work rounds on time.

How Much Information Should I Gather in the History and Physical?

Your history and physical should be complete on every patient you admit. Outstanding physicians take excellent histories and possess superior physical exam skills. The history provides information to make most diagnoses, and optimal patient care depends on the accuracy of this information and the strength of the physician-patient relationship created in the process. With practice and repetition, you will gain confidence in your ability to identify your patients' problems and become more efficient, but the medicine clerkship is not a place to cut corners.

What is a Good Presentation?

Many students approach case presentations as if their primary purpose was student evaluation. The main objective of the presentation is to convey the essentials of the patient's illness to team members so that all can learn and participate in subsequent discussions of management. This requires more than a simple recitation of what a patient told you; you need to provide a critical analysis of the information to produce a clear assessment and plan. At the end of a good presentation, your team should understand a patient's most pressing issues and your plan to address them. Being asked questions is a good thing. It means that your presentation held others' interest and they listened well enough to ask questions. Attributes of good work rounds presentations include the following:

- **Brevity:** The goal is 3–5 minutes for a new patient (less for daily progress reports). At first, you need to learn from your resident what information is appropriate; you only have time for crucial details. Expect questions and leave time for them.
- **Organization:** Practice on your on-call day. Don't freelance. People expect to hear information presented in a certain order. Disorganization creates confusion.
- **Eye contact:** Engage your team and they will listen. Presenting from memory greatly enhances your ability to achieve this goal. *Never* read from your written history and physical.

What Should I Include in My Write-ups?

Of all the notes in your patient's chart, yours should be the most complete. Initial write-ups generally average 3–6 pages and should succinctly review the history, exam, lab results, diagnostic reasoning, and plan. To avoid common pitfalls, pay attention to the following:

- **Chronology:** Use day of admission as a consistent point of reference: "3 days prior to admission (PTA), she noticed chest pain. One day PTA, she noted shortness of breath."
- **Pertinent negatives:** Include at the end of the HPI to reflect the differential diagnosis.
- **Abbreviations:** Use only familiar abbreviations; write everything else out.
- **Organization:** Use a bulleted outline for PMH, medications, exam, and plan so that details can be found at a glance.
- **Completeness:** Describe physical findings completely; be attentive to detail.

How do I Write a Good Assessment and Plan?

The assessment and plan section is probably the source of greatest confusion for most students. It's actually quite simple. First, state the problem (diagnosis, symptom, sign, or lab test result). Second, give a realistic differential diagnosis for that problem. Third, state which diagnosis is most likely and why others are not, incorporating data from your history and physical. It is good to list your differential in order of most likely to least likely. Remember to include "Can't Miss" diagnoses (diagnoses that may not be the most likely, but are life-threatening and should never be missed). Finally, for each problem, list the diagnostic and therapeutic plan so that readers can rapidly find and review your plan. By following this formula, you can avoid the two most common mistakes:

- **Don't ramble:** Rambling assessments that regurgitate textbook differentials and pathophysiology reflect poor synthesis of information and are not relevant to the case.
- **Don't be too brief:** Very brief assessments reflect poor understanding of the differential diagnosis and rationale for evaluation and treatment.

What Should I Try to Learn When Reading about My Patients?

To monitor your patients effectively and contribute to diagnostic and therapeutic decision making, begin by reviewing the following information:

- **Differential diagnosis**—for common presenting conditions
- **Pathophysiology**—disease processes of the major diagnoses in your patients
- **Typical signs and symptoms**—for the major conditions in the differential diagnosis
- **Diagnostic algorithm**—rationale for tests, sequence of testing, cost, and potential ramifications of test results on therapeutic options
- **Treatment algorithm**—rationale for choosing treatment options, including efficacy and cost
- **Drug side effects**—side effects or toxicities, drug interactions, and convenience

Which Reading Sources are Most Useful?

Anything you read in the attempt to provide excellent patient care will be better retained than information reviewed out of context, but different sources have different attributes. **Syllabus/spiral-bound manuals** provide concise reviews with practical management advice. **Texts** are strong on pathophysiology and typical disease signs and symptoms, but can be out of date regarding work-up and therapy. **Online texts** are updated frequently and often contain more practical and timely information. **MEDLINE** is a comprehensive guides to the medical literature. Being able to construct a literature search to answer a clinical question is an essential skill, but be sure that the articles you find are relevant to your patient.

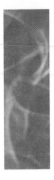

3

Day-to-Day Outpatient Skills

JOHN V. L. SHEFFIELD

How do I Prioritize the Outpatient Visit?

Inpatients often have a single problem leading to hospitalization, whereas outpatients usually present several issues for you to address in a brief period of time. Often you will not have time to deal with every issue and must determine which to address in a single visit. Each visit should begin with an attempt to set an agenda for that visit. Before entering the room, review the problem list and set some goals. When you see the patient, ask what goals he or she has: "What are your concerns today?" After you have heard the patient's list, try to cover key management goals, address special patient concerns, and avoid overlooking potentially serious new problems. You may respond: "Those are a lot of important issues. Let's cover your blood pressure and sore leg today. We probably won't have time to discuss the chronic shoulder pain, but let's do that carefully next time, okay?"

What is an Appropriate Exam?

Your exam should address the problems of the day. For a patient with a sore throat, vital signs, a good HEENT, neck, and lung exam should suffice. A complete exam is generally done only with new patients, patients with vague or troubling symptoms, and when patients request it specifically.

What Should I Present to My Attending?

In clinic, your presentations should clarify the issues you discussed and your plan for each. Let your attendings know when you are running behind and how they might help you most. One popular and effective format is as follows:

Identify the Patient and Frame a Question that You Want the Attending to Address:

Mr. K is a 45-year-old man with diabetes, hypertension, and depression. He is here for a new lesion on his leg and for a BP check. I'd like you to look at his leg with me, and I need your thoughts on his BP.

Give an Efficient, Problem-based History, Exam, and Plan:

Leg lesion. He noticed this lesion a few months ago, and it's gradually grown. He doesn't recall injuring himself, and it's nontender. He has not had fever or chills. On exam, the temperature is 37°C, and on his right anterior shin he has a smooth, shiny, well-demarcated plaque with central atrophy and telangiectasia. The surrounding leg and skin are normal in appearance, and sensation is intact. Because he's diabetic, I was originally concerned about infection, but there are no signs or symptoms of that. Could you look at it with me?

Blood pressure. He's had hypertension for 5 years, and it had been well controlled until recently when his medication doses have had to be increased. He's currently taking atenolol 50 mg, hydrochlorothiazide 25 mg, and lisinopril 20 mg. He does not drink and has always been compliant with his medications. Now his BPs at home range from 140s to 150s over 90s. In clinic today, his BP is 152/92 and pulse is 54. There is no edema. I am uncertain why his hypertension is becoming more difficult to control, and I'd like to review possible explanations and management with you.

Other issues. We didn't talk about his diabetes today. I'd like to schedule an appointment for follow-up in 2 weeks to go over that and his test results.

Get Feedback
Any suggestions for me?

What should I Include in my Notes?

When reviewing your clinic notes, a reader should be able to identify rapidly your patient's problems, medications, and management plan. With the exception of the assessment and plan section, clinic notes are generally much more concise than ward notes. Basic elements include the following:

- **Patient identification and chief complaint**—briefly frame the patient and purpose of the visit
- **Problem list**
- **Medications**
- **Current concerns**—concise histories of problems addressed
- **Exam**—detailed descriptions of exam performed that day
- **Lab test results**—summarize key findings only
- **Assessment and plan**—for each problem, discuss your rationale and plan

What is My Responsibility for Follow-up?

It is your responsibility to follow up on your patient's test results and to determine appropriate timing for a return visit. Before a patient leaves the clinic, review how they will learn of test results. You may need to devise a system to remind you to look up results. When tests are back, you should either send a letter or make a phone call to the patient.

In some clinics, patients can call in for results, but this may not be adequate for abnormal results. You also should discuss when the patient should return to the clinic. There are no clear guidelines to follow, so this can be difficult. Ask your attending if you are unclear. From the standpoint of your education, scheduling return visits to occur before you leave the rotation can enhance your experience significantly.

When Should I Read?

Some students find it difficult to incorporate reading into diagnostic and therapeutic decision making in clinic. Several little breaks in the clinic routine exist, and you can use each to advantage. Read **before the visit**, especially when you know the chief complaint and are unsure what an appropriate history and exam would entail. Ask your attending for guidance on what to read. A few minutes of advance preparation can save time in the room. Read **before the exam** to look up something during the minute a patient takes to disrobe, but be quick. Read **before your presentation** to clarify questions about diagnosis, elements of the story, exam, or lab test results before you present to the attending. Read **between visits**, to take advantage of any gaps in your schedule. Try to find at least one thing to read about on each clinic patient you see. If you don't have time in clinic to read, make a list and read about those issues when you have time.

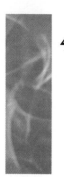

4

Communicating with Patients

LISANNE R. BURKHOLDER

What Do I Accomplish with a Good Patient Interview?

A good interview provides key diagnostic information in most cases. Verbal and nonverbal cues help establish a partnership of trust and mutual understanding, setting the stage for compliance with treatment decisions. A good interview elicits the patient's perceptions about the illness ("what does this illness mean to you"), about the role the patient expects the physician to play in his or her health care ("what do you hope I can do to help you?"), and sets patient expectations for future interactions.

How Should I Begin a Patient Interview?

Introduce yourself, and explain why you are seeing the patient. Also, establish with the patient how he or she would like to be addressed. If in doubt, use Mr. or Ms. and the patient's last name. Never assume you can call someone by their first name because this is offensive to some patients. Ask the patient about his or her health concerns ("why did you come to the hospital?" or "why did you want to see the doctor today?"). Listen, listen, listen!

What Barriers to Communicating with Patients Will I Encounter?

The biggest barrier to good communication is physicians' poor listening skills. Listening is probably the most important skill for any physician. Good listening transcends many cultural and power differences between patients and their physicians and helps patients feel heard, respected, and understood. Most physicians begin their careers with a good idea of how to listen and with the desire to convey caring and respect. These values and the listening skills that accompany them may atrophy during medical training unless specific attention is paid to practicing respectful patient interactions. Listening skills are not just innate features of some personalities—they can be learned (and forgotten). For example, physicians interrupt patients on average within the first 7-11 seconds of history. Allowing patients to tell their story without interruption gets the visit off to a much better start without actually lengthening the visit time. After several minutes, if you feel it is necessary, you can gently redirect patients with rambling stories: "now let's get back to your chest pain," or "we need to stay focused or I won't be very helpful to you." Patients' human stories may unfold in circuitous, unpredictable, and revealing ways. To the physician focused on gathering "the facts," this may seem frustrating. There is much to be learned, however, about the individual by allowing the patient to tell his or her story. Finding ways to appreciate the breadth of human expression while you are in the midst of gathering data during an interview greatly improves patient and personal satisfaction with the interaction.

What Can I Do to be a Better Listener?

One key listening tool is silence. Use silence to give patients time to answer questions. Use silence, or a simple nod of the head, to encourage patients to share more meaningful information. Another tool is open-ended questions ("tell me more about your pain ..."; "what has this been like for you ..."). This allows the patient to direct the interview. Closed-ended questions ("is your pain sharp or dull?") are less helpful in creating a good physician-patient interaction, although they can be useful when used near the end of the interview to flesh out a review of systems. Another tool is reflective statements that summarize what you have heard using the patient's words ("so you have a squeezing feeling around your chest when you walk uphill"). This validates the patient experience and lets the patient know you have listened. Summary statements also allow you to make transitions from one part of the history to another.

How Can My Nonverbal Cues Help Communicate Caring and Respect to Patients?

Nonverbal cues may be more important than your words. Sit at eye level to avoid the power difference implied by looming above a patient. Maintain good eye contact. You can take notes, but don't shuffle through the chart while the patient is talking. Practice respectful listening, an exercise in sharing rather than taking control of the conversation. The exam is another powerful venue for nonverbal cues. Don't poke and prod to extract information with your hands. Instead, listen gently, respectfully, and deliberately with your hands and stethoscope, while staying attentive to your patient for any signs of pain or concern. Your patients will feel the difference. Furtive glances at a watch signal you have other more important things to do. Instead, it is better to acknowledge time limits openly and plan with the patient for the best use of time. Stay on schedule, especially in clinic, respecting patients' busy lives.

What Can I Say During the Physical Exam?

Although silence during the history is a useful tool, silence during the exam can increase patient anxiety as the patient wonders what you are doing, what you are finding, and if he or she is going to be okay.

During the exam, keep the patient involved as a partner in the experience. Briefly explain what you are doing as you go ("I'll be tapping here to find your liver now"). Reassure patients as you perform the exam when things are normal. Briefly review your findings at the end of the exam. Give patients permission to stop you if the exam becomes uncomfortable.

How Do I Communicate Test Results?

Set patient expectations when you order tests for when, how, and with whom you will communicate results. Some patients do not want to hear news directly, but instead prefer you communicate with a family member. In the clinic, you may mail normal results, and call with abnormal results. In the hospital, you may want to come back in the afternoon with test results—if you promise to return with test results, follow through on your promise. Also explain what you are hoping to learn from the test. In the hospital, significant lab and other test results should be shared with patients daily, ideally as soon as they are available. Be brief. Use language the patient can understand to explain the meaning of the test. You may start by asking the patient if he or she remembers your earlier conversation about why the test was obtained. This helps you assess if they have understood prior discussions.

How Do I Give Bad News?

Often, it is effective to start with a screening question to assess patient understanding of why the test was obtained and what they think is likely to be found. This may make it easier to confirm their suspicions with the bad result ("do you understand why we got that CT scan of your abdomen?"). You also may want to establish how much the patient wants to know and if he or she is ready to hear results. Keep it simple, short, and direct ("I have bad news. The CT scan shows a growth that could be cancer."). Give patients time to absorb bad news—a pause or even a few minutes of silence are often very useful. Some patients become emotional. This is normal. There is no need to say anything or to try to skirt the emotions. Just being present is often helpful. Some patients have many questions. If you don't know the answer to a question, say so and offer to find out. Some patients are quiet. In general, it is best to keep the message simple and let patient questions guide how much more information you discuss. Offer to answer questions then and later after they have had time to absorb the news. Leave written information letting patients know how to reach you if they have questions later. Set a time to return for more discussions and come back at the agreed time. It is often reassuring for patients to hear that you are going to be there to see them through whatever happens next.

How Do I Do A Successful Bedside Presentation?

Bedside presentation is a tradition that has fallen out of favor. Bedside presentations work well as the format for daily morning work rounds. The entire team goes to the bedside each day, and the intern or student succinctly presents pertinent information regarding hospital course and discusses the plan for the day. Patients prefer hearing bedside presentations on work rounds, rather than hearing pieces of conversations about them (or other patients) from the hallway. Teams that do daily bedside rounds often grow to prefer them as well. Bedside presentations provide an efficient way of updating the patient and team simultaneously, including the patient as a partner in plans, making rounds professional and succinct, and allowing quick confirmation of findings. Specific approaches to bedside rounds may vary by team and teaching institution. Basic ground rules include introducing each team member on the first visit, using language the patient can understand, and orienting the patient to the goals of this daily routine ("I'm going to fill the team in on why you came to the hospital and share the information we've gathered about you overnight"). Most patients respond appropriately when encouraged to participate or edit the presentation. Presenters can speak to the patient or speak to the team. Attendings, residents, and students who object to bedside rounds often fear that unanswered questions may arise, or that the patient may see different opinions about how to proceed. This is also a strength of bedside rounds, however, because ambiguities and information gathering are a part of medical decision making. It is fine to say, "we don't know," and make a plan for how to find answers and when to get back to the patient with more information. Another fear is that patient questions and concerns may monopolize the conversation and interrupt or prolong rounds. In the rare case that this occurs, the team can acknowledge the need for longer discussion later in the day and plan a time for one team member to return. Most patients appreciate being involved in this patient-centered way of communicating about their care and benefit greatly from seeing the complex nature of the decision-making process of medicine. When patients hear the presentation, they know that you have listened to them and paid attention to all the details of their story.

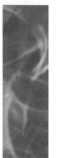

5

Ethics in Medicine

KELLY FRYER-EDWARDS

CONFIDENTIALITY

What Does the Duty of Confidentiality Require?

Confidentiality is one of the core tenets of medical practice. The obligation of confidentiality prohibits the physician from disclosing information about the patient's case to other parties without permission and encourages the physician to take precautions to ensure only authorized access to information occurs. Discussions about patients with other physicians are often crucial for patient care and are an integral part of the learning experience in a teaching hospital. These discussions are justifiable, so long as precautions are taken to limit the ability of others to hear or see confidential information.

What Kinds of Disclosure are Inappropriate?

The realities of communication in medical practice make it difficult to protect patient confidentiality. Inappropriate disclosure of information occurs when cases are discussed in the elevator or hallway; when extra copies of handouts with patient information on them are left out; or when patient family members are informed, even about minor care issues, against the patient's wishes. The patient's right to privacy is not being respected in these situations.

When Should Confidentiality be Breached?

Confidentiality is not an absolute obligation and may be broken if there is concern for the safety of specific individuals or for public welfare. Clinicians have a duty to protect identifiable individuals from any serious threat of harm if they have information that could prevent the harm. In the most clear-cut cases of limited confidentiality, physicians are required by state law to report to public health authorities certain communicable and infectious diseases, such as AIDS, hepatitis A and B, measles, and tuberculosis. Suspected cases of child, dependent adult, and elder abuse are reported, as are gunshot wounds. Local municipal code and institutional policies can vary regarding what is reportable and standards of evidence required. It is best to ask about your institution's policy.

INFORMED CONSENT

What is Informed Consent?

The most important goal of informed consent is to allow the patient to be an informed participant in health care decisions. It originates from the legal and ethical right of the patient to direct what happens to his or her body, and from the ethical duty of the physician to involve the patient in his or her health care. The term "basic consent" entails letting the patient know what you would like to do and asking for his or her permission. This is appropriate for simple procedures such as drawing blood. Decisions that merit this streamlined approach have a high level of community consensus and a low level of risk. A more formal process of informed consent should occur for more invasive procedures, such as lumbar puncture or thoracentesis. The more formal process includes a discussion of several aspects of the procedure (Box 5-1) and a consent form signed by the patient and filed in the chart.

What are My Responsibilities During the Informed Consent Discussion?

Consent is valid only if given voluntarily by a patient competent to make the decision. Patients often feel powerless and vulnerable, and it is easy for coercive situations to arise in this setting. To encourage voluntariness, the physician must make clear to the patient that he or she is participating in a decision, not merely signing a form. With this understanding, the informed consent process should be seen as an invitation to the patient to participate in decisions. The physician also is generally obligated to share the reasoning process and provide a

---

BOX 5-1

ELEMENTS TO DISCUSS WHEN OBTAINING FORMAL PATIENT CONSENT

- The nature of the decision or procedure
- Reasonable alternatives to the proposed intervention
- Relevant risks, benefits, and uncertainties related to each alternative
- Assessment of patient understanding
- Choice made by the patient

recommendation to the patient. Comprehension on the part of the patient is equally as important as the information provided. Consequently, the discussion should be carried on in lay terms, and the patient's understanding should be assessed along the way.

What Sorts of Interventions Require Informed Consent?

For a wide range of decisions, written consent is not required, but some meaningful discussion is needed. For instance, a man contemplating having a prostate-specific antigen screen for prostate cancer should know the relevant arguments for and against this screening test, discussed in lay terms. Most health care institutions have policies that state which health interventions require a signed consent form. Surgery, anesthesia, and other invasive procedures are usually in this category.

Is There Such a Thing as Implied Consent?

Consent can be implied, rather than obtained, in emergency situations when the patient is unconscious or incompetent and no surrogate decision maker is available. This type of consent is based on the principle of beneficence, which requires a physician to act on the patient's behalf when the patient's life is at stake. The patient's presence in the hospital ward, ICU, or clinic does not imply consent to undergo treatment or procedures.

 # DO-NOT-RESUSCITATE ORDERS

What is a DNR Order?

A DNR order means the patient will not receive CPR if he or she is found with no pulse or respirations. In some cases, a patient has a DNR order on the chart. In many cases, the question has never been addressed, and you need to discuss preferences with the patient regarding CPR. Deciding whether to forego future resuscitation involves a careful consideration of potential clinical benefit and the patient's preferences. Real or perceived differences in these two considerations make decisions to forego CPR difficult.

When can CPR be Withheld?

If the patient stops breathing or his or her heart stops beating in the hospital, the standard of care is to perform CPR in the absence of a valid physician's order to withhold it. CPR can be withheld when the patient, or the legal surrogate if the patient is not competent, clearly indicates that he or she does not want CPR should the need arise. It also can be withheld when CPR is deemed futile (judged to be of no medical benefit).

When is CPR Futile?

CPR is futile when it offers the patient no clinical benefit; in such cases, you are ethically justified in withholding it. CPR has been prospectively evaluated in a wide variety of clinical situations. Knowing the probability of success with CPR can help determine futility. CPR has virtually 0% probability of success in the following clinical circumstances: septic shock, acute stroke, metastatic cancer, and severe pneumonia. Even in other clinical situations, survival after CPR is extremely limited.

How Should the Patient's Quality of Life be Considered in Decisions about CPR?

CPR also might be judged futile when the patient's quality of life is so poor that no meaningful survival is expected even if CPR were successful at restoring circulatory stability. Judging "quality of life" tempts prejudicial statements about patients with chronic illness or disability. There is substantial evidence that patients with chronic conditions often rate their quality of life much higher than healthy people would. Nevertheless, many experts would agree that patients in a permanent unconscious state possess a quality of life that virtually no one would accept. CPR is usually considered futile for patients in a persistent vegetative state.

Are "Slow Codes" Ever Justified?

"Slow codes" are those in which a half-hearted effort at resuscitation is made. Physicians may be tempted to resort to using a slow code when there is disagreement between the patient and the physician about the utility of CPR. Slow codes are not ethically justified.

What if the Patient is Unable to Say What His or Her Wishes Are?

In some cases, the decision about CPR must be made when the patient is unable to participate. There are two general approaches to this dilemma. One is to use an existing advance directive, a document that indicates with some specificity the decisions the patient would like to be made should he or she be unable to participate. The other solution involves identifying a surrogate decision maker. The law recognizes a hierarchy of family relationships in determining which family member should be the official decision maker (Box 5-2), although ideally all close family members and significant others should be involved in the discussion and reach some consensus.

BOX 5-2

HIERARCHY FOR CHOOSING A SURROGATE DECISION MAKER

1. Legal guardian with health care decision-making authority
2. Individual given durable power of attorney for health care decisions
3. Spouse
4. Adult children of patient (all in agreement)
5. Parents of patient
6. Adult siblings of patient (all in agreement)

TERMINATION OF LIFE-SUSTAINING TREATMENTS

When is it Justifiable to Discontinue Life-sustaining Treatments?

Occasionally, you encounter patients who are receiving treatments or interventions that keep them alive, and you face the decision of whether to discontinue these treatments. Examples include dialysis for acute or chronic renal failure and mechanical ventilation for respiratory failure. In some circumstances, these treatments are no longer beneficial, whereas in others the patient or family members no longer want the treatment. If the patient has the ability to make decisions, fully understands the consequences of the decision, and states he or she no longer wants a treatment, it is justifiable to withdraw the treatment. Treatment withdrawal also is justifiable if the treatment no longer offers benefit to the patient.

Do Different Standards Apply to Withholding and Withdrawing Care?

Many clinicians believe that it is easier not to start (withhold) a treatment, such as mechanical ventilation, than to stop (withdraw) it. Although there is a natural tendency to believe this, there is no ethical or legal distinction between withholding and withdrawing treatment.

What if I'm not Sure Whether the Patient is Competent?

Patients must be "competent" to make treatment decisions. A better term is "decision-making capacity" to avoid confusion with legal determinations of competence. For example, an elderly man may be found incompetent to manage a large estate, but still may have intact capacity to make treatment decisions. The capacity to make treatment decisions, including withholding or withdrawing treatment, is considered intact if the patient satisfies all four basic criteria (Box 5-3). If the patient does not meet these criteria, his or her decision-making capacity should

---

BOX 5-3

CRITERIA INDICATING PATIENT COMPETENCE TO MAKE TREATMENT DECISIONS

- ◆ Understands the clinical information presented
- ◆ Appreciates the situation, including the consequences of refusing treatment
- ◆ Is able to display reason in deliberating about her or his choices
- ◆ Clearly communicates choice

be questioned, and the surrogate decision maker should be consulted. Sometimes patients are awake, alert, and conversant, but their decisions seem questionable or irrational. It is important to distinguish an irrational decision from simple disagreement. In these situations, talk with the patient to clarify his or her reasoning.

What About a Patient Whose Decision-making Capacity Varies from Day to Day?

Patients can move in and out of a coherent state from medication effects or underlying disease. You should do what you can to catch a patient in a lucid state, reducing medications if necessary, to include him or her in the decision-making process.

Does Depression or Other Mental Illness Impair a Patient's Decision-making Capacity?

Patients with active mental illness, including depression, should have their decision-making capacity evaluated carefully, usually by a psychiatrist. Patients should not be presumed to be unable to make treatment decisions. In several studies, patients voice similar preferences for life-sustaining treatments when depressed as they do after treatment of depression.

KEY POINTS

◆ With a few exceptions, patient information should be kept in confidence.

◆ The ethical principle of respect for individuals creates an obligation for physicians to foster patient participation in health care decisions.

◆ DNR orders should be written when the patient (or surrogate) states such a preference.

◆ Competent, fully informed patients have the right to refuse life-sustaining treatments.

Case 5-1

A 48-year-old man has severe end-stage liver disease and is admitted to the medical floor with a poor prognosis. He asks that you not share any of his medical information with his wife because he does not think she will be able to take it. His wife catches you in the hall and asks about her husband's prognosis

A. Will you tell his wife?
B. What are you required to do legally?

Ethics in Medicine

Case 5-2

A 60-year-old carpenter and heavy smoker presents with weight loss. On chest x-ray you see a mass. You believe a diagnostic thoracoscopic lung biopsy is warranted. After explaining the intervention, and the risks of not pursuing treatment, the patient refuses the treatment. He is clear that he understands the implications of letting his symptoms go unaddressed, but "doesn't want to go there," and gets up to leave.

    A. Can the patient refuse to give consent for this intervention?
    B. What are your professional obligations in this case?

Case Answers

5-1 A-B. *Learning objective:* **Recognize what actions the duty of confidentiality requires.** The duty to maintain confidentiality remains strong in this case because information about the patient does not directly concern others' health, welfare, or safety. There is no imminent danger to others here. The wife is certainly affected by her husband's health and prognosis, however. Every effort should be made to encourage sharing of information, although it remains his right to do so or not.

5-2 A-B. *Learning objective:* **Recognize effective ways to address patient participation and respect for individuals in decision making.** The patient seems to understand what is at stake with his treatment refusal. Because he is competent, you have a duty to respect his decision. You should explore his reasons for refusing treatment and consider alternative treatments or ways of reducing his risk. You can be clear that his treatment refusal will be honored, but that it is not the end of the discussion.

REFERENCE

Jonsen AR, Siegler M, Winslade WJ. Clinical Ethics: A Practical Approach to Ethical Decisions in Clinical Medicine, 5th ed. New York, McGraw Hill, 2002.

USEFUL WEB SITE

http://depts.washington.edu/bioethx/toc.html

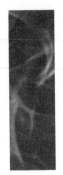

6

Practical Skills for the Medical Student

DOUGLAS S. PAAUW, LISANNE R. BURKHOLDER, MARY B. MIGEON, DAWN E. DEWITT, ANDREA A. CHUN, ERNIE-PAUL BARRETTE, LINDA E. PINSKY, SIANG Y. SOH, and ABHIJIT P. LIMAYE

 HOW TO READ ELECTROCARDIOGRAMS

How do I Report ECG Findings in my Notes?

A normal report covers the six key features of an ECG: rhythm, rate, axis, intervals, chamber sizes, and ischemic changes.

How do I Recognize Normal Sinus Rhythm?

Normal sinus rhythm (Figure 6-1) occurs when orderly depolarization begins in the sinus node, progresses through the atria (P wave), traverses the AV node (PR interval), then passes through the ventricles (QRS complex), causing a ventricular contraction. After depolarization is finished, there is a brief pause (ST segment), and then the ventricles repolarize (T wave). In normal sinus rhythm, every QRS complex is preceded by a P wave, and every P wave is followed by a QRS complex, with a constant PR interval for every beat.

How do I Calculate the Rate?

The heart rate is ventricular contractions per minute. On a standard ECG, a little box passes by in 0.04 second, and a big box passes by in 0.2 second. Estimate rate by counting the big boxes between each QRS complex and memorizing the corresponding rate (Table 6-1). Alternatively, use rate = 300/B, where B is the number of large boxes between each QRS.

Why is it Useful to Understand Vectors?

Understanding vectors in the limb and precordial leads allows you to localize heart muscle injury (Table 6-2). Also, with vectors you can calculate axis, which helps identify ventricular hypertrophy. You need to

Waves: P, Q, R, S, T

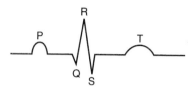

Intervals: PR, QRS, ST, QT

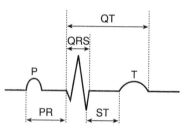

FIGURE 6-1 Components of a normal ECG tracing.

Table 6-1

Calculating Rate by the Number of Large Boxes between QRS Complexes

Boxes between QRS complexes	1	2	3	4	5
Rate (beats/min)	300	150	100	75	60

Table 6-2

Contiguous Leads That Localize Acute Myocardial Infarction

Location	Leads Affected (ST, T, Q Changes)
Anterior wall of LV	V1-4
Inferior wall of LV	II, III, aVF
Lateral wall of LV	I, aVL, V5, V6
Posterior wall of LV	V1-2 (large R waves)
Septal wall	V1-2
Right ventricle	Right-sided precordial leads

read an ECG text for details about vectors. Normal axis of the QRS reflects the LV's great muscle bulk, which points down and to the left between leads aVF and I. If QRS is upward in I and aVF, the axis is normal. LVH shifts the axis to the left and creates a negative QRS in lead aVF. Right ventricular hypertrophy shifts the axis down and to the right with a resultant negative QRS in lead I.

What Specific Changes would a Patient with Myocardial Damage Show on an ECG?

In general, ST segment changes and flipped T waves occur with early myocardial damage; significant Q waves appear 24-48 hours later. The spectrum of injury ranges from reversible subendocardial ischemia to irreversible transmural infarction (Figure 6-2). T wave inversions are a nonspecific sign of myocardial ischemia or early infarction. Normal T waves follow the direction of the QRS complex, but flip to the opposite direction with myocardial injury.

How do I Recognize Pericarditis on an ECG?

PR segment depression or ST elevation or both in multiple, noncontiguous leads suggests pericarditis. If pericarditis is accompanied by pericardial effusion, the voltages in all leads may be unusually low.

What are Intervals all About?

Prolonged intervals represent delays in conduction. A PR interval consisting of more than one big box (>0.2 second) indicates atrioventricular nodal block and can be caused by MI or medications such as digoxin or diltiazem. QRS widening to beyond three small boxes (>0.12 second) is caused by interventricular conduction delay such as a bundle branch block or with ectopic beats generated in the ventricle such as ventricular tachycardia or isolated premature ventricular beats. Detect left bundle branch block by the "rabbit ears" (RR') in leads V5-6. Right bundle branch block causes RR' in leads V1-2. QT prolongation is important because it can lead to torsades de pointes, a deadly ventricular arrhythmia. The QT interval depends on the heart rate and is normal if it is less than half the RR interval. QT prolongation occurs with tricyclic antidepressant overdose, hypomagnesemia, hypocalcemia, some antiarrhythmic drugs, and interactions of some medications (diltiazem and erythromycin).

How do I Detect Chamber Wall Hypertrophy or Enlargement?

LVH creates a leftward axis and large S waves in leads V1-2 and large R waves in aVL, V5, and V6 (Table 6-3). Right ventricular hypertrophy creates large R waves in leads V1-2. Left atrial enlargement is best seen in lead V1 as a late negative deflection in a biphasic P wave. The negative portion of the P wave must be >1 mm deep and one box wide. Right atrial enlargement creates a large peaked P wave >2.5 mm high best seen in lead II.

Practical Skills

Subendocardial ischemia

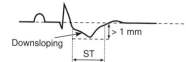

- Downsloping ST segment depression > 1 mm below baseline

Downsloping

ST

A

Transmural myocardial infarction
Early (minutes/hours)

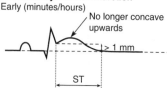

No longer concave upwards

> 1 mm

- ST segment elevation > 1 mm above baseline
- In 2 or more contiguous leads

ST

B

Transmural myocardial infarction
Late (hours/days)

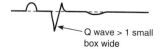

Q wave > 1 small box wide

- T wave inversion
- Q waves > 1 box wide and deep
- In 2 or more contiguous leads

C

Pericarditis

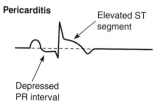

Elevated ST segment

- Diffuse ST segment elevation
- Diffuse PR segment depression

Depressed PR interval

D

FIGURE 6-2 A-D, ST segment, T wave, and Q wave changes with myocardial injury.

Table 6-3		
Criteria for Left Ventricular Hypertrophy Using Wave Amplitudes*		
R wave in aVL		>11 mm high
(S in V1 or V2) + (R in V5 or V6)		>35 mm high

*LVH can be confirmed by satisfying either criterion.

Practical Skills

HOW TO READ AN ABDOMINAL FILM

When should I Obtain Abdominal Films?

Not all patients with abdominal pain require x-rays, which are often nonspecific. Obtain films when they would aid diagnosis—for perforation, obstruction, or chronic pancreatitis (Figure 6-3).

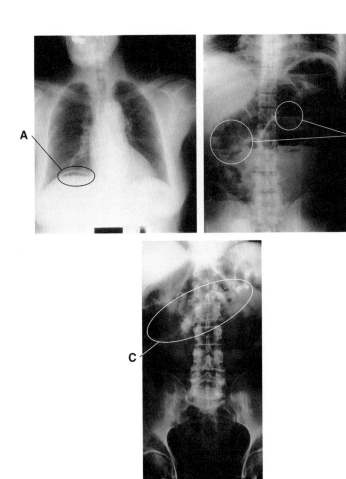

FIGURE 6-3 Key abdominal series findings. **A,** Free air indicates perforation. **B,** Air-fluid levels of bowel obstruction. **C,** Pancreatic calcifications are pathognomonic for chronic pancreatitis.

How do I Order Abdominal Films?

Order an abdominal series, which consists of supine and upright abdominal films and a CXR. The CXR shows the lung fields and diaphragms and screens for pulmonary pathology such as pneumonia presenting with abdominal symptoms and for free air in the abdomen.

What Key Findings should I Look for in an Abdominal Series?

Free air, a surgical emergency until proved otherwise, is best seen on CXR as a dark crescent under the right diaphragm in contrast to the radiodense liver. If the patient cannot stand, a cross-table lateral x-ray with the patient left side down would show free air. Common causes of free air are bowel wall perforation from duodenal ulcer, diverticula, or cancer. Another critical finding is dilated bowel from obstruction or ileus. If markedly dilated, toxic megacolon secondary to *Clostridium difficile* should be considered.

What Constitutes Dilation for Large and Small Bowel?

Roughly 3 cm for small intestine, 6 cm for large intestine, and 9 cm for the cecum constitute dilation. To discern between large and small bowel, use anatomy. The small bowel valvulae are circumferential and so create lines across the entire bowel; in the large bowel, haustrations only partially embrace the circumference and give a scalloped border. Additionally, the large bowel generally frames the edges of the abdomen, whereas the small bowel sits in the center.

How can I Tell the Difference Between Ileus and Bowel Obstruction?

In both conditions, air-fluid levels and dilation are seen. Air in the rectum suggests ileus. In true obstruction, no air passes from above, so the rectum collapses within 24 hours. Also, air-fluid levels the same height throughout the gut suggest obstruction, rather than the varying levels seen in ileus.

What Other Findings can be Helpful?

Extensive stool suggests constipation. Arterial calcification raises concern for mesenteric ischemia. Calcified gallstones or kidney stones may be seen. Pneumatosis, air in the bowel wall, is a grim indicator of mesenteric necrosis. Hepatomegaly, splenomegaly, or enlarged kidneys may be suggested. Bowel wall thickening from edema can be seen. Calcifications in the pancreas are diagnostic of chronic pancreatitis.

HOW TO READ CHEST X-RAYS

What is the Best Way to Read CXRs?

The key to reading CXRs is to proceed systematically through six major steps (Box 6-1). This ensures that you do not overlook anything. Remember the hardest lesion to see on x-ray is the second one.

BOX 6-1

KEY ELEMENTS OF READING A CHEST X-RAY

A = Airways and lung fields
B = Bones and soft tissue
C = Cardiac contour and mediastinum
D = Diaphragms and costophrenic angles
E = Examine technique
F = Foreign bodies, tubes, and wires

Why is Technique Important?

X-ray technique varies from film to film and must be taken into account. PA and lateral films are preferred, but require the patient to stand. If the patient is unable to stand, AP films are taken with the patient in bed, the film behind the patient's back. On such AP films, divergence of x-ray beams exaggerates heart size. Appropriate **exposure** on AP view barely reveals the vertebrae behind the heart. With overpenetration, darkened normal lungs may be mistaken for emphysema. Underpenetration or poor inspiration increases interstitial markings. Adequate **inspiration** is determined by counting at least 10 posterior (horizontal) ribs in the lung field. Patient **rotation** artificially widens the mediastinum; normally, the vertebrae line up between the clavicular heads (Figure 6-4).

What Can be Seen in Bones and Soft Tissue?

Look for fractures, dislocations, and lytic lesions from cancer. Severe osteoporosis can be seen as transparent bone or vertebral compression

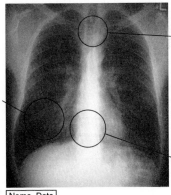

Alignment: Vertebrae aligned between clavicular heads

Inspiration: Count at least 10 posterior ribs behind lung fields

Penetration: Vertebrae are just barely visible behind heart

Details: Note patient name, whether PA or AP, and date

Name, Date

FIGURE 6-4 Elements of techniques important in evaluating a CXR. (Copyright © 1997, Mike Richardson.)

fractures (vertebral wedging on the lateral view). Examine the soft tissue for swelling or subcutaneous air (subcutaneous emphysema).

What Causes a Widened Mediastinum?

Patient rotation, thoracic aortic aneurysm, tumor, or lymphadenopathy can widen the mediastinum.

Why Should I Look at the Diaphragms and Costophrenic Angles?

Free air under the diaphragm occurs with bowel perforation. A blunted costophrenic angle, sometimes the only sign of pleural effusion, should prompt decubitus films (patient lying on the side, affected side down) or ultrasound to evaluate the amount of pleural fluid and if it is free flowing or loculated.

What is a Silhouette Sign?

The silhouette sign occurs when something of the same density (fluid or infection) in the lung is adjacent to and obliterates the border of the hemidiaphragm or heart. If the right heart border is poorly seen, this is a right middle lobe "silhouette sign," indicating a right middle lobe infiltrate (Figure 6-5). Similarly, left lower lobe pneumonia obliterates the left hemidiaphragm.

What does Pneumonia Look Like?

Pneumonia may have many appearances: a focal infiltrate (a white opacity where dark air in the lung should exist, suggesting inflammatory

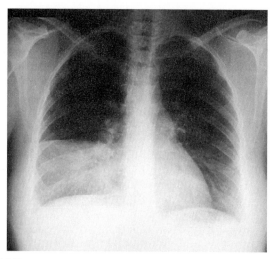

FIGURE 6-5 Loss of the right heart silhouette with right middle lobe pneumonia. Note: Right diaphragm is still clearly seen. (Copyright © 1997, Mike Richardson.)

Practical Skills

Table 6-4

Acute Catastrophes Not to Miss on Chest X-ray

Finding	Condition
Subdiaphragmatic "free" air	Bowel perforation
Widened mediastinum	Thoracic aortic aneurysm or dissection
Mediastinal air	Esophageal rupture
Mediastinal shift, air in pleural space	Pneumothorax

fluid filling alveoli and small airways), a silhouette sign, interstitial infiltrates (white opacity in a fine lacy pattern following the interstitial tissues lying between alveoli and small airways), and unexplained pleural effusions. In a volume-depleted patient, an infiltrate may be subtle. Apical infiltrates can occur with any form of pneumonia, but are classic for tuberculosis.

What Acute Catastrophes Should I not Miss on CXR?

Certain conditions should never be missed (Table 6-4).

What Causes Nodules in the Lung Parenchyma?

Cancer (primary or metastatic), arteriovenous malformations, focal infection or abscess, hamartomas, and granulomas all can appear as nodules.

What are Clues to Volume Overload or CHF?

Look for an enlarged cardiac silhouette, greater than half the width of the thorax on PA view, interstitial prominence, Kerley B lines, and cephalization of vessels. **Kerley B lines** are thin horizontal linear densities at the periphery of the lung fields caused by edema in the interlobular septa. **Cephalization** is abnormal engorgement of pulmonary vessels in the upper lung fields; normally, gravity makes vessels more prominent at the bottom of the lung field. **Blunting of the costophrenic angles** suggests pleural effusion.

HOW TO PERFORM BASIC PROCEDURES AND BODY FLUID ANALYSIS

What is the First Step for all Procedures?

All procedures require informed consent. The performing physician should explain the indication for the procedure, what the procedure involves, the risks (i.e., what a reasonable person would want to know), the alternatives to the procedure, and the consequences of not having the procedure performed. Patient competence is essential in this process. Patients should be able to reiterate the key points of the procedure and risks. Patients <18 years old and patients with altered mental status are not considered competent; a surrogate decision maker is needed in

Practical Skills

these cases. In an emergency, informed consent is unnecessary if the procedure is considered lifesaving. The informed consent discussion should be documented in the medical record.

What Habits Facilitate a Successful Procedure?

Before beginning, review your technique, collect all supplies, place a waste receptacle nearby, and carefully position the patient. Always observe universal precautions and use sterile technique. Clean up after the procedure, and dispose of all sharp implements appropriately. Check on the patient later to ensure that there were no complications from the procedure.

How do I Document a Procedure?

There is a standard format for procedure notes (Box 6-2).

LUMBAR PUNCTURE

What are the Indications for LP?

Any patient with unexplained fever and mental status changes should undergo LP to rule out CNS infection. Patients with new-onset "worst headache of their life" and a negative head CT scan require LP to rule out subarachnoid hemorrhage. LP is diagnostic for carcinomatous meningitis, Guillain-Barré, neurosyphilis, and normal pressure hydrocephalus. LP can be used to administer intrathecal chemotherapy or epidural anesthesia.

BOX 6-2

STANDARD PROCEDURE NOTE

Date and Time _____
Procedure   _____
Indication   _____
Operators   _____

   Verbal and written informed consents were obtained after explanation of indications, risks, benefits, and alternative treatments. The area (*describe where*) was prepped and draped in sterile fashion. ____ mL of 1% lidocaine was injected. ____ mL of (*type, description*) fluid were withdrawn without complication and sent for (*tests*). Wound cleansed and dressed. Patient tolerated the procedure well with ____ mL estimated blood loss. Follow-up studies (i.e., CXR after thoracentesis) were negative.
   Signature_____

When is LP Contraindicated?

Increased intracranial pressure is an absolute contraindication to LP because of the risk of precipitating uncal herniation. Risk factors for increased intracranial pressure are age >60 years, immunocompromised state, history of CNS lesion, recent seizure, mental status changes, and abnormal neurologic exam. If one of these risk factors is present, a CT scan before LP is mandatory. Coagulopathy is a relative contraindication to LP.

What are the Key Steps in Performing an LP?

Place the patient on his or her side with the head and spine parallel to the floor. A vertical line connecting the iliac crests crosses the spine at interspace L3-4: mark this area. To widen this interspace, have the patient curl up in a fetal position with the knees and head pulled into the chest. Prepare and drape the low back in sterile fashion, apply anesthesia to the skin as a wheal, and then apply anesthesia to the deep tissues, making sure you are not injecting a vessel by pulling back on the syringe plunger before injecting. Insert the spinal needle in the same hole used to administer anesthesia, aiming for the umbilicus. Obtain an opening pressure and collect several milliliters of CSF in each of four vials. Replace the stylet before removing the spinal needle.

What are the Complications of LP?

Complications of LP are post-LP headache, infection, hemorrhage, and uncal or tonsillar herniation.

What CSF Tests Should I Order, and How do I Interpret Them?

Order glucose, protein, cell count and differential, bacterial culture, and Gram stain. Glucose should be 60% of the simultaneous blood glucose. A low CSF glucose can be seen in bacterial, tuberculous, and fungal infections. High protein (>50 mg/dL) is nonspecific because it is seen in all CNS infections and inflammatory states. Normal CSF WBC is 0-5 cells/mm^3. Acute bacterial meningitis has a WBC >1000 cells/mm^3, with neutrophils predominant. Acute viral meningitis generally has a lower WBC of 5-300 cells/mm^3 with lymphocytes predominant, although early viral meningitis may have a neutrophilic predominance. Bloody CSF may indicate a traumatic spinal tap or recent CNS bleed. Traumatic taps show a decrease of the RBC from the first to the fourth vials of CSF. Subtract 1 WBC for every 700 RBCs to calculate the corrected WBC during a traumatic tap. Order cytology if malignancy is suspected, and order cryptococcal antigen, fungal stain, and culture in immunocompromised patients. Specific viral testing is available for herpes simplex, varicella zoster, West Nile, and other viruses.

THORACENTESIS

What are the Indications for Thoracentesis?

Patients with a new or unexplained pleural effusion require thoracentesis for diagnosis. Thoracentesis in CHF patients is unnecessary unless one of the following occurs: (1) asymmetric effusions, (2) pleuritic chest pain, or (3) fever. Effusion associated with pneumonia requires thoracentesis to rule out pleural space infection (empyema) requiring drainage. Thoracentesis also can be used therapeutically to remove large, symptomatic effusions.

When is Thoracentesis Contraindicated?

Relative contraindications to thoracentesis include coagulopathy, cutaneous infections at the puncture site, and uncooperative patients. Pleural fluid from small or loculated effusions may be obtained more safely with ultrasound guidance.

What are the Key Steps to Thoracentesis?

Position the patient sitting on the edge of the bed, leaning over a tray-table. Raise the bed to a comfortable height for you. Locate and mark the insertion site two intercostal spaces below where dullness to percussion begins. Needle insertion should be above the rib to avoid the neurovascular bundle at the inferior margin of each rib. Prepare with povidone-iodine (Betadine) and drape in sterile fashion. Apply anesthesia generously, especially at the periosteum and the parietal pleura. Advance a 22-gauge, 1½-inch needle over the top of a rib while pulling back on the plunger until fluid is obtained. A diagnostic thoracentesis requires about 30 mL of fluid. No more than 1.5 L of pleural fluid should be removed to avoid re-expansion pulmonary edema. Fluid collection devices vary; some thoracentesis needles have a catheter and stopcock system to prevent air entry into the pleural space and damage to the underlying lung. Combat negative intrapleural pressure by having the patient exhale any time you must open the system. A postprocedure CXR should be obtained routinely and ordered emergently if there is aspiration of air during the procedure, or if the patient develops dyspnea or hypotension.

What are the Complications of Thoracentesis?

Complications of thoracentesis are pneumothorax, hepatic or splenic puncture, infection, hemothorax, and re-expansion pulmonary edema.

What Pleural Fluid Tests Should I Order, and How do I Interpret the Results?

The first step in evaluating pleural fluid is to classify it as either a transudate or an exudate. Exudative effusions meet at least one of the criteria (Table 6-5). Transudative effusions are caused by CHF, cirrhosis, pulmonary embolism, nephrotic syndrome, or myxedema. There are multiple causes for exudative effusions, including infection, hemorrhage,

Table 6-5

Criteria for Exudative Pleural Effusion*

Pleural protein/serum protein	>0.5
Pleural LDH/serum LDH	>0.6
Pleural LDH/upper normal limits serum LDH	66%

*One or more are necessary.

Practical Skills

trauma, malignancy, pulmonary embolism, gastrointestinal disease, collagen vascular disease, and pericardial disease. To evaluate exudative effusions, send pleural fluid for cell count and differential; bacterial, fungal, and AFB culture; Gram stain; and cytology. To obtain a pleural fluid pH, you should send the fluid in a blood gas syringe on ice to the lab for an accurate result. Parapneumonic effusions have a predominance of polymorphonuclear cells. Pleural fluid lymphocytosis is seen in tuberculous pleurisy, malignancy, or autoimmune disease. An empyema may look like frank pus, have a low glucose level, and have a pH <7.2; these are indications for chest tube drainage. A chylothorax has a milky appearance and an elevated triglyceride level. A hemothorax is diagnosed by a pleural fluid HCT greater than one half of the serum HCT. Pleural fluid amylase may be elevated in esophageal rupture or acute pancreatitis. A pleural biopsy may be needed to diagnose TB pleuritis depending on the clinical scenario.

PARACENTESIS

What are the Indications for Paracentesis?

New-onset ascites requires paracentesis for diagnosis. Patients with chronic ascites and new abdominal pain, fever, unexplained increase in ascites, or admission to the hospital should undergo paracentesis to evaluate for SBP. Paracentesis also can be done to remove fluid for symptom relief.

When is Paracentesis Contraindicated?

Paracentesis is contraindicated if there is a cutaneous infection in the area of needle insertion. Coagulopathy is not a contraindication for paracentesis because risk of serious bleeding is low.

What are the Key Steps to Paracentesis?

Position the patient slightly upright to facilitate movement of fluid into the lower quadrant. Identify an insertion site in the lower quadrant, midway between the umbilicus and the anterior superior iliac spine; avoid the inferior epigastric vessels that run under the rectus abdominis muscles. An alternative site is in the midline below the umbilicus; ensure that the patient empties the bladder fully before the procedure to prevent bladder perforation. Prepare with Betadine, and drape in sterile fashion. Inject 1% lidocaine generously in a skin wheal and in the subcutaneous tissues. To avoid fluid leakage, advance an 18-gauge, 1½-inch needle through a zigzag

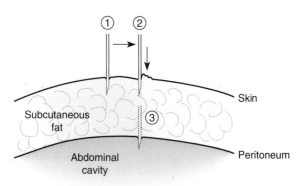

FIGURE 6-6 Zigzag path through the subcutaneous fat to prevent leakage after paracentesis. 1, Enter skin; 2, pull skin 1-2 cm away from original entry site with needle perpendicular to skin surface; 3, advance needle through peritoneum.

path in the subcutaneous tissue (Figure 6-6). Pull back on the plunger as you advance. As with thoracentesis, collection devices vary. After collection, withdraw the needle, and place a pressure dressing over the site.

What are the Complications of Paracentesis?

Complications of paracentesis are bowel perforation, bladder perforation, abdominal wall hematoma, and infection.

What Peritoneal Fluid Tests Should I Order, and How do I Interpret Them?

Order cell count and differential, albumin, protein, bacterial culture, and cytology. Diagnostic criteria for SBP are absolute neutrophils $>250/mm^3$ (total WBC $\times$ % neutrophils). WBC $>10,000/mm^3$ suggests peritonitis from perforated duodenal ulcer or colon and is an indication for an immediate CT scan and surgical consult. Calculate the SAAG: serum albumin $-$ ascites albumin. A SAAG >1.1 g/dL (>11 g/L) is consistent with ascitic fluid secondary to portal hypertension. A SAAG <1.1 g/dL (<11 g/L) is consistent with high protein peritoneal fluid secondary to TB or peritoneal carcinomatosis. Gram stains are rarely ever positive in patients with SBP. Bacterial cultures are best obtained by inoculating blood culture bottles at the bedside with ≥10 mL per bottle. Cultures for TB in peritoneal fluid are low yield. Protein <1 g/dL indicates higher risk for SBP, and prophylaxis should be considered.

ABNORMAL LABORATORY TESTS

My Clinic Patient has an Abnormal Lab Test Result. What Should I do Next?

In the outpatient setting, you have several options for follow-up of abnormal tests: call and ask the patient to return for more history or exam, order follow-up tests, refer for a diagnostic study or consultation, or simply observe over time.

What is the Role of Screening Lab Tests?

Some physicians routinely obtain screening panels of lab tests; patients also may request these. There is no evidence, however, that these "routine" lab tests are helpful in healthy patients. They generate false-positive results and unexpected abnormalities that worry patients, very rarely discover new diseases, and often perplex providers. Because the abnormal range for each test includes normal outliers at the high and low end, a random set of 20 lab tests would have, on average, one abnormal result just by chance. To avoid this trap, order tests only to pursue your evaluation of symptoms and signs of disease.

Are There any Lab Tests that I Should Order Routinely?

In a well adult with no symptoms and a normal exam, reasonable screening tests are total cholesterol, high-density lipoprotein, and glucose. Some physicians also check PSA in men >50 years old, HCT in menstruating women, and TSH in older women. These screening tests are not uniformly agreed on.

WHITE BLOOD CELL COUNT

What does an Elevated WBC (leukocytosis) Mean?

The most common causes of leukocytosis are infection and steroids. Bacterial infections usually cause elevation of the neutrophil count with "left shift" (an increase in immature forms of neutrophils). Toxic granulation also may be present with infection, a sign that neutrophils are actively producing digestive enzymes to fight intruding bacteria. Viral infection can cause elevated lymphocytes or atypical lymphocytes. In hospitalized patients, it is common to see a mild stress-related leukocytosis, a condition that usually rapidly resolves when the patient's condition is more stable, often within 24 hours. Leukemia is an infrequent cause of leukocytosis, usually with immature blast forms in the peripheral circulation.

My Patient has Elevated Eosinophils; what could be Causing This?

Eosinophilia may be due to neoplasm, allergy (includes drug reactions and asthma), Addison's disease, collagen vascular disease, or parasitic infection (mnemonic *NAACP*).

ERYTHROCYTE SEDIMENTATION RATE

When Should I be Concerned about an Elevated ESR?

The ESR increases with age. In general, an ESR greater than half the age is almost always pathologic and warrants evaluation. More specifically, normal values for men are < age/2, and for women are < (age + 10)/2. For example, an 80-year-old woman should have an ESR <(80 + 10)/2, or <45. With an ESR >100, the diagnosis is usually obvious during initial evaluation. An elevated ESR is the only hint of disease in 0.06% of cases—extremely rarely.

Is the ESR Helpful for Patients with Vague Symptoms or Positive Review of Systems?

A normal ESR makes the diagnosis of TA and PMR less likely, but is not helpful for other disorders. A normal ESR is not strong enough evidence to exclude a serious illness. The ESR is routinely normal in infectious mononucleosis and typhoid fever and in 10% of patients with active TB.

What Causes an ESR >100?

Infection is the most common cause of an ESR >100, followed by malignancy and collagen vascular disease. Infections that increase the ESR include TB, pulmonary infections, syphilis, chronic bacterial infections (osteomyelitis; endocarditis; septic arthritis; liver, spleen, or perinephric abscess), UTIs, and AIDS. Malignancy accounts for 15% of ESRs >100 and is almost always metastatic when the ESR is that high. The most likely cancers include multiple myeloma, lymphoma, breast cancer, lung cancer, and colon cancer. Rheumatologic diseases can cause a striking elevation in the ESR, especially TA, PMR, RA, and SLE.

What Evaluation Should I Pursue when the ESR is >100?

Perform a careful history and physical, including pelvic exam and stool Hemoccult. This should suggest a diagnosis. Blood tests and imaging studies do not substitute for a detailed history and physical. Pursue the laboratory tests and studies most likely to confirm the diagnosis. Consider CBC with differential and urinalysis to look for infection; electrolytes, BUN, and creatinine to check kidney function and acid-base status; and LFTs to look for hepatic injury. Because myeloma is more common with these extreme elevations in ESR, consider serum and urine electrophoresis (SPEP, UPEP). Obtain a chest radiograph to look for lung infection, vasculitis, or tumor. In 5%-10% of cases with an ESR of >100, no cause is found.

What about Less Extreme Values—ESR 35–75?

Many of these values are normal when rechecked in several weeks. This should be the extent of the work-up in an asymptomatic patient. Another option is to check a C-reactive protein. If the C-reactive protein is <0.2 mg/dL, the ESR elevation is likely a false positive. For persistently elevated values, a careful history, exam, and careful use of the aforementioned tests lead to the answer. In an asymptomatic patient with a benign exam, almost all elevated ESR results go unexplained.

LIVER FUNCTION TESTS

How do I Interpret LFTs (ALT, AST, and Alkaline Phosphatase)?

Elevations of the hepatic transaminases, ALT and AST, suggest parenchymal injury to the liver, with the highest values seen in severe viral hepatitis, toxin or drug injury, and severe hypotension. The most common causes of ALT and AST elevation include medications, alcohol, hepatitis B and C, fatty liver, and hemochromatosis. Increases in alkaline phosphatase and conjugated bilirubin suggest obstructive biliary pathology, either extrahepatic or intrahepatic cholestasis. ALT and AST may be normal or mildly elevated with cholestasis. ALT increases are more specific to liver injury because AST is found in many other tissues, most importantly muscle. ALT and AST tend to increase equally except in alcohol ingestion, where the AST/ALT ratio is usually >2.

How Should I Evaluate an Elevated Alkaline Phosphatase?

Biliary obstruction and bone diseases are the main causes of an elevated alkaline phosphatase. To sort out which is present, obtain a GGT or 5'-nucleotidase, either of which would be elevated with biliary tree pathology, but not with bone disease. Alkaline phosphatase isoenzymes also distinguish the source, but take several weeks. If biliary pathology is suggested, look for gallstones or tumor compressing the biliary tree (pancreatic cancer, cholangiocarcinoma) by abdominal CT scan. Also consider autoimmune disease, such as primary biliary cirrhosis, which is diagnosed by a positive anti–mitochondrial antibody test in >90% of cases. Alkaline phosphatase also can be elevated in hepatitis, cirrhosis, or late in pregnancy, although is rarely more than one to two times the upper limits of normal and not usually greater than the ALT. When bone disease is likely, consider fractures, Paget's disease, bone metastases, or infection.

TUMOR MARKERS

What are Tumor Markers?

Tumor markers are substances produced in excess by particular tumors and found in the blood (Table 6-6). Tumor markers are too nonspecific to use for diagnosis or general screening. They can be used to assess completeness of resection or recurrence after treatment. Occasionally, they can suggest a diagnosis when findings are nonspecific. In the case of a liver mass, elevated AFP suggests primary liver tumor, whereas an elevated CEA suggests colon cancer metastatic to the liver. Patients with cirrhosis at high risk for hepatocellular carcinoma (especially cirrhosis secondary to hepatitis B and C and hemochromatosis) may undergo annual AFP screening, although outcome data are lacking to support this practice. Germ cell tumors are classified based on β-HCG and AFP production.

Practical Skills

Table 6-6

Common Tumor Markers and Their Clinical Use

Tumor Marker	Associated Tumor	Clinical Use
AFP	Germ cell cancer, liver cancer	Classify tumor type, follow for recurrence; evaluate liver mass; screen high-risk cirrhosis patients
β-HCG	Germ cell tumor	Classify tumor type
CEA	Colon cancer	Follow for recurrence; evaluate liver mass
CA-125	Ovarian cancer	Follow for recurrence
PSA	Prostate cancer	Follow for recurrence; use for routine screening is debated.

HOW TO INTERPRET SENSITIVITY AND SPECIFICITY

What are Sensitivity and Specificity?

When diagnosing or treating a condition, we need to know "how accurate is this test?" In a screening test for cancer, we want a balance between a big net that catches all cancers (sensitivity) and yet has openings small enough to omit cases that are not cancer (specificity). Put another way, sensitivity is the proportion of individuals with the condition who test positive; specificity is the proportion of individuals without the condition who test negative. You can calculate a test's sensitivity and specificity by using a 2 × 2 table (Table 6-7).

How do Levels of Sensitivity and Specificity Affect How I Interpret a Test?

Some people find the mnemonics **SpPIN** and **SnNOUT** helpful. If a test has high **Sp**ecificity, a **P**ositive test rules the condition **IN**. If a test has

Table 6-7

Calculating Sensitivity and Specificity

Test	Disease	
	Present	**Absent**
Positive	A (true positive)	B (false positive)
Negative	C (false negative)	D (true negative)

Sensitivity	Specificity
$\frac{A}{A+C}$ or $\frac{\text{True positive test results}}{\text{All patients with disease}}$	$\frac{D}{D+B}$ or $\frac{\text{True negative test results}}{\text{All patients without disease}}$

high Sensitivity, a Negative result rules OUT the condition. For example, a peritoneal fluid wave on physical exam is 92% specific for ascites. If a fluid wave is present, you can rule ascites in (a highly specific test, positive finding, rule it in). In a study of patients at a Veteran's hospital, a history of ankle edema was 93% sensitive for the presence of ascites. If the patient has no history of ankle edema, you can rule ascites out (sensitive test, negative finding, rule it out).

If a Patient has a Positive Test, what is the Likelihood that He or She Actually has the Condition?

Sensitivity and specificity relate to characteristics of the test itself. The question of likelihood turns the focus to the characteristics of the patient being tested. We ask, "Given a positive test, what is the probability that this patient actually has the condition?" or "Given a negative test, what is the probability that the patient doesn't have this condition?" The statistical terms for these concepts are positive and negative predictive value (PPV and NPV). The predictive value depends on the estimated prevalence of a disease, or "pretest probability." To determine how likely it is that a positive test indicates disease, you must have an estimate of the patient's risk and the sensitivity and specificity of the test being applied.

What are the Steps to Calculate the Predictive Values?

Calculate predictive values using the 2×2 table (Table 6-8). Pick an arbitrary number of patients, such as 1000, and multiply the pretest probability to get the "disease present" and, conversely, "disease absent" totals. Then multiply the total "disease present" by the sensitivity to get A=true positives. For D=true negatives, multiply the "disease absent" by the specificity. To get C and B, subtract A from total "disease present" and D from total "disease absent." Finally, for PPV, divide the true positives, A, by the total positive tests, A plus B. For NPV, divide D by total negative tests, D plus C.

Table 6-8

Calculating Predictive Value*

	Disease		
Test	Present	Absent	
Positive	**A** (true positive)	**B** (false positive)	*Positive Predictive Value* $\frac{A}{A+B}$ or $\frac{\text{True positive test results}}{\text{All positive test results}}$
Negative	**C** (false negative)	**D** (true negative)	*Negative Predictive Value* $\frac{D}{D+C}$ or $\frac{\text{True negative test results}}{\text{All negative test results}}$

*Requires prior knowledge of sensitivity, specificity, and pretest probability (i.e., prevalence of disease).

How are Predictive Values and These Calculations Applied to a Real Clinical Scenario?

The renal artery duplex is a highly sensitive (92%) and specific (94%) test for renal artery stenosis as a cause of hypertension. Because the incidence of the disease is so low (2%) in the general population, the PPV is 23%, whereas the NPV is 99.8% (Table 6-9). So back to the question, "My patient has a positive renal artery duplex. Does she really have renal artery stenosis?" The answer is, "This patient, despite the positive test result, only has a 23% chance of truly having renal artery stenosis."

Is there a Method to Apply Test Characteristics Easily to various Patient Populations with different Pretest Probabilities?

Likelihood ratios (LRs) represent a method of calculating post-test probabilities in populations in which the prevalence of the disorder is different from that of the study population. The LR of any clinical finding or test is the probability of that finding being present or test being positive in patients with disease divided by the probability of the same finding or positive test in patients without disease:

$$LR = \frac{\text{probability of finding or positive test in patient with the disease}}{\text{probability of finding or positive test in patients without the disease}}$$

LRs may range from 0 to infinity. If the LR is 1, the test is equally likely to be positive whether or not the patient has the disease and is of no diagnostic value. As the LR increases, a positive test more convincingly suggests the presence of the disease. Tests with LRs between 0 and 1 argue against the diagnosis of interest; the closer the LR is to 0, the less likely the disease. Because LRs are calculated as odds, the pretest probability must be converted into odds and the post-test odds

Practical Skills

Table 6-9

Predictive Values of Renal Artery Duplex in Renal Artery Stenosis

Pretest probability = 2% prevalence of renal artery stenosis in general population. **Assume** 1000 patients, so 20 have disease, 980 do not.
Assume for renal artery duplex test sensitivity of 92% and specificity of 94%.

	Renal Artery Stenosis		
Duplex	Present in 20	Absent in 980	
Positive	*A*	*B*	*PPV*
Positive	18*	60	18 ÷ 78 = **23%**
Negative	*C*	*D*	*NPV*
Negative	2	920[†]	920 ÷ 922 = **99.8%**

*Calculated from known sensitivity of 92%—92% of 20 = 18 true positives.
[†]Calculated from known specificity of 94%—94% of 980 = 920 true negatives.

Table 6-10

Likelihood Ratio as Diagnostic Weight

Likelihood Ratio	0.1	0.2	0.5	1	2	5	10
Estimated Change in Probability	−45%	−30%	−15%	No change	+15%	+30%	+45%

Note: The estimated change in probability is added to the pretest probability, not multiplied. From McGee S: Simplifying likelihood ratios. J Gen Intern Med 2002;17:646.

converted back into probability. Another method involves the use of a nomogram to avoid these calculations. Clinicians use a method (Table 6-10) to estimate roughly the increased probability derived from the LR. The estimates derived in this manner are accurate to within 10% of the calculated answer for all pretest probabilities between 10% and 90%, with an average error of 4%.

HOW TO USE ANTIBIOTICS

How do I Choose and Dose Antibiotics?

Learning about all antibiotics is nearly impossible given the large number of choices available. To complicate matters, many antibiotics sound alike, especially cephalosporins. The decision to use an individual antibiotic is based on several factors, including coverage of the likely or cultured organisms, drug allergy history, formulary availability, cost, and oral versus parenteral formulations. When you decide which drug to use, consult a Pocket Pharmacopoeia, or Palm Pilot program such as ePocrates for dosing, and remember to adjust for renal function.

What is Empiric Therapy?

Empiric therapy is "best guess" therapy when a specific pathogen is unknown. Patients present with signs of infection, but definitive culture of blood, urine, or body fluid takes several days. In the interim before the pathogen is known, we frequently begin antibiotics. In many cases, especially with pneumonia or skin infections, we never isolate a specific pathogen, and our whole treatment course is based on the most likely pathogen in a given setting.

What is a Good Starting Point for Choosing Antibiotic Therapy?

Learn a few antibiotics appropriate for use with common bacterial pathogens, such as *Staphylococcus aureus,* gram-negative rods, anaerobes, and *Enterococcus,* and atypical organisms that cause community-acquired pneumonia (CAP), such as *Chlamydia, Legionella,* and *Mycoplasma* (Table 6-11).

Table 6-11

Antibacterial Spectrum of Commonly Used Antibiotics

Antibiotic	Excellent Activity (>85% Isolates Sensitive)	Fair Activity (70%-85% Isolates Sensitive)	Poor Activity
Penicillin	*Streptococcus* species except *Enterococcus* Oral anaerobes	—	Aerobic gram-negative rods *S. aureus* Atypical CAP organisms
Ampicillin	*Streptococcus* species Oral anaerobes	*H. influenzae* *Enterococcus*	Most aerobic gram-negative rods *S. aureus* Atypical CAP organisms
Trimethoprim-sulfamethoxazole	*Streptococcus* species except *Enterococcus* *E. coli** *S. aureus* including community-acquired MRSA	—	Anaerobes Hospital-acquired gram-negative rods
Clindamycin	*Streptococcus* species except *Enterococcus* Anaerobes *S. aureus*	—	Aerobic gram-negative rods Atypical CAP organisms
Quinolones: ciprofloxacin[†], ofloxacin	Aerobic gram-negative rods *S. aureus* Atypical CAP organisms	*Streptococcus* species	Anaerobes *Enterococcus*
Levofloxacin, moxifloxacin	Aerobic gram-negative rods *S. aureus/Streptococcus* Atypical CAP organisms	Anaerobes (moxifloxacin)	*Enterococcus*
Azithromycin, clarithromycin	*Streptococcus* species except *Enterococcus* *H. influenzae* *Chlamydia* (chlamydophila)	—	Most gram-negative rods

(continued)

Practical Skills

Table 6-11

Antibacterial Spectrum of Commonly Used Antibiotics (Continued)

Antibiotic	Excellent Activity (>85% Isolates Sensitive)	Fair Activity (70%-85% Isolates Sensitive)	Poor Activity
Azithromycin, clarithromycin	*Helicobacter pylori* *Legionella* species‡ *Mycobacterium avium* complex *Mycoplasma pneumoniae*		Most gram negative rods

CAP, community-acquired pneumonia (atypical organisms include *Chlamydia*, *Mycoplasma*, and *Legionella*); MRSA, methicillin-resistant *S. aureus.*
*Increasing resistance to *E. coli* approaching 15%. See Chapter 32.
†Ciprofloxacin superior in gram-negative coverage to levofloxacin, moxifloxacin, and inferior in *S. aureus* and *Streptococcus* coverage.
‡Intravenous therapy with high-dose erythromycin or azithromycin warranted for documented *Legionella* infections.

When should I Worry About *S. aureus* Infections?

S. aureus is a common pathogen, and its drug resistance makes it particularly troublesome. Typical situations for *S. aureus* infections include endocarditis in intravenous drug users, skin and wound infections (especially in patients with diabetes), and nosocomial pneumonia.

What are Good Drugs for Treating *S. aureus* Infections?

S. aureus infections are divided into methicillin-sensitive (MSSA) and methicillin-resistant (MRSA) infections. When MRSA is likely and the patient is seriously ill, as in frequently hospitalized or institutionalized patients, vancomycin is used for empiric coverage until sensitivities are available. Oral vancomycin is not absorbed, and should be used only for topical therapy of *Clostridium difficile* colitis. Community-acquired MRSA infections are becoming more common. The most common site of infection for community-acquired MRSA infections is the skin. Most community-acquired MRSA strains are sensitive to trimethoprim-sulfamethoxazole, clindamycin, or doxycycline (Box 6-3). Hospital-acquired MRSA infections are usually not sensitive to trimethoprim-sulfamethoxazole, clindamycin, or doxycycline. The best antibiotics for MSSA are first-generation cephalosporins and nafcillin (Table 6-12). Other drugs with good MSSA activity include clindamycin, certain quinolones, or combination penicillin products with beta-lactamase inhibitors such as ampicillin-clavulanate (Unasyn), piperacillin-tazobactam (Zosyn), or ticarcillin-clavulanate (Timentin).

BOX 6-3

BEST DRUGS FOR COMMUNITY-ACQUIRED* METHICILLIN-RESISTANT *STAPHYLOCOCCUS AUREUS*

- Trimethoprim-sulfamethoxazole
- Doxycycline
- Clindamycin
- Vancomycin

---

*For hospital-acquired methicillin-resistant S. aureus, use vancomycin until culture results are available.

Table 6-12

Best Drugs for Methicillin-Sensitive *Staphylococcus aureus*

Intravenous	Oral
Nafcillin	Dicloxacillin
First-generation cephalosporin: cefazolin	Cephalexin
Vancomycin	

How does Anyone Keep the Cephalosporins Straight?

The cephalosporins are confusing because they have similar names. Classify them by generation: First-generation drugs have better gram-positive coverage, and third-generation drugs have better gram-negative coverage.

- Gram-positives: first generation > second generation > third generation.
- Gram-negatives: third generation > second generation > first generation.

Other special features of cephalosporins are as follows: (1) Cefotetan and cefoxitin are the only cephalosporins with good anaerobe activity (both are second generation). (2) Ceftazidime and cefoperazone are the only third-generation cephalosporins with activity against *Pseudomonas aeruginosa*. Cefepime is a "fourth-generation" cephalosporin that has antipseudomonal activity. (3) Ceftriaxone is a third-generation cephalosporin that can be given once a day. (4) No cephalosporin covers *Enterococcus*.

When do I Worry About Gram-negative or Anaerobic Infections?

Gram-negative bacteria are generally seen with genitourinary tract infections (pyelonephritis, UTI) or infection from a bowel source (biliary tract disease or peritonitis from bowel wall perforation). In addition to gram-negative rods, the bowels can be the source of **anaerobes** or gram-positive cocci, such as *Enterococcus* or both. The oral gingiva is another common source of anaerobic infections (tooth abscess, aspiration pneumonia). A subcategory of less common gram-negative rods includes nosocomial, or hospital-acquired, gram-negative rods, such as *Klebsiella* or *Pseudomonas*.

What are the Best Antibiotics for Treating Gram-Negative Infections?

Aminoglycosides and the monobactam, aztreonam, provide narrow coverage of aerobic gram-negative rods only. They are useful for almost all gram-negative infections, although they usually are not used alone as empiric therapy because of their narrow spectrum. For situations in which multiple types of organisms are possible, choose broader spectrum empiric therapy, such as quinolones (superb gram-negative coverage), extended-spectrum penicillins (mezlocillin and piperacillin), third-generation or fourth-generation cephalosporins, imipenem, or meropenem. Of this group, imipenem and meropenem have the broadest spectrum of activity, including gram-positive organisms and aerobic and anaerobic gram-negative rods. Although it is tempting always to use the broadest antibiotics, this wipes out normal colonizing gut and vaginal flora and potentially predisposes to fungal superinfection. Choose the narrowest spectrum possible, and narrow therapy promptly when culture results are available.

What Antibiotics Provide Excellent Coverage for Anaerobic Infections?

Anaerobes can be either gram-negative or gram-positive and are distinguished by their inability to grow well in the presence of oxygen (Box 6-4). Their response to antibiotics is unique. Anaerobic infections of the mouth are generally sensitive to penicillin or ampicillin. By contrast, anaerobes of the gastrointestinal tract (especially *Bacteroides fragilis*) manufacture beta-lactamase and these "below the diaphragm" anaerobes are frequently resistant to penicillin. The best anaerobe drugs in

Practical Skills

BOX 6-4

BEST DRUGS FOR ANAEROBES

- Clindamycin
- Metronidazole
- Penicillin derivative with beta-lactamase
- Cefotetan/cefoxitin
- Meropenem/imipenem

this situation are clindamycin, metronidazole, a penicillin derivative/beta-lactamase inhibitor combination, cefotetan, cefoxitin, imipenem, or meropenem.

How do you Treat Enterococcal Infections?

Enterococcal infections are difficult to treat. Ampicillin, vancomycin, and linezolid are options. Ampicillin has the most activity, but resistance is growing. For enterococcal bacteremia, aminoglycosides are frequently combined with ampicillin or vancomycin for synergy. Only about one third of enterococcal strains are sensitive to aminoglycosides.

What Drugs are Best for the Atypical Organisms *Legionella*, *Chlamydia*, and *Mycoplasma*?

Erythromycin and tetracycline are the traditional drugs for these infections. Azithromycin and clarithromycin are newer medications in the same class as erythromycin and just as effective against atypical organisms with the benefit of less frequent dosing and fewer side effects, but the drawback of higher cost. Fluoroquinolones also have activity against these pathogens.

How do I know the Cost of Antibiotics?

In general, the drug cost of new antibiotics is greater than older antibiotics. For intravenous antibiotics, the number of doses is the biggest determining factor in cost. The administration cost of an intravenous antibiotic is $18-$24 per dose. Consequently, an expensive once-daily intravenous antibiotic would have a lower daily cost than a cheaper intravenous antibiotic, which needs to be given several times a day. For example, ceftriaxone 2 g intravenously every 24 hours = $50 (cost of 2 g of ceftriaxone) + $20 for 1 intravenous administration = $70 per day is cheaper than ampicillin 1 g intravenously every 6 hours = $6 (cost of four doses of 1 g of ampicillin) + $80 for four intravenous administrations = $86.

HOW TO INTERPRET PULMONARY FUNCTION TESTS

What are PFTs?

PFTs provide objective measures of lung function and help distinguish between obstructive and restrictive lung disease. Several different types of tests can be ordered (Table 6-13). For diagnostic purposes, patients can be sent to a pulmonary function lab to have all four categories of PFTs measured. For following progression of known disease, a subset of the full PFTs may be sufficient, as with office-based spirometry available in some physicians' offices. Indications for ordering PFTs are listed in Box 6-5.

Practical Skills

Table 6-13

Types of Pulmonary Function Tests

Pulmonary Function Test Type	Measures
Spirometry (air flow)	FEV_1 (forced expiratory volume in 1 second)
	FVC (forced vital capacity)
	FEV_1/FVC ratio (%)
	PEF (peak expiratory flow)
Lung volumes	TLC (total lung capacity; volume at end of maximal inhalation)
	VC (vital capacity)
Diffusing capacity	DLCO (diffusing capacity of carbon monoxide)
ABG	pH
	$Paco_2$
	Pao_2

BOX 6-5

INDICATIONS FOR ORDERING PULMONARY FUNCTION TESTS

♦ Screen high-risk patients (e.g., smokers, industrial/ environmental exposures such as asbestos)
♦ Diagnose patient with dyspnea or hypoxia or both
♦ Monitor disease progression or treatment outcome
♦ Assess preoperative risk
♦ Monitor for complications of treatments (e.g., with amiodarone, bleomycin, lung radiation)

How do I Tell the Difference between Obstructive and Restrictive Lung Disease?

In obstructive lung disease, such as asthma and COPD, FEV_1 and FVC may be decreased, with a concomitant decrease in the FEV_1/FVC ratio. Lung volumes may be normal with mild disease, but are usually increased as a result of air trapping as disease worsens. In restrictive disease, FEV_1 and FVC may decrease, but their ratio remains normal, whereas lung volumes decrease. DLCO may be decreased in obstructive and restrictive disease as a reflection of tissue destruction (Table 6-14). Patients with severe airway obstruction also may retain carbon dioxide, best measured with ABG testing.

How do I know if the PFTs are Normal?

PFTs are generally reported as a percentage of a predicted value. Predicted values are based on patient age, height, and gender. A normal

Table 6-14

Lung Diseases and Correlated Pulmonary Function Test Results

Type of Dysfunction	Common Causes	Typical Pulmonary Function Test* Abnormalities
Obstructive lung disease	Asthma COPD	$\downarrow\downarrow$FEV$_1$ when disease is active $\downarrow$ FVC $\downarrow\downarrow$ FEV$_1$/FVC Normal or $\uparrow$ TLC Normal or $\downarrow$ DLCO
Restrictive lung disease	Pulmonary fibrosis Silicosis Asbestosis Amiodarone Methotrexate Radiotherapy	May have $\downarrow$ FEV$_1$ and $\downarrow$ FVC FEV$_1$/FVC normal $\downarrow$ TLC $\downarrow$ DLCO
Neuromuscular weakness	Guillain-Barré syndrome Amyotrophic lateral sclerosis	May have $\downarrow$ FEV$_1$ and $\downarrow$ FVC FEV$_1$/FVC unchanged $\downarrow$ TLC Normal DLCO

*See Table 6-13 for definitions of pulmonary function tests.

FEV$_1$ for a 50-year-old man is 4 L, and a normal FEV$_1$ for a 50-year-old woman is 3 L. Patients with severe COPD may have an FEV$_1$ <1 L. Accuracy of results is an issue because results may be confounded by patient effort and ability to understand instructions. If multiple measures are reproducible, the results are likely to be more accurate. In addition, although general ranges of "normal" are given, individual patients' baseline values are the best reference in long-term monitoring. The FEV$_1$/FVC ratio is the one measure that is reported as a number, rather than a percentage of predicted value.

When do I do Special Maneuvers?

Postbronchodilator spirometry measures the reversibility of airway obstruction. Improvement in FEV$_1$ of >12% measured 10 minutes after the administration of a bronchodilator is considered a sign of acute bronchodilator responsiveness. When asthma is suspected, but baseline spirometry is normal, methacholine challenge can be used to precipitate underlying airway reactivity.

KEY POINTS – HOW TO PERFORM BASIC PROCEDURES AND BODY FLUID ANALYSIS

◆ Use your knowledge of indications, risks, and complications in obtaining patient consent.

◆ Proper operator preparation, patient positioning, and anesthesia are key for a safe procedure.

◆ Order appropriate tests on your specimens to facilitate your patient's evaluation.

KEY POINTS – HOW TO USE ANTIBIOTICS

◆ Vancomycin is the appropriate antibiotic for severe *S. aureus* infections until sensitivity results are available.

◆ In general, gram-positive coverage by the cephalosporins is first generation > second generation > third generation; gram-negative coverage is third generation > second generation > first generation.

◆ The best antibiotics for anaerobe coverage are clindamycin, metronidazole, penicillin derivatives plus beta-lactamase inhibitor, and cefotetan or cefoxitin and carbapenems (imipenem and meropenem).

Case 6-1

A 24-year-old woman requests an HIV test. She is monogamous with no risk factors (assume a pretest probability of 1/1000). Sensitivity and specificity are 98%.

A. Using a 2 × 2 table, calculate the predictive value of a positive test.
B. Calculate the PPV in an intravenous drug user who obtains drugs through prostitution. Assume a pretest probability of 25%. Sensitivity and specificity are still 98%.

Case 6-2

When using a CT scan to diagnose appendicitis, how can you increase the PPV of the test?

Case 6-3

A 22-year-old obese African American lineman on the UW football team comes to the primary care clinic with a 2-week history of a painful nodule on his left shoulder where he was scraped by his shoulder pad. On physical exam, he is found to have a 3 × 3 cm indurated erythematous area with purulent drainage centrally.

A. What are the most likely organisms causing this infection?
B. What treatment would you use if this were MRSA?
C. If this patient was an intravenous drug user or had been recently hospitalized, how would your treatment change?

Case Answers

6-1 A. *Learning objective:* **Recognize that a low pretest probability markedly decreases PPV.** When applied to high-risk patients, the HIV test has excellent PPV and NPV. The results are quite different when applied to low-risk populations (see following table). What is striking is that although this test is highly sensitive and specific, a positive test result in a low-risk patient has only a 5% likelihood of reflecting true disease (see table).

Predictive Value Calculations for HIV Test in a Low-Risk Patient

Pretest probability = 1/1000
Assume N = 1000

Test	Disease	
	Present in 1	**Absent in 999**
Positive	A 0.98	B 20
Negative	C 0.02	D 979

$$PPV = \frac{0.98}{20 + 0.98} = 5\%$$

$$NPV = \frac{979}{979 + 0.02} = 99\%$$

6-1 B. *Learning objective:* **Use sensitivity, specificity and pretest probability to generate a 2x2 table and to calculate positive predictive value.** Assume 1000 patients. Using pretest probability of 25%, 250 will have disease, and 750 will have no disease. Then, working backwards, use the sensitivity and specificity of 98% to calculate the number of true positives (A = 98% of 250 = 245) and true negatives (D = 98% of 750 = 735). Quadrant B is total disease absent − true negatives (750 − 735 = 15). Quadrant C is total disease present − true positives (250 − 245 = 5). With all quadrants filled in, you can calculate PPV and NPV. With a calculated PPV of 94%, we can say that with a positive test, this high-risk patient is 94% certain to have HIV infection (see the following table).

Predictive Value Calculations for HIV Test in a High-Risk Patient

Pretest probability = 25%
Assume N = 1000

| | Disease | |
Test	Present in 250	Absent in 750
Positive	A 245	B 15
Negative	C 5	D 735

$$PPV = \frac{245}{245 + 15} = 94\%$$

$$NPV = \frac{735}{735 + 5} = 99\%$$

6–2. *Learning objective:* **Understand that the pretest probability affects the predictive value of a test, and use this concept to select patients for testing carefully.** The predictive value of the test can be increased by carefully selecting in whom you use it. By choosing to test a population of patients who have an increased risk of having the condition you are suspecting, you increase the pretest probability and the predictive value of the test.

6-3 A. *Learning objective:* **This patient most likely has community-acquired MRSA presenting as a skin abscess.** His risk factors for this include obesity, African American ethnicity, playing a contact sport (including possibly sharing equipment), and skin trauma. Other possible, but less likely organisms include MSSA and group A streptococcus.

6-3 B. *Learning objective:* **The treatment for community-acquired MRSA is oral trimethoprim-sulfamethoxazole.** Other drug regimens include doxycycline, clindamycin, and minocycline. In patients thought to be chronic carriers of community-acquired MRSA, mupirocin ointment placed in the anterior nares three times a day for 3-5 days has been shown to decrease the carrier rate. Bathing in antimicrobial soap also has been suggested, but there have not been studies to support this theory.

6-3 C. *Learning objective:* **Patients who have been hospitalized, are injection drug users, or have been exposed to non–community-acquired MRSA are often resistant to the previously mentioned treatments and should be started on vancomycin.** The empiric treatment can be changed when sensitivities return. In patients who are resistant to vancomycin, other regimens, including linezolid and quinupristin-dalfopristin, can be considered.

REFERENCE

How to Interpret Pulmonary Function Tests
Crapo RO: Pulmonary function testing. N Engl J Med 1994;331:5.

USEFUL WEB SITES

How to Read ECGs
http://www.ecglibrary.com/ecghome.html
http://www.gwc.maricopa.edu/class/bio202

How to Read CXRs
http://rad.usuhs.mil/rad/chest_review/
http://www.rad.washington.edu/teachingfiles.html

How to Perform Basic Procedures and Body Fluid Analysis
http://en.wikipedia.org/wiki/Thoracentesis
http://medicine.ucsf.edu/housestaff/handbook/HospH2002_C15.html

How to Use Antibiotics
http://hopkins-abxguide.org/

Patients Presenting with a Symptom, Sign, or Abnormal Lab Value

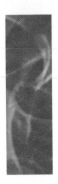

Abdominal Pain

LISANNE R. BURKHOLDER

 ETIOLOGY

How do I Categorize the Many Causes of Abdominal Pain?

The acuity, duration, and location of abdominal pain are most helpful in narrowing the differential diagnosis early in your history taking. The list of likely causes of acute abdominal pain, seen usually in hospitalized patients, is different from the list for chronic abdominal pain, occurring over weeks to months in outpatients (Tables 7-1 and 7-2). Diffuse abdominal pain is characteristic of many common conditions (Box 7-1). Focal pain should be approached geographically, with a differential diagnosis that includes pathology in organs located in the area involved (Figure 7-1). This chapter does not address the issue of functional abdominal pain, a common source of chronic abdominal pain without identifiable physical pathology.

What are some Abdominal Catastrophes I Shouldn't Miss?

Some causes of abdominal pain can lead to rapid clinical decline and death, especially if diagnosis is delayed (Box 7-2). Bowel perforation, cholangitis, and ischemic bowel can cause gram-negative sepsis. Aortic aneurysm rupture, splenic rupture, and ruptured ectopic pregnancy cause rapid volume depletion and shock.

What Important Extra-Abdominal Problems Masquerade as Abdominal Pain?

Angina may present atypically as epigastric pain. The other more typical characteristics of angina may still be present (e.g., pain worsened by exercise; relieved by resting; associated dyspnea, diaphoresis, or nausea). Lower lobe pneumonia or PE can irritate the diaphragm and cause upper quadrant abdominal pain, usually worsened by breathing. Abdominal wall pain from muscle strain, hernia, nerve entrapment,

57

Table 7-1

Causes of Acute Abdominal Pain, Associated Risk Factors, and Key Features

Causes	Risk Factors	Key Features
Common Causes		
Acute mesenteric infarction	Elderly, atherosclerotic risk factors, atrial fibrillation, or other embolic risk	Soft abdominal exam ("pain out of proportion to exam") Acidosis
Appendicitis	Generally young, but not always	Diffuse or periumbilical pain progresses over hours to RLQ pain Lying still with peritoneal signs if adjacent peritoneum inflamed Anorexia (severe) Steadily worsening fever, leukocytosis
Cholecystitis	"Fat, forty, female"; prior biliary colic or gallstone	RUQ postprandial pain Fever, nausea, vomiting, anorexia May radiate to right shoulder
Less Common Causes		
Bowel obstruction	Prior abdominal surgery, adhesions, hernia	Inability to pass stool or flatus Feculent emesis Distended, tympanitic abdomen
Cholangitis	Gallstone disease, pancreatic cancer, AIDS	Triad of high fever, RUQ pain, and jaundice
Diverticulitis	Elderly, prior diverticulosis	LLQ pain develops usually over days Fever
Ectopic pregnancy	Sexually active women, prior PID, IUD	Sudden, severe lower quadrant pain Significant pallor due to anemia
Obstipation	Elderly, narcotics, calcium channel blockers	Constipation Hard stool on abdominal/rectal exam
Pancreatitis	Gallstone disease, alcohol use or recent binge, high triglycerides, medications	Postprandial, midabdominal, or diffuse pain radiating to the back Nausea/vomiting in 90% Turner's or Cullen's signs if hemorrhagic, pain decreases with leaning forward
PID	Sexually active women, prior sexually transmitted disease, IUD, douching	Subtle to severe lower abdominal pain with fever, shortly after menses Cervical motion tenderness Purulent cervical discharge May have abnormal bleeding High ESR, elevated WBC
Renal stone	Crohn's disease, prior renal stone	Paroxysms of pain, writhing patient Pain radiating to genitals Hematuria

Abdominal Pain

(continued)

Table 7-1		
Causes of Acute Abdominal Pain, Associated Risk Factors, and Key Features (Continued)		
Causes	**Risk Factors**	**Key Features**
Ruptured aortic aneurysm	Elderly, atherosclerotic risk factors	Sudden-onset pain radiating to back May have loss of lumbar nerve functions Rapidly expanding abdominal size Pulsatile abdominal mass, shock

rectus sheath hematoma, or herpes zoster (shingles) may mimic an intra-abdominal process.

What Causes of Abdominal Pain have Associated Back Pain?

Cholecystitis can radiate to the back or right shoulder. Pain from pancreatitis and aortic aneurysm often radiates to the back. Pyelonephritis may cause flank pain and costovertebral angle tenderness. Lower thoracic or upper lumbar nerve irritation, as with herpes zoster (shingles), osteoporotic fracture, or a ruptured disc, can cause pain radiating from the back to the abdomen.

What Causes should I Think of in Elderly Patients Who have Abdominal Pain?

Cholecystitis, ischemic bowel, obstipation, diverticulitis, aortic aneurysm, and abdominal presentations of coronary artery disease are more common in elderly patients. Elderly patients may have a more subtle (altered mental status, vague symptoms), diffuse, or chronic presentation of a usually acute and focal process in the abdomen.

EVALUATION

What are some "Red Flags" I Shouldn't Miss in Evaluating Patients with Abdominal Pain?

A prolonged evaluation can delay urgent intervention in a very ill patient. It is wise to do a quick initial survey for abnormal vital signs and peritoneal signs to get a sense of the urgency of intervention. In an acutely ill patient, dyspnea, pallor, diaphoresis, cyanosis, hypotension, tachycardia, and a rigid abdomen are worrisome signs of severe illness and warrant rapid evaluation by the most senior member of your team available. In such patients, it also is wise to involve the surgery consult team early because some conditions, such as splenic or aortic rupture, may require urgent intervention even before imaging is obtained. In patients with chronic pain, symptoms of fever, sweats, weight loss, melena, and

Table 7-2

Common Causes of Chronic Abdominal Pain, Associated Risk Factors, and Key Features

Cause	Risk Factors	Key Features
Atypical angina	Hypertension, family history of early MI, hyperlipidemia, smoking	Worse with exercise, eating Associated dyspnea, diaphoresis, nausea
Biliary colic	"Fat, forty, female"	Intermittent episodes of RUQ pain Pain may radiate to right shoulder Postprandial pain, especially after fatty food often at night
Chronic mesenteric ischemia (ischemic bowel)	Atherosclerotic risk factors	Postprandial, diffuse abdominal pain (also called intestinal angina) Anorexia, weight loss
Gastroesophageal reflux	Obesity, calcium channel blocker use	Acid or food regurgitation Symptoms worse supine
Inflammatory bowel disease	None known	Nocturnal pain, intermittent bloody stool Extraintestinal manifestations—arthritis, gallstones, erythema nodosum, pyoderma gangrenosum, episcleritis, uveitis, thromboembolism, sclerosing cholangitis
Irritable bowel syndrome	Anxiousness, female, young to middle-aged	No nocturnal symptoms Improved with defecation Alternating constipation, diarrhea Mucus in stool
Obstipation	Elderly, narcotics, calcium channel blockers	Inability to pass stool Hard stool
Peptic ulcer	NSAIDs, prednisone, alcohol, caffeine	Improved with antacids Worse with acidic or spicy food, NSAIDs Melena

cachexia are worrisome for a serious illness and usually warrant imaging by CT or endoscopy or both.

How do I Approach History Taking When There are so Many Questions I Could Ask?

Initially, ask open-ended questions to get a description of the onset and location of the pain in the patient's own words (e.g., "tell me more about your pain"). Listen for key information (Box 7-3). If necessary, ask more pointed questions to get as clear a picture as possible. Along

---

BOX 7-1

CAUSES OF DIFFUSE ABDOMINAL PAIN

Bowel obstruction
Constipation
Early appendicitis
Ischemic bowel
Pancreatitis
Peritonitis

---

the way, keep a running list of possible diagnoses, and test them out by asking a few specific, key questions. If you are thinking about appendicitis as a possibility, ask about loss of appetite, fever, and change of symptoms over time because appendicitis usually causes profound anorexia and worsening fever and progresses from diffuse or periumbilical pain to focal RLQ pain over hours. Your write-up and presentations should reflect your differential diagnosis by pointing out the pertinent features on history and exam supporting and refuting the key illnesses you are considering. You can optimize your learning and improve your

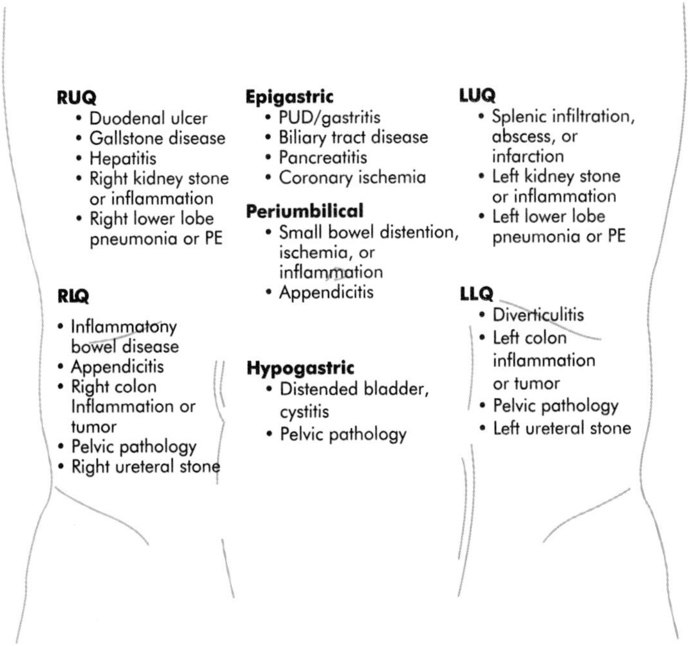

RUQ
- Duodenal ulcer
- Gallstone disease
- Hepatitis
- Right kidney stone or inflammation
- Right lower lobe pneumonia or PE

RLQ
- Inflammatory bowel disease
- Appendicitis
- Right colon Inflammation or tumor
- Pelvic pathology
- Right ureteral stone

Epigastric
- PUD/gastritis
- Biliary tract disease
- Pancreatitis
- Coronary ischemia

Periumbilical
- Small bowel distention, ischemia, or inflammation
- Appendicitis

Hypogastric
- Distended bladder, cystitis
- Pelvic pathology

LUQ
- Splenic infiltration, abscess, or infarction
- Left kidney stone or inflammation
- Left lower lobe pneumonia or PE

LLQ
- Diverticulitis
- Left colon inflammation or tumor
- Pelvic pathology
- Left ureteral stone

Abdominal Pain

FIGURE 7-1 Common causes of abdominal pain by location in the abdomen.

> ### BOX 7-2
>
> **POTENTIAL ABDOMINAL CATASTROPHES**
>
> Appendicitis
> Bowel perforation
> Cholangitis
> Ectopic pregnancy
> Ischemic bowel
> Ruptured abdominal aortic aneurysm
> Splenic rupture

differential diagnostic skills by consulting a text after taking a history and returning to the bedside to ask a few more questions based on what you learned from your reading.

What Specific Questions should I Ask When Patients have Diffuse Abdominal Pain?

To assess for the likelihood of pancreatitis, ask about risk factors, including gallstone disease, excessive alcohol use, hypertriglyceridemia, and certain medications (e.g., antiretrovirals, prednisone, hydrochlorothiazide). Also ask about worsening of symptoms with eating and radiation of pain to the back or flank. To assess for the likelihood of bowel obstruction, ask about inability to pass stool or flatus, feculent vomiting, and prior abdominal surgery. To assess for the likelihood of ischemic bowel or aneurysm, ask about atherosclerotic disease risk factors, such as personal history of hypertension, hyperlipidemia, smoking, diabetes, or family history of early MI. Ask about postprandial symptoms

> ### BOX 7-3
>
> **KEY INFORMATION TO GATHER ABOUT ABDOMINAL PAIN FROM THE PATIENT HISTORY**
>
> Onset and duration
> Character and severity of pain
> Location and radiation
> Progression of symptoms over time
> Associated symptoms
> Relation to meals, exercise, defecation
> Change in stool or flatus
> Exacerbating and relieving factors
> History of recent travel, infectious exposure, alcohol use
> Medications

and weight loss because these may accompany recurring episodes of ischemic bowel. When patients have postprandial abdominal pain, think of gallbladder disease, ischemic bowel, gastroesophageal reflux disease, pancreatitis, small bowel obstruction, and irritable bowel syndrome. Ask about risk factors for chronic liver disease (alcohol use, country of origin, unprotected sexual exposures, and intravenous drug use) because cirrhosis with ascites can present with diffuse pain and is a risk for SPB. Ask if the pain occurs at night. Pain caused by gallbladder stones and gastroesophageal reflux often occurs when individuals are sleeping.

What Risk Factors Exist for the Various Causes of Abdominal Pain?

Older men with BPH may have painful bladder distention secondary to outlet obstruction. Prior gallstones put patients at risk for cholangitis, pancreatitis, and gallstone ileus. NSAIDS, cigarettes, oral steroids, caffeine, and heavy alcohol use are risks for PUD. Cigarette and significant steroid use also are risk factors for atherosclerotic disease, increasing the risk of angina, bowel ischemia, or aortic aneurysm. Patients with heavy alcohol use are at risk for gastritis, PUD, liver disease, and pancreatitis. Patients having unprotected intercourse or sharing needles for injected drug use are at risk for hepatitis. Women with unprotected sexual exposures are at risk for PID or ectopic pregnancy. Depression, anxiety, or sexual or physical abuse may be risk factors for functional abdominal pain without identifiable physical pathology.

What are Helpful Findings on Physical Exam in Patients with Abdominal Pain?

Tachycardia or hypotension suggests a serious illness, requiring rapid assessment. Peritoneal signs of involuntary guarding or rebound tenderness are present when the peritoneal lining is irritated, usually by infection (e.g., with bowel rupture or appendicitis) or extravasation of blood into the peritoneum. Patients with peritoneal signs usually lie still to avoid irritating the peritoneum. Turner's and Cullen's signs are ecchymoses seen on the flank (Turner's sign) or around the umbilicus (Cullen's sign) in patients with retroperitoneal hemorrhage (usually as a result of hemorrhagic pancreatitis). Look for a hernia because a trapped piece of bowel can lead to bowel obstruction. Shifting dullness or a fluid wave may suggest ascites and a complication of liver disease. A Sister Mary Joseph nodule is an indurated nodule of metastatic cancer in the umbilicus and is seen occasionally in patients with GI malignancy. The pelvic exam is important in women with abdominal pain. Cervical motion tenderness and purulent cervical discharge suggest PID. Adnexal fullness or tenderness may accompany ectopic pregnancy or tubo-ovarian abscess. Finger point tenderness at McBurney's point is used to confirm appendicitis. This point is located 1.5 to 2 inches from the ASIS on a line drawn between the ASIS and the umbilicus.

Abdominal Pain

Carnett's sign is used to determine if an abdominal wall process is causing pain. It is performed by examining patients in a half sit-up position; in this position, intra-abdominal pathology is usually less painful to deep palpation, and abdominal wall pathology is more painful.

What Work-up should I Order in Acutely ill Patients with Abdominal Pain?

In patients with severe abdominal pain, standard lab work-up includes urinalysis, CBC, ABG, electrolytes, liver function tests, an amylase or lipase, and a pregnancy test. Blood cultures are warranted if fever is present. An abdominal x-ray series may detect bowel obstruction or perforation (see Chapter 6). Don't forget the bladder or kidney as a potential source of pain. Bladder catheterization or ultrasound may reveal a bladder outlet obstruction. Obtain a CT scan if you suspect cholecystitis, cholangitis, appendicitis, ischemic bowel, or abdominal aortic aneurysm, or if the cause remains unclear in a patient with severe abdominal pain. Ultrasound can be used to detect an ectopic pregnancy or biliary tree pathology. For patients with abdominal pain in shock (with unstable vital signs), urgent surgical exploration may need to be done before there is time for imaging. If you suspect an extra-abdominal source of pain, get a chest x-ray and ECG.

What Studies are Warranted in Patients with Mild or Chronic Abdominal Pain?

For younger patients with dyspepsia or reflux symptoms, a successful trial of antacid therapy can be used as a diagnostic test; patients >50 years old with dyspepsia or patients with alarm symptoms require gastroscopy (see Chapter 14). For patients with focal, episodic, RUQ pain unresponsive to antacids, an ultrasound or CT scan may reveal gallstones to suggest recent biliary colic. Gallbladder wall thickening or biliary dilation with acute ongoing pain indicates cholecystitis or cholangitis. In patients with worrisome weight loss, bloody stool, melena, or change in bowel habits and abdominal pain, general lab studies including CBC, electrolytes, glucose, and LFTs are reasonable along with referral for endoscopy. A large percentage of patients with chronic abdominal pain have functional disease, meaning pain not associated with a discoverable pathologic abnormality. Such patients often have already undergone a work-up without obtaining a clear diagnosis. A good psychosocial history is key and may reveal prior or current abuse or depression.

 TREATMENT

For specific treatments of common causes of abdominal pain, see other relevant chapters on dyspepsia, GI bleeding, gastroenterology, hematology and oncology, and infectious disease.

When Should I Hospitalize Patients with Abdominal Pain?

Reasons for admitting a patient with abdominal pain include severe pain of unclear cause, peritoneal signs, unstable vital signs, suspected cholangitis, cholecystitis, bowel obstruction or perforation, appendicitis, aneurysmal leak, splenic rupture, ectopic pregnancy, and tubo-ovarian abscess. Patients with pyelonephritis or PID with vomiting who need intravenous antibiotics also should be admitted. Part of treating a patient hospitalized for abdominal pain includes frequent serial examinations to assess for progression of disease, whether or not a diagnosis has been made. Patients with an unclear source of acute abdominal pain accompanied by peritoneal signs or shock may need urgent exploratory surgery, so it is important to involve a surgical consult team early.

KEY POINTS

◆ Narrow the differential diagnosis of abdominal pain by acuity and location of the pain.

◆ Order a pregnancy test and perform a pelvic exam in young women with lower abdominal pain of unclear cause.

◆ A painful but soft abdomen in an elderly patient is ischemic bowel disease until proved otherwise.

◆ MI and PE can masquerade as abdominal pain.

Case 7-1

A 15-year-old girl is brought to the emergency department by a friend. She reports 3 days of steadily worsening abdominal pain in her right lower abdomen with associated fevers and sweats at night. She has had unprotected sex with several different partners in the last few months, does not take any medications, and has been otherwise healthy without prior surgeries or hospitalizations. Her pulse is 110 beats/min, BP is 90/60 mm Hg, and temperature is 101.6° F. Rectal exam is unremarkable, with guaiac-negative tan stool.

   A. What is your differential diagnosis?
   B. What steps do you wish to take next in her evaluation and treatment?

Case 7-2

A 74-year-old man with a history of hypertension, diabetes, cigarette smoking, and alcohol use reports 3 days of worsening abdominal pain and constipation preceded by several months of anorexia and a 10-lb weight loss. His medications are hydrochlorothiazide, amlodipine, metformin, and aspirin. On exam, he is rotund and pale, with a protuberant abdomen. His heart rate is 112 beats/min, blood pressure is 90/60 mmHg, respiratory rate is 28, and temperature is 100.9° F. The abdomen is distended and tender, especially in the LLQ, with involuntary guarding. Rectal exam reveals a diffusely large prostate and guaiac-positive stool. Extremities are without edema, although dorsalis pedis pulses are markedly diminished.

A. What is your differential diagnosis for his abdominal pain?
B. What tests do you order to confirm your diagnosis and rule out other possibilities?

Case Answers

7-1 A. *Learning objective:* **List likely diagnoses for abdominal pain using all available clinical information.** Pain in the RLQ in a sexually active young woman could be an ectopic pregnancy, most concerning because of its potential for rapid blood loss and shock; or tubo-ovarian abscess, more likely in light of her fever; or UTI, such as pyelonephritis, although with this diagnosis you would expect some right flank pain and tenderness. Other pelvic pathologic conditions include ruptured ovarian cyst or ovarian torsion, although these usually have a more acute onset. Appendicitis usually presents more acutely as well with <24 hours of pain progressing to acute rupture within 24 hours. IBD, such as Crohn's ileitis, is possible, although less likely without change in bowel habit or bloody stool.

7-1 B. *Learning objective:* **Inform your senior resident before spending too much time figuring out what to do because this patient is quite ill.** Choose appropriate testing to confirm your diagnosis in a young woman with RLQ pain. Order a pregnancy test, CBC looking for blood loss or infection, ESR, chemistry panel with renal function, PT, PTT, urinalysis, and blood and urine cultures. Amylase and LFTs complete the "abdominal pain" blood tests, although these are less likely to contribute to the diagnosis in this case. Perform pelvic examination to look for a purulent cervical discharge or tender adnexal mass. Pelvic ultrasound may confirm an abscess or ectopic pregnancy.

7-2 A. *Learning objective:* **List likely diagnoses for abdominal pain using all available clinical information.** Pain in the LLQ with guaiac-positive stool and preceded by weight loss in an older man is likely a bowel cancer until proved otherwise. With constipation, there could be an associated bowel obstruction, and with associated fever, tachycardia, and hypotension, there may be an associated gram-negative sepsis owing to bowel perforation. Diverticulitis also is common in older patients and causes LLQ pain, GI bleeding, and bowel perforation; however, this diagnosis doesn't explain the weight loss. UTI or bladder distention or both are possible, especially given his large prostate, although these would not usually cause LLQ pain and wouldn't explain weight loss and GI bleeding. Ischemic bowel also is possible in light of his multiple risk factors for atherosclerosis, although a patient with ischemic bowel would usually present with a soft abdomen, unless infarction and peritonitis have set in. Aortic aneurysm also is possible with these atherosclerotic risk factors, although if it is causing pain, the pain is more diffuse and radiates to the back, and the patient is usually more catastrophically ill, rather than having pain for several days. With alcohol use, cirrhosis and ascites with SBP also is possible to explain a protuberant abdomen and fever, although it would not explain the focal nature of his tenderness or his pallor. Most patients with ascites and SBP also have leg edema, which he does not have. Obstipation or bowel obstruction also is possible, in light of his constipation and calcium channel blocker use, although this alone would not explain the weight loss and GI blood loss. Pancreatitis is unlikely given the LLQ pain, although he does use alcohol and take hydrochlorothiazide, two potential precipitants of pancreatitis.

7-2 B. *Learning objective:* **Order appropriate investigations to evaluate older patients with LLQ pain.** Inform your senior resident of this extremely ill patient with signs of septic shock as soon as possible. Blood work should include a CBC to detect blood loss and systemic infection; ESR, renal function, electrolytes, and ABG to detect any renal impairment and metabolic acidosis; liver enzymes and PT INR to assess liver function; urinalysis to look for UTI; and blood and urine cultures to look for bacterial infection. Although pancreatitis is unlikely, amylase can be obtained to be sure. An abdominal x-ray series should be obtained to rule out perforation or bowel obstruction. Bedside maneuvers, such as looking for shifting dullness or bulging flanks, may help rule out ascites. Ultrasound can be used to look for ascites or urinary retention. Abdominal CT may detect a mass or inflammation associated with diverticulitis. Colonoscopy can be performed to obtain a biopsy specimen of any suspicious lesion when the patient is no longer unstable or septic.

Abdominal Pain

REFERENCES

Orient JM: Sapira's Art and Science of Bedside Diagnosis, 3rd ed. Baltimore: Lippincott Williams & Wilkins, 2005.

Spiro HM: An internist's approach to acute abdominal pain. Med Clin North Am. 1993;96:163.

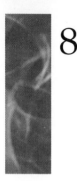

8

Anemia

DEBORAH L. GREENBERG

 ETIOLOGY

What is Anemia?

Anemia is a decrease in RBC mass. Because RBC mass is difficult to measure directly, we use hemoglobin or HCT as surrogate measures. Hemoglobin <12 g/dL (120 g/L) in women and <13 g/dL (130 g/L) in men defines anemia. HCT is roughly three times the hemoglobin. Hemoglobin and HCT measures are plasma volume dependent. They are falsely elevated in dehydration and falsely decreased in volume overload (e.g., cirrhosis or CHF).

How Does Anemia Occur?

Blood loss is the most common cause of anemia, usually from GI bleeding or menses. Any disruption in the RBC life cycle also causes anemia, including inadequate production or excessive destruction. Any of these causes may coexist. RBC **production** is abnormal if the bone marrow does not have necessary building blocks, such as iron or vitamin B_{12}, or if the marrow is damaged because of drugs, fibrosis, or cancer infiltration. **Destruction** occurs by hemolysis, either within blood vessels (intravascular) or in the spleen (extravascular).

How Do the Reticulocyte Count and MCV Help Determine Etiology?

The normal bone marrow responds to anemia by releasing more reticulocytes (immature RBCs). With hemolysis or acute blood loss, the reticulocyte count increases. A normal marrow response is reflected in a corrected reticulocyte index of >2-3. Lower values, no matter what the cause of anemia, suggest that the bone marrow is not functioning normally (i.e., there is a production problem). In this case, the MCV would help distinguish causes (Table 8-1).

Table 8-1

Causes of Hypoproliferative Anemia by Mean Corpuscular Volume

MCV	Common Causes	Less Common Causes
MCV <80		
Microcytosis	Iron deficiency	Thalassemia Anemia of chronic disease Hemoglobin E
MCV 80-95		
Normocytosis	Anemia of chronic disease Acute bleeding Anemia of renal disease	Bone marrow suppression, fibrosis, or infiltration
MCV >95		
Macrocytosis	Alcohol	Vitamin B_{12} deficiency Folate deficiency Hypothyroidism Reticulocytosis

What Causes the Changes in RBC Size Reflected in an Abnormal MCV?

Enlarged RBCs often develop when abnormal DNA synthesis delays nuclear maturation of erythrocyte precursors as in vitamin B_{12} or folate deficiency. Alcohol may be the most common cause of macrocytic anemia; 40%-90% of alcoholics have an MCV >100 fL, mostly owing to a direct effect of alcohol on the bone marrow, although occasionally as a result of folate deficiency. Small RBCs occur with problems in hemoglobin synthesis, as with iron deficiency or thalassemia.

How Do People Become Deficient of Folate or Vitamin B_{12}?

Folate deficiency generally results from inadequate nutritional intake of leafy green vegetables and citrus fruits and is especially seen in severely disabled patients and alcoholics. Deficiency also results from problems with absorption (as with small bowel disease or the use of phenytoin or phenobarbital) or increased demand (as in pregnancy, psoriasis, chemotherapy, or hemolytic anemia). The body stores only a 3-month supply of folate, so deficiency can develop after a short period of time. In contrast, the liver stores a 3- to 5-year supply of vitamin B_{12}, so a nutritional deficiency alone almost never occurs. Vitamin B_{12} requires binding to intrinsic factor from the stomach to be absorbed in the terminal ileum. Vitamin B_{12} deficiency usually is caused by pernicious anemia, an autoimmune destruction of the parietal cells, which make intrinsic factor in the stomach. Achlorhydria, or loss of stomach acid, is common in older patients and causes deficiency by preventing binding of vitamin B_{12} to intrinsic factor. Proton-pump inhibitors can decrease vitamin B_{12}

absorption by 90% by reducing stomach acid. Colchicine and neomycin also can block vitamin B_{12} absorption. Vitamin B_{12} deficiency can cause any combination of nausea, heartburn, vague abdominal pain, depression, or subacute neurologic disease (e.g., dementia, dorsal and lateral column defects).

Why Does Chronic Disease Cause Anemia?

Anemia of chronic disease, also known as inflammatory block, is a mild-to-moderate anemia resulting from an inability to use iron. Inflammatory mediators prevent the normal transfer of iron from bone marrow stores into hemoglobin. This type of anemia is associated with chronic conditions, such as RA, SLE, CHF, malignancy, and chronic infections such as osteomyelitis.

What Causes Hemolysis?

Hemolysis can be categorized according to where the hemolysis occurs. In **intravascular** hemolysis, RBCs are broken down directly in the blood vessels. Examples include RBC fragmentation across mechanical heart valves or over fibrin strands in DIC. In **extravascular** hemolysis, abnormal RBCs are lysed in the reticuloendothelial system of the spleen or liver. RBCs are recognized as abnormal by the reticuloendothelial system owing to attached antibodies, such as in autoimmune hemolysis or infection, or membrane or hemoglobin defects, such as sickle cell or thalassemia.

What Medications Cause Anemia?

Medications can cause anemia by a variety of mechanisms. Always review the medication list of a patient with unexplained anemia. Common drugs associated with anemia are anticonvulsants, colchicine, trimethoprim, chloroquine, and certain antibiotics. Pioglitazone and rosiglitazone can cause a dilutional anemia. Other medications cause macrocytosis by altering DNA synthesis directly (e.g., chemotherapy agents, anticonvulsants, trimethoprim, and sulfasalazine). Dapsone frequently causes hemolytic anemia.

EVALUATION

In Whom Should I Suspect Anemia?

Mild anemia is asymptomatic and is often discovered incidentally as part of routine blood work. Asymptomatic patients should not be screened for anemia. Symptoms of anemia are nonspecific and reflect inadequate oxygen delivery. Symptoms also depend on the abruptness of onset, severity, age, and cardiopulmonary reserve of the patient. In general, you should suspect anemia as a contributing factor in patients with fatigue, shortness of breath, dyspnea on exertion, dizziness, pallor, or tachycardia. Patients with iron deficiency anemia may present with the onset of restless legs syndrome.

Anemia

What Should I Look for When I Evaluate Patients with Anemia?

A history of chest pain, light-headedness, or shortness of breath indicates possible end-organ hypoxia and should prompt rapid evaluation. Exam findings in patients with significant anemia include tachycardia, cardiac flow murmur, pale conjunctivae, and pale palmar creases and nail beds.

What Tests are Key in Differentiating Types of Anemia?

Order an HCT or hemoglobin to confirm the diagnosis of anemia. Reticulocyte count, MCV, and peripheral smear suggest a diagnosis or direct further testing (Figure 8-1).

If I Suspect Hemolysis, What Tests are Helpful?

Peripheral smear differentiates between intravascular and extravascular hemolysis. Spherocytes are formed during extravascular hemolysis when abnormal RBC membrane is removed by the reticuloendothelial system. Irregularly shaped RBC fragments, called schistocytes, are formed as RBCs sheer across intravascular obstacles such as prosthetic valves and fibrin strands; they are seen only in intravascular hemolysis. Regardless of the site of hemolysis, RBC destruction results in reticulocytosis, elevated indirect bilirubin, elevated LDH, and decreased haptoglobin. Measurable haptoglobin decreases because it binds to the hemoglobin released from hemolyzed RBCs. A sudden unexpected "good" hemoglobin A_{1C} may be due to hemolysis in a patient with diabetes.

If I Suspect Iron Deficiency, What Else Should I Look for?

Ask about heavy menses, bloody or black stool, fatigue, restless legs syndrome, and pica (eating nonfood items, such as paper or clay). Pagophagia,

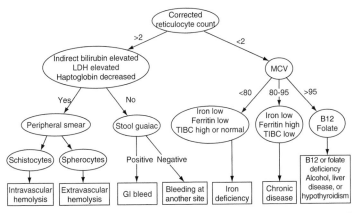

FIGURE 8-1 Diagnostic work-up for common causes of anemia. Sequence of testing may vary depending on the clinical situation.

or pica for ice, is considered a specific symptom for iron deficiency. Spoon nails (koilonychia) and a smooth red tongue (atrophic glossitis) are uncommon signs of iron deficiency. Obtain serum iron, TIBC, and ferritin. Iron deficiency initially results in a decreased ferritin. Subsequently, serum iron decreases, and TIBC increases. As deficiency progresses, hemoglobin decreases, and microcytosis develops, causing a decreased MCV. If the lab tests suggest iron deficiency, you need to find the source of blood loss. In addition to guaiac testing, endoscopy may be necessary.

What Should I Do Next if My Patient Has Normocytic Anemia (MCV 80-95 fL)?

Review the history and physical for symptoms or signs of inflammation, which might cause anemia of chronic disease: 75% of anemias of chronic disease are normocytic. Because normocytic anemia can result from early iron deficiency, iron studies are helpful in differentiating iron deficiency from the anemia of chronic disease. Review medications, which could suppress the bone marrow, such as antibiotics or chemotherapeutic agents. Additionally, check for signs or symptoms of neoplastic disease, including anorexia, weight loss, or night sweats. Peripheral smear may suggest hemolysis or sickle cell disease or may show teardrop-shaped RBCs in the case of marrow fibrosis or infiltration. Other specific studies for hemolysis, chronic renal failure, or thyroid disease may be warranted. Bone marrow biopsy can rule out myelodysplasia, infiltration, or bone marrow fibrosis.

The MCV Is Low and Lab Tests Have Ruled Out Iron Deficiency. What Do I Do Next?

Iron deficiency is the most common cause of a decreased MCV. If lab tests rule out iron deficiency, however, consider anemia of chronic disease or thalassemia. In anemia of chronic disease, the ferritin, an acute phase reactant, is often increased, whereas TIBC and serum iron are decreased. Despite low serum iron, iron replacement is of no benefit because of the inflammatory block. Thalassemia is a genetic disease of globin chains seen in patients with Mediterranean, African, or Asian heritage. Patients with thalassemia have a very low MCV in the 60–70 range, out of proportion to a mild anemia (Hct 33–40). Often target cells are seen on peripheral smear. Molecular methods can often be used to confirm beta-thalassemia and alpha-thalassemia. If the diagnosis remains unclear after full lab work-up, consider a bone marrow biopsy and iron stain.

What Tests Should I Order if My Patient Has Macrocytic Anemia (MCV >95 fL)?

Review the history for alcohol or medication use, risk factors for and symptoms of vitamin B_{12} deficiency (gastric surgery, vitiligo, paresthesias in the feet, memory loss), symptoms of hypothyroidism, or chronic liver disease. Also, look for signs or symptoms of acute bleeding or hemolysis because reticulocytes are larger than mature RBCs and increase the MCV. Examine the patient for signs of vitamin B_{12} deficiency, such as beefy red tongue and decreased peripheral vibratory or position sense, or for findings of end-stage liver disease. Review the smear for hypersegmented neutrophils and macro-ovalocytes, megaloblastic changes that are caused by abnormal DNA synthesis and delayed nuclear maturation of erythrocyte precursors. RBC folate and serum vitamin B_{12} levels may reveal the cause. If these tests are equivocal, methylmalonic acid and homocysteine levels can be drawn for confirmation. If no obvious diagnosis is apparent, consider getting a bone marrow biopsy.

 TREATMENT

In general, the underlying cause of the anemia should be identified and treated. Outpatients rarely need to be hospitalized or transfused for their anemia alone.

How Do I Treat Iron Deficiency Anemia, and What Response Should I Expect from Treatment?

The goals of treatment are to (1) identify and treat the cause of iron deficiency and (2) provide sufficient iron to correct the anemia and replenish stores. With few exceptions, replace iron orally. Compliance can be difficult because about 25% of patients have side effects when they take iron on an empty stomach (nausea, epigastric pain, constipation, and diarrhea). Although absorption is decreased 40% when iron is taken with food, this may be a necessary compromise. Start with 325 mg of ferrous sulfate once a day. You rarely need to give >325 mg/d. Ferrous gluconate and elixir preparations are available as well. Giving iron with vitamin C may help absorption. The HCT should increase by 2 points every 3-4 weeks. A reticulocytosis is the first sign of response and is evident after 10 days. An important drug interaction to know about is that oral iron can bind thyroid hormone and lead to malabsorption of thyroid hormone. Thyroid hormone and iron should not be given at the same time.

When Should I Hospitalize a Patient with Anemia?

Hospitalize patients with anemia when they have a declining HCT because of ongoing blood loss or rapid hemolysis, or when cardiac or pulmonary symptoms occur.

When Should a Patient with Anemia be Transfused?

General guidelines for blood transfusion are arbitrary because of lack of data. In general, transfusion is indicated when hemoglobin decreases to <7 g/dL (70 g/L) in otherwise healthy patients. In patients >65 years old or with cardiorespiratory diseases, transfusion may be required at higher hemoglobin levels. Patients with rapid or uncontrolled blood loss also may require transfusion at higher hemoglobin levels. For every unit of packed RBCs given, the hemoglobin generally increases by 1 g/dL (10 g/L).

Anemia

KEY POINTS

◆ Anemia is never normal—seek a cause in all patients who are anemic.

◆ History and physical are key in narrowing the differential diagnosis of anemia.

◆ Carefully review medications for a cause of anemia.

◆ Begin lab evaluation with an HCT, MCV, reticulocyte count, and smear.

◆ For iron deficiency anemia, start with low-dose iron replacement (325 mg orally daily)

Case 8-1

A 74-year-old woman with history of hypertension has new-onset fatigue. She is sleeping well and has no other concerns. She takes a diuretic and a beta blocker for her hypertension. Her HCT is found to be 33% with an MCV of 82. She has normal iron studies, including a normal ferritin.

A. What additional lab test would most likely reveal the etiology of her anemia?

B. What should you do next?

Case 8-2

A 32-year-old woman with heavy periods and fatigue is diagnosed with iron deficiency. Her initial HCT is 33% with a low serum iron, elevated TIBC, and a low ferritin of 7. She is started on iron therapy and returns 3 months later. She is taking her iron twice daily as instructed, but her HCT is now 32% with a ferritin of 6.

A. Why has she failed to respond to iron therapy?

B. What is the next step in your evaluation?

Case Answers

8-1 A.   *Learning objective:* **Recognize anemia of chronic renal disease as a common cause of anemia in the elderly.** Chronic renal insufficiency is the most likely cause of this patient's mild normocytic, normochromic anemia given her underlying hypertension and her normal iron studies. A creatinine should be ordered to evaluate

Anemia

for this etiology. Anemia of chronic renal disease is becoming more prevalent as the population ages.

8-1 B. *Learning objective:* **Patients with anemia of chronic renal disease should be treated with erythropoietin to maintain a hemoglobin of 11 g/dL (110 g/L).** Use of erythropoietin in this way has been shown to improve health outcomes, including quality of life. Because this patient has already reached that goal, her hemoglobin should be monitored periodically until the threshold for treatment has been reached.

8-2 A. *Learning objective:* **Understand that heavy bleeding, malabsorption, and nonadherence to medications are common reasons that patients with iron deficiency fail to respond to oral iron therapy.** Assuming that she is taking her iron and her bleeding has not increased in severity, malabsorption should be investigated as the cause of her failure to respond.

8-2 B. *Learning objective:* **If the patient has not had abdominal surgery, an IgA endomysial antibody assay would be an appropriate next step to assess for celiac sprue.** If this test is negative, referral to a gastroenterologist may be necessary for further evaluation of malabsorption.

REFERENCES

Brill JR: Normocytic anemia. Am Fam Physician 2000;62:2255.
Davenport J: Macrocytic anemia. Am Fam Physician 1996;53:155.
Joosten E: Strategies for the laboratory diagnosis of some common causes of anemia in elderly patients. Gerontology 2004;50:49.
Woodman R, Ferrucci L, Guralnik J. Anemia in older adults. Curr Opin Hematol 2005;12:123.

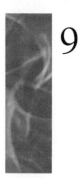

9

Chest Pain

THOMAS O. STAIGER

 ETIOLOGY

What are Common Causes of Mild-to-moderate Chest Pain in Clinic Patients?

Angina, esophageal reflux, and musculoskeletal pain (including costochondritis) are common. Less common causes are panic disorder, esophageal dysmotility, and viral or bacterial infection causing pleural irritation. Rarely, biliary, gastric, or pancreatic disease causes chest pain.

What are Life-threatening Causes of Chest Pain I Shouldn't Miss?

Acute aortic dissection, unstable or acute angina pectoris, MI, mediastinitis secondary to esophageal rupture, pericarditis, pneumothorax, and PE shouldn't be missed. Aortic dissection occurs when the aorta tears, allowing blood to dissect between layers of the vessel wall. Angina is chest pain that is due to insufficient oxygen supply to the heart muscle for the level of cardiac work (ischemia), seen particularly in patients with risk factors such as hypertension, diabetes, cigarette use, family history of early cardiac disease, or dyslipidemia. MI occurs if angina persists long enough to cause cell death (infarction). Mediastinitis is an infection of the mediastinum, usually caused by an esophageal rupture. Pericarditis develops if inflammation occurs in the pericardial sac. A pneumothorax involves air entering the pleural space. Pulmonary embolism occurs if a clot from the venous circulation lodges in a pulmonary artery.

 EVALUATION

What Pertinent History Helps Determine if Chest Pain is due to Angina?

Ask all patients with chest pain about cardiac risk factors, character and distribution of pain, and associated symptoms. Angina is a heavy, tight, or squeezing retrosternal or left chest discomfort, which can radiate to the neck, jaw, shoulders, or left arm. Associated symptoms may include dyspnea, diaphoresis, nausea, or lightheadedness. Most angina is brought on by exertion, although stress or large meals can sometimes precipitate angina. Angina typically is relieved by rest or by sublingual nitrates. Atypical presentations are common, especially in women, the elderly, and diabetics. Atypical angina may present as burning or pressure in locations such as the arm, neck, jaw, shoulder, or abdomen or as isolated dyspnea or nausea. Unstable angina refers to angina at rest, or to a substantial change in a previously stable angina pattern. MI causes similar but more severe pain and generally lasts >30 minutes. Pain that is pleuritic, sharp, positional, or exactly reproduced by palpation is unlikely to be due to ischemia. Pain lasting for only a few seconds is never due to ischemia. Findings that suggest specific noncardiac causes of pain are listed in Table 9-1.

Table 9-1

Clues to Nonischemic Causes of Chest Pain

Diagnosis	History	Physical Exam	Diagnostic Tests
Costochondritis	Recent viral illness	Tender to palpation just lateral to sternum	None
Mediastinitis	Dyspnea, vomiting, recent esophageal instrumentation	Subcutaneous emphysema, "Hammon's crunch"—crepitus with heartbeat	CXR: mediastinal air, pleural effusion (usually left-sided)
Musculoskeletal pain	Worse with motion or breath, history of trauma or cancer with metastasis	Pain reproduced by palpation	Physical exam, CXR
Pericarditis	Sharp pain improved by leaning forward, recent viral illness, autoimmune disease	Pericardial friction rub, jugular venous distention, pulsus paradoxus* (with large pericardial effusion)	ECG: diffuse ST elevation, PR depression
Pleurisy	Pleuritic pain, dyspnea, recent viral illness, autoimmune disease	Pleural friction rub	CXR: normal, ± small effusion

(continued)

Table 9-1

Clues to Nonischemic Causes of Chest Pain (Continued)

Diagnosis	History	Physical Exam	Diagnostic Tests
Pneumonia	Fever, cough, dyspnea, purulent sputum, pleuritic pain	Crackles, egophony over involved lung	CXR: pulmonary infiltrate
Pneumothorax	Pleuritic pain, dyspnea, history of asthma, COPD	Hyperresonance over one lung field, decreased breath sounds, tracheal shift	CXR: loss of lung markings outside sharp pleural line
PE	History of cancer, CHF, immobility, OCP use, pleuritic pain, dyspnea, syncope	Tachycardia, pleural friction rub, unilateral swollen leg	ABG, D-dimer test, ventilation-perfusion scan, venous duplex

*Pulsus paradoxus is a decrease in systolic BP of >10 mm Hg with inspiration, caused by pericardial fluid compressing the right ventricle. You can palpate this at the radial pulse in dramatic cases of tamponade. To measure it more exactly, inflate a BP cuff above systolic pressure, let air out slowly until you just begin to hear beats only during the patient's expiration, and remember that value. Let out more air until you hear all the beats through inspiration and expiration. Subtract this pressure from the first; if >10 mm Hg, pulsus paradoxus is present, indicating cardiac tamponade. Significant pulmonary obstructive disease also causes pulsus paradoxus.

How do Patients with Aortic Dissection Present?

Aortic dissection causes pain that is severe, sharp, or tearing and often begins abruptly. Tears distal to the left subclavian typically radiate to the back, whereas tears of the ascending aorta may radiate to the anterior chest, neck, or back. Pain also can radiate down the arms. Aortic dissection can cause neurologic deficits, decreased consciousness, or hoarseness. Complications can be life-threatening (Table 9-2).

Table 9-2

Complications of Acute Aortic Dissection in the Thorax

Complication	Mechanism
Acute CHF	Aortic insufficiency due to valve involved in dissection
Acute MI	Dissection disrupts opening from aorta to coronary artery
Cardiac tamponade	Blood fills pericardium and compresses heart
Neurologic deficits	Flow to innominate, carotid, or spinal arteries disrupted

What Pertinent Questions Should I Ask to Explore the Possibility of PE?

Ask about the triad of predisposing factors: (1) hypercoagulable states, such as cancer or family history of hypercoagulability; (2) prolonged stasis, as with airplane trips, surgery, or immobility; and (3) vessel injury with prior DVT, recent surgery, or trauma. Ask about unilateral leg swelling because this may reveal the embolic source. Massive embolism can stretch a pulmonary artery, mimicking angina or causing actual right ventricular ischemia. Smaller PEs may produce lung infarcts at the pleural surface, causing sharp pleuritic pains. Isolated dyspnea without pain is the most common presentation. Syncope occurs in about 10% of PEs and is a sign of a larger embolus.

What Pertinent History Should I Ask to Reveal an Esophageal Source of Pain?

Historical clues to esophageal pain from acid reflux include burning pain worsened with acidic or fatty foods or with lying down, relief with antacids, and absence of relation to exertion. Esophageal spasms may closely mimic angina and often reverse with nitroglycerin. Cardiac catheterization is sometimes needed to distinguish it from coronary vascular disease.

How does Pericarditis Differ from Angina in its Presentation?

Pain from pericarditis is classically worse lying down, better leaning forward, and unimproved by rest. Risk factors for pericarditis include recent viral syndrome, renal failure, connective tissue disease, and metastatic cancer.

What Should I Look for on Exam?

Assess the patient's general appearance; patients with chest pain who appear to be in significant discomfort are likely to have ischemia or some other serious cause for their pain. Hypertension, although nonspecific, often accompanies angina and aortic dissection. Hypotension can be seen in patients with extensive (or right ventricular) MI, large PE, or tension pneumothorax. Check for hypoxia because this suggests serious underlying pathology, such as PE, pneumonia, pneumothorax, or MI. Tachycardia may accompany PE, MI, or hypoxia of any cause. Check BP in both arms because they are unequal (>30 mm Hg) when a dissection interrupts vascular supply to one side. Listen for new murmurs: Aortic insufficiency (diastolic murmur at the sternal border) suggests dissection involving the aortic valve; MR (systolic murmur at the apex) suggests an MI involving the mitral valve papillary muscle. Listen for rubs: A pulmonary friction rub timed with inspiration suggests viral pleuritis or pulmonary infarct secondary to PE; a rub with each heartbeat suggests pericarditis. Palpate the chest wall to assess for tenderness, and ask if any tenderness exactly reproduces the patient's pain.

What Diagnostic Tests do I Order in an Outpatient with Chest Pain?

Obtain current and old **ECGs** and **CXRs** in all patients with acute chest pain. Look for the focal ST changes of angina or MI or the diffuse ST elevations and PR depressions of pericarditis. CXR can reveal CHF, pneumonia, pulmonary infarction, pneumothorax, rib fractures, or lytic bone lesions. A widened mediastinum on CXR is a sign of possible aortic dissection, although 20% of dissections have a normal mediastinal width. **Therapeutic trials** in the clinic or at home also may aid in making a diagnosis: Relief with antacids suggests GERD or PUD; relief with sublingual nitroglycerin does not change the likelihood of cardiac ischemia. Refer patients with stable episodes of angina-like symptoms for outpatient ETT to assess for fixed coronary artery narrowing. For women (in whom ETT has low sensitivity), a patient with left bundle branch block (which generally masks the ischemic changes on an ETT), or a patient unable to walk, alternatives to ETT include nuclear medicine tests or stress echocardiogram.

What Tests are Appropriate for Patients Hospitalized because of Chest Pain?

In addition to an ECG and CXR, obtain serial cardiac enzymes (see Chapter 26 for details). Because of the high mortality of acute aortic dissection, obtain TEE or chest CT scan if a dissection is suspected. CHF and MI can accompany aortic dissection. Thrombolytics for MI are likely fatal if given to patients with concurrent aortic dissection and can be fatal for patients with pericarditis. These diagnoses need to be carefully excluded before a patient is given thrombolytics. Obtain a CBC with differential to look for anemia or infection; platelets, PT, and PTT for coagulopathy; and a chemistry panel.

My Clinic Patient "Ruled-out" for MI, but Still has Pain. What Other Tests are Useful?

Patients "rule-out" for MI when serial enzymes and serial ECGs fail to reveal heart muscle damage. CAD is still possible even after "ruling-out" and can be diagnosed by ETT or other imaging (see Chapter 26). An outpatient GI evaluation may include a trial of PPIs (first choice), a more invasive EGD to look for esophageal or gastric lesions, or 24-hour esophageal pH monitoring to confirm GERD. Further evaluation for esophageal dysmotility may include barium swallow or esophageal pressure monitoring.

▉ TREATMENT

When Should Patients be Hospitalized for Chest Pain?

Patients with chest pain suspicious for ischemia or with atypical chest pain and ECG changes consistent with ischemia are generally admitted.

Table 9-3

Therapeutic Options for Noncardiac Causes of Chest Pain

Cause of Chest Pain	Treatment Options
Acute aortic dissection	BP control, surgical repair
Costochondritis	NSAIDs or acetaminophen, time
Gastroesophageal reflux	PPIs, lifestyle modification, surgical fundoplication
Esophageal spasm	Antacids, calcium channel blocker, nitroglycerin
Musculoskeletal pain	Rest, stretching, physical therapy, NSAIDs or acetaminophen
Pericarditis	NSAIDs
Pneumonia	Antibiotics, oxygen, chest physiotherapy
Pneumothorax	If tension pneumothorax, urgent decompression by angiocatheter, chest tube

Patients with atypical chest pain, with no ECG changes, and who have cardiac risk factors are admitted or transferred to a cardiac observation unit if there is concern that their pain could be due to ischemia. If vital signs are abnormal, or the presentation suggests PE or aortic dissection, patients are admitted for rapid evaluation and observation.

What Specific Treatments are Available for Common Causes of Chest Pain?

See Chapter 26 for treatment of ischemia and Table 9-3 for other causes.

What is the Prognosis for Patients with Noncardiac Chest Pain?

Normal angiography is associated with a 7-year cardiac mortality of <1%. Chest pain of unclear etiology can develop into a chronic pain syndrome, causing patients significant morbidity and cost. These patients are best managed by primary care physicians with continued vigilance for the possibility of CAD (especially in the elderly), selected evaluation for esophageal or psychiatric disease, judicious use of medications for symptom control, and reassurance. One third of patients with chest pain and normal coronary arteries on angiography have panic disorder as the cause of their recurrent chest pain.

KEY POINTS

◆ Consider life-threatening causes in all patients with chest pain and use focused history, physical, and studies to find or exclude them rapidly.

◆ After the initial evaluation, if ischemic cardiac chest pain is still a reasonable possibility, admit for monitoring and serial cardiac enzyme testing.

Continued

◆ Consider a PE in any patient with unexplained chest pain, especially with associated dyspnea, hypoxia, or pleuritic pain.

◆ Pericarditis causes diffuse ST elevation or PR depression on ECG and pain relieved by leaning forward.

◆ Aortic dissection causes pain that begins abruptly and radiates to the back or chest, unequal pulses, and a widened mediastinum and may have associated neurologic deficits, CHF, or MI.

Case 9-1

A 60-year-old man presents to the emergency department complaining of 48 hours of progressively increasing chest pain. The pain is 8/10, sharp, substernal, and pleuritic and is worsened by lying supine. He gives a history of 1 week of low-grade temperatures, sore throat, and a nonproductive cough. He reports mild dyspnea that he attributes to his pain. He denies calf pain or swelling. His past history includes a total knee replacement 1 month ago, hypertension, and hypercholesterolemia. His medications are hydrochlorothiazide and atorvastatin. He is sitting on a stretcher and looks uncomfortable. Vital signs are temperature 37.5° C, pulse 110 beats/min, BP 125/80 mm Hg, and respirations 18.

    A. What are possible causes for his pain?
    B. Which clinical features suggest pericarditis? Which features suggest a PE?
    C. A nurse hands you his ECG (Figure 9-1). What is the most likely diagnosis?
    D. What would you expect to find on physical exam?
    E. What is the most likely cause for this patient's syndrome? Are there any other causes it would be important to exclude?

Case 9-2

A 65-year-old woman presents with 4 hours of chest pain. The pain is a 5/10 substernal nonradiating pressure, associated with nausea and mild dyspnea. She has diabetes and hypercholesterolemia. Her father had an MI at age 54. She has no prior history of similar pain and denies dyspnea or tobacco use. Her medications are metformin and lovastatin. She appears moderately uncomfortable and diaphoretic. Vital signs are temperature 36.8° C, pulse 112 beats/min, BP 146/92 mm Hg, and respirations 22. Her chest is clear, and cardiac exam shows regular S_1S_2 without murmurs, rubs, or gallops.

    A. List this patient's CAD risk factors. What are other cardiac risk factors?
    B. What are the significant findings on this patient's ECG (Figure 9-2)?
    C. What are the most likely diagnoses in this patient? What are other possible diagnoses?

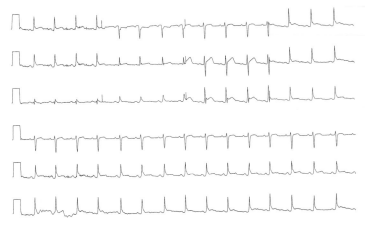

FIGURE 9-1 (From Chan TC, Brady W, Harrigan R, et al: ECG in Emergency Medicine and Acute Care. St Louis: Mosby, 2005, p 202.)

Case Answers

9-1 A.   *Learning objective:* **List causes of pleuritic pain.** The most likely causes of pain in this patient include pericarditis, PE, pneumonia, pleurodynia (pleuritis), costochondritis, or a rib fracture. Other causes to consider include angina and a pneumothorax.

9-1 B.   *Learning objective:* **Identify clinical features that support a diagnosis of pericarditis or PE.** Pericarditis is suggested by a recent viral illness and by pain worsened by lying down. PE is suggested by his recent surgery and his dyspnea. Pleuritic pain can occur with pericarditis or a PE.

9-1 C.   *Learning objective:* **Recognize clinical features and ECG findings of pericarditis.** The patient's pleuritic pain worsened by lying down, a recent viral illness, and ECG findings of diffuse ST elevation and PR depression (most visible in lead II) all suggest a diagnosis of pericarditis.

9-1 D.   *Learning objective:* **Recognize the pertinent exam findings of pericarditis.** The most helpful exam finding to support a diagnosis of pericarditis is the presence of a pericardial friction rub. This is a high-pitched, scratching sound heard best with the patient sitting up and exhaling. If a patient has a large pericardial effusion associated with pericarditis, the exam may reveal distant heart sounds, distended neck veins, and a pulsus paradoxus (see Table 9-1).

9-1 E.   *Learning objective:* **List the causes of pericarditis pertinent for this patient.** The most likely cause of pericarditis in this patient is

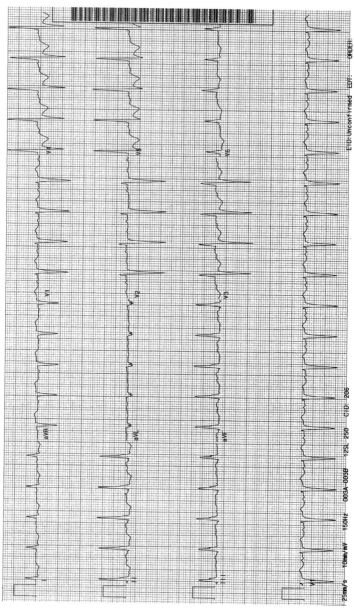

FIGURE 9-2 ECG for patient in Case 9-2.

his recent viral illness. Viral causes for pericarditis include coxsackie-virus, echovirus, adenovirus, and influenza. Pericarditis can occur after an MI, so excluding this with cardiac enzymes would be important, given his cardiac risk factors. Other causes include renal failure; autoimmune diseases; metastatic cancer; trauma; myx-edema; drugs; and bacterial, fungal, and tuberculous infections.

9-2 A.   *Learning objective:* **Identify cardiac risk factors.** This patient's cardiac risk factors include diabetes, hypercholesterolemia, and a family history of early CAD (present in a first-degree male relative <55 years old or a first-degree female relative <65 years old). Other risk factors include hypertension and tobacco use.

9-2 B.   *Learning objective:* **Recognize the ECG findings of ischemia.** This patient shows evidence for anterolateral ischemia, with ST segment depressions and T wave inversions in leads I and V3-6 and an isolated T wave inversion in lead II.

9-2 C.   *Learning objective:* **Create a differential diagnosis for chest pain appropriate to the patient's history and physical.** The most likely diagnoses in this patient are unstable angina and MI. If her ECG was unchanged from an old ECG (which is unlikely), other diagnoses to consider would include PE, esophageal reflux, esoph-ageal spasm, biliary colic, pneumonia, and chest wall pain.

REFERENCES

American College of Emergency Physicians: Clinical policy: Critical issues in the evaluation and management of adult patients presenting with suspected acute myocardial infarction or unstable angina. Ann Emerg Med 2000;35:521.

Panju AA, Hemelgarn BR, Guyatt GH, et al: Is this patient having a myocardial infarction? JAMA 1998;280:1256.

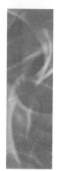

10

Cough

DAWN E. DEWITT

 ETIOLOGY

What are the Most Common Causes of Cough?

Acute cough, <3 weeks' duration, is almost always due to infection (usually viral) or irritants such as cigarette smoke. **Chronic cough** (>3 weeks) is most commonly caused by the conditions listed in Box 10-1. Chronic bronchitis is defined as productive cough on most days for at least 3 months of 2 consecutive years and occurs almost exclusively in smokers. After acute viral infection, 40% of patients have persistent cough for several weeks as a result of transiently reactive airways. Of cases of chronic cough, 62% have more than one cause. ACEIs cause cough in 10%-50% of patients, with the highest rates in Asian women.

What are the Serious Causes of Cough I Shouldn't Miss?

Cancer is a concern in patients with chronic cough, particularly in smokers >50 years old. Eighty percent of cancer patients have other symptoms, such as weight loss or hemoptysis. Patients with heart failure may present with cough. TB and pertussis, major public health risks, should always be considered. Serologies consistent with recent pertussis infection are found in 25% of adults with cough of >3 weeks' duration without another cause. Previous vaccination does not exclude pertussis. PE is an infrequent but serious cause of acute cough.

When Cough is Accompanied by Hemoptysis, What Should I Consider?

Acute bronchitis is the most common cause of bloody sputum in the U.S. Consider cancer in smokers or patients >50 years old. PE, TB, and pulmonary-renal syndromes are less common causes.

86

BOX 10-1

COMMON CAUSES OF CHRONIC COUGH

Cough-variant asthma	60%
PND	58%
Gastroesophageal reflux	41%
Chronic bronchitis/ bronchiectasis	5%-14%
Single cause	39%
Multiple causes	62%

EVALUATION

What Historical Points and Exam Findings are Important?

Table 10-1 lists pertinent history and physical findings to explore for each of the common causes of chronic cough. Note exacerbating medications such as ACEIs or beta blockers (think of reactive airways).

Table 10-1

History and Physical Findings in Common Causes of Chronic Cough

Cause	History	Physical
Asthma	Recent viral infection Cold/exercise provoke cough Aspirin or NSAID sensitivity Family or personal history of asthma/ allergies Wheezing	Eczema Wheezing (rare) Prolonged forced expiration
Postnasal drip	Nasal drainage Early morning productive cough Throat clearing	Conjunctival irritation Pharyngeal cobblestoning Pale and boggy nasal mucosa Mucus in posterior pharynx
GERD	Heartburn Acid or food regurgitation Cough after meals Symptoms worse when supine Obesity Hoarseness Calcium channel blocker use	Obesity Hoarseness

Cough

Review constitutional symptoms and risk factors for cancer and HIV. Obtain a history for hobby or work exposures, such as asbestos; risks for HIV, TB, or pertussis; and history of cat or bird contact.

What Tests Help Determine Benign Causes of a Chronic Cough?

There is no standard work-up. Office spirometry is reasonably specific for asthma if FEV_1 is <80% predicted or FEV_1/FVC ratio is >75%, but normal spirometry does not rule out asthma. Methacholine challenge to induce bronchospasm in patients with cough-variant asthma is the most sensitive test. Cough caused by GERD is almost always diagnosed by response to PPIs. In reality, most causes of cough are suggested by history and confirmed by response to an empiric trial of appropriate therapy.

How Can I Use Therapeutic Trials to Diagnose These Three Common Conditions?

Cough should improve significantly with appropriate therapy, but allow 4-6 weeks before you assess treatment impact. If you suspect upper airway cough syndrome, which is usually caused by postnasal drip or allergic rhinitis, try an antihistamine/decongestant combination such as diphenhydramine or chlorpheniramine plus pseudoephedrine, which promotes nasal mucosal drying. If there is only a partial response, and the patient still has nasal congestion, add a steroid nasal inhaler. For patients with symptoms suggestive of cough-variant asthma (exacerbation with cold or exercise), treat with beta-agonist inhalers. If the patient already uses beta-agonists, add a steroid inhaler. Steroid inhalers can irritate airways, so do not start them during acute infection. Also consider treating for asthma if the patient has no response to treatment for upper airway cough syndrome and no localizing signs for cause of the cough. If GERD is suspected, begin by eliminating substances that relax the gastroesophageal sphincter, such as cigarettes, alcohol, spicy foods, chocolate, and peppermint. Raise the head of the bed 6 inches with blocks or bricks (pillows don't work because bending at the waist increases pressure on the stomach). Prescribe empiric PPIs; H_2 blockers are acceptable, but often less effective. Combined measures may take 6 months to work.

When Should I Obtain a CXR or Other More Specialized Invasive Tests?

Get a CXR in patients with acute cough accompanied by fever, tachycardia, history concerning for pulmonary embolism, abnormal lung exam, or hypoxia on pulse oximetry. For patients with chronic cough, if history, exam, and empiric trial do not elucidate a cause, or if constitutional symptoms or cancer risk factors are present, get a CXR. Because of low sensitivity, sputum cytology cannot be used to rule out cancer. A CXR should be considered early in the work-up if the patient has a history of cigarette use, occupational exposure, or risks for TB or HIV.

TREATMENT

How do I Manage Acute Infectious Cough?

Antibiotics do not change outcomes or cough duration in sinusitis, bronchitis, and other viral respiratory infections except for sinusitis with worsening symptoms after 1 week. Community-acquired pneumonia should be treated with appropriate antibiotics (azithromycin, doxycycline, and levofloxacin are good choices).

What are Some Ways to Relieve Symptoms for Cough Patients?

Postviral cough may respond to beta agonists. Eliminate irritants, especially cigarette smoke. Counsel about smoking cessation. Advise adequate hydration and humidity. Many patients expect a prescription for cough syrup, but the efficacy of narcotic cough syrups is questionable. More recent reviews show no efficacy for codeine cough syrups. Over-the-counter preparations with only one or two active ingredients, such as guaifenesin (expectorant) or dextromethorphan (suppressant), are mildly helpful. "Cold" and "flu" preparations are best avoided because the active ingredients may double (acetaminophen) or interact with other medicines (e.g. SSRIs).

When Should I Refer?

Refer to a pulmonologist when the cause of cough is unclear or empiric therapy has not helped; when bronchoscopy is indicated to rule out TB, cancer, or other rare disease; or when specialized intervention is required (e.g., biopsy for interstitial lung disease, cancer). Reflux that does not respond to twice-daily PPIs should be referred to a gastroenterologist. In addition to your own counseling regarding cigarette use, smoking cessation clinics are helpful. If occupational exposure is possible, refer for occupational medicine evaluation.

> ## KEY POINTS
>
> ◆ The history and physical provide the key information for diagnosis.
> ◆ Acute cough is almost always infectious or due to airway irritants.
> ◆ Nonproductive chronic cough is often due to upper airway cough syndrome (PND), GERD, or bronchospasm (postinfectious or asthma). Empiric therapy is often helpful.

Case 10-1

A 25-year-old graduate student in animal behavior comes to see you about severe dry cough, right-sided sharp chest pain, and weight loss (4 kg) for

4 weeks. His cough has been keeping him awake, and he is afraid to eat too much because he has vomited with coughing after large meals on several occasions. He has been previously healthy and smokes only an occasional cigarette when out with friends. Several other graduate students in his lab have been sick with "coughs and colds," although no one has had symptoms as bad as his. He has had four sexual partners total, but none are ill. He has no tattoos or other HIV risk factors. His PhD is on bird behavior.

A. What is your differential diagnosis?
B. What additional history and physical would be most helpful?
C. How will you treat this patient?

Case 10-2

A 32-year-old woman comes in after 3 days of productive cough associated with rhinorrhea, sore throat, and fever to 38° C. Exam shows nasal discharge, pharyngeal cobblestoning, and several tender 0.8-cm cervical lymph nodes bilaterally. Her chest is clear. She asks for antibiotics and cough syrup because her cough is keeping her up at night.

A. What diagnoses and therapies should you consider?

Case Answers

10-1A. *Learning objective:* **Identify risk factors for causes of cough, and list the likely causes of prolonged cough in a young patient with several risk factors.** Most acute infections cause cough for 11 days, but many adults have cough lasting 17 days; 25% of adults with cough lasting ≥3 weeks have pertussis. This patient likely has pertussis based on severe dry cough for several weeks and vomiting. Pertussis immunity wanes after vaccination, and the incidence is increasing in teens and young adults in particular. Some countries now provide 10-year boosters for teens. You also should consider HIV-related illness and psittacosis or Q fever based on his bird exposure. Weight loss should always bring up consideration of TB (including laryngeal TB), HIV, and cancer. Pulmonary-renal syndromes are rarer, but should be considered. Smoking is a questionable risk factor based on his history, but he may be under-reporting his cigarette use.

10-1 B. *Learning objective:* **Evaluate cough using examination and tests.** An examination should focus on vital signs, HEENT exam (tympanic membranes, oropharynx), lymphadenopathy, heart and lungs, skin, and extremities. With the possibilities outlined previously, CBC, CXR, and serologies would be most helpful. An HIV test and one of several possible *Bordetella pertussis* tests (whichever is preferred by the clinic's lab) would help exclude HIV and evaluate for pertussis.

10-1 C. *Learning objective:* **Understand therapy for pertussis and pro-phylaxis for close contacts.** At this time, the patient probably would not benefit from therapy. Complications of pertussis can include rib fractures and other problems, including aspiration pneumonia from vomiting. Prophylaxis can be helpful in close contacts to prevent infection.

10-2 A. *Learning objective:* **Understand the difference between several main types of acute infection causing cough and the therapeutic implications.** This patient almost certainly has one of many common rhinoviruses. Studies have evaluated consequences of antibiotic prescribing or withholding in patients who present with a viral upper or lower respiratory infection. Symptoms such as cough duration are no different between treated and untreated groups. Patients who were not given antibiotics had slightly lower initial patient satisfaction and a slightly higher return rate to clinic. Patients were less likely to return, however, for another respiratory tract infection or to request antibiotics at a later date or both. Although over-the-counter cough syrups may reduce symptoms slightly, no benefit has been shown for narcotic cough syrups. A first-generation antihistamine plus a decongestant can help symptoms of acute cough and PND caused by colds. Studies are conflicting on whether use of beta agonists for viral-induced cough is helpful in patients without underlying asthma. A higher fever with more respiratory symptoms and myalgias might indicate influenza, which causes approximately 38,000 deaths in the U.S. every year. If influenza is likely, oseltamivir shortens symptom duration and is effective for prophylaxis. Antibiotics may be useful in patients with sinus symptoms such as discharge, pain (especially facial pain with bending), and fever that continue to worsen after 1 week. Antibiotics are useful in patients with demonstrable pneumonia (high fever, elevated WBC, and chest findings), whereas patients with COPD exacerbations (increase in productive cough without fever or CXR infiltrate) probably do not benefit from antibiotics. Patients with COPD exacerbations do benefit from intravenous or oral steroids and aggressive inhaler therapy (beta agonists and anticholinergics).

Cough

REFERENCES

Bolster DC: Cough suppressant and pharmacologic pertussive therapy: ACCP evidence-based clinical practice guidelines. Chest 2006;129:238.

Irwin RS, Boulet LP, Cloutier MM, et al: Managing cough as a defense mechanism and as a symptom: A consensus panel report of the American College of Chest Physicians. Chest 1998;114:133S.

Little P, Rumsby K, Kelley J, et al: Information leaflet and antibiotic prescribing strategies for acute lower respiratory infection: A randomized controlled trial. JAMA 2005;293:3029.

Pratter MR, Brightling CE, Boulet LP,, et al: An empiric integrative approach to the management of cough: ACCP evidence-based clinical practice guidelines. Chest 2006;129:222.

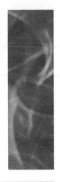

11

Chronic Nonmalignant Pain

MATTHEW F. HOLLON

 ETIOLOGY

What is Chronic Nonmalignant Pain?

Chronic nonmalignant pain is defined as pain not due to cancer, persisting for a minimum of 3 months. It is best thought of as a poorly understood disease state with little correlation between pain complaints, findings on physical exam, and results of diagnostic tests. Chronic pain is thought to be caused by a disruption in the balance of the nociceptive system and consequent neural remodeling. Evaluating and treating chronic pain is challenging because of its myriad contributing factors, including psychiatric comorbidity.

How Common is Chronic Nonmalignant Pain?

In the U.S., 50 million individuals have chronic pain. Nearly 10% of the adult population report that pain has a major impact on their lives. The prevalence of chronic pain in primary care ranges from 5%-33%.

What are the Principal Causes of Chronic Nonmalignant Pain?

Common causes include low back pain, arthritis, musculoskeletal pain secondary to previous trauma, neuropathic pain including diabetic and postherpetic neuropathy, and rheumatologic conditions such as fibromyalgia. Less common causes include headache syndromes, chronic abdominal pain including chronic pancreatitis, chronic pelvic pain, and reflex sympathetic dystrophy.

 EVALUATION

What are the Initial Steps in Evaluating a Patient with Chronic Pain?

Use the history and physical to detect reversible physical causes. Seek to understand how the pain affects the patient as a whole person, and validate the patient's experience. Review previous medical records carefully because most patients with chronic pain have had extensive previous evaluations.

What Elements of the Patient's History are Important?

Ask about location, quality, and intensity of pain over time using a scale from 1 (least severe) to 10 (most severe) and the frequency with which the pain reaches maximum intensity. Ask about substance abuse, mental health history, and work and living situations. A clear assessment of functional status (ability to perform household chores, work tasks, leisure interests, and sleep) is crucial because improving function, rather than pain, is a primary goal. Review previous treatments. Screen for depression because 85% of patients with chronic pain are depressed. Ask about history of sexual abuse in women with chronic abdominal or pelvic pain.

What Investigations are Warranted in Patients with Chronic Pain?

Consider further testing only if there are gaps in previous evaluations, a patient's symptoms have changed substantially, or a significant period of time (>1 year) has passed since previous testing. Follow a sequential rather than a "shotgun" approach, focusing diagnostic testing on the most likely cause of the pain.

TREATMENT

What are the Primary Treatment Goals in Managing Chronic Pain?

The goals are to improve quality of life, functional status, and to decrease pain intensity. A goal of complete resolution of pain is unrealistic.

What are General Strategies in Managing Chronic Pain?

Chronic pain requires a comprehensive approach that involves lifestyle modification, emphasis on coping skills, nonpharmacologic modalities, medications, and, for complex cases, the use of specialists in the management of chronic pain (Box 11-1).

What are the Principal Challenges in Managing Chronic Pain?

The numerous challenges in caring for patients with chronic pain are listed in Box 11-2.

What Nonpharmacologic Options Help Patients with Chronic Pain?

The mainstay of nonpharmacologic approaches is physical exercise, which is shown to be of particular benefit for patients with chronic

Chronic Nonmalignant Pain

BOX 11-1

STRATEGIES FOR DEVELOPING A TREATMENT PLAN FOR CHRONIC PAIN

1. Simultaneously address all components of the problem from the biopsychosocial perspective
2. Taper use of inappropriate medications to avoid polypharmacy
3. Correct misconceptions such as complete resolution of pain
4. Emphasize increasing physical activity
5. Avoid making a distinction between physical and psychological causes of pain
6. Encourage strategies for self-management
7. Encourage decreased reliance on the health care system
8. Establish a time line for achieving specific, realistic goals
9. Encourage return to a meaningful functional role in society
10. Consider use of complementary therapies such as acupuncture

---

BOX 11-2

CHALLENGES IN MANAGING CHRONIC PAIN

1. Absence of adequate, generalizable research
2. Lack of curative therapy
3. Lack of objective measures of pain or precise measures to gauge patient improvement
4. Concern on the part of physicians that they are being manipulated by patients to support prescription drug abuse
5. Presence of complex comorbidities
6. Presence of a sense of helplessness among patients with chronic pain

---

low back pain and fibromyalgia. Exercise may help by retraining the nervous system to re-establish normal neural connections affected by chronic pain. A patient diary of physical activity may be helpful in assessing adherence. Occupational therapy, behavioral therapy, and psychotherapy can be useful. Complementary medicine therapies such as acupuncture also may help some patients.

What Drugs Help Chronic Pain?

NSAIDs, acetaminophen, anticonvulsants, anesthetics, antidepressants, and opioids may help, although none result in dramatic improvement. Many patients work through trials of many different medications, often in combination. Polypharmacy is common and should be avoided by tapering or stopping all unhelpful medications.

What is the Role of NSAIDs in Treating Chronic Pain?

NSAIDs are limited by a ceiling analgesic effect and GI toxicity. Their efficacy for controlling chronic pain is not well established other than in the setting of RA and osteoarthritis. NSAIDs should be used with caution or not at all in patients with cirrhosis, kidney disease, heart disease, and previous GI bleeding. Acetaminophen's mild-to-moderate analgesic effect and low risk of toxicity at doses of 4 g/d make it a useful substitute for NSAIDs.

What is the Role of Antidepressant Medication in Treating Chronic Pain?

Depression is common and undertreated in patients with chronic pain. Additionally, TCAs and SSRIs have proven analgesic effects. Compliance is best with SSRIs compared with TCAs in the treatment of depression. It may be useful to try a TCA first, however, given the improvement in neuropathic and chronic pain. Watch for anticholinergic effects and arrhythmias. Venlafaxine works at multiple receptors (e.g., serotoninergic and noradrenergic) and may be more effective than other SSRIs.

What is the Role of Anticonvulsants or Anesthetics in Treating Chronic Pain?

Anticonvulsant medications, such as gabapentin, have established efficacy in treating neuropathic pain, such as diabetic neuropathy and post-herpetic neuralgia. Although many clinicians prescribe anticonvulsants for other types of pain, the benefit is unproven. Capsaicin cream applied topically can be used as an adjunct to other therapies for neuropathic pain or osteoarthritis. Avoid using capsaicin on the face near the eyes. Topical 5% lidocaine patches can be applied over areas of pain, although evidence of long-term efficacy is lacking.

What is the Role of Opioids in Treating Chronic Pain?

Anecdotal case series of carefully selected patients from pain clinics and approximately 15 randomized controlled trials have dispelled myths about opioid tolerance and addiction: Infinite escalations in dose and iatrogenic opioid addiction in patients with chronic pain are unlikely. Although existing randomized trials from specialty pain clinics have methodologic problems, they do show a 30% reduction in pain scores with the use of opioids, although no consistent improvement in functional status. There are no compelling studies supporting the long-term use of opioids in primary care settings.

Is it Reasonable to Consider a Trial of Opioids and, if So, for Which Patients?

Select patients for an opioid trial based on clear criteria (Box 11-3). Identify goals for improvement in function and decrease in pain, and plan monthly visits. Consider obtaining signed informed consent at

Chronic Nonmalignant Pain

BOX 11-3

CHARACTERISTICS OF PATIENTS WHO CAN BE CONSIDERED FOR OPIOID TRIAL

1. Pain complaint that is well defined and regional (e.g., spinal stenosis)
2. No history of substance abuse, including alcohol
3. Adequately treated depression (opioids may exacerbate depression)
4. Patient engages in regular physical activity
5. Patient has failed all other treatment strategies

---

the outset of a trial. Stop the trial if it does not meet explicit goals after a predetermined time period. If the opioid is to be taken on a daily basis, use long-acting opioids such as methadone. There is no role for "breakthrough" medication as is commonly and appropriately done in the treatment of pain resulting from malignancy.

What are the Important Legal Considerations in the Use of Opioids for Chronic Pain?

A patient care agreement signed by the physician and patient is wise in light of the growing problem of prescription drug abuse in the U.S. This agreement outlines the conditions for ongoing use of the controlled substance (Box 11-4). At every visit, carefully document the location and cause of the pain; the dose, frequency, and quantity of opioid medication prescribed; and the effect of the medication on functional status.

BOX 11-4

COMMON COMPONENTS OF A PATIENT CARE AGREEMENT FOR A TRIAL OF OPIOIDS

1. The patient will not adjust dose of medication without consulting with physician
2. The patient will not seek early refills of medication
3. The patient will not get medication for chronic pain from other providers, clinics, or emergency departments
4. The patient will not use illicit drugs and consents to random urine sample for drug test
5. The patient will attend all scheduled appointments for follow-up
6. If medications are lost or stolen, replacement is at the discretion of the physician; repeatedly lost or stolen prescriptions may result in discontinuation of opioid medication altogether
7. Any acute injury or illness that the patient believes necessitates additional pain medication requires medical evaluation

---

Chronic Nonmalignant Pain

When Should a Patient be Referred to a Multidisciplinary Pain Clinic?

Multidisciplinary pain clinics can provide a comprehensive and integrated approach to the care of patients with chronic pain. Complicated cases, including patients failing to respond to therapies, patients having significant disability or complex psychiatric comorbidity, patients with a history of substance abuse or requirements for high doses of medication, and patients failing to adhere to previous treatment plans, should be referred to a specialty pain clinic.

KEY POINTS

◆ Set realistic goals to improve quality of life and functional status and decrease pain, and recognize that complete resolution of pain is unlikely.

◆ The mainstay of nonpharmacologic treatment for chronic pain is physical exercise.

◆ Depression is common; consider using antidepressant medication in almost all patients, even if overt depression is not obvious.

◆ Long-term use of opioid analgesics may benefit a small subset of patients, although routine use of opioids in the primary care setting is unwarranted.

◆ Patients with complicated, refractory chronic pain should be referred to a multidisciplinary pain clinic.

Case 11-1

A 45-year-old woman presents with chronic abdominal pain of 12 years' duration. Her pain has been attributed to endometriosis and complicated by multiple abdominal surgeries (including hysterectomy). She recently "fired" her primary care provider because, despite trying antidepressant therapy in combination with oxycodone and acetaminophen, she continues to have pain and remains on disability. Which of the following is most important during the initial visit?

A. Begin a trial of anticonvulsant therapy by starting gabapentin at a dosage of 300 mg three times daily and asking her to increase it gradually.

B. Explain to her that because she has had a hysterectomy and no longer has endometrial tissue she should not be having any pain from endometriosis.

C. Advise her that although you are willing to try to help her, a goal of complete resolution of her chronic pain is unrealistic.

D. Stop her oxycodone and start her on methadone, increasing her dosage of methadone until she gets complete relief from her pain.

E. Encourage her to go back to work.

Case 11-2

A 58-year-old man with chronic low back pain of 5 years' duration that is believed to be due to degenerative changes seen on MRI 1 year ago returns for follow-up. He continues to have burning pain that radiates into his right leg and is often worse at night. He reports that he has been taking more of the hydrocodone with acetaminophen than you prescribed so that he can sleep. He notes that since starting the opioid he has been able to return to his work as a security officer, but sometimes feels no hope for the future. He is not on any other therapy currently. He was hospitalized 4 years ago for GI bleeding, but is otherwise in excellent health. What should you do next?

A. Refer the patient to a multidisciplinary pain clinic.
B. Begin a TCA such as nortriptyline, 25 mg at bedtime, increasing as tolerated.
C. Add a scheduled NSAID.
D. Stop the opioid because he has increased the dose on his own.
E. Repeat the MRI.

Case Answers

11-1 C. *Learning objective:* **Prioritize initial steps in the management of chronic pain, especially the establishment of reasonable expectations.** Although it may be reasonable to consider a trial of gabapentin, it is not the most important first action. At the initial visit, it is important that the physician validate the patient's experience of the pain rather than be dismissive: answer B is incorrect. Although methadone, as a long-acting pain reliever, may be the best option if she is to continue with opioid therapy, the physician needs additional history and the opportunity to outline the goals of therapy before deciding to continue opioids. If she has not had noticeable improvement from the oxycodone and acetaminophen, it may be more reasonable to taper this medication. Although going back to work is a reasonable long-term goal, it is more important to set short-term realistic goals for functional improvement, such as completing a household chore on a regular basis. The most important action is for the physician to educate the patient that complete resolution of her pain is unrealistic.

11-2 B. *Learning objective:* **Patient is an overall straightforward case of chronic low back pain that does not need evaluation in a specialty clinic.** The patient should avoid NSAIDs given his previous history of GI bleeding. The opioid has led to functional improvement, so it should not be stopped. He needs to be advised that if he thinks the dosage of opioid should be changed, he needs to discuss this with you first. Repeating any radiologic procedure should be done only if there is substantial change in his symptoms, such as new bowel or bladder incontinence. His feelings of hopelessness, the side effects of opioid therapy, and the neuropathic quality of his pain warrant a trial of TCA therapy. Screen for suicidality, however: If he is actively suicidal, use an SSRI, which, in contrast to TCA, is relatively safe in overdose.

REFERENCES

Bair MJ, Robinson RL, Katon W, et al: Depression and pain comorbidity—a literature review. Arch Intern Med 2003;163:2433.

Kalso E, Edwards JE, Morre A, et al: Opioids in chronic non-cancer pain: Systematic review of efficacy and safety. Pain 2004;112:372.

Marcus DA: Treatment of nonmalignant chronic pain. Am Fam Physician 2000;61:1331.

Stacey BR: Effective management of chronic pain—the analgesic dilemma. Postgrad Med 1996;100:281.

Chronic Nonmalignant Pain

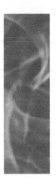

12

Diarrhea

DEBORAH L. GREENBERG

 ETIOLOGY

Does my Patient Really have Diarrhea?

Diarrhea is an increase in stool water or a stool weight >200 g/d. If stool takes the shape of the container it is in, the patient probably has diarrhea. Chronic diarrhea lasts >1 month.

Why does Diarrhea Occur?

Three main pathologic processes cause diarrhea (Table 12-1). In **secretory** diarrhea, intact intestinal cells produce excess fluid, usually from a toxin effect. In **osmotic/malabsorptive** diarrhea, malabsorption of osmotically active agents increases stool volume. In **inflammatory** diarrhea, intestinal lining cells are destroyed, so RBCs and WBCs are evident in the stool. Any of these may coexist. Inflammatory diarrhea can result in lactose intolerance (osmotic diarrhea), and rotaviruses create a malabsorptive and secretory diarrhea.

What are the Common Causes of Acute Diarrhea?

Viral infections cause most acute diarrhea in developed countries (rotaviruses in infants and enteric adenoviruses, calciviruses, and Norwalk-like viruses in all ages). Bacteria (*Campylobacter, Shigella, Salmonella*) or parasites are less common culprits. Transmission occurs via the fecal-oral route by person-to-person contact, ingestion of contaminated food or water, or sexual activity. Less common causes of acute diarrhea include leakage around a fecal impaction, narcotic withdrawal, diverticulitis, and medications (Box 12-1).

What Causes Bloody Diarrhea?

Bloody diarrhea indicates inflammation, most commonly from invasive enteric pathogens, such as *Campylobacter, Shigella, Salmonella,* and *E. coli* O157:H7. IBD (Crohn's disease and ulcerative colitis) also may

Table 12-1

Patterns Suggesting Underlying Pathologic Process in Patients with Diarrhea

Cause	Stool Pattern	Common Symptoms
Secretory		
Rotavirus	Watery	Low-grade fever, myalgias
Cholera	Watery, large volume	Severe dehydration
Hormone-producing tumors	Watery	Persists with fasting
Malabsorptive/Osmotic		
Lactose intolerance	Loose	Bloating, cramping, flatulence
Pancreatic insufficiency	Loose	Greasy (floats like oil in water)
Inflammatory		
Ulcerative colitis	Bloody	Tenesmus, weight loss
Enteric pathogens	Bloody	Higher fever, myalgias, cramping

manifest this way, usually in young adults. Other causes of bloody diarrhea include ischemic colitis, radiation injury, and rapid GI bleeding resulting from an ulcer or esophageal varices.

Is Antibiotic-associated Diarrhea always due to *Clostridium difficile* Overgrowth?

Antibiotic-associated diarrhea is generally mild, dose related, and without a causative agent and resolves when antibiotics are stopped. *C. difficile* causes 25% of antibiotic-associated diarrhea.

BOX 12-1

COMMON MEDICATIONS THAT CAN CAUSE DIARRHEA

Alcohol
Antibiotics
Antihypertensives: beta blockers, furosemide, hydralazine
Anti-inflammatory medications: ibuprofen, colchicine
Caffeine
Digoxin
Laxatives
Magnesium-containing antacids
Protease inhibitors
SSRIs
Sorbitol: cough drops, sugarless gum

What are the Common Causes of Chronic or Recurring Diarrhea?

The differential diagnosis of chronic diarrhea is broad. Lactose intolerance, indolent infection, and IBS are the most common causes. Lactose intolerance, an acquired lactase deficiency, occurs in >75% of African Americans and Asian Americans and 20% of whites. Undigested lactose after milk product ingestion causes flatulence, bloating, and diarrhea. Infections with *Giardia lamblia* or *C. difficile* may be recurrent or chronic. *Giardia* is most notable for foul-smelling flatulence and steatorrhea. None of these conditions cause nocturnal diarrhea or bloody stool, so evaluate further if these symptoms are present. Other causes to keep in mind are IBD and microscopic colitis.

What's the Difference between IBS and IBD?

IBS is a common alteration in intestinal motility with enhanced visceral sensitivity. IBS and IBD can cause intermittent abdominal pain, cramping, and alternating diarrhea and constipation over many years. IBS has specific clinical criteria (Box 12-2). IBD (Crohn's disease and ulcerative colitis) is due to bowel wall inflammation of unclear cause, with peak incidence in 15- to 35-year-olds. In addition to diarrhea, patients with IBD may have bloody stool, tenesmus (if rectum involved), or weight loss. Crohn's disease causes transmural inflammation and involves any part of the bowel from oral mucosa to rectum in discontinuous patches. Ulcerative colitis causes more superficial inflammation of the bowel wall, begins at the rectum, and affects a continuous section of colon. Patients with IBS rarely have nocturnal symptoms.

BOX 12-2

DIAGNOSIS OF IRRITABLE BOWEL SYNDROME

One of these for at least 12 weeks during the past year:

♦ Persistent or intermittent abdominal pain or discomfort relieved with defecation
♦ Persistent or intermittent change in stool frequency or consistency

Often also have two of the following:

♦ Altered stool frequency of more than three bowel movements per day or fewer than three per week
♦ Altered stool form, either hard or loose
♦ Altered stool passage with straining, urgency, or feeling of incomplete evacuation
♦ Passage of mucus
♦ Bloating or feeling of abdominal distention

Why is Malabsorption Important?

Clinically significant malabsorptive syndromes can cause deficiencies of nutrients or vitamins or both. This can occur with intestinal cell injury or loss of digestive enzymes. If fat is malabsorbed, owing to bile salt depletion or Crohn's ileitis, fat-soluble vitamins A, D, E, and K can become deficient, causing vision problems (vitamin A), bone thinning (D) or coagulopathy (K). Vitamin B_{12} deficiency also can develop with malabsorption in the terminal ileum.

EVALUATION

What Questions should I ask my Patient with Diarrhea?

Many patients cannot specifically characterize their diarrhea. Prompt them to describe frequency, volume, and appearance of the diarrhea to assess the severity of their illness and identify likely causes. Categorize the diarrhea as acute or chronic based on duration of symptoms. Try to characterize the diarrhea as inflammatory by the presence of blood and mucus, secretory by large volumes of watery stool, or malabsorptive by looseness without blood or water. Ask about exposures, including food consumption, medications, and sick contacts. Other pertinent details to ask about are presented in Table 12-2.

What History Suggests an Infectious Cause?

Acute onset, fevers, chills, or myalgias suggest infection. Patients at high risk include children in day care centers and their household contacts; travelers; patients institutionalized or hospitalized, immunocompromised, or recently on antibiotics; and individuals who have anal sex.

Table 12-2

Pertinent Questions Regarding Diarrhea

Question	Cause Suggested by Positive Answer
Bloody stool, mucus	Inflammatory cause
Fever	Infection (viral, bacterial), IBD
Greasy stools	Fat malabsorption (sprue, pancreatic insufficiency)
Nocturnal symptoms	Concerning for pathologic cause, IBD
Persistence with 24-h fast	Secretory cause (VIPoma)
Recent antibiotics, institutionalization	*Clostridium difficile*
Camping, day care exposures	*Giardia lamblia*

Diarrhea

What Diagnostic Tests Should I Order in a Patient with Acute Diarrhea?

Most episodes of diarrhea are self-limited and require no tests. Although many tests are available, their indiscriminate use is unproductive and costly. Routine stool cultures for enteric pathogens in patients with diarrhea are positive only 2% of the time. Consider further testing only when the patient has any of the following: symptoms >3 days, fever >38.5° C, bloody diarrhea, severe volume depletion, severe abdominal pain, or immunocompromise (Figure 12-1).

When Should I Test for *C. difficile* or *Giardia*?

Obtain *C. difficile* toxin in patients with recent antibiotic use, recently hospitalized patients, day care participants, and long-term care facility residents. *C. difficile* toxin testing identifies clinical disease; cultures are positive with asymptomatic colonization, as seen in 20% of inpatients. The test for *Giardia* antigen has good sensitivity (>92%) and specificity (95%) and should be obtained in campers and day care workers with persistent diarrhea.

What Diagnostic Tests should I Order for Chronic Diarrhea?

Confirm the presence of diarrhea with a 24-hour stool collection because 40% of patients referred for diarrhea have fecal weights <200 g/d. Discontinue loperamide before testing. Consider IBS in patients who do not have true diarrhea. Obtain a CBC to look for infection or blood loss, ESR, electrolytes, and albumin. Try to categorize the patient's diarrhea as inflammatory, watery, or malabsorptive, and pursue

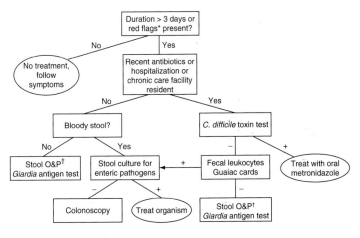

* Red flags: high fever, bloody diarrhea, severe volume depletion, severe abdominal pain, or immunocompromise. †In travelers.

FIGURE 12-1 Work-up of acute diarrhea.

further testing based on this categorization. Stool guaiac and fecal leukocytes should be ordered to look for inflammation, and *C. difficile* toxin and *Giardia* antigen should be ordered in patients at risk. If signs of malabsorption are present, such as weight loss, anemia, low albumin, ecchymoses, or neuropathy, obtain qualitative fecal fat, iron, and vitamin B_{12} studies and PT (for vitamin K deficiency). Consider the diagnosis of celiac sprue in patients with weight loss and malabsorptive diarrhea. Serologic tests for sprue are IgA tissue transglutaminase and IgA endomysial antibodies. A successful trial of a lactose-free diet diagnoses lactose intolerance. A 24-hour fast helps distinguish between malabsorption of ingested material (diarrhea abates) and secretory diarrhea (diarrhea continues). If parasitic infection is suspected, as in travelers or individuals engaging in anal sex, obtain three stool samples for ova and parasite studies.

How do I Test for IBS?

IBS is a functional disorder, meaning symptoms occur without objective abnormalities. Similar to many other clinical syndromes, there is no diagnostic test, and clinical criteria assist in making the diagnosis (see Box 12-2).

When Should I refer to a Gastroenterologist?

Refer patients when the etiology of documented diarrhea is unclear, for endoscopic procedures (indicated in malabsorption and inflammatory diarrhea without infectious cause), and for treatment of advanced cases of IBD.

▮ TREATMENT

Who needs Antibiotics?

Antibiotics are not required for most acute infectious diarrhea. Treat *Giardia* and *C. difficile* with oral metronidazole. Refractory or recurrent *C. difficile* may require oral vancomycin. Severe traveler's diarrhea, often caused by an enteric pathogen, can be treated with a fluoroquinolone to reduce severity and duration. In patients with high fever, leukocytosis, and frequent stool, test for enteric pathogens, and treat if indicated. Do not use antibiotics for known or suspected *E. coli* O157:H7 infection because antibiotics may increase the risk of hemolytic uremic syndrome. *Campylobacter jejuni* and *Giardia* relapse in about 20% of cases, so consider retreating for recurrent symptoms.

Which Medications Decrease the Symptoms of Diarrhea?

Treat volume depletion: For mild orthostasis, caffeine-free, glucose-containing beverages are adequate; for more severe depletion, use oral rehydration solutions, which also contain sodium and potassium. Bismuth subsalicylate can reduce by 50% the number of unformed stools

Diarrhea

through antibacterial, anti-inflammatory, and antisecretory action. Opiate derivatives, such as loperamide, slow intestinal motility and reduce the number of stools by 80%. Antimotility agents can prolong the course of invasive bacteria and are not used in IBD. Rule out *C. difficile* if this is a possibility before starting loperamide because of the risk of toxic megacolon and rupture.

How do I Treat IBS?

An effective physician-patient relationship is important for reassurance and for education about the chronic nature of symptoms, dietary modification (high fiber; low fat, caffeine, and alcohol), and exercise. Treat the predominant symptom—hyoscyamine for abdominal cramping, loperamide for diarrhea, and high fiber to even out alternating constipation and diarrhea. Newer drugs have been approved for treatment of certain subsets of patients with IBS. Alosetron, a 5-HT$_3$ receptor antagonist, can be used in women with severe diarrhea-predominant IBS, and tegaserod, a 5-HT$_4$ receptor agonist, helps women with predominant constipation.

When Should I Hospitalize a Patient with Diarrhea?

Hospitalize patients with severe dehydration (>20% of volume lost) or significant emesis preventing oral rehydration for intravenous fluids and electrolytes. Patients with severe GI bleeding, as from a flare of IBD, may need hospitalization for stabilization and initiation of intravenous nutrition or steroids.

KEY POINTS

◆ Acute diarrhea is usually self-limited, requiring rehydration without further work-up.

◆ Take a thorough history to identify risk factors for acute diarrhea.

◆ Confirm the presence of chronic diarrhea by measuring stool volume.

◆ Use history and physical to distinguish inflammatory, osmotic, or secretory chronic diarrhea.

◆ The presence of nocturnal symptoms suggests an organic, not functional cause of diarrhea.

◆ Always consider *C. difficile* in patients who were recently hospitalized or on antibiotics.

Case 12-1

A 28-year-old Vietnamese man reports intermittent loose stools over the past 9-12 months. His diarrhea is accompanied by abdominal bloating and excessive gas. He has a 2-year-old daughter in day care.

Diarrhea

A. What are the possible causes of this patient's diarrhea?
B. What would be your initial diagnostic approach?

Case 12-2

A 56-year-old man has had RLQ abdominal pain and weight loss over the past 4 months. He also has noted intermittent low-grade fever and occasional periods of bloody diarrhea, which sometimes occur six times a day. He has normal vital signs and minimal RLQ tenderness to palpation, but no palpable masses.

A. What is the most likely diagnosis in this patient?

Case Answers

12-1 A. The most common causes of this patient's *diarrhea* would be lactose intolerance, *Giardia*, and IBS.

12-1 B. Given the patient's possible exposure to *Giardia*, you might check a *Giardia* antigen as your initial step. If negative, a 2-week trial of a lactose-free diet would most likely have a significant impact given his ethnic background.

12-2 A. The patient presents with fairly classic symptoms of Crohn's disease in the terminal ileum. Other possible causes of chronic bloody diarrhea include ischemic colitis and vasculitis. Although patients most commonly present in their late 20s and early 30s, IBD can develop later in life.

REFERENCES

Ehrenpreis ED: Irritable bowel syndrome: 10% to 20% of older adults have symptoms consistent with diagnosis. Geriatrics 2005;60:25.

Fekety R: Guidelines for the diagnosis and management of Clostridium difficile-associated diarrhea and colitis. American College of Gastroenterology. Am J Gastroenterol 1997;92:739.

Musher DM, Musher BL: Contagious acute gastrointestinal infections. N Engl J Med 2004;351:2417.

Schiller LR: Chronic diarrhea. Gastroenterology. 2004;127:287–293.

Yates J: Traveler's diarrhea. Am Fam Physician 2005;71:2095.

Diarrhea

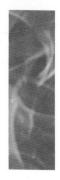

13

Dizziness and Syncope

C. SCOTT SMITH

ETIOLOGY

How do I Categorize Causes of Dizziness?

It is most useful to characterize dizziness into one of three broad categories—vertigo, presyncope, or other. You can accomplish this by asking the patient to describe the sensation without using the word dizzy. **Vertigo** is an illusory sense that either the room or the patient is moving; this implicates the central or peripheral vestibular system. **Presyncope** is often described as lightheaded, "seeing stars," "blacking out," or impending faint. This sensation implies cerebral dysfunction resulting from decreased perfusion, such as from low BP or arrhythmia. One large study found that nearly half of patients complaining of dizziness had more than one cause.

What are the Causes of Vertigo?

Vertigo is the most common type of dizziness, accounting for 40%-60% of all patients presenting with the complaint. Causes of vertigo are divided by anatomic source: *peripheral,* located in cranial nerve VIII or the inner ear, or *central,* located in the cerebellum or brainstem (Table 13-1). Peripheral causes are common and usually benign; central causes are more worrisome. Certain features can help distinguish peripheral from central causes, including pattern of onset, latency (the time to onset of symptoms after an aggravating maneuver such as head movement), whether the symptoms are fatigable (get better with repeated maneuvers), and whether nystagmus is prominent (Table 13-2).

What are the Causes of Presyncope and Syncope?

Presyncope and syncope are caused by decreased cerebral perfusion. The main classes are **decreased intravascular volume**, from bleeding, diarrhea, or diuretic overuse; **cardiac**, from intrinsic heart disease or

Table 13-1

Clinical Features and Frequency of Selected Causes of Vertigo

Location/ Cause	Clinical Features	Frequency
Peripheral		
BPV	Moderate to severe Brief spells (often <1 min) Most pronounced with position changes Occurs in patients >50 years old; younger if history of head trauma Resolves in 3-10 days, but may recur	25%-30% of all vertigo

Meniere's disease	Episodes with a triad of:
	  Vertigo
	  Tinnitus
	  Hearing loss
	Episodes last minutes to hours, not days
		10% of all vertigo

Central		

Brainstem ischemia or lesion	Usually accompanied by other
	  brainstem deficits:
	  Diplopia
	  Weakness
	  Facial numbness or weakness
	  Dysarthria
		Rare

Cerebellar hemorrhage	**Life-threatening**
	Abnormal finger-to-nose or heel-to-shin exam
	May have other associated symptoms:
	  Gaze palsy
	  Facial weakness
	  Occipital headache
	  Vomiting
	  Neck stiffness
		Very rare

Central and Peripheral		

Acoustic neuroma	Unilateral hearing loss
	Tinnitus, headache
	Presents similarly to peripheral causes initially,
	  then insidiously progresses to central pattern
	May involve cranial nerves V and VII with facial
	  weakness or numbness
		Very rare

arrhythmia; and **neurally mediated**, from loss of vascular tone or brady-cardia or both. Neurally mediated causes may be triggered by micturi-tion or a vasovagal response to pain. Common in patients <60 years old, these reflex-mediated problems often have associated nausea and warmth before lightheadedness or syncope. Elderly patients have a dif-ferent set of neurally mediated causes, including an exaggerated carotid

Table 13-2

Features That Help Distinguish Peripheral from Central Causes of Vertigo

Findings	Peripheral	Central
Initial onset of symptoms	Sudden	Insidious
Fatigability (Decreases with successive trials)	Yes	No
Latency (Delay in onset of vertigo after exacerbating maneuver i.e., moving the head)	3-20 sec	None
Nystagmus	Minimal Decreases with fixation	Marked Increases with fixation

sinus reflex and autonomic neuropathy. Elderly patients also are more sensitive to medications (nitroglycerin, antihypertensive agents, and antidepressants), which can lead to chronic postural lightheadedness or syncope.

What Suggests a Cardiac Cause of Syncope?

When symptoms occur without warning or with exertion, cardiac syncope is more likely. Cardiac syncope is more common in patients >60 years old. Syncope may be due to ischemia, arrhythmia, or structural problems such as critical aortic stenosis or hypertrophic cardiomyopathy. A PE can suddenly decrease left ventricular filling and cardiac output, resulting in syncope. Consider PE when syncope occurs in patients with low cardiac risk or high DVT risk or both (e.g., pregnant women or OCP users).

What are Some Other Important Causes of Dizziness?

Three other causes to keep in mind are early pregnancy, hyperventilation, and multiple sensory deficits. Hyperventilation is a common cause of a dysphoric lightheadedness, often accompanied by perioral or extremity tingling and numbness. Reproducing the symptoms after forced hyperventilation confirms the diagnosis and reassures the patient. *Ill-defined lightheadedness* is a term used to describe the vague feeling of dizziness associated with panic disorder and other psychiatric conditions. A common mixed condition is hyperventilation exacerbating benign positional vertigo. Multiple sensory deficits are common in elderly patients with dizziness. Minor dysfunction in two or three of the spatial orientation systems (vestibular, visual, and proprioceptive) can cause significant lack of confidence and an unsteady sensation. In addition, polypharmacy can exacerbate problems with dizziness.

EVALUATION

What Questions Should I ask the Patient with Dizziness or Syncope?

- Timing, chronicity, onset, and prior episodes
- Effect of physical factors (position, movement, stress, or micturition)
- History of ear infections, head, or barotrauma (suggests BPV)
- Medications causing hypotension or arrhythmias (nitroglycerin, antihypertensive agents, antidepressants) or ototoxicity (aminoglycosides, loop diuretics, salicylates, quinine, or quinidine)
- Hearing loss, tinnitus (suggests Meniere's disease or acoustic neuroma)
- Brainstem ischemic symptoms (double vision, dysarthria, facial weakness or numbness)
- Palpitations, chest pain, or shortness of breath (suggest cardiac cause or hyperventilation)
- Pregnancy risks

What Should I Look for on the Physical Examination?

Vital signs: irregular pulse, tachypnea, postural hypotension

HEENT: ear canals, carotid bruit, and upstrokes; carotid sinus massage if age >60 to look for excessive bradycardic response from an exaggerated carotid sinus reflex (*do not* perform carotid massage in patients with a bruit, a history of ventricular tachycardia, or recent MI or cerebrovascular accident)

Lungs: rales suggesting CHF

Heart: murmur, S_1/S_2, gallop, displaced PMI, JVP

Genitourinary: occult blood if patient appears volume-depleted

Neurologic: *cranial nerves,* especially hearing, visual acuity, diplopia, facial sensation and symmetry; *cerebellar function* with finger-to-nose, rapid alternating movement, heel-to-shin; ~~gait~~, especially ~~~~

Other: 3 m~~~~
    tion; Dix-Hallpike~~~~
    distinguishes peripheral ~~~~
    13-1)

What Tests Should be Obtained Routinely?

Obtain an ECG when patients present with syncope or when you suspect a cardiac cause of dizziness. Echocardiogram, treadmill testing, or cardiac monitoring also may be warranted. Obtain HCT in patients with tachycardia, volume depletion, or guaiac-positive stool. Obtain audiology if vertigo is accompanied by hearing loss. Obtain head MRI if documented sensorineural hearing loss accompanies vertigo.

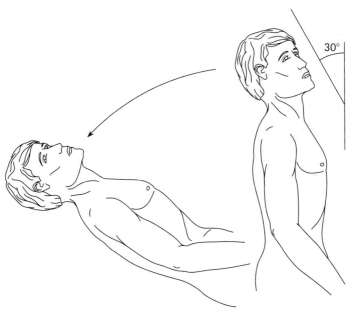

FIGURE 13-1 The Dix-Hallpike (or Nylen-Bárany) maneuver. Have the patient sit up with the head tilting back 45 degrees and to the side 45 degrees. Lay the patient rapidly backward while maintaining the same head position relative to the body (i.e., so the head ends up hanging off the edge, tipped 45 degrees below the plane of the table). Have the patient keep eyes open. Look for nystagmus and reproduction of symptoms. Repeat the test tilting the head to the other side. The side down when nystagmus is elicited is the affected side. Nystagmus onset is immediate with the postural change for central causes and delayed by a few seconds for peripheral causes of vertigo. Nystagmus from a peripheral cause is fatigable, meaning it decreases with repetition of the test (although the patient may think you are deliberately making them feel worse!).

 TREATMENT

What Can I Try before Using Medications?

Almost 50% of vertigo is from a benign peripheral cause, either BPV or vestibulitis. These conditions are fatigable, that is, get better with repeated provocation. You can ask your patient to repeat whatever physical maneuver reproduces the vertigo until they no longer get symptoms (5-10 repetitions) about four times per day. If the patient can tolerate this, it is an excellent therapy. Repositioning maneuvers can help move debris to the utricular cavity. The most successful of these maneuvers is the Epley maneuver. Hyperventilation is made better by breath-holding or bag-breathing exercises and therapy for underlying depression or anxiety. Particularly in the elderly, treat sensory deficits with eyeglasses, hearing aids, or a cane as needed. Wearing loose-necked shirts and avoiding neckties may help individuals with overactive carotid sinus reflexes. Consider PT for balance training.

What are Useful Medications for Vertigo?

Antivertigo drugs treat symptoms and generally fall into four categories: neuroleptics (prochlorperazine, droperidol, promethazine), antihistamines (meclizine and cyclizine), anticholinergics (scopolamine and dimenhydrinate), and sympathomimetics (pseudoephedrine). Pseudoephedrine is useful in combination with antihistamines or anticholinergics because it helps to counter their sedation. Occasionally, a patient might need benzodiazepines (diazepam) for severe vertigo, antidepressants for hyperventilation, or thiazide diuretics for Meniere's disease.

When Should I Admit or Refer Patients with Dizziness?

Consider hospital admission of a patient any time you suspect one of the five life-threatening causes of dizziness: arrhythmia, critical cardiac outflow obstruction, cerebellar hemorrhage, PE, or significant blood loss (Table 13-3). This includes patients who have a first syncopal episode. Patients with a suspected central cause of vertigo need admission when very ill or clinically unstable; these patients will likely need HEENT or neurosurgery referral depending on audiology and MRI findings. Outpatients with vestibulitis or BPV can be managed symptomatically and do not require referral, unless the symptoms endure and do not improve over several weeks. If the patients are having severe problems with BPV, or it

Table 13-3

Potentially Life-threatening Causes of Dizziness or Syncope

Condition	Findings
Cardiac arrhythmia	History of palpitations
	Irregular pulse
Cardiac outflow obstruction	Exercise-induced syncope
(e.g., aortic stenosis or hypertrophic cardiomyopathy)	Systolic murmur
	Delayed carotid upstrokes
	Abnormal splitting of S_2
Cerebellar hemorrhage	Abnormal cerebellar exam
PE	Risk for DVT
	Tachycardia and hypoxia
	Loud S_2
Significant blood loss	History of bleeding
	Orthostatic hypotension
	Guaiac-positive stool
	Low hematocrit

persists despite home exercises, referral to a physical therapist to perform the Epley maneuver is appropriate. Some patients with hyperventilation, especially patients with associated panic symptoms, may benefit from psychiatric referral.

KEY POINTS

◆ Dizziness is common; is usually self-limited; and should be categorized by history as vertigo, presyncope/syncope, or other.

◆ Quickly screen dizzy patients for life-threatening causes, including arrhythmia, cardiac outflow obstruction, cerebellar hemorrhage, PE, or significant blood loss.

◆ Use nonpharmacologic measures and medications such as meclizine to decrease symptoms of vertigo.

◆ Ask patients to call if symptoms get worse, if new symptoms develop, or if the symptoms have not resolved in 2 weeks.

Case 13-1

A 20-year-old man comes in for evaluation because of a recent episode of syncope while playing basketball. He relates some spells in the past of lightheadedness with strenuous exercise. He has no other significant history. On exam, BP and pulse are normal. His apical impulse is hyperdynamic and displaced to the left. He has a grade III/VI systolic murmur best heard at the left sternal border. The murmur gets louder after standing from a squatting position.

A. What is the likely cause of his syncope?
B. What test would you obtain to confirm your suspicion?

Case 13-2

A 67-year-old man comes to the office complaining of dizziness. He describes it as a feeling that the room is spinning. It began when he got out of bed this morning. It lasted about 1-2 minutes and has recurred on and off all morning, especially when he moves his head. He denies trouble speaking, weakness, numbness, or headache. He has never had this before. On exam, he has normal pulse and BP. His carotid pulses are normal, and he has no bruit. Cardiac exam is normal. He has no edema. Finger-to-nose and heel-to-shin are normal bilaterally. You lay him rapidly down from a sitting position on the exam table. After about 4 seconds, his symptoms are reproduced, and he has mild horizontal nystagmus. The symptoms are less the second time you perform this maneuver.

A. What is the most likely diagnosis?

B. What test should you do to confirm this?

Case Answers

13-1 A.   *Learning objective:* **Recognize a cardiac cause of syncope, hypertrophic cardiomyopathy.** Syncope with exertion in a young adult suggests cardiac outflow obstruction or arrhythmia. When the patient goes from squatting to standing, the ventricular chamber size gets smaller. The relative obstruction as a result of hypertrophy gets more severe, and the murmur of hypertrophy gets louder. Virtually all other systolic murmurs (except some mitral valve prolapses) get softer. This is a potentially serious cause of dizziness. This patient should be told not to participate in strenuous exercise until further evaluation is obtained. Many athletes have died as a result of this abnormality.

13-1 B.   *Learning objective:* **Identify echocardiogram as the appropriate test for evaluation of a patient with syncope and significant murmur on exam.** This abnormality is best confirmed with a cardiac echocardiogram. CXR and ECG are nonspecific. If the echocardiogram is normal, a Holter monitor is the next step to evaluate for a significant arrhythmia.

13-2 A.   *Learning objective:* **Diagnose BPV.** The type of dizziness the patient is describing is vertigo, and the most common cause is BPV. This is a classic presentation for BPV. Features include: (1) it occurs in older people, (2) it is worse with head movement, (3) symptoms and nystagmus show latency and are fatigable with repeated confrontation, and (4) cerebellum is not involved (important to rule out a rare cerebellar hemorrhage).

13-2 B.   *Learning objective:* **Recognize that the diagnosis of BPV is confirmed by history and exam alone.** We don't always need another test! This presentation, with positive Dix-Hallpike maneuver (see Figure 13-1) is very specific for this disease. The patient can be treated with fatiguing exercises (repeatedly doing head movements that bring on symptoms to hasten recovery), mild antidizziness medication (e.g., meclizine), and reassurance. He should be told the expected course of the illness (slowly better over 3-10 days) and to report back if he's not better or he gets worse.

REFERENCES

Derebery MJ: The diagnosis and treatment of dizziness. Med Clin North Am 1999;83:163.

Kroenke K, Lucas C, Rosenberg ML, et al: One-year outcome for patients with a chief complaint of dizziness. J Gen Intern Med 1994;9:684.

Dizziness and Syncope

USEFUL WEB SITE

www.nlm.nih.gov/medlineplus/ency/article/003093.htm
The Medline plus website has easy-to-read articles on many topics (including this one on dizziness) that are suitable for patients and clinicians.

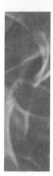

14

Dyspepsia

MELISSA M. HAGMAN

 ETIOLOGY

What is Dyspepsia?

Dyspepsia is recurrent pain or discomfort in the mid upper abdomen. It may be associated with other symptoms, such as bloating, early satiety, or heartburn (substernal burning). Dyspepsia is common and is one of the most frequent reasons for adult medicine outpatient visits.

What Causes Dyspepsia?

GERD, PUD, and functional dyspepsia are the most common causes of dyspepsia. Uncommon causes include chronic pancreatitis, biliary disease, gastroparesis, and gastric or pancreatic cancer. Many medications can cause dyspepsia, including NSAIDs, iron, antibiotics, and potassium supplements. Functional (or nonulcer) dyspepsia is the diagnosis given when no organic abnormality can be found to explain the dyspepsia. Sixty percent of patients with dyspepsia have functional disease.

 EVALUATION

What Aspects of the Patient's History Help to Identify the Cause of Dyspepsia?

Obtain a history of the character, location, and alleviating and precipitating factors of the pain or discomfort. Patients who have regurgitation and heartburn most likely have GERD. GERD is often exacerbated by smoking, alcohol, large meals, and supine position. Classic biliary colic, caused by a gallstone blocking the cystic duct, is characterized by isolated attacks of moderate-to-severe epigastric or RUQ pain, sometimes precipitated by a fatty meal. The pain may radiate to the right shoulder. With progression, the pain may become steady and severe and is often accompanied by

BOX 14-1

ALARM FEATURES OF SERIOUS CAUSES OF DYSPEPSIA

History

New onset at >55 years old
Dysphagia or odynophagia
Early satiety
Persistent vomiting
Anemia or signs of bleeding
Unexplained weight loss

Past Medical History

PUD
Malignancy
Gastric surgery

Family History

GI malignancy

Exam

Lymphadenopathy
Abdominal mass

nausea. Biliary colic is especially common at night, within hours of lying down to sleep. Angina sometimes can be confused with dyspepsia. Ask about diaphoresis, jaw pain, arm pain, shortness of breath, or changes in pain with exertion that may suggest angina. Upper GI bleeding or iron deficiency anemia or both may be present in PUD. Otherwise, PUD and functional dyspepsia cannot be differentiated based on history alone. "Red flags" or alarm features (Box 14-1) help identify patients who may have serious problems, such as complicated PUD or malignancy.

What Evaluation is Warranted for Patients with Alarm Features?

Patients with alarm features should undergo prompt EGD to rule out cancer and PUD. If normal, consider CT, labs.

What Evaluation is Appropriate for Patients with Classic GERD Symptoms?

Patients with uncomplicated GERD do not require further testing and should be treated empirically (see later). Patients who do not improve on empiric therapy should be considered for EGD and, if indicated, a 24-hour pH monitor in the esophagus. EGD also should be considered in patients who present with uncontrolled GERD symptoms for >5-10 years to screen for Barrett's esophagus, a premalignant lesion.

What Evaluation is Appropriate for Patients with Biliary Symptoms?

For patients with classic biliary symptoms, order an abdominal ultrasound scan. If gallstones are found, refer the patient to surgery for cholecystectomy (see Chapter 29).

When Should I Test for *Helicobacter pylori* Infection?

When evaluation of dyspepsia has excluded alarm features, classic GERD or biliary symptoms, and NSAID use, many experts recommend testing patients for *H. pylori* with a noninvasive test before beginning an empiric trial of a PPI (Figure 14-1). Although most patients with ulcers have *H. pylori* infection (or use NSAIDs), the converse is not true: Most patients with *H. pylori* infection do not develop ulcers. Ideally, experts recommend testing for *H. pylori* only if the patient comes from a population with a baseline prevalence of *H. pylori* $\geq$10%. Prevalence rates vary by age and living situation. In the U.S., the prevalence is approximately 50% in individuals >60 years old, 25% in individuals 30-60 years old, and 5% in children. Individuals from developing countries have a higher prevalence of 80%-95%.

How Should I Test for *H. pylori* Infection?

EGD with gastric mucosa biopsy is the "gold standard" for *H. pylori* diagnosis. Noninvasive methods to document infection are usually preferred, however, because of risks associated with EGD, such as perforation. Noninvasive test options include a serum antibody test (most common), Urease breath test (UBT), and stool antigen. Serology may remain positive for 6-12 months after eradication of the organism. Serologies may be less reliable in elderly patients and patients from areas of high *H. pylori* prevalence. The UBT and stool antigen may be falsely negative in individuals treated with PPIs or antibiotics within the prior 2 weeks. These tests are generally more costly and are less widely available than serology.

Why Test for *H. pylori* in Patients with Dyspepsia?

Some patients with dyspepsia have PUD. The most common causes of PUD are *H. pylori* infection and NSAID use. Eradication of *H. pylori* in patients with PUD leads to healing of the ulcer and dramatic reduction in the risk of recurrent PUD. *H. pylori* eradication also is helpful in some patients with functional dyspepsia.

What Evaluation is Appropriate for Dyspepsia When There are no Alarm Symptoms, There is no Clear Cause by History, and *H. pylori* Serology is Negative?

These patients should receive reassurance and a limited trial of antisecretory therapy, such as an H_2 receptor antagonist (H2RA) or PPI. If they have persistent symptoms, they should be offered endoscopy.

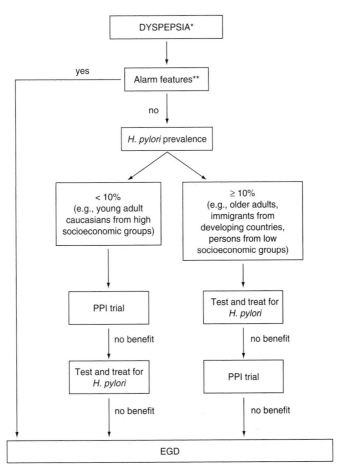

*consider concurrent workup for angina, biliary colic, or other diseases in patients with suggestive clinical presentations
**treat patients who have alarm features with a PPI while awaiting EGD

FIGURE 14-1 Dyspepsia work-up and therapeutic algorithm.

What are the Complications of GERD?

Asthma, pneumonia, bronchiectasis, chronic cough, laryngitis, and sinusitis are potential extraesophageal manifestations of GERD. GERD can lead to esophageal ulceration and stricture formation. Chronic GERD can lead to formation of Barrett's esophagus, in which the squamous epithelium of the distal esophagus is replaced by columnar epithelial cells. Barrett's esophagus is a precancerous condition that can develop into esophageal adenocarcinoma. Most experts suggest that patients with long-standing GERD be screened with EGD for the presence of Barrett's esophagus; some individuals with Barrett's esophagus may warrant routine endoscopic surveillance.

What are the Complications of PUD?

GI bleeding is the most common complication of PUD. In patients with upper GI bleeding, prompt endoscopy is indicated for diagnosis and therapy. Rarely, gastric outlet obstruction and perforation can occur as a result of PUD.

TREATMENT

What are the Treatment Options for GERD?

Lifestyle modifications (Box 14-2 and Figure 14-2) or antacids or both are the first line of therapy for milder symptoms. Patients with persistent symptoms require an H_2RA (e.g., ranitidine) or PPI (e.g., omeprazole). PPIs are the most effective treatment for symptoms and healing of erosive esophagitis. Start with a 2-week trial of a twice-daily PPI. The morning dose should be taken 30 minutes before breakfast. If symptoms resolve, continue the PPI at the lowest effective dose (usually daily) for 8 weeks and then stop. If symptoms recur, restart the PPI. Nissen fundoplication is a surgical alternative for patients who prefer not to take medications indefinitely. Many patients who undergo surgery still require medication for GERD symptoms, however.

What are the Treatment Options for PUD?

NSAIDs should be discontinued. Treat patients who are positive for *H. pylori* with multidrug therapy (Table 14-1). Some *H. pylori* is resistant to metronidazole or clarithromycin. If a patient fails an initial course of therapy containing one of these medications, try a second course with a different antibiotic. A total of 8 weeks of PPI therapy should be given to heal the ulcer. Bleeding secondary to PUD should be evaluated and treated endoscopically. If endoscopy fails to control the bleeding, surgical resection may be necessary.

Dyspepsia

BOX 14-2

LIFESTYLE MODIFICATIONS FOR TREATMENT OF GASTROESOPHAGEAL REFLUX DISEASE

- ◆ Avoid caffeine, mints, and fatty foods
- ◆ Avoid eating 2-4 hours before bedtime
- ◆ Avoid tobacco and alcohol
- ◆ Elevate the head of the bed
- ◆ Lose weight if obese

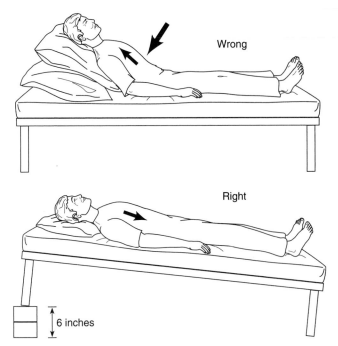

FIGURE 14-2 Appropriate bed elevation for GERD prevention.

What are the Treatment Options for Functional Dyspepsia?

Management of functional dyspepsia is challenging. A supportive physician-patient relationship is important for patients with functional dyspepsia. Education and reassurance often lead to symptom improvement. A trial of H$_2$RA, PPI, or metoclopramide (a promotility agent) can be initiated. Without clear improvement in symptoms, the medication

Table 14-1

Two Possible Treatment Regimens for *H. pylori*

Drugs	Doses
PPI of choice	Standard dose po bid × 10 d
Amoxicillin	1 g po bid × 10 d
Clarithromycin	500 mg po bid × 10 d
or	
PPI of choice	Standard dose po bid × 14 d
Bismuth subsalicylate	525 mg po qid × 14 d
Metronidazole	250 mg po qid × 14 d
Tetracycline	500 mg po qid × 14 d

bid, two times a day; qid, four times a day; po, orally.

should be discontinued. Some patients with functional dyspepsia improve with antidepressant therapy.

KEY POINTS

◆ Dyspepsia is defined as pain or discomfort in the upper abdomen with or without associated symptoms.

◆ Dyspepsia may be due to PUD, GERD, functional dyspepsia, biliary disease, angina, and less common causes such as gastric cancer.

◆ Noninvasive testing for *H. pylori* is commonly recommended as an initial approach to dyspepsia without alarm symptoms in patient groups with ≥10% prevalence of *H. pylori* infection.

◆ Prompt endoscopy should be performed in patients with dyspepsia and associated alarm features.

Case 14-1

A 60-year-old man presents with a 2-month history of epigastric pain. He denies NSAID use or heartburn. His examination and lab tests are normal.

A. What is the differential diagnosis?
B. What investigation is warranted?

Case 14-2

A 43-year-old woman complains of long-standing heartburn. She reports smoking two packs of cigarettes and drinking 2 glasses of wine each day. Her heartburn is typically worse at night, particularly after eating a late meal. She sleeps on three pillows to reduce her heartburn.

A. What lifestyle modifications and medications do you recommend?
B. Is any testing indicated?

Case Answers

14-1 A. *Learning objective:* **List the differential diagnosis for epigastric pain.** The differential diagnosis includes PUD, functional dyspepsia, gastroparesis, and gastroesophageal or pancreatic malignancy. It is difficult to distinguish between these diseases on history alone, but in older patients the recent onset of symptoms should raise concern over serious organic pathology.

14-1 B. *Learning objective:* **Design an appropriate evaluation for epigastric pain in a patient with alarm features.** Given his age, >55 years, the patient should have a prompt EGD to rule out complicated PUD or gastroesophageal cancer. Any patients with alarm symptoms (e.g., dysphagia, bleeding, weight loss, new-onset symptoms >55 years old) should have endoscopy, labs, and/or CT scan. The "test and treat" for *H. pylori* strategy is reserved for patients without alarm features.

14-2 A. *Learning objective:* **List lifestyle modifications for treatment of patients with GERD.** The patient should avoid smoking, alcohol, and late meals because these can exacerbate reflux. Sleeping on pillows increases intra-abdominal pressure and worsens GERD. Instead, she should raise the head of her bed by tilting the whole frame about 6 inches. Weight loss and looser waistbands decrease intra-abdominal pressure and decrease symptoms. If the patient's dyspepsia is refractory to lifestyle modifications, prescribe H_2RAs or PPIs.

14-2 B. *Learning objective:* **Refer patients with long-standing GERD for EGD to look for Barrett's esophagus.** Because long-standing GERD may be associated with a premalignant lesion, Barrett's esophagus, the patient should undergo endoscopy.

REFERENCE

Talley NJ, Vakil N, and the Parameters Commmittee of the American College of Gastroenterology: Guidelines for the management of dyspepsia. Am J Gastroenterol 2005;100:2324.

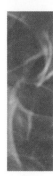

15

Dyspnea

THOMAS O. STAIGER and GEORGE NOVAN

 ETIOLOGY

What Causes Dyspnea?

A combination of mechanical receptors in the upper airway, lungs, and chest wall and chemoreceptors in the carotid arteries, aorta, and medulla seem to mediate the uncomfortable sensation of breathing experienced as dyspnea. Hypoxia, hypercapnia (elevated P_{CO_2}), and increased work of breathing all can contribute to dyspnea.

What are Common Causes of Chronic Dyspnea?

Although there are numerous causes for dyspnea, four conditions cause 70% of chronic dyspnea: asthma, COPD, CHF, and interstitial lung disease (Box 15-1). Deconditioning is another frequent cause for chronic exertional dyspnea. Less common causes for chronic dyspnea include anemia, neoplasms, hyperthyroidism, and recurrent PE.

What are Common Causes for Dyspnea of Recent Onset?

Patients with recent-onset dyspnea often have exacerbations of one of three chronic conditions—asthma, COPD, or CHF—or are found to have pneumonia (Box 15-2). Patients with bronchitis or other upper respiratory infections sometimes report dyspnea. This dyspnea is generally mild, unless the patients have an underlying pulmonary problem, such as asthma or COPD. Dyspnea is commonly associated with chest pain in patients with angina. Important and potentially life-threatening causes for acute dyspnea include PE, tachyarrhythmia, silent myocardial ischemia, and pneumothorax (Box 15-3). Dyspnea without chest pain can occur during myocardial ischemia or MI and is called silent ischemia; this is more common in women and in patients with diabetes. Recurrent dyspnea associated with anxiety is often due to panic attacks. Tachyarrhythmias also can produce symptoms similar to panic attacks. Anemia may present as dyspnea.

BOX 15-1

COMMON CAUSES OF CHRONIC DYSPNEA

- Asthma
- COPD
- CHF
- Interstitial lung disease

BOX 15-2

COMMON CAUSES OF ACUTE DYSPNEA

- Asthma exacerbation
- COPD exacerbation
- CHF exacerbation
- Pneumonia
- PE

BOX 15-3

LIFE-THREATENING CAUSES OF DYSPNEA

- Arrhythmia
- MI
- Pneumothorax
- PE
- Cardiac tamponade

Dyspnea

EVALUATION

How Helpful is the History in the Evaluation of Dyspnea?

In one study of 146 patients admitted with dyspnea, 74% were correctly diagnosed after a 5- to 15-minute history. Important historical features in a dyspneic patient include character, duration, severity, exacerbating and relieving factors, and associated symptoms; medication use, with special attention to whether medications such as diuretics or inhalers have been used as prescribed; past medical history, particularly cardiac or pulmonary disease or environmental exposures; and any history of trauma. Pay close attention to any risk factors for PE (OCP use, airplane travel, malignancy, recent surgery). Pleuritic chest pain associated with dyspnea suggests PE, pneumonia, or pneumothorax. It can be helpful to ask a patient how far they can walk or how many flights of stairs they can climb currently and compare this with their exercise tolerance at some time in the past. Patients who have dyspnea caused by panic attacks frequently have a family history of panic attacks or depression or both.

Which Symptoms are Commonly Associated with Important Causes of Dyspnea?

Table 15-1 summarizes symptoms that provide clues to diagnosis of causes of dyspnea.

Table 15-1

Symptoms and Exam Findings in Important Causes of Dyspnea

Condition	Symptoms	Exam Findings
CHF	Orthopnea (dyspnea when supine) PND (awakening short of breath) Increase in leg edema Pink, frothy sputum	Elevated JVP Crackles at lung bases Leg edema S_3
Asthma or COPD exacerbation	Productive cough Wheezing Chest tightness	Increased expiratory-to-inspiratory ratio Wheezing Supraclavicular retraction
Pneumonia	Fever Productive cough Pleuritic chest pain	Tachycardia Decreased breath sounds Rales or egophony or both
PE	Abrupt-onset dyspnea Calf pain or swelling Pleuritic chest pain	Pleural rub Unilateral calf swelling Tachycardia
Cardiac ischemia	Chest pressure, heaviness, or discomfort Nausea or diaphoresis	Tachycardia and hypertension Diaphoresis
Pneumothorax	Abrupt-onset dyspnea Pleuritic chest pain	Deviated trachea Hyper-resonance and decreased breath sounds on affected side
Hyperventilation	Anxiety Palpitations Paresthesias, distal extremities or perioral	Normal exam Depressed or anxious-appearing

Dyspnea

What are Typical Symptoms in a Patient Whose Dyspnea is Due to Panic Attacks?

Patients with panic attacks experience episodes in which they have some combination of dyspnea, chest pain, palpitations, dizziness, and anxiety. During an acute episode, patients often benefit from reassurance and from advice to slow their breathing. Patients who fail to respond to this can be asked to breathe into a paper bag to increase the P_{CO_2} level that has been reduced by hyperventilation. Patients may have underlying symptoms of anxiety or depression, so screen for these conditions. Patients with tachyarrhythmias may have similar symptoms; an event monitor, which records a tracing of a patient's heart during a period of symptoms, can be a useful way of distinguishing between the two.

Which Elements of the Physical Exam are Most Important in Evaluating a Patient with Dyspnea?

General appearance provides excellent information about the severity of the condition, including how hard the patient is working to breathe, the presence or absence of cyanosis, and the ability to speak a full sentence before taking a breath. Check vital signs for information about hemodynamic stability and the likelihood of infection. Measure the respiratory rate because this is frequently recorded incorrectly. Inspect the conjunctiva and nails for evidence of anemia. Inspect the chest, looking for intercostal, subcostal, and supraclavicular retractions; for abnormalities of the chest wall; and for abnormal prolongation of the expiratory phase. Percuss, listening for dullness secondary to effusion or consolidation, or for the hyper-resonance of a pneumothorax. Auscultate for wheezes, rales, rhonchi, or rubs and for symmetry of breath sounds. Patients with an exacerbation of CHF may have wheezes or "cardiac asthma" rather than rales. The absence of wheezes in an acutely dyspneic patient with asthma or COPD may be an ominous sign of a serious limitation of airflow. Listen for murmurs and extra heart sounds, such as the S_3 gallop of severe CHF. Inspect the neck veins to determine the JVP. Assess for edema and for unilateral calf swelling or tenderness.

Which Tests are Most Helpful in Evaluating a Patient with Dyspnea?

Select appropriate tests to investigate your diagnostic hypotheses generated from the history and physical. Routine blood tests to order include a CBC and a basic metabolic panel. A serum brain natriuretic peptide (BNP) level can provide useful data to assist in assessing whether heart failure is causing or contributing to dyspnea. Oximetry at rest or with exercise, or both, can detect hypoxia, but does not detect hypercarbia. ABG provides accurate information about oxygen and carbon dioxide levels, which is especially useful in patients with suspected serious airflow obstruction or PE. A CXR is useful in patients with moderate or severe dyspnea and in mildly symptomatic patients in whom the reason for their dyspnea is unclear. Measures of airflow (spirometry or peak flow) provide information about the presence and severity of airflow obstruction. Pulmonary diffusion capacity (DLCO) can be used to determine if a patient has interstitial lung disease. Obtain an ECG in any patient who might have a cardiac cause for their dyspnea. Order an echocardiogram when valvular heart disease or CHF is a concern. Cardiopulmonary exercise testing can be useful in some patients to clarify the cardiac and pulmonary components of their dyspnea and to determine the relative contribution of deconditioning. PE can mimic many cardiac and pulmonary problems. Dyspnea is the most common symptom in patients with large PE, but patients with small emboli may present with pleuritic chest pain, tachycardia, or hemoptysis. See Chapter 37 for work-up when PE is suspected.

Why do I Need an ABG When I Can Get Pulse Oximetry?

ABG gives a more accurate assessment of oxygenation, allows calculation of an alveolar/arterial oxygen gradient (see formula on the back cover), and identifies patients at risk for cardiac or neurologic compromise secondary to hypoxia. Normal pulse oximetry in patients with obstruction does not exclude retention of carbon dioxide from obstruction and respiratory fatigue. In addition to the oxygen level, ABG measures carbon dioxide, which indicates severity of airflow obstruction and likelihood of respiratory arrest in patients who are becoming fatigued from the work of breathing. pH gives acidemia/alkalemia information.

 TREATMENT

How do I Treat Dyspnea?

Identify and treat the underlying cause. See relevant chapters for further details of treatment. Asthma and CHF often respond well to treatment directed at the underlying problem. Other causes of dyspnea, such as COPD or interstitial lung disease, may have a limited response to treatment. Opiates and benzodiazepines have been shown to reduce the feeling of dyspnea (without improving ventilation or oxygenation); they should generally be avoided because of the risk of dependence and of respiratory depression except for palliation.

Which Patients with Dyspnea should Receive Supplemental Oxygen?

Supplemental oxygen has been shown to improve survival for patients with chronic dyspnea and a Po_2 ≤ 55. Medicare currently pays for supplemental oxygen if patients have the following:

- Po_2 on ABG ≤ 55
- Po_2 ≤ 60 and a condition worsened by hypoxia, such as cor pulmonale (right heart failure associated with hypoxia)
- Oxygen saturation by oximetry $\leq 88\%$

Patients with acute dyspnea who are moderately to severely symptomatic or who have oxygen saturations $>90\%$-91% should receive

Dyspnea

supplemental oxygen pending further evaluation and treatment. In chronic COPD, use oxygen cautiously because the respiratory drive in these cases is driven by hypoxia.

Which Patients with Dyspnea Should be Hospitalized?

Patients with chronic dyspnea can be evaluated as outpatients unless the vital signs are unstable or the hypoxia significant. Patients with acute dyspnea requiring supplemental oxygen or patients who have a potentially unstable cardiac or respiratory status should be hospitalized. Patients with acute dyspnea resulting from an exacerbation of asthma or COPD can be treated with inhaled bronchodilators and often improve sufficiently to avoid hospitalization. These patients are often given a short course of steroids to decrease airway inflammation.

KEY POINTS

◆ Most patients with dyspnea can be correctly diagnosed by taking a careful history.

◆ Common causes of chronic dyspnea are asthma, COPD, CHF, and interstitial lung disease.

◆ Common causes of acute dyspnea are exacerbations of asthma, COPD, and CHF and pneumonia.

◆ Consider PE in any patient with recent-onset dyspnea who doesn't have a clear explanation for his or her symptoms.

Case 15-1

A 58-year-old man presents to the emergency department with a 2-week history of worsening dyspnea on exertion, substernal chest heaviness, and nonproductive cough. Past history includes diabetes mellitus, hypertension, hyperlipidemia, and a long smoking history. A previous CXR 3 years earlier revealed aortic knob calcification and a reticular pattern in the lung bases thought to be chronic. On exam, vital signs are temperature 36.7° C, pulse 90 beats/min, BP 144/92 mm Hg, and respirations 28. At rest, the patient is comfortable, but can't speak in long sentences because of shortness of breath. JVP is normal. Coarse crackles are heard in both lungs, and heart sounds are regular without murmurs, gallops, or rubs. There is no peripheral edema, calf swelling, or clubbing. Pulse oximetry is 78% on room air and 95% on 4 L/min of oxygen. ECG shows nonspecific lateral wall ST-T wave changes. CXR shows a hazy, reticulonodular interstitial pattern from midlung field to the bases bilaterally.

A. List likely diagnoses for this patient from most to least likely.
B. What studies would you order and in which sequence?

Case 15-2

A 60-year-old woman presents to the emergency department with dyspnea. She became dyspneic while walking last night and since this morning has noted dyspnea at rest. She has had several days of a nonproductive cough, but denies fevers, chest pain, unilateral calf swelling, missing her medications, or smoking. Medications are metformin, enalapril, and furosemide. Past history is notable for diabetes, hypertension, CHF, and a knee replacement 2 months ago. On exam, vital signs are temperature 37° C, pulse 110 beats/min, BP 150/100 mm Hg, and respirations 24. Oxygen saturation is 86% on room air. She is speaking in 6- to 8-word phrases. Chest exam reveals bibasilar crackles and no wheezes. Cardiovascular exam shows regular S_1 and S_2 without murmurs, gallops, or rubs. JVP is 10 cm. Extremities show 1+ edema to her midcalves bilaterally.

A. Which diagnoses are most likely in this patient? What other diagnoses would you consider?
B. Which clinical features support each of these diagnoses?
C. Which diagnostic tests would you order?

Case Answers

15-1 A. *Learning objective:* **List a differential diagnosis of dyspnea for your patient using all of the available data.** Although this patient has risk factors for CHF secondary to ischemic heart disease and for COPD, there are elements from his history and physical that indicate another explanation. The patient has no JVD, pedal edema, or gallop to support a cardiac etiology for the dyspnea. His previous CXR 3 years earlier raises the strong probability of a previous and as yet undiagnosed interstitial process. Although not as common as CHF or COPD, progression to an accelerated phase of usual interstitial pneumonitis, also known as idiopathic pulmonary fibrosis or fibrosing alveolitis, should be highest in your differential listing. Your list would be completed by concomitant causes of dyspnea that could be adding to his breathing burden, including CHF, COPD, PE, or, less likely given lack of fever, acute pneumonia.

15-1 B. *Learning objective:* **State the value of obtaining pre-existent abnormal CXR and ordering appropriate other tests to establish a diagnosis in patients with dyspnea.** One of the first things to do in evaluating this particular patient is to obtain the old CXR to identify progression of pre-existent disease. While waiting for the old x-rays, you would obtain baseline studies such as CBC with differential, complete metabolic panel, and ABG. In addition, you might obtain a BNP level to try to identify whether CHF was contributing. Echocardiogram would identify ventricular dysfunction (left or right). High-resolution CT scan with contrast would assess the interstitial process and would detect PE. Finally, lung biopsy might be required to detail an interstitial process further.

Dyspnea

15-2 A. *Learning objective:* **State the causes of recent-onset dyspnea.** The most likely diagnoses in this patient are an exacerbation of CHF or PE. Worsening CHF could be due to cardiac ischemia, poorly controlled hypertension, or excessive salt intake. Pneumonia and cardiac ischemia without an exacerbation of underlying heart failure are possible, although less likely.

15-2 B. *Learning objective:* **Identify key clinical features associated with different causes of recent-onset dyspnea.** Worsening CHF is supported by the patient's prior history of CHF and by exam findings suggesting volume overload (elevated JVP, crackles, and edema). Her recent surgery increases her likelihood of having a PE. Pneumonia would be a consideration given her recent cough, although a cough also is seen in about one third of patients with a PE. The absence of fever or sputum production makes pneumonia less likely. Diabetes and female gender are risk factors for silent ischemia.

15-2 C. *Learning objective:* **Order appropriate diagnostic tests to evaluate a patient with acute dyspnea.** Order ECG to assess for ischemic changes; CXR to look for evidence of volume overload or pneumonia; and blood work, including a CBC, cardiac enzymes, metabolic panel, and BNP level. Further evaluation for a PE with D-dimer or imaging or both might be indicated, depending on the results of her initial studies.

REFERENCES

Jobe K: Dyspnea. In Fihn S, DeWitt D, (eds): Outpatient Medicine, 2nd ed. Philadelphia: Saunders, 1998, p 79.

Meek PM, Schwartzstein RM, Adams L, et al: Dyspnea: Mechanisms, assessment, and management. ATS consensus statement. Am J Respir Crit Care Med 1999;159:321.

Dyspnea

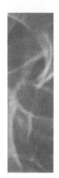

16

Ear, Nose, and Throat Symptoms

KARNA GENDO

 ETIOLOGY

What Causes Hearing Loss?

Conductive hearing loss is caused by abnormalities in the middle or external ear, which impair the passage of sound to the inner ear. Cerumen impaction, cholesteatoma, middle ear effusion, otosclerosis, and ossicle disruption are examples of such abnormalities. Sensory hearing loss results from abnormalities of the cochlea, such as loss of hair cells from the organ of Corti. Presbycusis, a progressive high-frequency loss that occurs in aging individuals, is a prime example of sensory hearing loss. Other examples are excessive noise exposure, head trauma, or systemic conditions such as diabetes or accompanying autoimmune disease. Neural hearing loss results from abnormalities of cranial nerve VIII, auditory nuclei, ascending tracts, or auditory cortex. Examples include acoustic neuroma, multiple sclerosis, and cerebral ischemia. Ototoxic drugs include certain antibiotics and anticancer drugs, loop diuretics, and anti-inflammatories. Sudden loss of hearing in one ear is usually the result of an occlusion of the internal auditory artery or a viral infection. A family history of hearing loss before age 50 suggests that genetic factors are involved.

What Causes Nasal Congestion?

Allergic rhinitis is the probable cause of congestion when there is a history of animal or pollen triggers or a family member with an allergic condition. The presence of pain, bleeding, fever, cough, unilateral symptoms, purulent discharge, and headache suggests other etiologies, such as sinusitis, polyps, foreign bodies, tumors, or granulomas. Non-allergic rhinitis, hypothyroidism, pregnancy, and medication side effects also can cause nasal congestion.

What Pathogens Cause Pharyngitis?

The major causes of pharyngitis are viruses, most commonly influenza, coronavirus, rhinovirus, and adenovirus. Group A streptococcus is the most common bacterial cause of exudative pharyngitis and is suggested by the presence of features known as the Centor criteria: fever >38°C, tender anterior cervical lymphadenopathy, lack of cough, and a pharyngotonsillar exudate.

 DIAGNOSIS

How do you Perform and Interpret the Weber and Rinne Tests?

For the Weber test (Table 16-1), a 512-Hz tuning fork is applied to the skull on the midline. In conductive loss, the sound is louder in the poorer hearing ear, and in sensorineural loss, the sound is louder in the better hearing ear. For the Rinne test (see Table 16-1), the tuning fork is first placed on the mastoid bone until the sound disappears, and then it's placed in front of the ear canal. Normally, the sound returns, but in conductive hearing loss, the sound does not return because bone conduction is greater than air conduction. In sensorineural loss, air conduction and bone conduction are decreased, but air conduction is still relatively superior.

What Studies are Indicated for Hearing Loss?

An audiogram is indicated for all patients. If the etiology is unclear, consider CBC, ESR, thyroid function, hemoglobin A_{1C}, and tests for syphilis and Lyme disease. An acoustic tumor should be ruled out with MRI in cases of sensorineural hearing loss, especially if the loss is unilateral or associated with tinnitus or cranial nerve V and VII palsies. Imaging is indicated for trauma. Consider an otolaryngology consult in all cases of confirmed hearing loss.

Table 16-1

Weber and Rinne Tests in Hearing Loss

Condition	Weber Test	Rinne Test—Right	Rinne Test—Left
Normal	Midline	Air conduction > bone conduction, about 60 sec	Air conduction > bone conduction, about 60 sec
Right conduction loss	→ R	Bone conduction > air conduction	Air conduction > bone conduction
Partial right sensorineural loss	→ L	Air conduction > bone conduction, about 10 sec	Air conduction > bone conduction, about 60 sec

ENT Symptoms

Table 16-2

Four-Item* Clinical Score for Diagnosing Acute Bacterial Sinusitis

No. Items	Sensitivity (%)	Specificity (%)
1	99†	49
2	96	77
3	81	89
4	24	97

*Unilateral purulent rhinorrhea, bilateral purulent rhinorrhea, unilateral pain, presence of pus in the nasal cavity.

†The presence of any one of the criteria has a very high sensitivity (99%), but also a very high false-positive rate (51%).

What Tests can be Considered for Nasal Congestion?

Allergy testing (skin tests or specific IgE blood tests) is indicated for patients who have a low pretest probability of allergic rhinitis, fail to respond to empiric allergy medication, or have symptoms that are severe enough to warrant avoidance therapy or immunotherapy. The use of imaging in acute sinusitis is limited because it is preferable to make the diagnosis of sinusitis clinically (Table 16-2). A limited CT scan of the sinuses can be considered when symptoms are vague or atypical, physical findings are equivocal, or the response to initial management is poor.

When Should I Obtain a Rapid Antigen Streptococcus Test for a Sore Throat?

First, classify the patient's symptoms using the Centor criteria. One strategy is to treat empirically patients who have all four criteria with antibiotics and not test or treat patients with zero or one criterion. Patients with two or three criteria receive rapid antigen testing and are treated for positive results.

How do I Confirm Infectious Mononucleosis in a Patient with Sore Throat?

Marked adenopathy, shaggy white-purple tonsillar exudates often extending into the nasopharynx, and abnormal LFTs suggest mononucleosis. Obtain a CBC looking for atypical lymphocytes and a monospot or heterophil test. Evaluate for accompanying streptococcal infection because one third of patients have streptococcal tonsillitis. The major alternative diagnosis for the same symptoms is acute HIV infection. Ask about HIV risk factors to assess whether testing for HIV (check HIV viral load to diagnose acute HIV) is appropriate.

How Sensitive and Specific are the Various Tests used in Ear, Nose, and Throat Symptoms?

Sensitivities and specificities are listed in Table 16-3.

ENT Symptoms

Table 16-3

Sensitivities and Specificities of Various Tests for Ear, Nose, and Throat Symptoms

Test	Sensitivity (%)	Specificity (%)
Allergy skin testing	79	91
Rapid antigen streptococcus test	80–90	95
Throat culture for group A streptococcus	90–95	>95
Monospot	~90	~90
Heterophil antibody	83–87	91–97
Sinus CT, limited	N/A*	N/A*
Sinus x-rays	90	61

*No comparison against sinus puncture, the "gold standard."

TREATMENT

How can I Treat Allergic Rhinitis?

An initial 2-to 4-week course of empiric nonsedating antihistamines and nasal steroids can be considered for patients with a family or personal history of allergy or symptoms triggered by animals or pollens. Antihistamines are effective for sneezing, rhinorrhea, itch, and eye symptoms. Nasal steroids are effective for all symptoms, including congestion. Unresponsive, moderately severe, or persistent rhinitis can be referred for allergy testing to confirm the diagnosis and proceed with allergen avoidance treatment or immunotherapy.

How can I Treat Acute Sinusitis?

Symptomatic therapy consists of mucolytic agents to reduce the viscosity of secretions, decongestants, antihistamines, or nasal steroids. Patients at high risk for bacterial sinusitis include those with at least two of the following: URI >7 days, facial pain, or purulent discharge. Antibiotics are considered for high-risk patients with less severe symptoms that do not improve after 7 days of symptomatic therapy or patients with severe symptoms. Amoxicillin (500 mg orally two to three times a day) and trimethoprim-sulfamethoxazole (Double Strength orally twice a day) are adequate and cost-effective first choices. If there is no significant improvement in 3 days, a different antibiotic should be prescribed, such as high-dose amoxicillin-clavulanate, cephalosporin, quinolone, macrolide, or ketolide. If a patient improves after 3–5 days of treatment, the antibiotic can be continued for 7 days after the patient feels well to prevent relapse.

Why Should I Treat Strep Throat with Antibiotics?

Reasons to consider treating streptococcal pharyngitis with antibiotics include a desire to ameliorate symptoms and prevent rheumatic fever, acute glomerulonephritis, suppurative complications, and transmission. In North American adults, these reasons are less compelling, however, because rheumatic fever and peritonsillar abscesses are very rare, early antibiotic treatment shortens the illness duration by only 1 day, and transmission prevention is more relevant in pediatric patients.

How do I Treat Strep Throat?

Use penicillin V potassium (250 mg orally three times daily or 500 mg orally twice daily for 10 days) or cefuroxime axetil (250 mg orally twice daily for 5–10 days). Erythromycin is an alternative in penicillin-allergic patients. A single injection of benzathine penicillin (1.2 million U) is the best choice if compliance is an issue. Amoxicillin has a risk of rash development if the patient actually has mononucleosis. Ancillary treatment includes analgesics and anti-inflammatory agents, salt water or anesthetic gargling, and anesthetic lozenges.

KEY POINTS

◆ Obtain an audiogram to document hearing loss, and refer patients with confirmed hearing loss to an otolaryngologist.

◆ Clinical features associated with group A streptococcal pharyngitis include fever >38° C, tender anterior cervical lymphadenopathy, lack of cough, and pharyngotonsillar exudates.

◆ Clinical features of acute bacterial sinusitis include purulent rhinorrhea, local pain with unilateral predominance, and nasal cavity pus on examination.

◆ Amoxicillin and trimethoprim-sulfamethoxazole for 10 days are adequate first choices in treating acute bacterial sinusitis.

◆ Clinical features associated with allergic rhinitis include a family or personal history of allergy or symptoms triggered by animals or pollens.

Case 16-1

An 18-year-old woman presents with severe sore throat for 2 days. She denies cough or fever, but does have some nasal congestion. She has no exudates on her tonsils, and her neck is supple without lymphadenopathy.

   A. What is her likely diagnosis?
   B. What further testing should you do?

ENT Symptoms

Case 16-2

A 40-year-old man reports chronic nasal congestion that makes it difficult for him to sleep. He reports he sleeps under a down comforter and has two dogs and a cat. His daughter has allergies. He has tried diphenhydramine (Benadryl), but it makes his mouth dry. The nasal stuffiness and itchy eyes are present year-round now.

   A. What is his most likely diagnosis?
   B. What treatment would you recommend?

Case Answers

16-1 A.   *Learning objective:* **Recognize viral pharyngitis.** A viral cause is most likely because she has only one of the four Centor criteria, sore throat, without cough or fever, and she has concurrent nasal congestion.

16-1 B.   *Learning objective:* **Recognize that patients with viral pharyngitis do not require any testing.** Patients with viral pharyngitis do not require blood or throat swab testing and can be treated with anti-inflammatory medication for symptom relief.

16-2 A.   *Learning objective:* **Identify allergic rhinitis.** With pet exposure and family history and constancy of symptoms, this is a case of allergic rhinitis until proved otherwise.

16-2 B.   *Learning objective:* **Outline initial treatment plan for allergic rhinitis.** Begin with a nonsedating antihistamine. With pronounced nasal congestion, a nasal steroid spray also would be a good choice. Consider allergy skin testing and environmental controls (removing rugs, keeping pets out of bedroom, or finding a new home for pets if symptoms are severe enough).

REFERENCES & WEB SITES

Bartlett J: Approach to acute pharyngitis in adults. In Rose BD (ed): UpToDate. 2005. http://www.patients.uptodate.com/topic.asp?File=pc_id/4421

Gardner G: Hearing loss. In Dambro M (ed): Griffith's: 5 Minute Clinical Consult 2005. Philadelphia: Lippincott Williams & Wilkins, 2005.

Gendo K, Larson EB: Evidence-based diagnostic strategies for evaluating suspected allergic rhinitis. Ann Intern Med 2004;140:278.

The diagnosis and management of sinusitis: A practice parameter update. J Allergy Clin Immunol 2005;116:S13.

ENT Symptoms

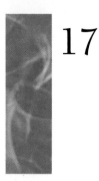

17

Fatigue

SARAH L. CLEVER

 ETIOLOGY

How Common is Fatigue?

Twenty-five percent of primary care patients report fatigue, and 5% of all office visits to primary care physicians are for a chief complaint of tiredness.

What Causes Fatigue?

More than half of cases of fatigue are due to a psychological cause, usually depression. Thirty percent of cases are due to a diagnosable medical illness. No cause is found in about 20% of cases. Common physical causes include viral infection, metabolic disorders, and medications (Box 17-1). Duration is important: Fatigue present for >4 months has a psychiatric cause determined in 75% of cases, whereas fatigue present for <4 weeks has a physical cause determined in 70% of cases.

What are Dangerous Causes of Fatigue I Shouldn't Miss?

Fatigue can be the presenting symptom for a vast array of diseases, including depression, infection (TB, HIV, hepatitis), hematologic/oncologic diseases (anemia, cancer), renal failure, endocrine disorders (diabetes, thyroid disease), neuromuscular diseases (multiple sclerosis), inflammatory diseases (sarcoidosis, rheumatoid arthritis), and sleep disorders (sleep apnea, restless legs syndrome).

What is Chronic Fatigue Syndrome?

Chronic fatigue syndrome is a symptom complex whose main feature is chronic or recurrent debilitating fatigue. Only 5% of chronically fatigued patients meet diagnostic criteria. To make the diagnosis, exclude known causes of fatigue. The diagnosis is made with the presence of clinically evaluated, unexplained persistent or relapsing chronic fatigue that is of new or definite onset (i.e., not lifelong); is not the result of ongoing

BOX 17-1

COMMON CAUSES OF FATIGUE

Endocrine and metabolic disorders
    Uncontrolled diabetes
    Cardiopulmonary disease
    Renal failure
    Thyroid disease
Hematologic/oncologic disorders
    Anemia
    Cancer
Medications
    Beta blockers
    Diuretics
    Sedatives
    Antidepressants
Pregnancy
Psychiatric disorders
    Anxiety
    Depression
    Somatization
Viral infections
    Hepatitis viruses
    HIV
    Mononucleosis
Sleep disorders
    Sleep apnea
    Substance abuse

exertion; is not substantially alleviated by rest; and results in substantial reduction in previous levels of occupational, educational, social, or personal activities. There also must be one of four or more of the following symptoms: impaired memory or concentration, sore throat, tender lymph nodes, muscle pain, multijoint pain without swelling or redness, headaches, unrefreshing sleep, and postexertional malaise lasting >24 hours. The cause is unknown, and many etiologies have been proposed, including chronic viral infection, hypothalamic dysfunction, and disordered autonomic regulation. A significant psychiatric component is often present confounded by the fact that chronic fatigue can be depressing in itself.

EVALUATION

What are the Key Parts of the History?

Ask the patient to describe what he or she means by fatigue, and ask what he or she thinks is the cause. This provides useful clues and the opportunity to allay fears. Question the duration and progress of symptoms. Ask a careful review of systems to identify new constitutional, neurologic, pulmonary, cardiac, or gastrointestinal symptoms. Patients who are short of breath sometimes refer to this symptom as "tiredness"; question patients about changes in their exercise tolerance. Pay particular attention to fevers, night sweats, or unexplained weight loss that suggest infection or tumor. Review medications, especially recent additions. Take a good sleep history, including initiation and maintenance of sleep, history of snoring (sleep apnea), and energy on awakening. In contrast to fatigue from physical causes, fatigue from psychological causes is unimproved by sleep, is worse in the morning, and improves through the day (Table 17-1). The one exception to this is sleep apnea, in which patients note unrefreshing sleep with persistent tiredness throughout the day, and bed partners may witness snoring or apneic spells.

Obtain a thorough social history, including work, substance use, sexual history, history of physical or sexual abuse, and recent major stressors (e.g., career changes, deaths, or relocation). When patients answer yes to most questions, review again for abuse because a significant proportion of patients with multiple complaints have a history of domestic violence. After you have reviewed physical symptoms, address possible depression in a direct and open manner. For example, you could say, "Many times fatigue is a sign of depression. I'd like to ask you about some of the other physical signs of depression." Ask about decreased libido and appetite, loss of the ability to enjoy anything (anhedonia), sadness, feelings of guilt or loss, thoughts about death or suicide, and difficulty concentrating as other clues to depression.

What is an Appropriate Physical Exam?

Perform a complete exam, with special attention to the most bothersome associated symptoms. Although the diagnostic yield compared

Table 17-1

Features of Fatigue from Psychological versus Physical Causes

	Psychological	Physical
Diurnal Pattern	Worse in morning	Better in morning
	Improves as day progresses	Worsens as day progresses
Duration	Chronic	Recent onset, parallels course of underlying disease
Effect of Sleep	Sleep is nonrestorative	Relieved by sleep
Onset	Coincides with stress, psychological disruption, conflict	Coincides with onset of a physical disease (e.g., respiratory infection)
Progression	Fluctuates; worse with distasteful activity or stress; may not progress	Progresses as disease worsens

with the history is low, the exam may confirm suspicions raised by the history, and a thorough exam itself reassures patients that their concerns are being taken seriously.

What Studies Should I Order?

Blood tests are appropriate to evaluate fatigue lasting <2–3 months or worsening symptoms. Order a CBC with differential, basic chemistry panel of electrolytes with glucose and renal function, ESR, liver transaminases, and TSH; consider vitamin D or B_{12} levels. Other tests may be indicated (chest x-ray, ECG, urinalysis, other endocrine tests) as suggested by history and exam. EBV titers are not useful and should not be ordered. When risk factors such as unprotected sex or intravenous drug use are present, test for HIV, hepatitis viruses, and syphilis (VDRL or RPR). For homeless, incarcerated, or HIV-infected patients, look for TB by placing a PPD with controls, and consider ordering a chest film. Consider a pregnancy test in premenopausal women. Consider a sleep study in patients with signs of sleep apnea.

What if the Results do not Point to any Specific Abnormality?

Emphasize the positive, that there is no evidence of a life-threatening disease. Reassure the patient that you still are concerned about his or her symptoms and want to see him or her again. Help problem solve to improve coping with symptoms. If there is personal turmoil, empathize that these upheavals can be exhausting. If you think the patient is depressed, find out what he or she thinks about this assessment. If the patient has trouble accepting this diagnosis, acknowledge that because depression can have stigma associated with it, and the symptoms may show up in the body before individuals recognize its effect on their mood. Finally, recognize that you have begun to address a problem whose solution may be beyond the time frame of a single visit. You can ask patients to keep a diary of symptoms, activities, and degree of fatigue for review at the next visit.

 TREATMENT

How do I Treat my Patient with Fatigue?

Treat any underlying psychiatric, endocrine, cardiac, pulmonary, or GI disorders uncovered by your evaluation. If no diagnosis is suggested, emphasize that the patient has gotten a thorough physical exam and testing, and that a life-threatening illness is unlikely. If you suspect depression, you may wish to recommend antidepressant therapy or psychiatry referral, emphasizing that even if depression is not the foundation of the problem, having fatigue for such a long time could by itself result in depression. Cognitive-behavioral therapy has been shown to be helpful in many somatic disorders. Set reasonable expectations: The goal of the chosen therapy will be to help the patient function with his or her symptoms, although the symptoms may not resolve entirely. For patients with chronic fatigue syndrome, treatment includes adjustment of maladaptive coping strategies, antidepressants, and a low-level exercise program.

KEY POINTS

◆ The duration, associated symptoms, progression, effect of sleep, and diurnal variation of fatigue help indicate whether the fatigue has a physical or psychiatric cause.

◆ Fatigue of recent onset or with new associated symptoms is concerning for physical disease.

◆ A trusting therapeutic relationship is the cornerstone of therapy for fatigue of unclear origin.

Case 17-1

A 26-year-old woman reports 2 months of fatigue. She says in addition that she sometimes feels "chilly," but has never taken her temperature, has had mild lower abdominal pain, and feels out of breath when she goes up stairs. On further questioning, she says that she has had unprotected sex with two men.

A. What features in this history are concerning for physical causes of her symptoms?
B. What other history would you seek?
C. What is your initial work-up?

Case 17-2

A 45-year-old man presents with feeling "tired all the time" for the past 5 years. He has been to many physicians and has a folder with his records. Since the onset of his tiredness, he has had headaches and joint aches, has had "ups and downs" in his temperature between 96.4° F and 99.2° F, feels unrefreshed after sleep, and feels "completely worn out" for more than a day after exercising. His records show that extensive lab, imaging, and cardiopulmonary evaluations have been done, all within normal limits. He says that he is "tired of being told it's all in his head" and hopes that you'll find out "what's really going on."

A. What further history should you take?
B. What should be the focus of your physical exam?
C. What is your initial work-up?

Case Answers

17-1 A. *Learning objective:* **Recognize "red flags" in a patient complaining of fatigue.** The relatively short duration of the patient's fatigue, the association with exertional dyspnea, and history of unprotected sex all are concerning for physical disorders.

17-1 B. *Learning objective:* **Ask appropriate history questions of patients with fatigue.** Ask about menstrual history, weight loss or gain, symptoms of thyroid disease such as temperature intolerance and changes in bowel habits, orthopnea, cough, symptoms of sexually transmitted diseases such as rashes or vaginal discharge, and history of exposure to TB.

17-1 C. *Learning objective:* **Select appropriate testing for patients with fatigue based on clues from history and exam.** Order CBC, electrolytes, renal function, glucose, TSH, bilirubin, and hepatic transaminases. With the patient's knowledge and consent, also order a pregnancy test, and consider syphilis, HIV, and HBV tests. Order chest x-ray and consider PPD testing and cervical swabs for gonorrhea and chlamydia.

17-2 A. *Learning objective:* **Obtain appropriate history in patients with fatigue, including looking for key features of chronic fatigue syndrome.** Take a more thorough sleep history, focusing on symptoms of sleep apnea such as snoring or apneas noted by a bed partner and daytime somnolence. Also ask about symptoms of depression and social stressors. Ask the patient what he is most concerned that his symptoms might represent, how it has affected his life, and what further evaluation he might like. Acknowledge that these symptoms are worrisome and frustrating. Tell him that his symptoms are real, and that even though the tests so far show no evidence of physical disease, there are things that can be done to help him cope with how he's feeling, although this may take time.

17-2 B. *Learning objective:* **Recognize the role of the physical exam in patients with fatigue in establishing rapport and reasonable patient expectations.** A thorough physical exam indicates to the patient that you take his concerns seriously. Because he has mentioned headaches and joint pain, do a good neurologic and joint exam, and tell the patient what you are checking as you do it.

17-2 C. *Learning objective:* **Recognize when further testing is unlikely to reveal a physical cause of fatigue.** Patients with fatigue of >4 months' duration, combined with no worrisome features on history or physical exam and previous blood tests do not require further testing. If you have difficulty with this conversation, consult with your supervisor for help. You may want to discuss the possibility of chronic fatigue with your supervisor before discussing your thoughts with the patient.

Fatigue

REFERENCE

Wessely S: Chronic fatigue: Symptom and syndrome. Ann Intern Med 2001; 134 (9 Pt 2): 838.

USEFUL WEB SITE

The National Center for Infectious Diseases Chronic Fatigue Syndrome: http://www.cdc.gov/ncidod/diseases/cfs/index.htm

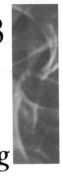

18

Gastrointestinal Bleeding

LISANNE R. BURKHOLDER and
DOUGLAS S. PAAUW

 ETIOLOGY

What are the Most Common Causes of Acute GI Bleeding?

GI bleeding is divided into upper and lower (Table 18-1), based on whether the bleeding originates above or below the ligament of Treitz in the distal duodenum. **Upper GI bleeding** occurs more often than lower GI bleeding, with PUD the most common cause. *Helicobacter pylori* infection and NSAID and alcohol use are common precipitants of PUD. Esophageal varices occur in patients with cirrhosis-induced portal hypertension and are potentially fatal because of how rapidly they bleed. Mallory-Weiss tear is a gastric mucosal tear that occurs after vomiting. **Lower GI bleeding** is usually due to a colonic lesion, such as diverticulosis or angiodysplasia, both of which are especially common conditions in older patients. In angiodysplasia, disordered and fragile vessels grow in the bowel wall. Colonic neoplasms and polyps account for a few lower GI bleeds, although bleeding tends to be low grade or occult. In patients <50 years old, bright red blood per rectum is often from hemorrhoids. Small intestinal bleeding is quite rare and may be due to angiodysplasia, tumors, or Meckel's diverticulum.

 EVALUATION

What Pertinent History should I Elicit when a Patient has GI Bleeding?

Use the history to distinguish whether the source of bleeding is from the upper or lower GI tract. Generally, patients with upper GI bleeds present with hematemesis, coffee-ground emesis, or melena (black, tarry stool owing to oxidation of blood during the prolonged transit time through the bowel). The sensitivity for melena for upper GI bleeding

Gastrointestinal Bleeding

Table 18-1	
Common Causes of Gastrointestinal Bleeding	
Upper GI Bleeding	**Lower GI Bleeding**
Gastritis	Angiodysplasia
Mallory-Weiss tear from retching	Brisk upper GI bleeding
Nosebleed	Colitis—infectious, inflammatory, or ischemic
Peptic ulcer disease	Colon cancer or polyp
Varices—esophageal, gastric	Diverticulosis
	Hemorrhoids

is 71% with a specificity of 88%. By contrast, lower GI bleeding produces hematochezia (maroon or bright red blood per rectum). The sensitivity for bright red blood per rectum for lower GI bleed is about 50% with a specificity of 90%. These are only general rules because occasionally a brisk upper GI bleed can cause hematochezia owing to the cathartic effects of fast bleeding, and right colon or small bowel bleeds can cause melena. Patients with rapid, severe bleeding may report dizziness, weakness, confusion, or syncope related to volume depletion. A slow or chronic bleed from any source can lead to fatigue and dyspnea on exertion as anemia progresses. Most GI bleeding is painless, although bleeding from peptic ulcers may be preceded by days to weeks of burning epigastric pain. Risk factors for PUD include NSAID, steroid, or alcohol use. The use of an SSRI may increase the risk of bleeding with coexistent NSAID use. If tenesmus is present, rectal inflammation is likely, as from ulcerative colitis. Weight loss or family history of colon cancer (especially if early onset) suggests neoplasm. Fever suggests infectious or inflammatory disorders. Alcohol use and chronic liver disease are risks for esophageal varices. Older age is a risk factor for angiodysplasia or diverticulitis. Patients with diverticular bleeds may have a history of prior episodes of painful diverticulitis.

How does the Physical Exam Help Me Evaluate a Patient with Bloody Stools?

Use the exam to judge the severity of bleeding. Tachycardia and hypotension are worrisome for rapid blood loss. Orthostasis (i.e., an increase in pulse or decrease in BP of >20 points from lying to standing) indicates volume loss of ≥20%. Pallor, cool skin, and poor capillary refill also are signs of severe blood loss and volume depletion. Conjunctival pallor and pale palmar creases indicate a hematocrit in the low 20s or less. Suspect esophageal varices if signs of chronic liver disease are present, such as spider telangiectasias, ascites, jaundice, asterixis, hepatomegaly or splenomegaly or both, palmar erythema, Terry's nails, or gynecomastia. Parotid or lacrimal gland enlargement, testicular atrophy, or Dupuytren's contractures of flexor tendons in the hand suggest alcohol abuse, which increases the risk for gastritis, PUD, and cirrhosis-related esophageal varices.

When are Anoscopy and NG Lavage Helpful?

Perform digital rectal exam and anoscopy in patients with bright red blood per rectum to distinguish hemorrhoidal bleeding from other, more proximal sources. Hemorrhoids on anoscopy do not rule out other sources of bleeding, especially in older patients, because 20% may have another more proximal lesion. Patients with signs of upper GI bleed or brisk hematochezia should have an NG tube placed. NG lavage can confirm ongoing gastric bleeding. The amount of saline lavage required to clear all blood from the NG aspirate correlates with the rapidity of bleeding. Clear NG aspirate rules out a gastric bleed, but not a duodenal bleed because without bile you cannot be sure if the duodenum has been sampled. NG aspirate with bile and no blood rules out active UGI bleed.

What Studies are Standard in a Patient with a GI Bleed?

Order serial hematocrits every 4 hours to gauge whether blood loss is ongoing, although a decrease in hematocrit may lag behind blood loss by several hours. Order blood type and crossmatch, and order 2–4 U of blood to be kept "in house" in the event of catastrophic bleeding. Check chemistry panel for renal function and electrolytes; BUN may increase with upper GI bleeding as a result of absorption of blood in gut. Glucose may be low with severe liver disease and may provide a clue to the presence of varices or gastritis. Check LFTs to screen for liver dysfunction, and check PT, PTT, and platelets for a coagulopathy, which could worsen blood loss. Follow calcium in patients receiving transfusions because the citrate preservative may cause calcium to decrease. In stable outpatients who have unexplained iron deficiency anemia or guaiac-positive stools, refer to a GI consultant for endoscopy. In patients with risks for cardiac disease, consider ECG and cardiac monitoring.

What Other Diagnostic Testing is Useful?

Plain films are relatively unhelpful except to rule out perforation with an upright view. Upper endoscopy for suspected upper GI bleed often identifies the cause of bleeding, identifies patients at high risk of rebleeding, can be used to take biopsy samples for diagnosis of *H. pylori* or tumor, and may be used therapeutically to stop bleeding from a variety of causes. Urgent colonoscopy after bowel preparation identifies the cause in more than half of patients with acute lower GI bleeds, although it can be challenging in the setting of ongoing blood loss. Selective arteriography or nuclear medicine labeled RBC scan may identify the source GI bleeding if the rate of bleeding is brisk in patients who are not candidates for endoscopy or in whom endoscopy is unrevealing.

TREATMENT

What Should be my General Approach to Treating GI Bleeding?

Treat the underlying cause of bleeding (Table 18-2).

Table 18-2

Presentation, Diagnosis, and Treatment Options of Common Causes of Gastrointestinal Bleeding

Cause	Presentation	Diagnosis	Treatment Options
Angiodysplasia	Elderly patients Slow occult bleeding Anemia and fatigue	Colonoscopy; Angiography if bleeding brisk	Surgical removal of involved bowel
Colon cancer	Elderly patients Slow occult bleeding Anemia and fatigue Weight loss Change in caliber of stool, new constipation	Colonoscopy; CT scan for staging disease, if lesion extensive	Surgical removal for cure if cancer isolated to the bowel; for palliation of obstructive symptoms if cancer is metastatic
Diverticulosis	Acute, rapid bleed Painless Prior diverticulitis	Colonoscopy, Selective arteriography or Labeled RBC scan if bleeding brisk	80% of bleeding resolves with bowel rest alone; surgical excision if persists
Ischemic bowel	Elderly patients Risk factors for atherosclerosis or emboli Midabdominal pain Postprandial pain Pain out of proportion to exam Acidemia	Plain radiographs or CT scan to identify edematous bowel and to rule out perforation	Surgical excision of infarcted bowel
PUD/gastritis	Preceding episodes of epigastric pain NSAIDs, alcohol, caffeine, steroids, cigarette use	Upper endoscopy with biopsy or serology for *H. pylori* depending on age and presence of alarm symptoms	PPI, H_2 blocker, Antibiotics for *H. pylori;* Stop NSAIDs, caffeine, alcohol
Mallory-Weiss tear	Retching preceding hematemesis Heavy lifting Usually painless	Upper endoscopy	Antiemetics, Supportive care
Varices	Hematemesis in patient with cirrhosis and portal hypertension Usually painless	Upper endoscopy	Variceal banding, Octreotide, Sengstaken- Blakemore tube, Beta blockers for prophylaxis, TIPS

My Patient is Hypotensive with Large Amounts of Bloody Stool. What Should I Do?

Patients with acute GI bleeding often require urgent resuscitation to restore intravascular volume. Obtain rapid intravenous access, usually two intravenous catheters, 16-gauge or larger, or a central line. Administer normal saline to maximize the portion that stays in the intravascular compartment. Packed RBCs or whole blood are better than saline for expanding the intravascular volume, but take longer to obtain. Replace factors or platelets as indicated by severe coagulopathy. Order 2–6 U of typed and crossmatched blood in house (determine the number of units based on severity of bleeding), so you can quickly transfuse rapidly bleeding patients. Place an NG tube (see earlier). Obtain GI and surgical consults early. GI consultants can assist with diagnostic and possibly therapeutic endoscopy. Surgical colleagues prefer knowing as early as possible about patients who may require surgery if bleeding is refractory to medical therapy. Revisit your patient frequently to review his or her clinical status and keep track of how much bleeding has occurred. Generally, if >3–4 U of blood are required in 24 hours, or >10 U overall, the patient should be considered for an urgent surgical intervention.

Gastrointestinal Bleeding

KEY POINTS

◆ Determine if GI bleeding is from the upper or the lower GI tract to guide your differential diagnosis and further work-up.

◆ Call GI and surgical consultants early.

◆ Obtain adequate intravenous access, type and crossmatch, and serial hematocrits, and perform frequent reassessment.

Case 18-1

A 55-year-old man is brought to emergency department vomiting blood after several weeks of epigastric discomfort. He smokes and drinks alcohol daily and has been using prednisolone for a COPD exacerbation, ibuprofen for chronic back pain, and diazepam for anxiety. On exam, he is pale, BP is 80/60 mm Hg, pulse 130 beats/min, and skin is cool and clammy. Heart exam reveals a 2/6 systolic murmur at the right upper sternal border without radiation. The abdomen is soft with mild epigastric tenderness. Rectal exam reveals bloody stool. Hematocrit is 22.

  A. Does this patient have an upper or lower GI bleed?
  B. What are his risk factors for GI bleeding?
  C. What other investigations would be useful?
  D. How should you manage this patient?

Case 18-2

A 75-year-old woman with a history of hypertension and hyperlipidemia who takes aspirin, atorvastatin, and an ACEI presents with painless rectal bleeding. She denies fevers, sweats, weight loss, anorexia, or altered bowel habit beyond her usual constipation. She is pale, with pale palmar creases. Heart rate is 120 beats/min and irregular, BP is 100/60 mm Hg; heart, lungs, and abdomen are normal; and rectal exam reveals bright red blood without tenderness or mass lesion.

    A. What are likely causes of this woman's bleeding?
    B. How would you manage this patient's care?

Case Answers

18-1 A.   *Learning objective:* **Recognize clinical features that distinguish upper from lower GI bleeding.** The patient's hematemesis and preceding epigastric discomfort suggest upper GI bleeding, as do his risk factors. Usually frank blood per rectum suggests lower GI bleed, although this also can occur with a brisk upper GI bleed.

18-1 B.   *Learning objective:* **List risk factors for upper GI bleeding.** Steroid, alcohol, cigarette, and NSAID use are risks for PUD. Heavy alcohol use also is a risk for cirrhosis, which may lead to variceal bleeding. You might need to revisit the exam to look for signs of chronic liver disease. Vomiting is a risk for Mallory-Weiss tear.

18-1 C.   *Learning objective:* **Order appropriate investigations for a patient with an upper GI bleed.** Serial blood counts, PT INR, urea, creatinine, electrolytes, liver enzymes, and type and crossmatch for blood products all would be useful. The patient also needs upper endoscopy for diagnostic and therapeutic purposes.

18-1 D.   *Learning objective:* **Appropriately manage patients with severe GI bleeding.** This patient first needs urgent placement of two large-bore peripheral intravenous access sites or a central venous catheter and resuscitation with normal saline to replace lost blood and improve hypotension and tachycardia. GI and surgical consultants should be called to arrange urgent upper endoscopy and notify of potential surgical need.

18-2 A.   *Learning objective:* **List likely causes of lower GI bleeding in an older woman.** The most likely cause is a diverticular bleed. Angiodysplasia, colonic neoplasm, and polyp also are possible.

18-2 B.   *Learning objective:* **Appropriately manage a patient with a lower GI bleed and cardiovascular comorbidities.** The patient is hypotensive relative to her usual diagnosis of hypertension and tachycardic with an irregular rhythm. An ECG should be done to assess her rhythm and assess how well her heart is tolerating the stress of the GI bleed. With her pale palmar creases, you are likely concerned about a very low hematocrit. Perform urgent resuscitation with placement of appropriate intravenous access and administration of saline and blood products when they are available, with a close eye on her fluid balance and cardiac function. Blood testing should include CBC, chemistry, coagulation status, and liver enzymes. She should be prepped for urgent colonoscopy, and the surgical consultant should be made aware of her progress, in case bleeding does not stop.

REFERENCES

Fallah MA, Prakash C, Edmundowicz S: Acute gastrointestinal bleeding. Med Clin North Am 2000;84:1183.

Zuccaro G: Management of the adult patient with acute lower gastrointestinal bleeding. Am J Gastroenterol 1998;93:1202.

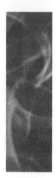

19

Headache

LINDA E. PINSKY

 ETIOLOGY

What Causes Headaches?

Approximately 99% of all headaches are recurrent benign headaches and are tension type, migraine, or cluster headaches. Rare causes not to miss are subarachnoid hemorrhage (SAH), meningitis, subdural hematoma, and cancer.

What Features are Associated with Chronic Daily Headaches?

A subset of headache patients has chronic daily headaches. Chronic daily headaches (Figure 19-1) are often associated with the following features: family history of headaches (90%), sleep disturbance (close to 100%), analgesic overuse (NSAIDs, ergotamine, barbiturates, and particularly narcotics such as codeine), and depression.

What are Cluster Headaches?

Cluster headaches occur predominantly in middle-aged men who smoke cigarettes and are severe, unilateral, retro-orbital, and often described as stabbing in quality. Cluster headaches often are accompanied by ipsilateral nasal congestion or lacrimation. These headaches recur over consecutive days to weeks and then remit—hence the term cluster headaches.

 EVALUATION

My Patient has Recurring Headaches. What Questions Should I Ask?

The basic goal of evaluation is to determine the type and severity of the headache. History should be directed at pattern and location, previous headaches and treatment, preceding and accompanying symptoms (nausea, vomiting, visual changes, photophobia, neurologic deficits),

154

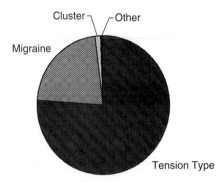

FIGURE 19-1 Common causes of chronic benign headaches. Relative frequency can be converted to chronic daily headache by repeated use of analgesics.

triggering factors, severity and progression, medication use, and family history.

What Distinguishes Tension Type and Migraine Headaches?

Patients with tension-type headaches classically describe a "bandlike pressure" around the skull that is mild to moderate in severity, but does not prevent daily activities (Box 19-1). Migraines are usually unilateral and throbbing; may be associated with nausea and vomiting; and may be disabling, with sufferers often retiring to bed in a dark, quiet room. Common migraine is frequently mild to moderate in intensity and may not be disabling. The major difference is that tension headache isn't disabling, whereas migraine headache can be disabling. An aura may precede a migraine headache, most commonly visual scintillations. Effective clinical criteria make the diagnosis (Box 19-2).

What are Clues to Ominous Headaches Versus Benign Ones?

Although the etiology of most headaches is benign, it is important to recognize signs that suggest an ominous cause for headache (Box 19-3).

BOX 19-1

FEATURES OF TENSION-TYPE HEADACHE

- Mild-to-moderate tightness, bandlike pressure
- Lasts 30 minutes to 7 days
- Not worsened by daily activity
- Lacks photophobia and phonophobia (one may be present)
- Ten previous episodes

BOX 19-2

CLINICAL DIAGNOSIS OF MIGRAINE HEADACHE

Requires any two of the following:

Unilateral site
Throbbing quality
Nausea
Photophobia or phonophobia

BOX 19-3

DANGER SIGNS SUGGESTING AN OMINOUS CAUSE OF HEADACHE

History

First headache, or marked change in chronic headache
Onset after age 50
Onset during exertion
Sudden onset or worst headache ever

Exam

Abnormal neurologic exam/mental status
Fever
Neck stiffness

What Should I Look for on Exam?

Perform a good general exam, with a complete neurologic evaluation including cranial nerve testing and mental status assessment. Conduct additional examination as suggested by the patient's history. If you suspect meningitis, check vital signs, mental status, and nuchal rigidity. If you are concerned about sinus infection, look for maxillary tenderness, purulent discharge, and poor transillumination of the sinuses. If you are concerned about temporal arteritis, palpate the temporal arteries.

My Patient Requests a CT Scan or MRI. Should I Order Imaging?

Headache is, for the most part, a clinical diagnosis. Several studies have shown that imaging does not add anything to the diagnosis, as long as the person with a headache doesn't have any of the warning signs mentioned earlier and has a normal neurologic exam. Longitudinal care helps with diagnosis; if the patient develops suspicious symptoms, has a mental status change, or doesn't get better as you expect, go back and revisit your original diagnostic assumptions, and reconsider further evaluation.

What Test do I Order if I Suspect SAH?

SAH usually presents suddenly, often as "the worst headache ever." The purpose of imaging is to detect the blood. The sensitivity of the CT scan depends on the presence of fresh bleeding. In the first 24 hours, CT detects 95% of SAH. If the CT scan is negative, and you still suspect SAH, order LP to detect the 5% of bleeds missed by CT scan. Look for xanthochromia, a yellow pigmentation to the spinal fluid indicating the breakdown of blood in the CSF. If the suspected bleed occurred >1 week before, MRI is more sensitive.

How will I know if my Patient has a Brain Tumor?

Patients with headache often fear they have a brain tumor; it is good to ask patients what they are worried about to address this concern directly. Although the headache of a brain tumor has been described as a morning headache associated with nausea and vomiting, in reality most brain tumor–associated headaches do not fit this or any other typical picture. Use warning signs for ominous cause of headache to prompt further evaluation. If no warning signs are present, longitudinal care is the key to monitor for any progression of symptoms or neurologic changes, which would warrant further evaluation.

TREATMENT

How Should I Treat Migraine and Tension-type Headaches?

Before adding a medication, make sure your patient isn't using any medications that might induce headaches, including OCPs, caffeine, alcohol, antidepressants, H_2 blockers, nitrates, and many more. Headaches also can be due to daily withdrawal symptoms from medications initially used to treat headaches, including NSAIDs, acetaminophen (Tylenol), and aspirin. Have the patient look for other triggers (wine, cheese, too much sleep) and remove them. Tension-type headaches respond well to NSAIDs.

What Medications are Useful for Treating Migraine Headache?

Medications to treat recurrent migraine headaches fall into two categories: abortive and prophylactic (Box 19-4). Abortive treatment is given at the time of the headache to try to stop it. Prophylactic treatment is used for headaches occurring more than four times a month. For abortive therapy, many people respond to aspirin, NSAIDs such as naproxen (500–1000 mg), or acetaminophen. Oral triptans are successful in 70% of cases with response rates of 80% with injectable sumatriptan, although relapse is common. Addition of naproxen to sumatriptan can improve efficacy and decrease relapse rates. Sumatriptan is available in injectable, nasal, and oral formulations. Cafergot, a combination of ergotamine and caffeine, is effective 60% of the time. Because of frequent GI upset, this medication is not commonly used. Ergotamines and triptans can cause vasoconstriction and may induce angina or

BOX 19-4

THERAPIES FOR MIGRAINE HEADACHE

Abortive Therapy

NSAIDs, aspirin
Acetaminophen
Ergotamines (dihydroergotamine, Cafergot)
Triptans (sumitriptan, others)
Narcotics (last resort)

Prophylactic Therapy

Beta blocker (propranolol)
Calcium channel blocker (verapamil)*
TCA (amitriptyline)
Riboflavin
Antiseizure medications (valproate, gabapentin, topiramate)

Management of Concurrent GI Symptoms

Antinausea agent (prochlorperazine)
Promotility agent (metoclopramide)

_____

*Calcium channel blockers have been used historically, but there are limited data to support their efficacy.

myocardial infarction, so do not use these in patients with atherosclerotic disease. Because gastroparesis accompanies headache, particularly migraine, concomitant use of promotility agents, such as metoclopramide, can improve the absorption and the effect of the analgesic medication.

If Abortive Therapy for Migraine is not Effective, What Next?

Patients with severe migraines often come to the emergency department or the physician's office having failed to get relief from the above-mentioned therapies. For these patients, consider the following: Sumatriptan is 80% effective when given subcutaneously, but headaches recur in 50% of patients. Intravenous prochlorperazine is particularly suited to patients with associated nausea, improving nausea and aborting 80% of headaches. Dihydroergotamine (intravenous or subcutaneous) is as effective as sumatriptan, but may cause nausea. If a patient has received a triptan in the past 24 hours, he or she should not receive dihydroergotamine. Narcotics, such as intravenous meperidine (Demerol), should be reserved as a last resort.

What Should I do If the Headaches are Frequent?

If your patient has bothersome headaches more than four times a month, ensure that basic measures have been taken, as follows: Regulate sleep patterns, avoid food triggers, and eliminate caffeine. Review medications to detect causes for withdrawal headaches. If these measures are to no avail, consider prophylactic treatment. A 4-month trial using the B vitamin riboflavin in high doses (400 mg) showed a marked effect on headache frequency (number needed to treat = 3), but less effect on severity, similar to effects seen with other prophylactic agents. Its favorable risk-to-benefit ratio and tolerability make it a good initial choice. Low-dose TCAs are especially effective for tension-type headaches, but also work for migraines. Beta blockers, especially nonselective propranolol and nadolol, are effective for preventing migraine headaches. If possible, choose a medication that treats a concurrent medical condition. In a patient with hypertension, beta blockers might be your first choice. The antiseizure drugs valproate gabapentin, and topiramate are options in patients who have failed beta blockers or TCAs.

How do I Treat Chronic Daily Headaches and Cluster Headaches?

The only treatment for chronic daily headache is to get the patient off all analgesics and start from scratch. Unmedicated patients with chronic daily headaches may respond to TCAs. For cluster headaches, lithium, ergotamine and 100% oxygen are effective.

How Often Should my Patient Follow Up, and What Should I Review at Appointments?

Headaches are a chronic condition. Have your patient keep a headache diary to track symptoms, medication use, response, and triggers. When you are initiating or changing therapy, follow up every 4 to 6 weeks. When stable, the frequency is dictated by the frequency of symptoms. At each appointment, review the headache diary for the type and frequency of headaches, triggers, compliance, and side effects. Strategize with the patient regarding avoidance or elimination of triggers. Review the treatment plan, and change medications if the current regimen is ineffective. If a compliant patient is not getting better as you would expect, or develops a new, different headache, reassess your diagnosis, and consider further evaluation or referral to a neurologist.

Headache

KEY POINTS

- ◆ Most headaches are benign.
- ◆ The diagnosis of a headache is based on accurate history and physical.
- ◆ Look for warning signs suggesting an ominous etiology.
- ◆ Always review patients' medications for those causing headache as a side effect or by withdrawal reactions.

Case 19-1

A 25-year-old woman reports right-sided headache, nausea, and phonophobia for 24 hours. She has had three previous episodes in the past 2 years. She has partial relief with extra-strength acetaminophen. Her neurologic examination, including mental status, is normal.

  A. What is your differential diagnosis?
  B. What imaging technique do you recommend?
  C. What treatment do you recommend?
  D. If her symptoms recur every week, what treatment would you recommend?

Case 19-2

A 72-year-old writer with a stressful year including the end of a 30-year relationship presents with a tingling headache over the right temple. She recently began exercising and eating a healthier diet. Despite these efforts, she reports muscle aches and increasing fatigue. She has difficulty getting out of bed in the morning.

  A. Does she have any warning signs for ominous headache?
  B. What testing will you order?

Case 19-3

A 26-year-old orthopedic surgery resident presents with a sudden severe headache while weightlifting. Neurologic exam, including CT, is normal. He is fine until his next call night when he collapses with a severe headache.

  A. What is his most likely diagnosis?
  B. What testing do you recommend?

Case Answers

19-1 A.   *Learning objective:* **Diagnose migraine headaches based on history.** This young woman's unilateral throbbing headache accompanied by nausea and phonophobia is classic for migraine. No "red flags" are present for an ominous cause.

19-1 B.   *Learning objective:* **Imaging is not required for headache with benign history and physical.** Studies have shown that with a normal neurologic exam and no "red flags" for an ominous cause, imaging (CT or MRI) is unnecessary.

19-1 C. *Learning objective:* **Identify abortive treatment for migraine.** Given her infrequent symptoms, an NSAID, such as naproxen (Naprosyn), is a reasonable choice at the first sign of headache. There may be gastroparesis, so consider adding a promotility agent, such as metoclopramide. Warn the patient of overuse of analgesics and the propensity to cause withdrawal headaches. If she develops more severe symptoms that do not respond to the naproxen (i.e., unable to work for more than a day, vomiting), consider a triptan. Before you prescribe a triptan, review risk for cardiovascular disease. In a young person, cardiovascular disease is unlikely.

19-1 D. *Learning objective:* **Recognize the importance of prophylactic treatment for frequent headaches.** With the increased frequency of her headaches, consider prophylactic treatment. The first choice would be riboflavin or naproxen taken daily. If this doesn't work, beta blockers are a reasonable choice.

19-2 A. *Learning objective:* **Identify warning signs for headache from a worrisome cause.** Age >50 and new headache is a concerning combination in this woman. Her fatigue and diffuse muscle aches raise further questions about overall health.

19-2 B. *Learning objective:* **Know appropriate work-up for concerning headache history.** This woman gives a history consistent with PMR and associated TA. On exam, she likely has tenderness with palpation over the temporal artery and diffuse muscle pain with normal strength. In one study, TA was as common as migraine in this age group. The most targeted test for PMR is ESR, and if elevated in this setting, it is diagnostic. If TA is a concern, obtain a temporal artery biopsy because steroid dose is higher in this condition than in PMR alone. If the diagnosis is unclear, screen with basic lab tests including CBC, electrolytes, and LFTs. Also consider contrast CT scan, looking for structural disease, such as tumors, in this age group.

19-3 A. *Learning objective:* **Recognize presentation of SAH.** This patient has a subarachnoid hemorrhage until completely proven otherwise. The sudden onset, association with weightlifting, and severity all point to this diagnosis.

19-3 B. *Learning objective:* **Outline the appropriate testing for SAH.** Although his CT scan is negative, there is still a 5% chance of a missed bleed. You must perform LP for xanthochromia.

REFERENCES

Colas R, Munoz P, Temprano R, et al. Chronic daily headache with analgesic overuse: Epidemiology and impact on quality of life. Neurology 2004;62:1338.

Pryse-Phillips WE, Dodick DW, Edmeads JG, et al. Guidelines for the nonpharmacologic management of migraine in clinical practice. Can Med Assoc J 1998;159:47.

Silberstein SD, for the US Headache Consortium: Practice parameter. Evidence-based guidelines for migraine headache (an evidence-based review). Neurology 2002;55:754.

Headache

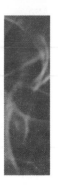

20

Healthy Patients

LINDA E. PINSKY and JOHN V. L. SHEFFIELD

 DISEASE PREVENTION AND SCREENING

What is Preventive Medicine?

Preventive medicine attempts to decrease disease and increase health. Prevention assumes that clinical disease is a cumulative process, and that interventions can prevent, stop, or slow that process. The process includes three stages: (1) health before disease; (2) preclinical disease, in which biologic changes have occurred, but disease isn't apparent; and (3) clinically overt disease. Examples of preventive interventions include screening tests, immunizations, counseling and behavioral changes, and chemoprophylaxis (e.g., bisphosphonate therapy to prevent osteoporosis).

Why is Prevention Important?

Many common diseases can be prevented. It has been estimated that half of the deaths in the U.S. are related to preventable external factors, including diet and activity habits; tobacco, alcohol, or illicit drug use; sexual behavior; and motor vehicles. Smoking alone contributes to one fifth of all U.S. deaths. In 1992, 41,000 deaths were attributed to not using a seat belt and driving while intoxicated.

What are Primary and Secondary Prevention?

The terms *primary prevention* and *secondary prevention* refer to the stage of the disease process during which the intervention occurs. In **primary prevention**, interventions are begun in asymptomatic patients before disease is present to alter susceptibility or reduce exposure. Examples are classes for smoking prevention or cessation, nutrition counseling, and immunization. **Secondary prevention** attempts to detect disease in preclinical or beginning stages. Examples include screening programs for cervical or breast cancer (Pap smears and mammography). **Tertiary prevention** attempts to restore function and alleviate disability from

---

BOX 20-1

CRITERIA FOR JUDGING WHETHER SCREENING IS WORTHWHILE

Disease Characteristics

Prevalent or responsible for high burden of suffering
Detectable before symptom onset
Effective treatment available
Early detection improves outcomes

Test Characteristics

Accurate (good sensitivity, specificity, and predictive values)
Acceptable to patients
Benefits outweigh risks

Population Characteristics

Sufficient incidence to justify cost
Population screened will live long enough to benefit
Intervention acceptable to and used by population

---

disease (e.g., with cardiac rehabilitation after heart attack). The distinction is important because the risk-to-benefit ratio and cost-effectiveness of an intervention differ depending on the stage of disease it targets. Reducing cholesterol in individuals who already have had an MI may be worth the cost and potential side effects of cholesterol-lowering drugs. In comparison, primary prevention with medications in healthy individuals may be too costly or may cause too many side effects for the smaller benefit gained.

Why do We Screen for Some Diseases and Not Others?

Certain criteria must be met before screening is considered worthwhile. These criteria vary according to the treatment of the disease, the test, and the patient population (Box 20-1).

Why are Some Screening Tests Controversial?

PSA is a screening test for prostate cancer that was clinically available before the implication of its use was clearly understood. There are several problems with it as a screening test. First, PSA has poor sensitivity and specificity: It can be elevated in the absence of prostate cancer or can be normal in the presence of cancer. Second, cancer identified by an elevated PSA may not be clinically significant—that is, the patient may have cancer, but may die from another cause. Third, the effectiveness of treatment for prostate cancer is debated. A Swedish study suggests that watchful waiting has the same mortality rates as surgery, without the perioperative risk or common postoperative complications of urinary incontinence or impotence.

Preventive Health Practices Differ for Age and Gender. How Can I Know What To Do?

In general, address the health issues specific to that age and gender. Some preventive measures apply to all adults, including tetanus immunization; BP screening; and counseling for healthy diet and exercise, smoking cessation, and use of seat belts. Other interventions are based on age or gender, such as Pap smears, mammography, and fecal occult blood testing. Certain measures are directed only to high-risk populations (e.g., aspirin for heart disease). For more specific guidance, consult available references. One of the most widely used is the U.S. Preventive Services Task Force (USPSTF) Guide to Clinical Preventive Services (Table 20-1). This guide provides evidence-based recommendations for groups of people based on age, gender, and risk factors. The need to base recommendations on well-designed outcome studies is especially important in preventive medicine because you are recommending interventions to healthy patients and do not want to cause harm.

How do I Track Health Maintenance and Promotion?

One approach is to have a health maintenance/promotion section in the problem list or in the assessment/plan to prompt you. The use of reminders or prompts, especially computer-based, has been shown to increase the rate at which providers address health maintenance issues with their patients.

Table 20-1

Suggested Preventive Health Care for Adults Based on Recommendations of the U.S. Preventive Services Task Force 2005

a. Periodic Health Exam

Height, weight, BP, and symptom-focused examination	Age 18–39: Every 3–5 y Age ≥40: Annual

b. Screening

Disease	Intervention	Recommended Schedule	Strength of Evidence
Breast cancer	Mammography	Annual for women age 40 or 50–69 Reasonable to continue beyond age 69	Good
Cervical cancer	Papanicolaou smear	Every 1–3 y from age 21 or onset of sexual activity Stop after hysterectomy for benign disease Stop at age 65 if repeatedly normal	Good

(continued)

Table 20-1

Suggested Preventive Health Care for Adults Based on Recommendations of the U.S. Preventive Services Task Force 2005 (Continued)

b. Screening (continued)

Disease	Intervention	Recommended Schedule	Strength of Evidence
Colorectal cancer	Fecal occult blood testing (FOBT)	Screen beginning at age 50 (in the presence of family history of early colon cancer, may screen earlier)	Fair
	Flexible sigmoidoscopy	Annual FOBT *and/or* sigmoidoscopy every 3–5 y *or*	
	Colonoscopy	Colonoscopy every 10 y, every 3–5 y if polyps	
High blood cholesterol	Total cholesterol	Men age 35–65 Women age 45–65	Fair
Osteoporosis	Bone mineral density (DXA)	Postmenopausal woman at risk and all women at age 65 (see Chapter 40 for further discussion)	Fair
PID	Chlamydia screening	One-time screening at a minimum; women age <25 with multiple sexual partners at highest risk	Fair
Prostate cancer	PSA	Discuss possible benefits and known risks of screening with patient before testing Men age 50–69 most likely to benefit	Poor

c. Counseling

Injury prevention	Use car lap/shoulder belts
	Wear bicycle helmets
	Install smoke detectors
Diet and exercise	Decrease fat and cholesterol intake
	Adequate calcium and vitamin D intake
	Exercise aerobically regularly
Sexually transmitted disease prevention	Use safe sex practices
Substance use	Abstain from or stop smoking
	Moderate alcohol use
	Abstain from illicit drug use

Healthy Patients

(continued)

Table 20-1

Suggested Preventive Health Care for Adults Based on Recommendations of the U.S. Preventive Services Task Force 2005 (Continued)

d. Routine Adult Immunization

Disease	Recommendation
Tetanus-diphtheria (Td)	Td boosters every 10 y throughout life
Tetanus-diphtheria pertussis (Tdap)	Adults substitute Tdap for one booster of Td
Measles-mumps-rubella	Single dose for adults born after 1956 without proof of immunity or documentation of previous immunization Second dose for college students, health care workers, and foreign travelers
Hepatitis B	Recommended for all young adults and older adults at high risk Assess serologic response in adults age >30
Hepatitis A	Recommended for adults at risk—foreign travelers, injection drug users, adults with multiple sexual partners, day care workers, adults with chronic liver disease
Influenza	Annually to all adults age ≥50, younger if at risk (e.g., COPD, CHF, asthma, cancer, health care worker) Consider for all healthy adults
Invasive pneumococcal disease	Recommended for all adults at age 65, younger if at risk Reimmunization recommended for high-risk adults at age 65 who received vaccine >5 years earlier, and asplenic and immunocompromised adults 5 years after first dose
Human papillomavirus (HPV)	Recommended for girls and women 9-26

Case 20-1

A 22-year-old, apparently healthy man comes for a routine visit.

A. What general counseling should you offer?
B. What specific immunizations are indicated?
C. Is prostate screening needed?

CHANGING HARMFUL HEALTH HABITS

What are General Guidelines to Changing Harmful Health Habits?

Studies of how people change provide a model that divides the process into clinically useful stages: (1) precontemplation, (2) contemplation, (3) preparation, (4) action, and (5) maintenance. Relapse often occurs, reinitiating the cycle (Figure 20-1). By identifying which stage the patient has achieved, you can target your efforts to help the patient reach the next stage. The focus is on moving the patient closer to change, rather than an "all or nothing" outcome.

What is an Example of Using This Model In Patient Care?

This example follows a patient through smoking cessation.

Stage 1: **Precontemplation.** In this stage, the patient is not consciously thinking of quitting. Studies show that simple physician advice and encouragement to consider quitting have an effect, although the results are not immediately obvious. Maintain an empathetic and nonjudgmental approach while making a clear statement: "I think it is important for you to quit smoking. In fact, this is the most important thing you can do for your health."

Stage 2: **Contemplation.** The patient is now considering quitting smoking. Ask questions at each visit to help the patient identify reasons and barriers to quitting. Personalize the motivation: "You have had one heart attack already; if you stop smoking, chances are higher you will be around to enjoy your new promotion." Make sure the motivation fits the particular age, gender, and individual. For example, adolescents tend to "bum"

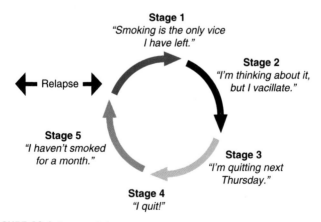

FIGURE 20-1 Stages of change.

Healthy Patients

cigarettes, so arguments about cost are ineffective. Rather, it may work to say, "If you quit smoking, you may be able to breathe better and that will help your soccer game."

Stage 3: Preparation. The patient has decided to quit smoking. Problem solve with the patient about what has worked in the past and what led to failure to quit. Address the patient's concerns about possible negative consequences of quitting, including weight gain, bad moods, and issues of peer nonsupport or other barriers. Offer a support system, such as an intensive smoking cessation program; nicotine replacement therapy such as gums, patch, or nasal spray; or other pharmacologic aids, such as bupropion.

Stage 4: Action. The patient quits! Schedule a series of biweekly or monthly visits, beginning 1 week after the quit date. Express continuing care and support.

Stage 5: Maintenance and Relapse. Congratulate the patient on successes, and reinforce the benefits of not smoking. Anticipate relapses; reframe these as positive learning experiences, and plan how to restart the cessation process.

What Techniques Can You Use to Help Patients Move from One Stage to the Next?

Different techniques that facilitate patient change are described in Figure 20-2.

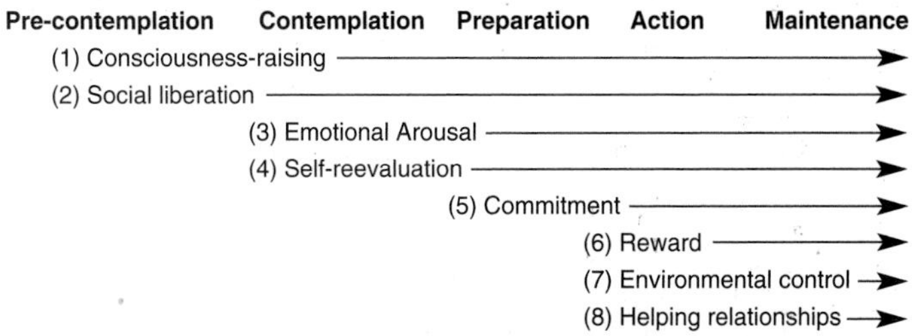

FIGURE 20-2 Model and strategies effective in eliciting change according to stages of change. *(1)* Consciousness-raising has the goal of increasing information about self and problem and using techniques such as observations, confrontations, interpretations, and bibliotherapy (guidance in the solution of personal problems through directed reading). *(2)* Social liberation uses the technique of advocating for rights, empowering, and policy interventions. *(3)* Emotional arousal involves experiencing and expressing feelings about one's problems and solutions. *(4)* Self-evaluations involve value, clarification, and corrective experiences. *(5)* Commitment is choosing and committing to an act or the belief in the ability to change. *(6)* Environmental control includes restructuring the environment. *(7)* Rewards encompass overt and covert reinforcement. *(8)* Helping relationships provide social support for one's actions.

What are Specific Guidelines in the Use of Medication and Nicotine in Smoking Cessation?

Physician counseling, group counseling, and extended support groups all assist patients in smoking cessation and long-term maintenance. Nicotine replacement and the antidepressant bupropion, started 1 week before the quit date, double the successful smoking cessation rate to 35%. Given the great difficulty patients have in stopping smoking, this is encouraging. Nicotine can be administered by gum, inhaler, or, most commonly, transdermal patch. For the patch, a dose of 21 mg for 10 to 12 weeks has shown the greatest success. Patients are advised not to smoke concurrently with the nicotine replacement, but studies of the patch have not revealed adverse cardiovascular outcomes. Extended-release bupropion is dosed at 150 mg daily for 3 days, then increased to twice daily. This staggered start minimizes the initial agitation that many patients experience on this medication. Additionally, the quit date should be set for 1 week after starting bupropion to ensure effective blood levels. Bupropion lowers the seizure threshold and so should not be used in patients with past history of seizure, alcoholism, or ongoing eating disorders. A benefit of bupropion that may encourage patients in its use is that it may offset the weight gain and depression that can follow smoking cessation.

Is this Model of Change Applicable to All Behavioral Changes?

Yes. Ambulatory medicine offers you a longitudinal relationship with a patient, allowing you to address these issues repeatedly, a little bit at a time. As you get to know your patients, you can help them recognize opportunities for and benefits of prevention that matter to them, whether it is being able to breathe easier when playing with their grandchildren since they quit smoking or their improved job performance since they quit drinking. Seeing the benefits of change is reinforcing for patients and physicians.

Case 20-2

A 35-year-old man wants to lose weight. He has tried several times in the past but failed and states he's "given up."

   A. What stage of change is he in?
   B. What questions should you ask?
   C. He decides to try to lose weight. What follow-up should you plan on?

KEY POINTS – DISEASE PREVENTION AND SCREENING

◆ Prevention saves lives, decreases disease, and increases health.

Healthy Patients

◆ Because prevention is aimed at healthy people, the evidence must be compelling that the benefits outweigh the risks.

◆ Evidence-based recommendations geared to specific age and gender are available, most notably in the USPSTF Guide to Clinical Preventive Services.

KEY POINTS – CHANGING HARMFUL HEALTH HABITS

◆ There is a cycle of change that occurs in predictable stages: precontemplation, contemplation, determination, action, and maintenance.

◆ Providers can assist patients in moving from one stage to the next.

◆ Providers should inquire about harmful health habits, advise patients to change them, and offer continuing support in a nonjudgmental, empathetic manner.

Case Answers

20-1 A. *Learning objective:* **Know what preventive health counseling is appropriate for young healthy men.** The leading cause of death in this age group is MVAs and other unintentional injuries, homicide, suicide, malignant neoplasms, and heart disease. General screening considerations are height, weight, activity level, BP, and assessment for substance abuse. Counseling is directed at injury protection, such as seat belt use, motorcycle helmets, safe use of firearms; avoidance of the use of tobacco, excessive alcohol intake, and illicit drug use; safer sex practices; healthy diet and adequate physical activity; use of sunscreen protection; and good dental health.

20-1 B. *Learning objective:* **Identify key immunizations for this age group.** Immunizations include tetanus (Tdap), hepatitis B, and measles-mumps-rubella (MMR) if not previously immunized. Other interventions may be indicated if, by history, he is in a high-risk population.

20-1 C. *Learning objective:* **Recognize that prostate screening has no role in young men.** There is no indication for prostate cancer screening in this age group.

20-2 A. *Learning objective:* **Apply the model for change to the patient's own process.** This man is in stage 2, contemplation. Although he is discouraged, he is still contemplating trying again.

> *20-2 B.*   *Learning objective:* **Design an approach to help the patient move through stages of change.** Focus questions on what barriers interfered with success in his last attempts. Work to increase motivation by helping him identify personal benefits of weight loss.
>
> *20-2 C.*   *Learning objective:* **Recognize and support the determination stage.** Now that he has determined to lose weight again, work on specific plans of action. Explore what medical and social supports are available to him. Readdress barriers and motivations. Make explicit plans for a date to start and follow-up appointments.

REFERENCES

Agency for Healthcare Research and Quality: Guide to Clinical Preventive Services, 3rd ed. AHRQ Publication No. 05–0570. Rockville, MD, Agency for Healthcare Research and Quality, 2005. http://www.ahrq.gov/clinic/pocketgd.htm

Prochaska JO: Changing for Good. New York, William Morrow, 1994.

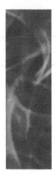

21

Joint and Muscular Pain

MARY B. MIGEON

 ## JOINT PAIN

ETIOLOGY

What Causes Joint Pain?

The causes of joint pain can be divided into two categories—mechanical and inflammatory (Figure 21-1). Osteoarthritis is the most common mechanical arthritis and occurs with age-associated wear and tear on the joint. Frequently, a single joint is affected. Inflammatory causes of joint pain are autoimmune disease, crystal-induced disease, and infection. These can involve few or multiple joints, often in a characteristic pattern. The autoimmune arthropathies, SLE and RA, affect small and large joints and multiple organs. In gout, typically few joints are involved. Septic arthritis usually affects a single joint, unless disseminated gonococcal infection is present. Occasionally, patients and physicians confuse muscular pain with joint pain.

What Serious Causes of Joint Pain Should I not Miss?

Don't miss septic arthritis, malignancy, or osteonecrosis. Clues to these include rest pain; delayed response to therapy; risk factors such as prior malignancy; or systemic signs, such as fever, chills, or weight loss. Osteonecrosis (death of bone owing to vascular insufficiency) is seen most commonly in the hip, particularly with long-term steroid use, sickle cell anemia, or vasculitis.

Why is Septic Arthritis Important?

Septic arthritis can cause joint destruction and is a medical emergency requiring rapid diagnosis and treatment, including possible surgical débridement. Onset is acute, with marked synovitis, effusion, and extreme pain with movement. Eighty percent of cases involve one joint, usually the knee. Infectious agents in adults are *S. aureus,* other gram-positive organisms, and *Neisseria gonorrhoeae* (a gram-negative coccus).

173

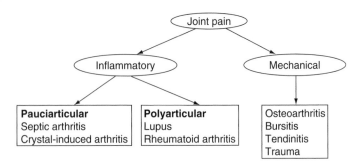

FIGURE 21-1 Classification of joint pain.

S. aureus is especially common in septic arthritis superimposed on RA. This is particularly tricky because a clinician may believe the inflammation is due to RA alone. In young sexually active adults, suspect gonorrhea, and remember that disseminated infection can affect multiple joints, albeit rarely.

What is Osteoarthritis?

Synonyms for osteoarthritis include *degenerative arthritis* and *mechanical arthritis*. This condition occurs as a consequence of wear and tear on the joints, which generates chronic low-grade inflammation. Prevalence is high in patients >55 years old, or when joints are heavily used, such as hip degenerative arthritis in a construction worker. Obesity or prior trauma also predisposes to early osteoarthritis.

Does Patient Age Change the Likely Cause of Joint Pain?

Patients >55 years old are much more likely to have degenerative arthritis, gout, or bursitis. Autoimmune arthropathies are more common in younger patients, as are trauma and overuse syndromes, such as ligament injury or tendinitis.

For Major Joints, what are the Common Causes of Joint Pain?

Degenerative arthritis occurs predominantly in high-use joints, such as the hands, and in weight-bearing joints, such as the knees and hips; the shoulder and elbow are often spared. Tendinitis and bursitis commonly occur secondary to overuse of any of the major joints (Table 21-1 and Figure 21-2). Psoriasis and hemochromatosis can have associated joint pain.

What is Rotator Cuff Tendinitis?

The rotator cuff comprises four muscles that rotate and stabilize the humeral head. The subacromial bursa lies between the cuff muscles and the acromial process. Various terms are used to describe a spectrum of disorders that affect this cluster of muscles and surrounding structures, including *rotator cuff tendinitis, subacromial bursitis, frozen shoulder syndrome,* and *impingement syndrome.* A biceps tendinitis can

Table 21-1

Common Conditions Affecting Major Joints

Location	Condition	Findings
Hip	Degenerative arthritis	Pain in groin, medial thigh
		Pain with internal and external hip rotation
	Trochanteric bursitis	Pain in lateral thigh
		Point tenderness on greater trochanter
Knee	Degenerative arthritis	Pain deep to patella
		Joint line tenderness
		Effusion without heat
	Prepatellar bursitis	Pain over patella when kneeling
		Heat, swelling anterior to patella
	Patellofemoral syndrome	Pain with deep knee bend, walking upstairs, prolonged sitting with knees bent
	Baker's cyst	Fullness behind knee, lower extremity swelling if ruptures
Shoulder	Rotator cuff tendinitis	Weakness if rotator cuff tear present
		Pain rolling onto shoulder at night
		Pain limits abduction and external rotation
	Frozen shoulder	Pain as above, markedly limited range of motion
	Trauma	Point tenderness, history of trauma, deformity with dislocation or fracture
Elbow	Lateral epicondylitis (tennis elbow)	Lateral elbow pain with wrist supination or extension
	Olecranon bursitis	Swelling and tenderness over olecranon process

occur simultaneously with any of these conditions. The primary symptoms of all of these conditions are shoulder pain and limited range of motion.

EVALUATION

How can I Distinguish Mechanical from Inflammatory Causes of Joint Pain?

The presentation of these conditions can overlap. Aside from acute trauma, mechanical causes of joint pain tend to be gradual in onset with minimal obvious inflammation. By contrast, inflammatory causes of joint pain come on rapidly or slowly, but synovitis is usually present with joint erythema, pain, swelling, and loss of function. These findings indicate either a vigorous inflammatory arthritis, such as gout or SLE, or possibly septic arthritis. Another key historical distinction is "gelling" and prolonged morning stiffness. In inflammatory arthritis, symptoms worsen with rest as the joint "gels" resulting in prolonged stiffness for >1 hour after a period of rest; in mechanical arthritis, the pain improves with rest, and stiffness is worked out of the joint over minutes.

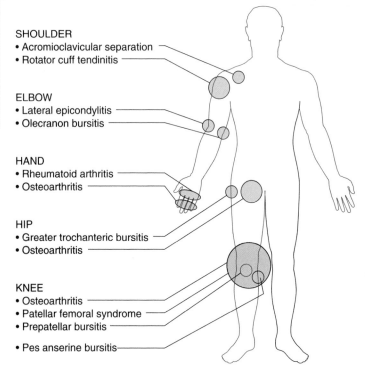

SHOULDER
• Acromioclavicular separation
• Rotator cuff tendinitis

ELBOW
• Lateral epicondylitis
• Olecranon bursitis

HAND
• Rheumatoid arthritis
• Osteoarthritis

HIP
• Greater trochanteric bursitis
• Osteoarthritis

KNEE
• Osteoarthritis
• Patellar femoral syndrome
• Prepatellar bursitis

• Pes anserine bursitis

FIGURE 21-2 Location of pain in major joint pathology.

How is Degenerative Arthritis Different from Bursitis or Tendinitis on Exam?

The primary distinction is the anatomic location of the pain. A good example is the knee. In degenerative arthritis, the pain is localized behind the patella within the joint space. In prepatellar bursitis, the pain is localized anterior to the patella. Similarly, in the hip, degenerative arthritis symptoms are deep in the groin and anterior thigh and are reproduced with hip range of motion. Greater trochanteric bursitis produces point tenderness over the bursa with deep palpation over the lateral aspect of the hip. With a tendinitis, the tendon is tender to palpation and stretch, and active use of the tendon exacerbates pain.

When Evaluating Joint Pain, what are Key Points on the Physical Exam?

Nothing replaces a solid knowledge of the musculoskeletal system, with particular attention to the location of bursae. Focus on the following items:

Joints: Tenderness, range of motion, synovitis (heat, spongy synovial hypertrophy), deformity, crepitus, effusions
Ligaments: Tenderness, laxity, pain with use against resistance
Tendons: Tenderness, laxity
Bursae: Tenderness, swelling, redness
Muscle: Tone, bulk, symmetry, strength, tender points (for fibromyalgia)
Cartilage: Locking, clicking
Skin: Scales of psoriasis

How can I Evaluate Shoulder Pain for Presence of Bursitis Versus Rotator Cuff Tear?

Rotator cuff tendinitis and subacromial bursitis present with shoulder pain in the deltoid distribution, exacerbated at night when rolling over onto the affected shoulder. On exam, pain is reproduced with arm abduction in an arc between 80 and 120 degrees and with internal or external rotation (reaching hands behind the back). Range of motion is limited focally by maneuvers that cause impingement of the subacromial bursa, especially shoulder abduction and external rotation. In frozen shoulder, calcification of the tendon limits motion passively and actively, and pain is more severe with any motion of the shoulder. Rotator cuff tear is distinguished by weakness, particularly with abduction. Pain and an inability to relax may make it difficult to assess strength. A lidocaine injection into the subacromial bursa may be necessary to allow evaluation for true weakness. Rotator cuff tears rarely occur in patients <40 years old; patients can often identify a specific injury.

Is X-ray Helpful in the Diagnosis of Joint Pain?

Degenerative arthritis causes joint space narrowing and sclerosis (focal bone thickening seen as a bright whiteness at the joint surface). RA and gout cause characteristic erosions, which may be absent in the initial phases of disease (see Chapter 38). If the evaluation is consistent with a chronic mechanical cause, x-rays do not add much information. If recent trauma or concern for cancer is present, however, an x-ray can help rule out fracture or lytic disease. For suspected rotator cuff tear, obtain ultrasound or MRI to confirm the diagnosis.

When is Arthrocentesis Required?

A synovial fluid tap is imperative if septic arthritis is suspected by the presence of fever, monarticular synovitis in a young person, or worsening monarticular inflammation in the setting of stable polyarticular disease. Any patient with undiagnosed synovitis should have arthrocentesis. Send the fluid for culture, cell count, crystal evaluation, and glucose. This distinguishes between gout (birefringent crystals), inflammatory arthritis (WBC 2000–75,000), and septic arthritis (low glucose, WBC >75,000, although lower counts of 30,000–60,000 can occur).

What Other Tests Should I Order for Patients with Joint Pain?

Given a history and physical consistent with a mechanical cause of joint pain, no further blood tests are needed. For suspected gout, obtain a serum uric acid, although this may be normal. For any acutely inflamed single joint, or if disseminated gonococcal infection is suspected, obtain a CBC (elevated WBC in infection, anemia in autoimmune disease), electrolytes, creatinine (looking for abnormal renal function in autoimmune disease or gout), uric acid (gout), and C-reactive protein or ESR (general assessment for inflammation). If disseminated gonorrhea infection is suspected, swab the throat, cervix or penile urethra, and rectum for gonococcal cultures to confirm the infection. Use of ANA reflexive panel and RF is outlined in Chapter 38. Check ferritin and percentage of saturation for hemochromatosis. For persistent unexplained pain or dysfunction, consider an MRI.

TREATMENT

How are Bursitis and Tendinitis Treated?

Maintaining range of motion and function is the overall goal. Instructions in strengthening exercises are helpful, either by handout or through personal instruction from a physical therapist. Short-term use of NSAIDs diminishes pain and inflammation. Most medication failures are due to insufficient or erratic dosing; NSAIDs must be taken at anti-inflammatory doses around the clock (e.g., ibuprofen 600–800 mg every 8 hours). For severe cases, consider steroid injection into the inflamed bursa or tendon. Do not inject more often than every 3 months for a total of three shots because this can weaken tendons and muscles.

What is the Appropriate Treatment for Osteoarthritis?

Avoid aggravating activities. Physical therapy and low-impact strengthening exercise have proved effective. Acetaminophen is the first-line treatment for pain and inflammation with fewer side effects than NSAIDs. The most common error is inadequate dosing; aim for up to 4000 mg/d, assuming normal liver function and minimal alcohol use. NSAIDs are second-line therapy and have more side effects, particularly GI bleeding. More recent data are mixed for cartilage derivatives chondroitin sulfate and glucosamine. As "nutritional supplements," these are not monitored by the FDA. Dosing depends on manufacturer's recommendations. Effects take 6 to 8 weeks, so warn patients to expect a delayed response. If symptoms are moderate despite consistent use of NSAIDs, another possible treatment is intra-articular injections of glucocorticoid or hyaluronic acid. These are temporizing measures; glucocorticoid effects last <6 weeks, and injections should be done >3 months apart at least. Although clinical trials of hyaluronic acid injections showed significant benefit, a meta-analysis cast some doubt on these results. This, combined with clinical experience showing moderate results only infrequently, has made these injections less readily adopted. For severe pain at rest or severe limitation of daily activities, refer to an orthopedist for joint replacement.

When Does Joint Pain Require Referral?

Refer for orthopedic evaluation any patient with joint dysfunction, such as locking or giving way, joint instability, or inability to bear weight. These symptoms suggest significant meniscal tear, ligamentous injury, unsuspected fracture, or osteonecrosis. Suspected septic arthritis requires immediate orthopedic evaluation and treatment. For patients with degenerative arthritis and pain significantly limiting daily activities, an orthopedic evaluation for joint replacement is indicated. Rheumatologists are expert in the management of systemic arthropathies, particularly RA and SLE. In any patient with persistent, unexplained symptoms, a subspecialty referral is indicated.

How Should the Inflammatory Causes of Joint Pain be Treated?

Septic arthritis is a surgical emergency. Treatment includes broad-spectrum antibiotics and joint space drainage. When an organism is identified, the antibiotic coverage can be narrowed. Repeated aspiration may be adequate, but often surgical drainage is required. For autoimmune processes such as SLE and RA, the standard of care is to treat aggressively before joint damage occurs by reducing inflammation with methotrexate or azathioprine. Acute gout responds to NSAIDs, prednisone, or colchicine. Allopurinol is effective for prophylaxis against repeat attacks, but may exacerbate an acute attack and so should not be started until several weeks after an attack is resolved.

When Should I Hospitalize a Patient with Joint Pain?

Any patient with acute monarticular synovitis with high fever needs immediate evaluation with a synovial arthrocentesis. If the patient is very ill, or if arthrocentesis confirms septic arthritis, the patient should be admitted.

Case 21-1

A 64-year-old obese woman presents with right hip pain, worse with walking and worse at night lying on her right side. Bilateral exam of knees shows mild arthritic deformity and small effusions, but no redness or heat. Fingers show swelling in her distal interphalangeal joints. She does not have groin pain with full range of motion of her hip, but notes some pain on the outside of her thigh when pressed there.

A. What is the most likely diagnosis?
B. What further evaluation do you recommend?
C. What treatment can you offer her?

Case 21-2

A 27-year-old female physician's assistant comes in with fatigue and joint pain. She reports her fingers, in particular the metacarpophalangeal joints, have been hot and swollen for several weeks. They improve when she is working, but after she has watched an hour or more of TV, her hands tighten up. She needs at least an hour to loosen up each morning. Exam reveals a tired-appearing woman with marked synovitis in the fingers, feet, and wrists bilaterally.

A. What is your differential diagnosis?
B. What tests will you order?

MUSCULAR PAIN

ETIOLOGY

What Causes Diffuse Persistent Muscular Pain?

Common causes are fibromyalgia, polymyalgia rheumatica (PMR), and hormonal conditions such as cortisol excess and thyroid aberrations. Less commonly, myositis with primary muscle inflammation is caused by autoimmune disease. Myalgias due to HMG CoA reductase inhibitors (statins) are common.

EVALUATION

How are Fibromyalgia, PMR, and Polymyositis Different?

All three conditions manifest with muscle pain and aching. Muscle weakness and elevated CPK are present in myositis only. **Fibromyalgia** is a syndrome of diffuse muscle and joint pain without any identifiable underlying pathology or inflammation. Criteria for diagnosis include widespread pain and the presence of at least 11 of 18 tender points on exam (Figure 21-3). Stiffness and sleep disturbances are common. **PMR** also manifests with diffuse muscle pain, particularly in the proximal limb muscles. In contrast to fibromyalgia, PMR occurs in patients >50 years old, causes elevated ESR, and can be associated with temporal arteritis (TA), a vasculitis that can cause blindness or stroke. In fibromyalgia and PMR, the muscle fibers themselves are not damaged, so muscle strength and enzymes are normal. **Myositis**, as the name implies, results in inflammation and destruction of muscle fibers with resulting weakness and elevated CPK and aldolase. When polymyositis occurs with a heliotrope rash (violaceous discoloration of the eyelids) and Gottron's papules (scaly, plaquelike eruptions over the finger joints), the condition is called dermatomyositis. All three conditions are distinguished from arthritis by normal joint exams and tender muscles. Myalgias are common in patients taking HMG CoA reductase inhibitors. Only a few of these patients have measurable elevations of CPK warranting discontinuation of the medication, although symptoms may be bothersome enough to necessitate stopping or switching.

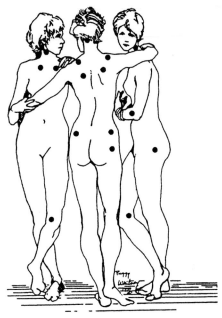

FIGURE 21-3 Tender points of fibromyalgia.
(From Wolfe F: Arthritis Rheum 1990;33:160.)

TREATMENT

Treatment depends on the underlying disorder (Table 21-2).

Table 21-2

Diffuse Muscular Pain: Common Causes, Findings, and Treatment

Cause	Findings	Treatment
Cushing syndrome	+/− Muscle weakness CPK may be elevated Plethora, central obesity	Identify and remove source
Fibromyalgia	Nonrestorative sleep Tender points Normal blood tests Normal strength	Exercise NSAIDs TCAs Improved sleep
Hypothyroidism	Myalgias, cramps Dry skin and hair Delayed reflexes Elevated TSH	Thyroid hormone

(continued)

Table 21-2

Diffuse Muscular Pain: Common Causes, Findings, and Treatment (Continued)

Cause	Findings	Treatment
Myalgias of "statins" (HMG CoA reductase inhibitors)	Myalgias variable CPK may be elevated	Trial off medication
Polymyalgia rheumatica (PMR)	Diffuse aches, worse in AM Elevated ESR Tender temple Jaw claudication	Low-dose prednisone High-dose if TA present
Polymyositis	Muscle weakness Muscle tenderness Elevated CPK and aldolase	Prednisone Methotrexate if needed

Case 21-3

A 65-year-old, forgetful woman with CHF and depression is taking carvedilol, simvastatin, and levothyroxine. She presents with muscle aching and difficulty standing up from the toilet. She has not been recently ill and has had no change in medications. On exam, she has symmetric proximal muscle weakness, lower extremities more than upper extremities. Neurologic exam is normal.

   A. What is your differential diagnosis?
   B. What initial lab tests would you order to help sort this out?

Case 21-4

A 75-year-old man cannot get out of bed in the morning. With his wife's assistance, he is able to get up and get dressed, but he is aching all over. On reflection, he thinks this has been getting gradually worse for 3 months or more. He has lost 10 lb, but has no other systemic or focal findings. Exam reveals a thin man, normal heart and lung sounds, normal extremities, and normal strength.

   A. What is your differential?
   B. What other history do you want?
   C. What lab findings would you expect?

KEY POINTS – JOINT PAIN

◆ Mechanical causes of joint pain generally occur gradually and with minimal inflammation.

◆ Inflammatory causes of joint pain cause prolonged stiffness after rest and marked synovitis.

◆ Septic arthritis is a medical emergency.

KEY POINTS – MUSCULAR PAIN

◆ Fibromyalgia has no laboratory abnormalities and is based on clinical criteria.

◆ Fibromyalgia and PMR have normal muscle enzymes and strength.

◆ PMR occurs in elderly patients, has elevated ESR, and may be associated with TA.

◆ Myositis results in elevated CPK and muscle weakness.

Case Answers

21-1 A. *Learning objective:* **Identify trochanteric bursitis.** The patient's history and exam findings are classic for trochanteric bursitis with incidental findings consistent with osteoarthritis in the knees.

21-1 B. *Learning objective:* **Recognize the diagnosis can be made by exam only.** Her findings are classic for trochanteric bursitis; she does not need further testing unless she does not improve.

21-1 C. *Learning objective:* **Describe treatment options for bursitis.** She can take NSAIDs around the clock, aided by physical therapy if she or you think it is warranted, or undergo lidocaine/corticosteroid injection in her trochanteric bursa.

21-2 A. *Learning objective:* **Recognize signs of inflammatory arthritis and list possible causes.** This is most likely RA with gelling and symmetric involvement of small joints, especially the metacarpophalangeal joints. Lupus also could manifest in this manner, but would require other features (rash, oral ulcers, anemia) to make the diagnosis. A reactive arthritis with viral infections such as parvovirus B19 also might manifest this way, but would resolve over time.

21-2 B. *Learning objective:* **List appropriate tests for acute polyarthritis.** Appropriate tests include CBC to look for anemia or high WBC that might suggest infection, C-reactive protein or ESR for inflammation, and ANA and RF to evaluate the likelihood of lupus or RA. If fever or monarthritis were present, an arthrocentesis of the joint would be indicated, but not in this scenario.

21-3 A. *Learning objective:* **Identify potential causes of muscle weakness in this scenario.** This patient presents with a picture consistent with myositis: She has pain and weakness. This could be a primary muscle disorder, such as polymyositis; it might be due to her simvastatin. With her forgetfulness, she may not be taking or appropriately absorbing her thyroid replacement. Muscle pain is a common side effect of the statin drugs. Many patients with pain resulting from statin use do not have an elevated CPK.

21-3 B. *Learning objective:* **Outline lab tests to work up myositis.** Most importantly, obtain a CPK and aldolase to look for muscle damage. Obtain a CBC for signs of inflammatory block and anemia and TSH to confirm appropriate thyroid replacement, send ESR and C-reactive protein, and consider anti-Jo and ANA. If the lab tests do not reveal a cause, consider a trial off simvastatin and re-evaluation after several weeks.

21-4 A. *Learning objective:* **List differential diagnosis for achiness without weakness.** Differential diagnosis includes PMR (which often has weight loss), malignancy, thyroid abnormality, fibromyalgia, and depression.

21-4 B. *Learning objective:* **State the symptoms associated with PMR and TA.** Ask about any jaw claudication, any visual changes, and any temporal headache or tenderness.

21-4 C. *Learning objective:* **Identify key lab findings in PMR** The ESR would be notably elevated, and the CPK would be normal. There may be an accompanying anemia, but WBC should be normal.

REFERENCES

American College of Rheumatology Subcommittee on Osteoarthritis Guidelines: Recommendations for the medical management of osteoarthritis of the hip and knee: 2000 update. Arthritis Rheum 2000;43:1905.

Arroll B, Goodyear-Smith F: Corticosteroid injections for osteoarthritis of the knee: Meta-analysis. BMJ 2004;328:869.

Felson DT, Anderson JJ: Hyaluronate sodium injections for osteoarthritis: Hope, hype, and hard truths. Arch Intern Med 2002;162:245.

Goldenberg DL. Fibromyalgia syndrome a decade later: What have we learned? Arch Intern Med 1999;159:777.

Watson MC, Brookes ST, Kirwan JR, et al: Non-aspirin, non-steroidal anti-inflammatory drugs for osteoarthritis of the knee. Cochrane Database Syst Rev 2000;CD000142.

Wolfe F: American College of Rheumatology 1990 Classification of Fibromyalgia: Report of multicenter criteria committee. Arthritis Rheum 1990;33:160.

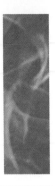

22

Low Back Pain

MARY B. MIGEON

ETIOLOGY

What Causes Acute Low Back Pain?

More than 95% of all low back pain arises from relatively benign changes to musculoskeletal structures in the low back. Degenerative arthritis, lumbosacral strain, bulging vertebral discs, sciatic nerve irritation, and spinal stenosis are common causes of low back pain. Pinpointing the anatomic source of the pain is often difficult and does not correlate with prognosis. Most low back pain resolves with a conservative approach of brief rest, anti-inflammatories, and gradual return to previous activity. Your job is to reassure the patient and yourself that a more serious condition doesn't exist and to monitor the patient's progress.

What is Sciatica?

Sciatica refers to pain radiating in the sciatic nerve distribution down the back of the leg. The sensitivity of sciatica for herniated disk is 90–95%. Although classically associated with a herniated disc, other conditions can cause this pain syndrome, such as spinal stenosis and sacroiliitis. Sciatica has a specificity of 88% for herniated disk.

What are the "Red Flags" for Dangerous Causes of Low Back Pain?

Warning signs for potentially serious causes of back pain are listed in Table 22-1.

EVALUATION

Is the Patient's Description of the Pain Helpful?

Most back pain is nonspecific and does not lead reliably to a diagnosis. The following generalizations may be useful. **Radicular pain** (i.e., pain

Low Back Pain

Table 22-1

"Red Flags" for Dangerous Causes of Low Back Pain	
Risk of cancer	Age >50
	History of cancer
Risk for infection	Intravenous drug use
	Immunosuppression, including diabetes and corticosteroid use
Risk for fracture	Osteoporosis, primary or secondary to corticosteroid use
	Trauma, "severe" in all patients or "mild" if patient age >50
Unusual course	Not improving as you would expect
	Progressive symptoms
Focal neurologic signs	History of weakness, numbness, bowel or bladder dysfunction or symptoms
	Exam findings of weakness, numbness, or diminished reflexes

in a nerve distribution) extends from the back and buttock past the knee and suggests impingement of a nerve as it exits the spinal canal. In contrast, back pain that extends to the thigh or hip but not past the knee is **radiating**, not radicular, pain and is less suggestive of a neuropathic cause. Rest pain or progressive pain may indicate cancer or abscess. Pain with cough, bowel movement, or sneeze is consistent with disc herniation because increased pressure through Valsalva worsens this condition.

How is the History for Spinal Stenosis Different from Other Causes of Low Back Pain?

Spinal stenosis is a narrowing of the spinal canal usually associated with arthritis. Walking or standing causes pain in the thighs and buttocks, which is relieved by sitting. Some patients with spinal stenosis have numbness in the legs or footdrop without much pain; pain is relieved by sitting. In contrast, back pain from herniated disc or musculoskeletal strain worsens with hip and lumbar flexion, for example, when sitting in the car.

What is an Appropriate Neurologic Exam for Low Back Pain?

For the evaluation of low back pain, a focused neurologic exam is your best tool. This does not mean an exhaustive exam. Greater than 90% of neurologic sequelae of back disease occur in the L5-S1 region, so your exam can focus primarily on the foot. The exception is a patient with bowel or bladder symptoms, symptoms of possible acute cord compression. In those cases, you need to check perianal sensation and rectal tone. The top of the foot allows you to test the three sensory distributions L4-S1. A helpful mnemonic is L4 = Large toe, S1 = Small toe. Reflexes are technically difficult to reproduce. Continued practice with reflex testing will improve your testing, but realize the results are not always accurate. Motor weakness should be obvious; a good screening test is great toe dorsiflexion (L5) and plantar flexion (S1) (Figure 22-1).

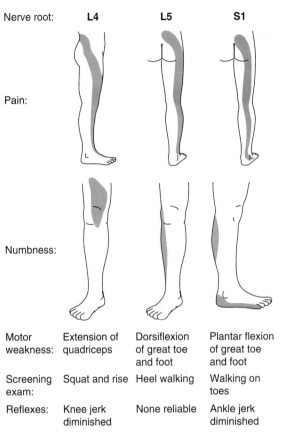

Nerve root:	**L4**	**L5**	**S1**
Motor weakness:	Extension of quadriceps	Dorsiflexion of great toe and foot	Plantar flexion of great toe and foot
Screening exam:	Squat and rise	Heel walking	Walking on toes
Reflexes:	Knee jerk diminished	None reliable	Ankle jerk diminished

FIGURE 22-1 Findings localizing lumbar nerve root compromise.

Which Physical Exam Test Best Identifies Nerve Impingement as the Cause of Acute Low Back Pain?

The best examination maneuver is the straight leg raise. With the patient lying on his or her back, elevate the straight leg. A positive test reproduces radicular pain with the leg 70 degrees or less from horizontal, indicating tension in the L5-S1 nerve root. If raising the contralateral leg reproduces pain on the affected side, this is most specific for a disc herniation and is called a positive crossed straight leg raise, (specificity = .90). Pain produced in the low back or hip does not qualify as a positive test.

If the Neurologic Exam is Abnormal, What Should I Do?

This is a "red flag." Major motor weakness, such as absent dorsiflexion of the great toe, particularly if it is acute, requires imaging. Even if the results of MRI indicate mild disc herniation, however, some patients with slight numbness or even weakness by history and physical can be managed conservatively for 2 to 4 weeks. If there is no improvement, or if there is any sudden decline in the patient's function, referral for potential surgery is warranted. A further evaluative tool is the EMG, which provides an objective measure of nerve damage.

How do "Red Flags" Help Me Decide What Further Studies to Order?

If no "red flags" are present, no further work-up is needed. When any "red flag" is present, start with obtaining an ESR and lumbosacral spine film. If history suggests infection, obtain a CBC or urinalysis or both. Although you may be tempted to obtain a CT or MRI scan early in your evaluation, remember that CT and MRI are very sensitive modalities, but they are quite nonspecific. These studies reveal disc bulging in 60% of the normal population. In asymptomatic elderly individuals, frank disc herniation is seen in 30%. Reserve these studies for symptoms and signs of cord compression (see later), when you suspect spinal stenosis, when there is an abnormal x-ray or ESR, or for preoperative evaluation.

What are Potential Low Back Pain Emergencies?

The spinal cord sits within a confined space, defined by the surrounding vertebral bone structure. If the cord is compressed, paralysis can occur. The main causes of acute spinal cord compression are epidural abscess (an infection in the epidural space surrounding or next to the cord), encroaching tumor, and, rarely, massive disc herniation. Acute neurologic change or progressive neurologic symptoms, particularly in high-risk patients with injection drug use or known cancer, should alert you to this possibility. If you suspect one of these conditions, the patient requires emergent imaging and neurosurgical evaluation. The quicker the treatment, the more complete the recovery.

What is the Cauda Equina Syndrome?

The cauda equina is the "horse's tail" of sacral nerves that travel in the distal spinal canal. This syndrome describes acute cord compression of these distal sacral nerves, causing bowel and bladder dysfunction of either marked constipation or incontinence, and sacral nerve numbness in the "saddle" distribution.

TREATMENT

How do I Treat Acute Low Back Pain?

When "red flags" are absent, conservative therapy is indicated. First, prescribe NSAIDs on scheduled three-times-a-day dosing; no evidence exists that any one NSAID is better than another. Second, have the patient return to previous activities as soon as tolerated, with the exception of

---

BOX 22-1

ELEMENTS OF CONSERVATIVE THERAPY FOR ACUTE LOW BACK PAIN

◆ NSAIDs
◆ Return to previous activities after minimal bed rest
◆ Physical therapy/back exercises

---

heavy lifting. Initially, some patients may require 2–3 days of bed rest, but with longer inactivity, outcomes worsen. Third, physical therapy and back exercises should be started as soon as tolerated (Box 22-1).

Do I Manage Acute and Chronic Low Back Pain Differently?

A repeat episode of acute low back pain is managed similarly to a first episode. Chronic back pain present for several months is a different problem. First, review your history and physical for "red flags," and consider further studies if the patient has not responded as you would have expected. Second, screen your patient carefully for depression. This condition is common among patients with chronic pain. Antidepressants serve a dual function in these cases, improving chronic pain and depression. Pending legal action predicts poorer prognosis.

How do I Fill out Disability Forms?

Describe objectively what you see on exam. You do not have to determine disability; that is the job of the Department of Labor and Industry. Often there is a section asking how many pounds the patient can lift. A general guideline follows symptom severity (Table 22-2).

Is There a Role for the Chiropractor? Is There a Role for Acupuncture?

In a nonblinded study, 400 men with acute back pain improved over controls with chiropractor intervention in the first 2 weeks after acute back pain. There is no evidence supporting more frequent weekly chiropractic intervention or acupuncture. Nonetheless, many patients anecdotally report relief from chiropractors and acupuncture.

Table 22-2

Weight Lifting Limitations by Symptom Severity

Symptom Severity	Women	Men
Moderate to severe	20 lb	20 lb
Mild	35 lb	60 lb
None	40 lb	80 lb

Low Back Pain

BOX 22-2

CRITERIA FOR SURGICAL INTERVENTION IN BACK PAIN PATIENTS

◆ Epidural abscess
◆ Cauda equina syndrome
◆ Cord compression
◆ Persistent nerve root compromise
◆ Severe spinal stenosis

What if My Patient has a True Disc Herniation?

If the patient has acute radicular pain and a positive straight leg raise, and none of the historical "red flags," he or she most likely has a herniated disc. Eighty percent to 90% of patients with disc herniation are back to normal after 1 month without any specific intervention. So unless the patient has significant neurologic symptoms or signs, you can watch and wait. If symptoms persist, it is reasonable to obtain CT or MRI and refer to a neurosurgeon. In some cases, epidural steroid injection targeted to the impaired nerve root may forestall surgery and provide temporary pain relief.

What Surgeries are Done for Back Pain? Do They Work?

With the exception of catastrophic herniations, most disc herniations resolve on their own. Although initial response to surgery may be good, at 4 years, there is little difference in conservative versus surgical management. Various surgical techniques have been developed, ranging from open discectomy, where the surgeon exposes the disc space and removes herniated disc material, to endoscopic discectomy (analogous to laparoscopic gallbladder removal—less invasive, leaves smaller scar). Outcomes have been mixed. Surgery should be considered only if the patient meets appropriate criteria (Box 22-2). For compression fractures, kyphoplasty is promising. Under radiographic guidance, cement is injected into the collapsed vertebra. This procedure can provide significant pain relief and potentially preservation of height. Side effects include subsequent fracture in adjacent vertebrae.

KEY POINTS

◆ Most back pain, although bothersome to patients, is benign and self-limited.
◆ "Red flags" for pathology dictate when to get further studies.
◆ With few exceptions, conservative therapy is the appropriate first step.

Case 22-1

A 37-year-old construction worker has severe low back pain after lifting a heavy stack of boards. He has never had back pain before. He smokes and takes no medications. On exam, he has paraspinal tenderness and normal lower extremity strength and sensation. He has pain in his lower back with the straight leg maneuver.

A. Do you want any further tests, and if so, what tests?
B. What do you recommend for treatment?
C. When can he return to work, and does he require any lifting limitations?

Case 22-2

A 68-year-old man with history of chronic back pain with prior back surgery 10 years ago comes in with low back pain after steelhead fishing over the weekend. His pain has been significant, and he has been unable to sleep or function. Previously he has required steady low-dose methadone to manage his back pain. His other medical problems include coronary artery disease and hypogonadism.

A. What are the "red flags" in his history?
B. Do you want any further tests?

Case Answers

22-1 A-C. *Learning objectives:* **Identify acute low back pain in a low-risk patient, outline a treatment plan, and prescribe a safe return to work plan.**

22-1 A. No further tests are warranted at this time. His exam is consistent with nonspecific low back pain. He has a negative straight leg test: He has pain only in his back, not in the radicular pattern down the back of his leg to the foot. He has no risk factors for worrisome causes.

22-1 B. Conservative management consists of NSAIDs, brief bed rest, and physical therapy.

22-1 C. He can return to work as soon as possible with light duty of lifting <20 lb as he has moderate back pain at this time.

22-2 A. *Learning objective:* **Recognize "red flags" suggesting more serious causes of back pain requiring further investigation.**

"Red flags" include the patient's age and his hypogonadism, which predisposes him to osteoporosis and fracture. His fishing activity might be a "red flag" if he sustained some trauma such as falling. His history of CAD puts him at increased risk for an abdominal aortic anuerysm. Finally, he has been stable for years, so this is an unexpected deterioration in his status.

22-2 B. *Learning objective:* **Identify plain x-ray as first appropriate screen.** A plain film is a good first step and would show fracture or any change in his hardware, which can occasionally break down. Consider MRI or CT. MRI may be difficult to read because of artifact from the metal.

REFERENCES

Atlas SJ, Deyo RA: Evaluating and managing acute low back pain in the primary care setting. J Gen Intern Med 2001;6:120.

Bigos S, Bowyer O, Braen G, et al: Acute Low Back Problems in Adults. Clinical Practice Guideline No. 14. AHCPR Publication No. 95–0642. Rockville, MD, Agency for Health Care Policy and Research, Public Health Service, US Department of Health and Human Services, 1994. http://text.nlm.nih.gov

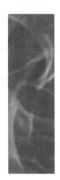

23

Lower Extremity Pain, Swelling, and Ulcers

HEIDI S. POWELL

 LOWER EXTREMITY PAIN

ETIOLOGY

What are Common Causes of Lower Extremity Pain?

Common causes of lower extremity pain are peripheral vascular disease (PVD, also known as arterial insufficiency), peripheral neuropathy (PN), radiculopathy, venous obstruction (also called venous stasis), and nocturnal cramps. Restless leg syndrome is a common cause of nocturnal leg discomfort.

Are there Any Emergencies that Cause Lower Extremity Pain?

Compartment syndrome and arterial occlusion from thromboembolism are rare emergencies. Compartment syndrome occurs when tissue swelling or hematoma in a muscle compartment increases pressures above arterial pressure, occludes blood flow, and causes tissue necrosis. Arterial occlusion causes acute onset of the five "P's": pain, paresthesias, paralysis, pulselessness, pallor.

EVALUATION

How do Symptoms Distinguish Between the Common Causes of Leg Pain?

Patients with PVD report claudication with exertion—muscle aching or cramping that occurs predictably with exercise and resolves with rest. Pain from spinal stenosis, also called neurogenic claudication, can be similar. In contrast to vascular claudication, spinal stenosis may be accompanied by back pain; it does not resolve with standing still, but requires sitting for several minutes. PN pain occurs in a stocking-glove distribution and is described variably as burning, tingling, perceived swelling, "pins and

193

needles," or numbness. It is often worse at night. Radiculopathy is often worse with sitting and relieved by standing. Pain from venous obstruction may be worse when legs are dependent and improved with leg elevation. Nocturnal muscle cramps occur only at night and are sudden, nonexertional, and relieved with massage or stretching.

What Physical Findings Help with Diagnosis?

With PVD, you may hear bruits, find weak or absent pulses, see loss of leg hair, dependent rubor, pallor with elevation, or delayed capillary refill. With PN, look for decreases in proprioception, light touch, sharp sensation, and deep tendon reflexes. PVD and PN are usually bilateral, although they may be worse on one side. Radiculopathy is usually unilateral and may give focal loss of a reflex or strength or shooting pain down the leg with straight leg raise (see Chapter 22).

What is the ABI?

The Ankle Brachial Index (ABI) assesses severity of PVD, as estimated by ankle systolic pressure divided by brachial artery systolic pressure. To measure ankle systolic pressure, inflate a cuff around the calf, and palpate the systolic pressure at the dorsalis pedis or posterior tibialis artery. Normal ABI values are 0.9–1.2. An ABI >0.9 generally rules out arterial insufficiency. An ABI of 0.6–0.8 usually correlates with one-block claudication. An ABI <0.4 indicates limb-threatening ischemia; these patients often have leg pain at rest or ischemic nonhealing ulcers or both. Obtain an arterial duplex study when the ABI is <0.9. ABIs may be falsely elevated and unreliable in diabetic patients because of noncompressible, calcified arteries.

What Tests are Appropriate for Patients with PN?

Most patients with PN have diabetes and require no further work-up. If diabetes is absent, you need to consider other causes (Box 23-1).

> ### BOX 23-1
>
> **CAUSES OF PERIPHERAL NEUROPATHY**
>
> **Common Causes**
>
> Metabolic—diabetes, alcohol use
> Medications—zalcitabine, stavudine, didanosine, isoniazid (if vitamin B_6 not replaced), amiodarone
>
> **Less Common Causes**
>
> Metabolic—malnutrition, hypothyroidism, renal insufficiency, vitamin B_{12} deficiency
> Medications—metronidazole, pyridoxine, simvastatin, hydralazine, colchicine
> Infections—HIV, Lyme disease, syphilis, leprosy
> Immunologic—multiple myeloma, paraneoplastic syndromes, vasculitis
> Toxins—lead, arsenic, solvents (toluene, hexane)

Table 23-1

Treatment Strategies for Common Causes of Lower Extremity Pain

Cause	Treatment
PN	Tight glycemic control in diabetes
	TCAs, SSRIs
	Anticonvulsants (gabapentin, carbamazepine)
	Topical capsaicin
	Foot care for prevention (shoes, lanolin to prevent cracks)
	Lidocaine patches
PVD	Risk factor reduction (smoking, hypertension, lipids, diabetes)
	Antiplatelet drug
	Exercise
	Angioplasty or surgery for claudication at rest
Nocturnal cramps	Quinine, calf stretching during day

A complete history, including alcohol use, diet, toxic exposures, medications, and family history, helps direct evaluation. In patients without diabetes, start with a CBC, vitamin B_{12}, TSH, creatinine, serum protein electrophoresis, and ANA (looking for vasculitis). EMG and nerve conduction studies confirm PN and assess its severity. Nerve biopsies are rarely indicated.

TREATMENT

How do I Treat Lower Extremity Pain?

Table 23-1 lists treatment strategies for common causes of lower extremity pain.

LOWER EXTREMITY SWELLING

ETIOLOGY

What Causes Swelling in the Lower Extremities?

Swelling is due to edema, the accumulation of fluid in the interstitial tissue. Edema is pitting when skin remains indented after pressure has been applied. Nonpitting edema does not indent and implies inflammation, infiltration, or chronic edema of any cause. Edema may signal significant systemic illness.

What Diseases Cause Unilateral Lower Extremity Edema?

This depends on how rapidly the edema develops. Acute edema occurring over hours to days is often associated with pain and inflammatory signs, such as increased warmth and erythema. Common causes of acute unilateral edema are DVT, cellulitis, Baker's cyst rupture, superficial thrombophlebitis, and trauma. Chronic unilateral edema accumulates over weeks to months without accompanying inflammatory signs and is usually caused by venous insufficiency or lymphatic obstruction. Lymphatic obstruction, also called lymphedema, may be idiopathic or secondary to tumor, infection, or scarring from previous surgery or radiation.

What is a Baker's Cyst?

A Baker's cyst is accumulation of excess synovial fluid in a pouch of synovium that extrudes from the knee joint into the popliteal fossa. It is related to underlying joint inflammation (osteoarthritis, RA, meniscal tear, trauma, or crystalline arthropathy).

What Diseases Cause Bilateral Lower Extremity Edema?

Causes of bilateral edema are venous insufficiency or systemic diseases that cause fluid retention or decreased albumin. Medication is a common cause of edema unresponsive to diuretics (Box 23-2).

BOX 23-2

SYSTEMIC CAUSES OF BILATERAL LOWER EXTREMITY EDEMA

Conditions Associated with Fluid Retention

CHF
Cushing's disease
Hypothyroidism
Menstrual cycle fluid retention
Pregnancy
Renal insufficiency
Chronic venous insufficiency
Idiopathic

Conditions Associated with Hypoalbuminemia

Hepatic cirrhosis
Malnutrition
Nephrotic syndrome
Protein-losing enteropathies

Medications

Clonidine
Corticosteroids
Estrogen, progesterone, testosterone
Hydralazine
Nifedipine, felodipine, amlodipine (common)
NSAIDs
Pioglitazone, rosiglitazone (common)
Proton pump inhibitors

EVALUATION

What Features of the History and Physical and Work-Up Distinguish a DVT?

All causes of acute unilateral edema can manifest exactly the same way (erythema, swelling, and pain developing over hours). Because DVT can cause life-threatening pulmonary embolism, it is imperative to exclude this first. Ask about DVT risk factors (OCPs, recent period of prolonged inactivity, pregnancy, postpartum, recent major surgery, family history of hypercoagulability, paresis, history of DVT, recent trauma). On exam of the leg, look for a palpable cord (indurated vein) or positive Homan's sign (pain elicited in popliteal region with ankle dorsiflexion and a flexed knee), although neither finding is sensitive or specific. The exam may be normal or reveal only mild unilateral calf swelling confirmed by measuring bilateral calf diameters. A negative D-dimer in outpatients at low risk for DVT has a high negative predictive value (99%). Duplex ultrasound can be highly sensitive (98%) and specific (>97%) for clots above the knee.

How do I Distinguish Baker's Cyst, DVT, Cellulitis, and Superficial Thrombophlebitis?

A Baker's cyst presents as a bulge on the medial aspect of the popliteal fossa and often is diagnosed by exam alone. Cyst rupture may create ankle or foot ecchymoses differentiating it from a DVT. With cellulitis, pain, lymphangitis (red streaking along a lymph vessel), ipsilateral groin lymphadenopathy, chills, or fever may be present. About 50% of the time, a portal of entry for bacteria can be identified, usually maceration from tinea pedis infection. Superficial thrombophlebitis causes a localized tender vein, without lymphangitis, adenopathy, or palpable cord. If you are not convinced that it isn't a DVT, obtain a D-dimer in a patient at low risk or a duplex ultrasound for all other patients to make sure.

When Should I Look for a Systemic Cause of Edema?

Bilateral lower extremity or generalized edema suggests a systemic cause. Perform a thorough history and physical. Ask about symptoms of CHF, including fatigue, dyspnea on exertion, orthopnea, and PND. Exam findings suggesting left heart failure include tachypnea, tachycardia, rales, and S_3. Signs of right heart failure include distended neck veins and hepatojugular reflux (see Chapter 26). Renal insufficiency and nephrotic syndrome may not be apparent from history or physical. Hypothyroidism and low albumin states such as nephrotic syndrome can cause periorbital edema. Hypothyroidism is usually accompanied by other symptoms, such as fatigue; weight gain; cold intolerance; and hair, voice, or skin changes (see Chapter 28).

What Lab Tests or Imaging Studies are Helpful?

Obtain a serum TSH, creatinine, BUN, Urinalysis, and albumin looking for hypothyroidism, renal insufficiency, or low albumin states in patients with new bilateral edema. If creatinine is increased, obtain a renal ultrasound scan to distinguish acute from chronic insufficiency. If albumin is decreased, obtain a urinalysis to screen for nephrotic syndrome. A decreased albumin without proteinuria suggests malnutrition, malabsorption, or liver disease, so re-examine for ascites, and consider LFT's, abdominal imaging, or a GI referral (to exclude a protein-wasting enteropathy). If you suspect heart failure, obtain CXR, ECG, brain natriuretic peptide, and echocardiogram. Obtain a 24-hour urine cortisol when you suspect Cushing's syndrome.

TREATMENT

How do I Manage Fluid Retention in the Legs?

General treatments include lower extremity elevation, salt restriction, elastic support stockings, and low-dose diuretics (hydrochlorothiazide 12.5 mg/d). Avoid medications that cause edema. Treat underlying Cushing's disease, CHF, thyroid disease, renal disease, or liver disease when present.

How do I Treat a DVT?

Clot at or above the popliteal fossa increases risk for PE. Identify and address any underlying risk factors, and if none are found, screen for a hypercoagulable state before starting anticoagulants (see Chapter 31). Warfarin is given orally for long-term dosing, but takes several days to become therapeutic. Intravenous or intramuscular heparins act rapidly and are used initially alongside warfarin until the warfarin is therapeutic. LMWH is used in patients without contraindications (e.g., no increased risk for bleed, no renal failure). LMWH can be used at home without monitoring, so it eliminates hospitalization. The goal of warfarin is to increase the PT INR to a therapeutic range of two to three times normal. For other patients, hospitalize for intravenous heparin, and start warfarin. Continue anticoagulation for 6 months. Longer duration of treatment depends on the underlying cause or presence of thrombophilia. Clot isolated to the calf can be treated with anticoagulation for 3 months or monitored for proximal migration with serial duplex ultrasound scans over several weeks.

How do I Treat a Baker's Cyst?

Observe smaller cysts. Aspirate cysts when large or interfering with knee function. Submit synovial fluid for crystal analysis and cell count. NSAIDs and intra-articular steroids can decrease inflammation. Recurrent problems may warrant MRI to look for a meniscal tear.

Is There an Effective Treatment for Lymphedema?

Address treatable obstructive processes (pelvic mass, infection). Treatment options are limited when lymphedema is idiopathic or due to postsurgical scarring or radiation. Compression garments and home lymphedema compression pump machines may be helpful. Diuretics are ineffective. Cellulitis worsens lymphatic obstruction, so prevent it by moisturizing skin and treating tinea.

How do I Treat Cellulitis and Superficial Thrombophlebitis?

Treat cellulitis with oral dicloxacillin or cephalexin. Patients with diabetes may need broader coverage. Arrange close follow-up. Consider intravenous antibiotics if response is inadequate. Treat superficial thrombophlebitis with warm compresses, elevation, and NSAIDs. Symptoms should resolve or improve significantly within 1 week. If not, obtain a duplex ultrasound.

LOWER EXTREMITY ULCERS

ETIOLOGY
What Predisposes Patients to Ulceration?

Main causes of lower extremity ulcers are venous insufficiency (90%), sensory PN, and arterial insufficiency secondary to PVD. Pyoderma gangrenosum is an unusual cause associated with IBD.

EVALUATION
What Distinguishing Exam Features Help with Diagnosis?

Venous insufficiency ulcers usually are painless; abrupt in onset; located on the medial malleolus; and accompanied by edema, stasis dermatitis, and superficial varicosities. Neuropathic ulcers are painless, sharply marginated, and found at plantar pressure points (metatarsal heads, distal phalanges, heels). Ulcers from arterial insufficiency or ischemia occur distal to the ankle joint (often at the tips of the toes), have a punched-out appearance, and are exquisitely painful. Associated findings include dependent rubor, nonpalpable pulses, delayed capillary refill, and loss of hair growth. Pyoderma gangrenosum ulcers are sharply demarcated, are exudative, and have heaped-up, boggy, violaceous edges that are often undermined.

How do I Know if the Ulcer or Underlying Bone is Infected?

Determining whether the ulcer or underlying bone is infected can be difficult. All ulcers are colonized with bacteria, and swab cultures are unhelpful. A yellow-green discharge is common, even in noninfected wounds. Débride and probe all ulcers to determine their depth. If the bone can be probed, osteomyelitis is likely. If there are systemic symptoms and signs (fever, chills, sweats, leukocytosis) or local signs of cellulitis (warmth, pain, erythema, and swelling), presume the ulcer is infected, and give antibiotics. X-ray may be helpful to screen for a foreign body, gangrene (gas), or late osteomyelitis (periosteal elevation). If you are highly suspicious that osteomyelitis is present, check sedimentation rate and obtain MRI, bone scan, or bone biopsy.

Table 23-2

Treatments for Common Lower Extremity Ulcers

Cause	Treatment
Ischemic ulcers	Vascular surgery referral
PN and neuropathic ulcers	Non–weight bearing
	Good shoes
	Avoidance of foot trauma
	Meticulous foot care
Venous insufficiency and stasis ulcers	Edema reduction (improves healing)
	Elevation
	Compressive stockings
	Skin lubrication (prevent cracks, cellulitis)
	Topical steroids for stasis dermatitis
Pyoderma gangrenosum	Oral steroids

TREATMENT

Are all Ulcers Treated the Same?

Some general wound care measures pertain to ulcers of many causes, such as saline wet to dry dressings, sharp débridement, synthetic occlusive dressings (Duoderm), or Unna boots. Ulcers caused by PN require non–weight bearing to heal. Other specific treatment depends on the cause (Table 23-2).

KEY POINTS

◆ Rule out DVT in a patient with acute unilateral peripheral edema.

◆ Bilateral lower extremity edema warrants an investigation for systemic diseases.

◆ Patients with diabetic PN and ulcers require non–weight bearing to heal.

◆ Lymphedema does not respond to diuretic therapy.

Case 23-1

A 48-year-old woman with type 2 diabetes, hypertension, and hyperlipidemia presents with a painless ulcer at the head of the first metatarsal. She has had it for more than a month and has been applying a topical antibiotic and a sterile dressing without any improvement. She has bilateral ankle edema and a callus with a 2-cm ulcer without exudates or erythema at the head of the first metatarsal. Peripheral pulses are palpable.

    A. What is the cause of her ulcer?

    B. How would you manage her?

Case 23-2

A 42-year-old woman with a history of depression presents to the clinic with 3-day history of right lower extremity edema and pain. There is no history of trauma or unusual physical activity. Her review of systems is unremarkable. On exam, she has a moderate amount of swelling around the ankle with a large ecchymosis on the medial malleolus extending to the dorsal aspect of the foot. There is some tenderness in the popliteal fossa and posterior calf. There is no significant calf swelling. Peripheral pulses are palpable. Lower extremity muscle strength is normal.

    A. What could be causing her symptoms?

    B. Would you order any tests?

Case Answers

23-1 A. *Learning objective:* **List common causes of lower extremity ulcers.** Peripheral arterial disease, PN, and venous stasis are the three main causes of lower extremity ulcers. It is important to determine the cause of an ulcer to treat it appropriately. This patient's ulcer is painless and on a metatarsal head (a point of pressure), which are typical features of a neuropathic ulcer. Peripheral arterial disease is unlikely in this patient given the lack of usual physical findings (e.g., violaceous toes, absence of hair on toes) and the presence of palpable pulses. Also, peripheral arterial disease ulcers often are on the tips of toes or distal ankles and are painful. Venous stasis ulcers are usually on the medial malleolus and painful.

23-1 B. *Learning objective:* **State the proper management of a neuropathic ulcer.** It is important first to assess if there are signs or symptoms of infection. The patient's ulcer is not infected because she does not have any localized erythema, increase in warmth, fevers, chills, or night sweats. She should undergo sharp débridement of the callus and any necrotic tissue if present. The key to healing for a neuropathic ulcer is non–weight bearing; a total contact cast best achieves this, but a nonremovable cast is another option. These ulcers heal slowly, if at all, even if there is only a minimal amount of weight bearing.

23-2 A. *Learning objective:* **List the differential diagnosis for acute-onset lower extremity pain and edema.** DVT, cellulitis, ruptured Baker's cyst, trauma, superficial thrombophlebitis, and compartment syndrome all can cause acute lower extremity swelling and pain. The patient has an ecchymosis around her ankle joint that makes a ruptured Baker's cyst the most likely diagnosis. There were no other physical findings to suggest a cellulitis (erythema, increased warmth), superficial thrombophlebitis (tender, erythematous vein), or compartment syndrome (pulselessness, pallor, paresthesias, paralysis).

23-2 B. *Learning objective:* **Recognize signs of ruptured Baker's cyst, and refrain from testing when the diagnosis is obvious.** The finding of an ecchymosis on the foot coinciding with the popliteal pain differentiates a Baker's cyst from a DVT. If she did not have the ecchymosis, it would be reasonable to evaluate for a DVT. In a low-risk individual, a negative D-dimer essentially rules out a DVT. In a moderate-risk to high-risk individual, a venous duplex study is the appropriate test.

REFERENCES

Bouton AJM, Kirsner RS, Vileikyte L: Neuropathic diabetic foot ulcers. N Engl J Med 2005;351:48.
Cho S, Atwood E: Peripheral edema. Am J Med 2002;113:580.
Lesho EP, Manngold J, Gey DC: Management of peripheral arterial disease. Am Fam Physician 2004;69:525.

Lower Extremity Pain

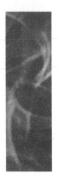

24

Lymphadenopathy

ERNIE-PAUL BARRETTE

 ETIOLOGY

Is Lymphadenopathy Always Pathologic?

Lymph nodes increase in size in response to infection, inflammation, medications, and cancer. Some lymphadenopathy can be normal. In the neck and groin, small "shotty" nodes <1 cm are common and are of no consequence in someone who feels well. Reactive nodes, which occur in response to infection, are tender, enlarge quickly, and regress in 4–6 weeks. Some reactive nodes do not regress completely; they may remain small and palpable, but are nonetheless benign.

When Should I be Concerned About Pathologic Causes of Lymphadenopathy?

Node size and risk factors for cancer and infection help determine whether lymphadenopathy is likely to be pathologic (Box 24-1). Nodes >1.5 × 1.5 cm^2 suggest malignancy in an adult. Lymphadenopathy is more likely to be pathologic in patients who have risk factors or symptoms suggesting malignancy or protracted infection, including weight loss, night sweats, fatigue, fevers, tobacco abuse, family history of cancer, excessive alcohol use, high-risk sexual activity, or TB exposure. Although age is a risk factor for most malignancies, the preponderance of lymphadenopathy is likely to be benign even at later stages of life. Although malignancy is found in 60% of patients >50 years old who are sent for node biopsy, these numbers reflect a selection bias in that the patients had been referred for biopsy. A retrospective study of a family practice clinic looked at unexplained lymphadenopathy in patients >40 years old; cancer was detected in only 4%. In patients <40 years old, cancer was found in 0.4%.

What is Meant by Generalized or Localized Lymphadenopathy?

Generalized lymphadenopathy is present when two or more noncontiguous sites have enlarged nodes (e.g., right neck and left axilla). The

BOX 24-1

LYMPHADENOPATHY REQUIRING FURTHER EVALUATION

♦ Node >1.5 cm
♦ Age >40–50 years
♦ Smoking or drinking history
♦ Constitutional symptoms (fever, sweats, weight loss)

most common causes are infectious (Table 24-1). Localized nodes occurring contiguously suggest an inflammatory process or malignancy in the corresponding area of drainage. A single source of infection may explain several clusters of nodes (e.g., a chronic nonhealing ulcer of the left hand causing forearm, epitrochlear, and axillary lymphadenopathy).

What Causes Lymphadenopathy in the Neck?

The neck is the most common site of lymphadenopathy. Unilateral cervical lymphadenopathy in a younger patient is most likely to be mononucleosis or pharyngitis. Bilateral cervical lymphadenopathy in younger patients is due to infectious mononucleosis, pharyngitis, or dental infections. Other, less common causes of cervical lymphadenopathy with a mononucleosis-like illness (fever, fatigue) include primary HIV infection, CMV infection, toxoplasmosis, primary herpes simplex infection, and secondary syphilis. Although cervical lymphadenopathy in a young patient is likely to be benign, more than half of patients with Hodgkin's disease present initially with lymphadenopathy in the neck. In older patients, cancer is more likely. Submandibular and anterior cervical nodes suggest head and neck cancer. Anterior cervical nodes also can arise from metastatic lung, breast, or thyroid cancer. Preauricular lymphadenopathy is seen with conjunctivitis and cat-scratch disease

Table 24-1

Causes of Generalized Lymphadenopathy

Commonly Seen	Less Commonly Seen
Infection	Drugs
Mononucleosis	Phenytoin
HIV or AIDS	Hydralazine
TB	Allopurinol
Hodgkin's lymphoma	Sarcoidosis
Non-Hodgkin's lymphoma	Secondary syphilis
Leukemia	SLE
	RA
	Serum sickness
	Hyperthyroidism
	Castleman disease

Lymphadenopathy

(a self-limited disease seen mostly in children), where postauricular lymphadenopathy is common with scalp infections or inflammation, such as seborrheic dermatitis.

What is Virchow's Node?

Supraclavicular nodes are often pathologic, and the side of presentation suggests the cancer of origin. Virchow's node refers to any left supraclavicular node and is usually due to a GI, renal, testicular, or ovarian malignancy. A right supraclavicular node may herald a pulmonary, mediastinal, or esophageal tumor.

What are the Common Causes of Axillary Lymphadenopathy?

The most common cause is ipsilateral injury or infection in the arm or hand. The axilla is a common spot for lymphadenopathy owing to cat-scratch disease because the hands and arms are the most common site for cat scratches. In a woman with unilateral axillary lymphadenopathy, breast cancer must be considered. Lymphomas such as Hodgkin's disease also manifest in the axilla. When a linear inflamed set of nodes leads from an open wound, group A streptococcal skin infection is the usual cause.

What Causes Epitrochlear Lymphadenopathy?

Unilateral epitrochlear nodes suggest infection in the hand. Bilateral epitrochlear lymphadenopathy is uncommon, but is a clinical clue suggesting lupus, secondary syphilis, or sarcoidosis.

What Causes Hilar Lymphadenopathy on CXR?

Causes of bilateral hilar lymphadenopathy on CXR include lymphoma; bronchogenic carcinoma; sarcoidosis; and infection such as primary TB, coccidioidomycosis, and histoplasmosis. If a mediastinal mass, pleural effusion, or pulmonary mass is associated with bilateral or unilateral lymphadenopathy, a diagnosis of cancer should be pursued. If a patient has bilateral hilar lymphadenopathy and is asymptomatic, the diagnosis is sarcoidosis.

What Causes Inguinal Lymphadenopathy?

Chronic, shotty, inguinal lymphadenopathy is common. This may be due to subclinical or low-grade infections in the lower extremities or perineum. A femoral hernia may masquerade as a single large inguinal node. More marked inguinal lymphadenopathy often accompanies acute lower extremity infection or sexually transmitted diseases, such as herpes, syphilis, gonorrhea, chancroid, and lymphogranuloma venereum. A persistent or large node can result from rectal, vaginal, or cervical cancer or melanoma.

What Causes Lymphadenopathy in Patients with HIV Infection?

In HIV infection, persistent generalized lymphadenopathy occurs often before the CD4$^+$ counts decrease to <200. Nodes are rarely >1.5 cm. Larger nodes or asymmetric distribution should be evaluated further.

Non-Hodgkin's lymphoma, Hodgkin's disease, Kaposi's sarcoma, and TB are more common in HIV-positive patients. They can occur when the $CD4^+$ count is only modestly suppressed (i.e., 200–500). If the $CD4^+$ count is <100, *Mycobacterium avium* complex, fungal, and suppurative infections need to be ruled out.

EVALUATION

Is This Lump a Lymph Node?

The exam for lymphadenopathy must include careful palpation of the occiput, around the ears, the entire neck, the supraclavicular fossa, the axillae, the epitrochlear space, the abdomen, and the groin. Pay attention to the quality of the node—size, mobile or matted, tender or painless, rock-hard or rubbery. Cancer tends to be painless and may or may not be matted. Infection is tender, mobile, and occasionally rubbery. The cervical node exam may be most problematic because of overlying muscle, tendon, thyroid, carotids, and salivary glands. The parotid and submandibular salivary glands can be nodelike. If their respective ducts are obstructed, inflammation or infection can occur. Parotid gland enlargement can occur with many conditions, including pregnancy, eating disorders, Sjögren's syndrome, sarcoid, diabetes mellitus, alcoholism, mumps, and HIV. Any distinct mass should be referred for biopsy. Similarly, submandibular glands may be the site of infection, but masses here are even more likely to be cancer. Other findings may mimic lymphadenopathy, such as rheumatoid nodules, lipomas, sebaceous or ganglion cysts, and less commonly thyroglossal and branchial cleft cysts.

If I Suspect an Acute, Self-Limited Infectious Cause of Lymphadenopathy, How can I be Sure?

A follow-up exam is required, particularly in patients with constitutional symptoms, such as ongoing fever, weight loss, or fatigue; risk factors for prolonged infection or cancer; or nodes >1.5 cm. For self-limited causes, the nodes are shrinking, and the symptoms should be resolved in several weeks. If not, further evaluation is required. Empiric antibiotics are not recommended for lymphadenopathy in the absence of a definite bacterial infection (e.g., streptococcal pharyngitis).

What are Pertinent Clues from the History in Patients with Generalized Lymphadenopathy?

The causes of generalized lymphadenopathy are limited, so a focused history can quickly narrow the differential diagnosis. Epidemiologic clues may provide the diagnosis before any lab tests return. Ask about symptoms of acute viral syndrome versus longer term weight loss, night sweats, and fatigue. Explore risk factors for HIV exposure. Patients with secondary syphilis have constitutional symptoms and a history of a painless genital ulcer that has healed. Review drug or serum exposure,

Lymphadenopathy

symptoms of hyperthyroidism, RA, and SLE. In Hodgkin's disease, some patients report pain in the nodes after ingestion of alcohol.

What Physical Exam Findings are Useful in the Evaluation of Generalized Lymphadenopathy?

The following findings are useful:

Skin: Rash on the palms and soles (syphilis), erythema nodosum (tender subcutaneous nodules seen on the lower extremities in sarcoidosis or TB), malar rash (SLE)

Oropharynx: Erythema or exudate of pharynx (mononucleosis), oral hairy leukoplakia (HIV)

Abdomen: Splenomegaly (lymphoma, leukemia, sarcoidosis, or mononucleosis)

Musculoskeletal: Synovitis (SLE, RA, serum sickness), tremor (hyperthyroidism)

What Lab and Imaging Tests are Helpful?

When the clinical picture is confusing, order a CBC, WBC differential, ESR, PPD (tuberculin skin test), and CXR. The presence of hilar lymphadenopathy points to granulomatous disease in a young patient and malignancy in an older patient. Atypical lymphocytes suggest mononucleosis, other viral infections, or toxoplasmosis. A CT scan is helpful to confirm lymphadenopathy, identify other nodal enlargement, or seek associated masses or abscesses. Extensive testing is rarely needed (Table 24-2). The list of causes of lymphadenopathy includes many

Table 24-2

Recommended Testing According to Clinical Presentation of Lymphadenopathy

Clinical Scenario	Recommended Testing
Cervical adenopathy and pharyngitis	Throat culture for strep ± gonorrhea Monospot
Cervical adenopathy and mononucleosis-like syndrome	Monospot (negative in 10% of EBV mononucleosis); if negative, consider EBV IgM, HIV RNA, CMV, and *Toxoplasma* serology
Cervical adenopathy in a patient age >40 or with history of tobacco or alcohol use	Refer for biopsy
Adenopathy and HIV risks	HIV test
Inguinal adenopathy, marked	HIV test, RPR Culture for herpes simplex and gonorrhea Chlamydia LCR Culture for *Haemophilus ducreyi*
Hilar adenopathy	PPD testing

uncommon causes, however. For persistent lymphadenopathy or unusual symptoms, refer to one of the references.

When Should I Pursue a Biopsy?

If no cause is found, and the node is enlarging, refer to a surgeon. Do not delay if cancer is suspected. When history and physical suggest a viral infection, a biopsy may be confusing because the histology may mimic lymphoma. In this case, watchful waiting for 4 to 6 weeks is advisable before referral for biopsy.

KEY POINTS

◆ A complete history and careful physical exam narrow the differential diagnosis for lymphadenopathy.

◆ Laboratory testing need not be extensive.

◆ When the diagnosis is uncertain, and the risk for malignancy is low, careful observation for 1 month is appropriate.

Case 24-1

A 48-year-old man presents with anorexia, fatigue, nasal congestion, rhinorrhea, and a sore throat. He has no past medical history. He has smoked one pack per day since age 16. On exam, a single firm 1.5-cm node is palpated just posterior to the left midclavicle. No other nodes are found.

   A. Would you recommend conservative management, observation, and a follow-up visit?

   B. What is your differential diagnosis?

   C. What work-up is indicated?

Case 24-2

A 22-year-old woman is admitted with low-grade fevers, arthralgias, rash, and an abnormal CXR. She is from Puerto Rico, but has lived in New York City for 10 years. She was well until 2 weeks ago, when she noted the onset of progressive discomfort in her knees, ankles, and wrists. She developed a rash 1 day ago and was barely able to walk today because of pain. On exam, she looks well. Her temperature is 38.3° C. Skin exam reveals tender red, flat, nodular lesions up to 6 cm over both shins. The remainder of her exam is unremarkable. Her CXR shows bilateral hilar lymphadenopathy.

Lymphadenopathy

A. What is your differential diagnosis?
B. How would you confirm the diagnosis?
C. What is her prognosis?

Case Answers

24-1 A. *Learning objective:* **Recognize that supraclavicular nodes are at high risk of representing malignancy, and order appropriate rapid evaluation to look for an associated tumor.** The presence of a left supraclavicular node is concerning for malignancy, especially with the patient's tobacco history and constitutional symptoms. Although his constitutional symptoms may be due to URI, URI would not account for a supraclavicular node.

24-1 B. *Learning objective:* **State the differential diagnosis of supraclavicular lymphadenopathy.** Left supraclavicular lymphadenopathy is associated with GI (gastric, gallbladder, pancreas), renal, testicular, and ovarian malignancies. Right supraclavicular lymphadenopathy is associated with mediastinal, pulmonary, and esophageal malignancies. Lymphomas and breast cancer may be seen on either side. Non-neoplastic etiologies are possible (e.g., TB or toxoplasmosis), but one would expect nodes in other areas also.

24-1 C. *Learning objective:* **Order appropriate work-up for supraclavicular lymphadenopathy.** Careful examination of the abdomen and testes may provide further clues. Immediate CBC with differential, CXR, and CT scan of the abdomen and pelvis are needed. If a mass is confirmed, a biopsy is needed to confirm the diagnosis. A consult with medical oncology would help direct further work-up (e.g., FNA versus excisional biopsy of the supraclavicular nodes versus biopsy of the primary mass). Even if the imaging and lab tests are normal, a biopsy of the supraclavicular node would be recommended. The rationale for imaging is that the work-up would proceed differently if a renal, gastric, or other primary mass were found.

24-2 A. *Learning objective:* **State the differential diagnosis of hilar lymphadenopathy and erythema nodosum.** Bilateral hilar lymphadenopathy is seen in sarcoidosis, endemic fungal infections (coccidioidomycosis, histoplasmosis), lymphoma, TB, berylliosis, and lung malignancy. The differential diagnosis of erythema nodosum includes infections (e.g., streptococci, TB, cat-scratch disease, coccidioidomycosis), drugs (e.g., sulfonomides), systemic illnesses (sarcoidosis, IBD, and Hodgkin's disease), and pregnancy. The overlap includes sarcoidosis, coccidioidomycosis, and TB. Coccidioidomycosis can be excluded because she has not been to an endemic area (San Joaquin Valley, CA, or southwest U.S.). TB is less likely in the absence of a known contact and with her limited symptoms. The constellation of bilateral hilar lymphadenopathy, arthralgias, and erythema nodosum (Löfgren's syndrome) is a common presentation of sarcoidosis, especially in Scandinavian, Irish, and Puerto Rican women.

24-2 B.   *Learning objective:* **Plan an appropriate work-up for a patient with hilar lymphadenopathy and erythema nodosum.** Consult a pulmonologist. Hilar node biopsy is required to confirm the diagnosis of sarcoidosis, usually by bronchoscopy

24-2 C.   *Learning objective:* **State the prognosis of sarcoidosis.** In general, the prognosis of sarcoidosis is good. More extensive lung involvement and multiple organ system involvement predict a poorer outcome. Acute onset of sarcoidosis presenting with bilateral hilar lymphadenopathy, erythema nodosum, and arthralgias is called Löfgren's syndrome. This syndrome predicts a particularly good outcome.

REFERENCES

Habermann TM, Steensma DP: Lymphadenopathy. Mayo Clin Proc 2000;75:723.
Pangalis GA, Vassilakopoulos TP, Boussiotis VA, et al: Clinical approach to lymphadenopathy. Semin Oncol 1993;20:570.

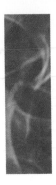

25

Sleep Disorders

ELIZA L. SUTTON

 ETIOLOGY

What is a Sleep Disorder?

Sleep disorders are a heterogeneous group of conditions (Table 25-1) in which sleep is abnormal or disrupted. **Insomnia**, defined as self-reported dissatisfaction with the quality, quantity, or timing of sleep obtained, is common. People with sleep disorders other than insomnia are typically unaware that their sleep is abnormal and often do not recognize feeling chronically sleep-deprived. Several medical conditions and medications can impair sleep (Table 25-2).

How Common are Sleep Disorders?

Sleep disorders are common, but underdiagnosed, particularly obstructive sleep apnea (OSA), (see Table 25-1). In middle-aged adults studied for sleep apnea, 24% of men and 9% of women showed impaired airflow, but not all were symptomatic. The prevalence of OSA increases with age and BMI. More than a third of primary care patients in the U.S. report two or three of the following: snoring, daytime fatigue, and obesity or hypertension. Of that group, 86% meet criteria for OSA in sleep studies. The condition has gone undetected in >80% of men and 90% of women with moderate-to-severe OSA.

 EVALUATION

How do Patients with Sleep Disorders Present?

Consider the possibility of a sleep disorder in a patient with fatigue or nonspecific problems with mood, memory, or cognition. A pattern of job loss or accidents can suggest a sleep disorder (or substance abuse). People with undiagnosed OSA have MVAs two to seven times more than the general population. Patients with severe OSA and obesity-hypoventilation

Table 25-1

Features of Selected Sleep Disorders

Disorder	Common Presentation	Prevalence in Adults	Causes, Contributing Factors
Insomnia (includes multiple disorders)	Difficulty falling asleep or staying asleep	Up to 19% chronically; 67% episodically	Multiple; can become self-perpetuating (conditioned insomnia)
OSA	Daytime somnolence, hypertension, leg edema, polycythemia Can present as insomnia	24% of men; 9% of women	Increases with BMI and age, supine sleep position
RLS	Difficulty falling asleep or staying asleep owing to leg restlessness or discomfort Symptoms include pain, pulling sensation, burning, "crawling, creeping" Symptoms relieved by movement	5%–15% Up to 20% of patients >80yo	Primary familial, idiopathic Secondary (see Box 25-4)
PLMD	Daytime somnolence, repeated sleep disruption owing to repetitive flexor movements of legs Sleep study makes diagnosis	Prevalence unknown Significant overlap with RLS	Similar to RLS (see Box 25-4)
Narcolepsy	Unplanned daytime sleep (sleep "attacks")	0.04%–0.09%	Familial; associated features—cataplexy, sleep paralysis, hypnagogic hallucinations

syndrome have morbid obesity, obvious somnolence and apneas, chronic pedal edema and hypoxemia, and respiratory acidosis. People with milder OSA may have unrecognized effects on daytime functioning, including mood and quality of life. Some patients report being told that they snore

Table 25-2

Medical Conditions and Substances That Can Impair Sleep

Medical Conditions	Psychiatric Conditions	Medications	Substances
Asthma or COPD	Anxiety or panic	Antidepressants—	Alcohol
CHF	disorder	bupropion, SSRIs	Caffeine
Cough	Bipolar disorder	Beta blockers	Nicotine
GERD	Depression	(nonselective)	Stimulants
Hyperthyroidism	Post-traumatic stress	Bronchodilators	
Menopause	disorder	Corticosteroids	
Nocturia (e.g.,		Decongestants	
BPH)		Quinolones (some)	
Pain		Stimulants	
Pregnancy		Theophylline	

loudly, choke, or stop breathing during sleep. OSA may manifest with sequelae of nocturnal hypoxia and increased sympathetic activity (Box 25-1). Insomnia does not result in daytime sleepiness. A second common sleep disorder, RLS, also is underdiagnosed. The patient and physicians may not have heard of it, resulting in a significant delay in diagnosis.

What Aspects of the History May be Helpful?

Take a screening sleep history (Box 25-2). If possible, query the sleep partner about loud snoring, apneas, and movements during sleep.

What are Helpful Findings on Physical Exam?

Most sleep disorders are not associated with abnormalities on exam. OSA can contribute to hypertension, a common finding among internal

BOX 25-1

SIGNS AND SYMPTOMS OF NOCTURNAL HYPOXIA AND INCREASED SYMPATHETIC ACTIVITY IN OBSTRUCTIVE SLEEP APNEA

- Edema
- Headache on awakening
- Hypertension
- Nocturia
- Nocturnal arrhythmias
- Nocturnal angina

BOX 25-2

SCREENING SLEEP HISTORY

1. How have you been sleeping lately?
   How well have you been sleeping?
   How much sleep have you been getting? Is it enough?
2. How is your energy level during the day?
   Do you feel refreshed when you wake up?
   Do you nod off during the day? Ever do so while driving?
3. Have you been told that you snore?
   Do you know if you snore loudly and often?
   Have you ever been told that you choke or stop breathing?
4. Do your legs bother you at night?
   What do you do to relieve it?
   What happens if you try to sit or lie still?

medicine patients. Physical examination of the neck, face, and oropharynx (Box 25-3) can suggest a predisposition to OSA.

Is Blood Testing Useful?

Most sleep disorders are not associated with lab abnormalities. Severe OSA may cause a mild polycythemia owing to chronic nocturnal hypoxia. RLS and PLMD can arise in the setting of several common medical conditions (Box 25-4), for which blood work can be helpful.

What is the Next Step if a Sleep Disorder Seems Likely?

If you suspect a sleep disorder, but the history and physical do not strongly suggest OSA, screen for depression. Order blood work to

BOX 25-3

PHYSICAL FINDINGS SUGGESTIVE OF OBSTRUCTIVE SLEEP APNEA

Neck circumference >17 inches (43 cm) in men or >16 inches (41 cm) in women
Crowded posterior oropharynx
    Large or high-riding tongue, large tonsils, long soft palate
    Difficulty seeing posterior oropharyngeal opening without
        a tongue blade
Micrognathia (small, recessed mandible)
Hypertension
Obesity, especially central obesity

BOX 25-4

MEDICAL CONDITIONS ASSOCIATED WITH RESTLESS LEGS SYNDROME AND PERIODIC LIMB MOVEMENT DISORDER

Iron stores low or low-normal (ferritin <50 μg/L)
Folate level low or low-normal
Vitamin B_{12} deficiency
Medications—SSRIs, OCPs, others
PN—diabetic neuropathy, lumbosacral radiculopathies
Pregnancy
Renal failure
RA
Sjögren's syndrome

---

evaluate for other causes of fatigue and for medical conditions that might cause RLS or PLMD (see Box 25-4). If the patient is not allowing adequate time for sleep, advise more. If the exam suggests OSA, ask about symptoms of snoring or daytime fatigue. If symptoms persist despite adequate sleep time, arrange consultation with a sleep medicine specialist, who may evaluate further with sleep studies. Advise anyone with daytime sleepiness to avoid driving when tired.

What is a Sleep Study?

An overnight sleep study, or nocturnal PSG, quantitates the time spent in each sleep stage (by EEG and by measurement of eye movements and chin muscle tone), respiratory effort and airflow, oxygen saturation, and limb movements (by leg EMG). PSG can be diagnostic for a variety of disorders, including OSA. A multiple sleep latency test (MSLT) monitors the patient by sleep EEG while he or she attempts to nap four to five times over the course of a day. The MSLT gives an objective measure of daytime sleepiness and can be diagnostic for narcolepsy. Sleep studies can be influenced by numerous factors, including recent sleep deprivation, alcohol or benzodiazepine use, psychiatric disorders, and medications. They are rarely used to evaluate insomnia. Sleep studies may not be diagnostic on the first attempt and may need to be repeated for diagnosis or to assess response to treatment.

 ## TREATMENT

What are Some Treatment Approaches for Insomnia?

For acute insomnia, sedative-hypnotics help and may lessen the chance that insomnia will become a long-term problem. For chronic insomnia, after RLS has been excluded, cognitive-behavioral therapy is as effective as medications in the long-term. Beyond educating the patient on good

---

BOX 25-5

SLEEP HYGIENE MEASURES

Keep the same bedtime and wake time every day.
Sleep in comfortable conditions in a quiet, darkened room.
Use the bedroom only for sleep and sex.
Get up out of bed if unable to sleep after 20 minutes; return
  when sleepy again.
Avoid alcohol, caffeine, and nicotine 4–6 hours before bedtime.
Exercise daily, but not within 4–6 hours of bedtime.
Get exposure to daylight or other bright light each morning.
Avoid daytime napping (or, if elderly or narcoleptic, keep stable
  nap schedule).
Keep clocks facing away from bed.

---

sleep hygiene (Box 25-5), this approach can include reducing the time
the insomniac spends in bed and addressing unrealistic expectations
about sleep. Melatonin can help with jet lag and in "night owls" to
encourage the brain's preferred sleep time to coincide with local expectations. Trazodone is commonly prescribed, but little studied. Dependence
and tolerance limit the usefulness of long-term benzodiazepines. Zale-
plon, zolpidem, and eszopiclone are more specific for inducing sleep
and seem safe, but are more expensive.

What are Some General Medical Treatment Approaches for OSA?

Obese patients with OSA benefit from weight loss. All patients with
OSA should avoid sedatives and alcohol, which worsen airway
obstruction. Apneas occur more in the supine (rather than lateral
decubitus) sleep position; you can suggest that the patient attach a
small ball to the back of his or her nightclothes, to encourage side
sleeping. CPAP, the preferred medical treatment for symptomatic
patients, provides a pneumatic splint to the posterior pharynx and
reduces fatigue, snoring, MVA risk, and possibly BP. Some patients
do not tolerate CPAP, however. For mild OSA, an oral appliance fitted
by a dentist can reduce apneas. Palate surgery reduces snoring, but not
apneas.

What are Some Treatments for RLS And PLMD?

Treat the underlying cause, if one is found, including iron supplementation if ferritin is <50 µg/L. Ropinirole is the only Food and Drug Administration–approved treatment for RLS, but other dopamine agonists also
are effective. Gabapentin may help. Clonazepam and other benzodiazepines reduce sleep loss, but not limb movements. Opiates are effective,
but should be reserved for refractory cases.

KEY POINTS

◆ Sleep disorders are common, but under-recognized, under-diagnosed, and under-treated.

◆ Take a screening sleep history when patients report fatigue or daytime sleepiness or when physical findings suggest OSA is likely.

◆ RLS is a common, treatable cause of insomnia that can be diagnosed by history and that may be due to an underlying medical condition.

Case 25-1

A 38-year-old woman presents with insomnia and fatigue. She has been falling asleep at work, at her desk, and in meetings. She describes feeling sleepy in the evenings, but then becoming anxious as bedtime approaches. She lies down but then feels agitated, has to get up again, and simply can't fall asleep for several hours.

    A. What do you think could be causing her anxiety at bedtime?

    B. What further history might you ask?

    C. Read the answer to B. What do you think is causing these symptoms?

    D. What approach would you suggest?

Case 25-2

A 57-year-old man with obesity and poorly controlled hypertension comes in for BP follow-up and requests referral to an otolaryngologist for "that laser surgery" to reduce snoring.

    A. What contributing medical condition should be considered in this patient?

    B. What further questions might you ask the patient or his wife?

    C. Read the answer to B. What advice might you give him?

    D. Would you refer him for any further evaluation or treatment?

Case Answers

25-1 A. *Learning objective:* **Develop a differential diagnosis for anxiety at bedtime.** This patient might have anxiety disorder or post-traumatic stress disorder, RLS, or conditioned (learned) insomnia.

25-1 B. *Learning objective:* **Recognize important aspects of history in evaluating insomnia.** On specific questioning, the patient describes uncomfortable "jittery" sensations in her legs that worsen significantly if she tries to be still (in bed or any other position) and that are relieved only by pacing the floors or by shaking her legs.

25-1 C. *Learning objective:* **Identify RLS by history.** Her history described in answer B describes RLS.

25-1 D. *Learning objective:* **Approach RLS by evaluating for underlying cause and by offering appropriate treatment.** Check ferritin (and other lab values). If her ferritin is <50, start an iron supplement. A dopamine agonist (e.g., ropinirole) also may help, either short-term until her ferritin increases or long-term if her iron stores are already adequate (and no other reversible cause is found).

25-2 A. *Learning objective:* **Recognize the potential for OSA in patients with certain characteristics.** This man is at high risk for having OSA because he has obesity, hypertension, and self-reported snoring.

25-2 B. *Learning objective:* **Pursue clues to OSA by taking further history.** You should ask about daytime sleepiness or impaired function and about witnessed apneas. This patient denies any daytime sleepiness or other problems, but his wife is present and reports that he commonly falls asleep when he is sitting in front of the TV. In addition, she's concerned that he often stops breathing for several seconds during sleep, then resumes breathing with a loud gasp. He has had two low-speed fender-benders in the past year but thinks that's normal.

25-2 C. *Learning objective:* **Identify key pieces of advice for a patient with probable OSA.** This patient should be advised not to drive if he is not feeling completely alert. He should avoid sedatives and alcohol before bedtime, and he should try to sleep on his side. Weight loss, although difficult, would help.

25-2 D. *Learning objective:* **Refer a patient with probable OSA for further evaluation and treatment.** This patient should undergo sleep testing to determine if he has OSA and CPAP therapy if so. In addition to suppressing his snoring, CPAP may improve the daytime sleepiness and might reduce his likelihood of further motor vehicle collisions.

REFERENCES

Caples SM, Gami AS, Somers VK: Obstructive sleep apnea. Ann Intern Med 2005;142:187.

Silber MH: Clinical practice: chronic insomnia. N Engl J Med 2005;353:803.

Thorpy MJ: Approach to the patient with a sleep complaint. Semin Neurol 2004;24:225.

Patients Presenting with a Known Condition

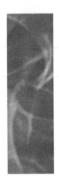

26

Cardiology

ANNELIESE M. SCHLEYER, DAWN E. DEWITT, CAROLINE S. RHOADS, and KAREN STOUT

 COMMON CARDIAC ARRHYTHMIAS

ETIOLOGY

What are Arrhythmias, and How should I Categorize Them?

Arrhythmias are abnormal heart rhythms that are categorized by (1) their ventricular rate and (2) the origin of the rhythm disturbance. Rhythms with a rate >100 beats/min are called *tachycardias*; rhythms <60 beats/min are called *bradycardias*. Rhythm abnormalities may originate in the atria, sinoatrial or atrioventricular nodes, or ventricles. Close inspection of the ECG usually allows specific localization (Figure 26-1).

What are the Types of Tachycardias?

Tachycardias can originate anywhere within the heart. Fast rhythms that arise in the atria or atrioventricular node are collectively referred to as SVT. Common causes include sinus tachycardia and atrial fibrillation. Less common are atrial flutter, re-entrant tachycardia, and multifocal atrial tachycardia. VT originates below the atrioventricular node within abnormally functioning ventricular tissue.

What is Sinus Tachycardia, and What Causes It?

In sinus tachycardia, the rate is >100 beats/min, but the rhythm originates in the atria and is conducted through regular channels. ECG shows a normal P wave before each QRS (Figure 26-2A). Causes include fever, pain, hypovolemia, hypoxia, anemia, and hyperthyroidism. Unexplained sinus tachycardia requires a search for a cause.

What is the Cause of Other Atrial Tachycardias besides Sinus Tachycardia?

Atrial fibrillation results from disorganized electric activity in the atria causing atrial muscle to quiver or fibrillate. On ECG, atrial fibrillation

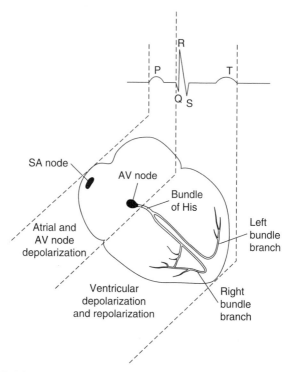

FIGURE 26-1 How the ECG reflects the normal sequence of heart muscle depolarization. Normal depolarization begins in the sinoatrial (SA) node and travels through the atria, causing a P wave. There is a slight delay as depolarization funnels through the atrioventricular (AV) node, reflected in the PR interval. The QRS reflects rapid depolarization via the bundle of His and bundle branches. The T wave reflects ventricular repolarization to resting potential.

shows an irregularly irregular rhythm without identifiable P waves (see Figure 26-2B). Atrial fibrillation may have a normal ventricular rate of 60–100 beats/min; however, often the ventricular rate is >100 beats/min. Atrial fibrillation may exist in isolation ("lone afib"), but usually occurs in the setting of long-standing hypertension, heart failure, hypoxia, valvular or structural heart disease, hyperthyroidism, alcohol or cocaine use, electrolyte abnormalities, or high catecholamine states such as MI or surgery. Incidence increases with age. Atrial flutter, a related rhythm, occurs when an organized circuit of electric activity causes a fast atrial rate. ECG shows a regular oscillating ("saw-tooth") baseline (see Figure 26-2C). Atrial flutter can degenerate into atrial fibrillation. Atrial flutter is seen in patients with underlying cardiac or pulmonary disease. A third atrial rhythm, multifocal atrial tachycardia, (26-2D) may be confused with atrial fibrillation because it also causes an irregularly irregular rhythm. In contrast to atrial fibrillation, the ECG in

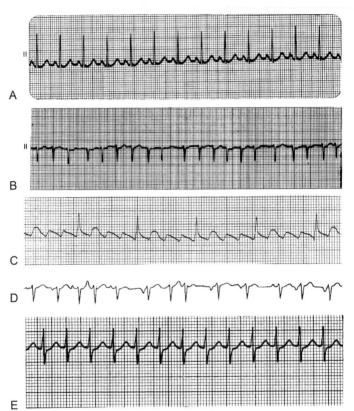

FIGURE 26-2 Atrial arrhythmias. **A**, *Sinus tachycardia*: rate >100 and regular, QRS is narrow, each P wave is associated with a QRS, each QRS has a P wave, PR interval is normal in length. **B**, *Atrial fibrillation*: most common cause of an irregularly irregular rhythm, QRS is narrow, P waves are absent or slow, depending on how refractory the atrioventricular node is to conducting the erratic atrial electric activity to the ventricles. **C**, *Atrial flutter*: regular rate with a saw-toothed baseline of P waves going at a rate of about 300/min (one per large box), conducting every fourth P through to the ventricles (4:1 conduction). Atrial flutter can be associated with a fast or slow ventricular rate depending on refractoriness of the atrioventricular node. **D**, *Multifocal atrial tachycardia*: a less common cause of an irregularly irregular rhythm with a P wave before each QRS and at least three different P wave morphologies reflecting three or more atrial foci initiating beats. **E**, *SVT*: rate >100 and regular, QRS is narrow, P waves may be absent so PR interval cannot be determined. Cause is likely atrioventricular nodal re-entry loop (see text).
(From Goldberg AL: Clinical Electrocardiography: A Simplified Approach, 6th ed. St. Louis: Mosby, 1999.)

multifocal atrial tachycardia shows P waves before each QRS. To be diagnostic, there must be at least three different P wave morphologies reflecting multiple atrial foci (see Figure 26-2D). Multifocal atrial tachycardia often occurs in patients with pulmonary disease or electrolyte abnormalities.

What is a Re-entrant Tachycardia?

Re-entrant tachycardias are another type of SVT created by a cyclic loop of electric activity in or around the atrioventricular node that is conducted simultaneously to the ventricles and the atria from the atrioventricular node area. It produces a regular tachycardia usually 160–240 beats/min (see Figure 26-2E). P waves may occur within or just after the QRS complex as the electricity travels backward from the re-entrant loop to the atria. Although not a sign of heart disease, re-entrant tachycardias may produce ischemia, hypotension, or heart failure because of their fast rates.

What Causes Bradycardia?

Sinus bradycardia is common and is seen with advanced age, athletic training, MI, hypokalemia, hypothyroidism, and drugs (beta blockers, calcium channel blockers, and digoxin). Less common causes of bradycardia are atrioventricular nodal block or sinoatrial node failure. In complete atrioventricular block and sinoatrial node failure, an ectopic ventricular focus (idioventricular rhythm) or area in the atrioventricular node (junctional rhythm) may take over pacing the ventricular beats.

What is Atrioventricular Block?

Atrioventricular block occurs as a result of impaired conduction of atrial impulses through the atrioventricular node. Atrioventricular block is categorized into first, second, or third degree based on the severity of the abnormality (Figure 26-3A-C). Cardiac ischemia and medications such as beta blockers, calcium channel blockers, and digoxin are the most common causes. Placement of a permanent pacemaker is indicated if there is a type II second-degree block or third-degree/complete heart block (see Figure 26-3C).

What are VT and Ventricular Fibrillation?

VT is a potentially lethal rhythm requiring rapid identification and intervention. In VT, the fast ventricular rhythm originates from an ectopic focus in a ventricle, while the sinoatrial node may continue to produce independent P waves at a different rate. These P waves may be buried or appear as irregularities superimposed on the wide QRS complexes. The rate is usually 160–200 beats/min and regular (see Figure 26-4B). VT often occurs with cardiac ischemia, but also is seen with electrolyte abnormalities (particularly K and Mg), cardiomyopathy, and drug intoxication (Table 26-1). Sustained VT can deteriorate rapidly

Cardiology

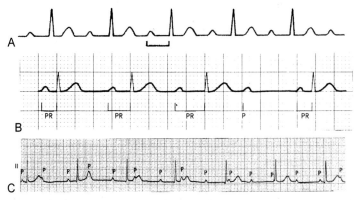

FIGURE 26-3 Atrioventricular node blocks. **A**, *First-degree block*: PR interval uniformly prolonged longer than one big box (>0.2 sec). **B**, *Second-degree block type 1 (Wenckebach)*: a cycle of PR widening culminates in a dropped QRS, then cycle begins again. **C**, *Third-degree block*: no atrial impulses pass through the atrioventricular node, causing complete atrioventricular dissociation. Atrioventricular node or ventricle may beat independently, usually at a rate far slower than 60/sec giving atrioventricular dissociation as seen above. (From Goldberg AL: Clinical Electrocardiography: A Simplified Approach, 6th ed. St. Louis: Mosby, 1999.)

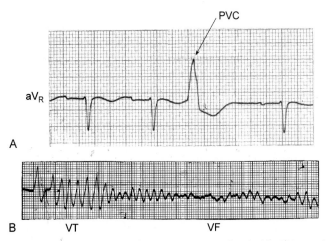

FIGURE 26-4 Ventricular arrhythmias. **A**, *PVC*: an isolated wide QRS superimposed on the baseline sinus rhythm. **B**, *VT*: a rapid regular rhythm >100/sec with wide QRS.

Cardiology

Table 26-1

Causes and Types of Tachyarrhythmias

	Common Causes	Less Common Causes
SVT Originates above or in atrioventricular node	Sinus tachycardia Atrial fibrillation	Atrial flutter Multifocal atrial tachycardia Atrioventricular node re-entry
VT Originates below atrioventricular node	Cardiac ischemia	Electrolyte abnormalities ($\downarrow$ Mg, $\downarrow$ or $\uparrow$ K) Cardiomyopathy Drug intoxications TCAs Quinolones

into ventricular fibrillation, completely disorganized electric impulses causing the ventricles to "fibrillate" (Figure 26-4).

What Could be Causing "Extra Heart Beats" or Palpitations?

Commonly, patients' reports of "palpitations" are due to PACs or PVCs, although these ectopic beats occur without symptoms in most patients. Atrial fibrillation, atrial flutter, or nonsustained VT also can be felt as palpitations. PACs occur when atrial tissue outside of the sinoatrial node initiates an early beat and do not indicate cardiac pathology. In PACs, ECG shows an early P wave that is different from preceding beats. PVCs result from the same phenomenon, but the beat starts in the ventricle. The ECG shows episodic wide QRS complexes without associated P waves (see Figure 26-4A) superimposed on the baseline rhythm. When frequent (more than five consecutive), PVCs can indicate ischemic or structural heart disease. If a patient has a history of infarction and an EF of <40%, frequent PVCs indicate a high risk of sudden cardiac death.

What is Wolff-Parkinson-White Syndrome?

Wolff-Parkinson-White syndrome, also called pre-excitation syndrome, results when an accessory pathway bypasses the atrioventricular node and transmits electric current directly to the ventricle without the usual delay through the atrioventricular node. The resulting PR interval is shortened to <0.12 second. The initial portion of the QRS has a more gradual rise, called a delta wave, representing the electricity passing through the bypass tract. This delta wave also may cause the QRS interval to look slightly wider than usual. Most patients with Wolff-Parkinson-White syndrome are asymptomatic and require no intervention.

Other bypass tracts exist without causing a delta wave, but the common feature of any bypass tract is a shortened PR interval. Atrial fibrillation and flutter occur more commonly in patients with Wolff-Parkinson-White syndrome.

EVALUATION

What Symptoms Suggest a Cardiac Arrhythmia?

Some patients are asymptomatic, and an arrhythmia is identified only when an abnormal pulse is noted. In general, however, arrhythmias cause the heart to function poorly or work harder resulting in syncope, dizziness, chest pain, palpitations, dyspnea, or exercise intolerance.

How do I Evaluate an Abnormal Pulse?

First, ensure stability with a quick vital sign assessment. Look for evidence of cardiac ischemia or shock. Get help immediately if the patient is unstable. If the patient is stable, ask about prior heart problems and symptoms. Characterize the pulse by rate and pattern, and obtain an ECG.

Now that I have an ECG, How do I Identify the Rhythm?

First, determine the *rate*: Is it normal, tachycardic, or bradycardic? Second, measure the *QRS width* to help determine the rhythm origin. A narrow QRS (less than three small boxes or 120 msec) indicates a rhythm that originates in the atria or atrioventricular node and travels to the ventricles via the His-Purkinje system. Conversely, a wide QRS indicates a ventricular origin. Occasionally, very rapid supraventricular rhythms do not conduct normally through the His-Purkinje system owing to incomplete recovery of bundle tissue between rapid beats. This is called aberrancy, or intraventricular conduction delay, and can make distinguishing VT from SVT difficult. Third, compare *RR intervals* to decide if the rhythm is regular. Regular rhythms have equal RR intervals. An irregular rhythm with no pattern is almost always atrial fibrillation. Fourth, look for *P waves*. If absent, and the rhythm is irregular, atrial fibrillation is likely. If P waves occur in no relation to the QRS complexes, consider atrioventricular dissociation with VT (fast wide QRS) or atrioventricular block (with a slow ventricular escape rate). Examine the *PR interval* for prolongation, variability, or intermittently dropped QRS complexes suggestive of atrioventricular block. Figures 26-5 and 26-6 are algorithms to aid in identifying rhythm disturbances.

How do I Evaluate an Irregularly Irregular Rhythm?

Atrial fibrillation is most likely, but confirm with an ECG. If ECG shows atrial fibrillation, obtain oxygen saturation, electrolytes, cardiac enzymes, TSH, and a CXR to look for pulmonary disease or heart failure. Consider a stress test if you are concerned about underlying ischemic heart disease and an echocardiogram to identify valvular or structural heart disease or ventricular dysfunction. Pulmonary

Cardiology

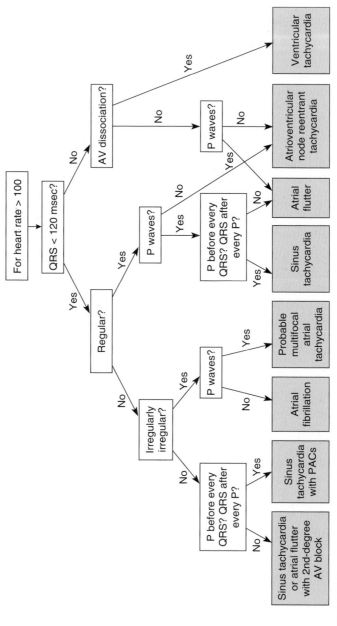

FIGURE 26-5 Algorithm for identifying tachycardias. AV, atrioventricular.

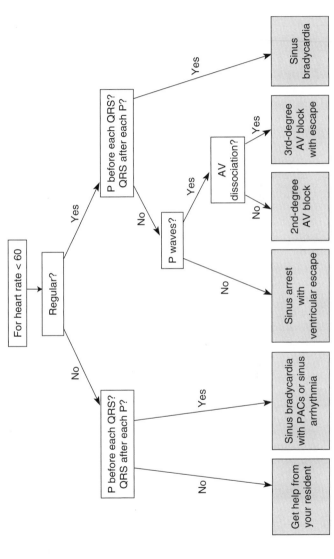

FIGURE 26-6 Algorithm for identifying bradycardias. AV, atrioventricular.

Cardiology

embolism is a possible cause of atrial fibrillation, so ask about risk factors (prior clots, estrogens use, smoking, prolonged immobility, recent surgery), and look for clinical signs (unilateral leg swelling, dyspnea, hypoxia).

How do I Evaluate Bradycardia?

Study the ECG to identify the rhythm. If ischemia is suspected or the patient had syncope or presyncope, hospitalize the patient for monitoring, cardiac enzyme testing, and possible pacing. A medication list may identify possible precipitants (digoxin, calcium channel blockers, beta blockers). Prior ECGs may help identify the patient's baseline heart rate.

How do I Evaluate a Patient with Palpitations?

Get a clear description. Ask about prescription and nonprescription medications, caffeine, and substance abuse. "Extra beats" without symptoms are usually PACs or PVCs. ECG may be adequate evaluation. Associated dizziness, syncope, chest pain, or dyspnea are concerning for SVT, VT, ischemia, or structural problems and require electrolytes, TSH, and cardiac monitoring, and may require stress testing and echocardiogram.

TREATMENT

How do I Treat my Patient with Chronic Atrial Fibrillation?

The three main treatment goals for patients with stable chronic atrial fibrillation are rhythm control, rate control, and anticoagulation. In the past, there was more emphasis on chronic rhythm control with antiarrhythmics, such as amiodarone or sotalol, although more recent studies suggest patients receiving rate control and anticoagulation do better without the addition of agents for rhythm control. Many patients with atrial fibrillation have enlarged atrial size, which makes it unlikely that they can be maintained in normal sinus rhythm, even with long-term antiarrhythmic therapy. Rate control is accomplished with drugs that slow conduction through the atrioventricular node to keep ventricular rate slow: beta blockers, nondihydropyridine calcium channel blockers such as diltiazem and verapamil, or digoxin. Digoxin does not keep heart rate controlled during activity so is less desirable. Anticoagulation is key to prevent development of clot in the fibrillating atria and subsequent systemic embolism. The risk of thromboembolic events in patients with atrial fibrillation without anticoagulation is about 5% per year. Even on long-term antiarrhythmic therapy, patients experience clots if they are not anticoagulated.

How do I Treat my Patient who Presents with New Atrial Fibrillation and a Rapid Ventricular Response?

The same three goals exist: restore and maintain normal sinus rhythm, control rate, and anticoagulate. Unstable patients with hypotension, active cardiac ischemia, or heart failure should be urgently cardioverted (e.g., given a shock to change the rhythm acutely from atrial fibrillation to normal sinus rhythm). Stable patients with rapid ventricular response can be electively cardioverted with electricity or medications if onset of atrial fibrillation is clearly within 48 hours. Patients with atrial fibrillation for >48 hours have a significant risk of atrial clot and embolism; they should receive anticoagulation for 3–4 weeks before cardioversion and 4 weeks after. If a transesophageal echocardiogram shows no evidence of atrial thrombus, cardioversion can occur sooner followed by 4 weeks of anticoagulation. Pharmacologic agents for chemical cardioversion include amiodarone (drug of choice in recurrent atrial fibrillation and structural heart disease), propafenone, sotalol, ibutilide, dofetilide, and flecainide. As before, elective cardioversion may not be useful if echocardiogram shows dilated atria because atrial fibrillation is likely to recur. In stable patients, hospitalization for new-onset atrial fibrillation is not required. Give a beta blocker or calcium channel blocker to bring the ventricular rate to <100 beats/min. Digoxin may be used especially in patients with heart failure, but not as the sole agent because it does not maintain rate control with activity. Initiate anticoagulation with warfarin if there are no contraindications.

How do I Treat SVT?

Unstable patients require immediate electric cardioversion to restore sinus rhythm. In stable patients, adenosine is the agent of choice to terminate SVT and help diagnose the underlying arrhythmia. Vagal maneuvers also may abort the rhythm. Long-term use of beta blockers or calcium channel blockers may decrease recurrence. Refer patients with recurrent episodes of re-entry to a cardiologist for consideration of catheter-directed ablation of abnormal conduction pathways.

How do I Treat Wolff-Parkinson-White Syndrome?

Patients with Wolff-Parkinson-White syndrome and a narrow complex tachycardia can be treated the same way as patients with any SVT. In patients with Wolff-Parkinson-White syndrome with acute atrial fibrillation or flutter, never treat with beta blockers, calcium channel blockers, or digoxin because these can completely block the atrioventricular node, allowing direct transmission of impulses via the bypass track. Instead, treat with intravenous procainamide or ibutilide. Shock if the patient is unstable. Patients with Wolff-Parkinson-White syndrome and arrhythmias usually can be cured with radioablation.

How do I Treat VT?

Cardiovert any patient with sustained VT to prevent deterioration of the rhythm into ventricular fibrillation. Usually synchronized electric cardioversion is required, although occasionally patients with sustained monomorphic VT who have stable BP and no chest pain can be chemically cardioverted with antiarrhythmic drugs (amiodarone). SVT with aberrancy may look like VT. In the setting of instability or chest pain, assume the rhythm is VT, and electrically cardiovert immediately.

How do I Treat Bradycardias?

In patients without symptoms, intervention is unnecessary. Associated dizziness or syncope usually requires hospitalization to initiate cardiac pacing. Stop medications likely to slow the rate. Unstable patients should be given atropine and considered for cardiac pacing.

Case 26-1

In the hospital, you are called to see a 57-year-old man with acute-onset shortness of breath. The patient had initially been admitted 3 days prior after an MVA in which he sustained multiple orthopedic injuries; he is now status post surgical repair. The patient reports shortness of breath and palpitations, but denies associated chest pain, diaphoresis, or nausea. On exam, he is an uncomfortable-appearing man, speaking in two- to three-word sentences. BP is 170/100 mm Hg; heart rate is fast and irregular. Oxygen saturation is 90% on room air. His rhythm strip is shown in Figure 26-7.

   A. What is the rhythm?
   B. What are the possible etiologies of this arrhythmia?
   C. How will you treat this patient, and what testing will you do?

Case 26-2

A 59-year-old woman with a long history of depression and recent antibiotic treatment for a UTI comes to the emergency department and reports two "fainting spells" earlier in the day. She has had some associated chest pain. On exam, she is pale and diaphoretic; BP is 85/54 mm Hg. Her rhythm strip is shown in Figure 26-8.

   A. What is the rhythm?
   B. How should this patient be treated?
   C. What are the possible etiologies of her arrhythmia?

Answers appear on page 254.

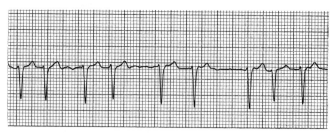

FIGURE 26-7 ECG for patient in Case 26-1.

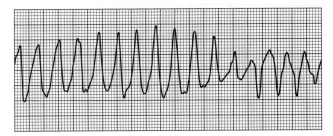

FIGURE 26-8 ECG for patient in Case 26-2.

HEART FAILURE

Cardiology

ETIOLOGY

What is Heart Failure, and What are the Common Causes?

Heart failure, also commonly called CHF, is a clinical syndrome including dyspnea, fatigue, and fluid overload that occurs as a final pathway in various cardiac diseases. The left ventricle (LV) or right ventricle (RV) or both may be involved. Heart failure affects 1% of all people in the U.S. and 10% of individuals >70 years old. Hypertension and CAD cause 50%-75% of left ventricular failure. Right ventricular failure is usually caused by left ventricular failure (Table 26-2).

Table 26-2

Causes of Systolic Dysfunction in Left and Right Heart Failure

	Common Causes	Less Common Causes	Rare Causes
Left Ventricular Failure	Left ventricular ischemia Hypertension Valvular disease Idiopathic dilated cardiomyopathy	Chronic alcohol use Hypothyroidism Toxins (chemotherapy)	Viral myocarditis including HIV Chest irradiation Hemochromatosis* Amyloidosis*
Right Ventricular Failure	Left heart failure Right ventricular ischemia COPD	Sleep apnea Recurrent PE	Interstitial pulmonary diseases Primary pulmonary hypertension

*Commonly present with diastolic dysfunction.

How do I Classify a Patient's Heart Failure?

Heart failure is classified as right or left ventricular failure, with systolic or diastolic dysfunction. In systolic dysfunction, EF is low owing to poor ventricular contraction. In diastolic dysfunction, EF is normal, but cardiac output is low owing to poor filling of a stiff ventricle during diastole. Functional status is classified as I-IV (Table 26-3). These functional categories guide treatment and prognosis.

EVALUATION

What are Classic Findings in Left Ventricular Failure?

Left ventricular failure increases pulmonary venous pressure and causes pulmonary manifestations (Table 26-4), including decreased exercise tolerance (dyspnea on exertion), shortness of breath while supine (orthopnea), or awakening from sleep short of breath (paroxysmal nocturnal dyspnea [PND]). You may hear an S_3, an early diastolic filling sound over the left ventricular apex, and crackles in the lungs secondary to pulmonary edema. Characteristic CXR findings include enlarged heart, pulmonary edema, redistribution of pulmonary blood flow against gravity to upper lung zones (called cephalization), Kerley B lines, or pleural effusion. Left ventricular failure can overload the right ventricle and cause right ventricular failure.

What are Classic Findings in Right Ventricular Failure?

Right ventricular failure increases systemic venous pressure. Isolated right ventricular failure does not cause lung symptoms, but because most right ventricular failure is due to left ventricular failure, fluid overload in the lungs suggests left ventricular failure as the cause. Pertinent findings are listed in Table 26-4. To evaluate jugulovenous pressure (JVP), elevate the head of the bed to 30–45 degrees, and observe for venous pulsations in the neck. Measure the height of the pulsations vertically up from the angle of Louis (where second rib meets the sternum). Convention in the U.S. is to add 5 cm to your measurement to estimate the vertical height in cm H_2O above the right atrium. To evaluate for abdominojugular reflux,

Cardiology

Table 26-3	
New York Heart Association Functional Classification	
Functional Class	**Symptoms**
I	No limitation with ordinary physical activity
II	Mild symptoms, slight limitation with ordinary activity
III	Marked symptoms of fatigue, dyspnea, palpitations, or angina with minimal activity
IV	Symptoms at rest; symptoms increase with any activity

Table 26-4

Symptoms and Signs of Left and Right Ventricular Failure

	History	Exam
Left Ventricular Failure	Orthopnea Dyspnea on exertion PND Cough Frothy hemoptysis	Leg edema Rales (crackles, fine crepitations) S_3 over left ventricle PMI >3 cm and displaced laterally Cool, mottled lower extremities Abnormal abdominojugular reflux
Right Ventricular Failure	Exercise intolerance Dyspnea Increasing abdominal girth RUQ pain Anorexia	Leg edema JVP >8 cm H_2O Right ventricular parasternal heave S_3 over right ventricle Abnormal abdominojugular reflux Ascites

apply pressure to the abdomen for 10 seconds while you watch the JVP. If JVP rises >4 cm for the duration of pressure, this implies high right heart filling pressures.

What Diagnostic Tests Should I Order in a Patient with Signs of New Left Ventricular Failure?

Standard work-up includes CBC (anemia can cause CHF), chemistry panel (to assess baseline electrolytes and creatinine before starting medications), fasting cholesterol and glucose, ECG, CXR, and echocardiogram. Chest films may reveal underlying lung disease (causing pulmonary hypertension). Echocardiogram estimates EF and evaluates ventricular wall motion and valve function. An EF <40% is considered systolic dysfunction. An EF >40% does not rule out CHF because left ventricular diastolic dysfunction, seen in one third of patients with clinical CHF, manifests with normal EF. Focal wall motion abnormalities suggest ischemic injury. If ischemia is likely by presence of risk factors and symptoms, angiogram is warranted. Otherwise, noninvasive stress test should be performed. If standard work-up does not reveal a diagnosis, review the history for alcohol use, consider further testing for thyroid disease, hemochromatosis, amyloidosis, or HIV. Finally, if the cause of dyspnea is uncertain (e.g., versus pulmonary causes of dyspnea), a plasma brain natriuretic peptide (BNP) >100 pg/mL can be helpful, but is not needed when heart failure is obvious or previously established.

Cardiology

TREATMENT

What are the Treatment Goals in CHF Patients?

Management goals are to reduce symptoms, prevent complications, and improve survival.

What can Patients do to Improve Symptoms?

Patients can restrict salt intake to 3–4 g/d, stay as active as possible, and avoid cigarettes and alcohol. They can follow home BPs and daily weights, and notify their physician of major changes so medications can be adjusted. Nonadherence with medications is common in CHF patients (20%-60%), so counsel patients to take medications as prescribed.

What Medicine is Best for Left Ventricular Systolic Failure?

ACEIs are the first-line agents for left ventricular systolic dysfunction. They reduce left ventricular afterload and decrease morbidity and mortality, particularly in patients with decreased EF from recent MI. Increase the ACEI dose as tolerated to maximum dose or systolic BP 90–100 mm Hg. Monitor serum creatinine and the potassium frequently because both may increase with initiation of ACEI therapy. Common side effects include hypotension, worsening renal function, hyperkalemia, cough, rash, or taste disturbance. The side effect of angioedema is an absolute contraindication to continuing ACEIs. About 10% of patients develop intolerable ACEI cough. Cough is common from CHF itself, but if it is clearly due to ACEI therapy, consider changing to angiotensin II receptor blockers. Angiotensin II receptor blockers also decrease afterload and mortality, but do not cause cough. The combination of hydralazine and isosorbide, also used to decrease afterload, is less effective in reducing mortality, but should be used when angiotensin-blocking agents are not tolerated.

When do Patients Need Diuretics?

Most patients with heart failure have sodium and water overload. Start a diuretic if ACEI alone does not resolve volume overload. Titrate diuretics to achieve a JVP <8 cm H_2O. Give diuretics once a day unless high doses are required (e.g., furosemide >160 mg/d). Hypokalemia requires replacement if the potassium level is <4 mEq/L; use potassium cautiously in patients on ACEI therapy. Low-dose aldosterone antagonists, spironolactone or eplerenone (newer with fewer side effects), decrease mortality and the need for potassium supplementation. Hyperkalemia is a concern with aldosterone antagonists, especially if prescribed with an ACEI.

When Should I use Beta Blockers for Heart Failure?

Increased plasma norepinephrine levels in patients with heart failure are strongly associated with worsening heart failure and increased mortality.

Beta blockers block this effect and improve left ventricular function, decrease hospitalization, and delay need for heart transplant. Most importantly, beta blockers decrease heart failure mortality significantly, especially in post-MI patients. Use carvedilol (an alpha and beta blocker with antioxidant properties), metoprolol, or bisoprolol. Because of negative inotropy with these agents, symptoms may initially worsen; start with low doses, and monitor for fluid overload suggesting the need for a temporary increase in diuretics.

When Should Digoxin be Used?

Add digoxin when patients remain symptomatic on full-dose ACEIs and diuretics, and when beta blockers are not an option. Digoxin is a good choice for patients with atrial fibrillation and CHF. Digoxin increases exercise tolerance and improves functional class; withdrawal of digoxin results in worsening heart failure and increased risk for hospitalization. Digoxin has not been shown to decrease mortality, however. Digoxin toxicity causes arrhythmias, confusion, visual disturbances, anorexia, nausea, and vomiting. Levels do not reflect clinical digoxin toxicity, so follow symptoms and ECG changes. Renal insufficiency, hypokalemia, hypothyroidism, and drug interactions increase the risk of digoxin toxicity.

How is Treatment for Diastolic Dysfunction Different?

The main aims of treatment are to control hypertension and to increase cardiac output by increasing diastolic filling time for patients with diastolic dysfunction. Beta blockers and calcium channel blockers slow ventricular rate (especially in atrial fibrillation) and are first-line therapy; use diuretics as needed. ACEIs are second-line therapy. Revascularization should be considered early if CAD is the cause.

What are the Major Prognostic Indicators in Patients with Heart Failure?

Poor prognostic signs include symptoms at rest, poor EF, hyponatremia, high brain natriuretic peptide levels (>500), and ventricular arrhythmias. Major causes of death include progressive heart failure (40%) and sudden death (40%). One-year mortality for patients with class IV heart failure exceeds 50%.

What Complications are Common?

Ninety percent of CHF patients have complex ventricular ectopy. Amiodarone suppresses ventricular arrhythmias. Automatic implantable cardiac defibrillating devices can resuscitate patients with frequent ventricular fibrillation. Implantable defibrillators are recommended for patients with nonischemic cardiomyopathy, EF <35% and NYHA Class II or III failure. Thromboembolism is more common when left ventricular EF is ≤25%, so warfarin is often used. Depression decreases medication adherence. Because TCAs increase the risk of arrhythmias, use an SSRI.

When Should I Hospitalize Patients with Heart Failure?

Hospitalize patients with newly diagnosed heart failure of unclear etiology to rule out ischemic disease and begin work-up and treatment. Admit patients for clinical exacerbations with hypoxia or hypotension, or if ECG suggests new ischemic injury. Admission orders should include daily weights, records of fluid intake and output, and a low-salt (2–4 g) diet. Monitor clinical volume status using daily exam, serum chemistries, and renal function. Daily exam should include vital signs (including orthostatics), weight, JVP, cardiovascular exam for S_3, lung exam for crackles or effusions, and extremity exam for edema. For significant volume overload, give oxygen, intravenous diuretics, or a furosemide drip if necessary. Swan-Ganz catheters are used in refractory CHF for careful volume management or when inotropic agents are used. Intravenous dobutamine, an inotropic agent, may be used to increase cardiac output and decrease afterload. Some patients require intermittent hospitalization for intravenous dobutamine therapy while they await cardiac transplant.

Cardiology

Case 26-3

A 72-year-old woman presents with increasing dyspnea on exertion so that she now can barely walk to the end of her driveway. She has had hypertension for 30 years and has been treated with hydrochlorothiazide for most of that time. Her BP today is 160/94 mm Hg, and her pulse is 92 beats/min and regular. Her JVP is normal; cardiac exam reveals a focal but prominent PMI and an S_4; she has a few lung crackles at both bases and trace pedal edema

  A. Describe her heart failure (right/left; systolic/diastolic)?
  B. What would you expect to see on her ECG and echocardiogram?
  C. What medication would you add to her thiazide?

Case 26-4

A 55-year-old man with ischemic heart disease and known class II heart failure comes to the clinic. He has increasing dyspnea on exertion and swelling in his ankles. He says that he is not sleeping well and has lost his appetite. His wife reports that he just hasn't been himself lately. He says his arthritis has gotten worse, so he has given up his weekly golf game, and he has not seen any of his friends for weeks. He does not smoke, but has increased his alcohol intake from his usual 2 drinks per week to 2 drinks nightly. Medications include daily lisinopril, furosemide, atorvastatin, and aspirin with ibuprofen as needed for arthritis pain. Exam confirms an elevated JVP and an S_3 and crackles in his lungs. His CXR shows cephalization of the vessels, Kerley B lines, and an enlarged heart. ECG is unchanged from previous.

  A. What has precipitated this patient's exacerbation of his heart failure?

B. What counseling should he have?
C. How would you treat his condition?

Answers appear on page 254.

ISCHEMIC HEART DISEASE

ETIOLOGY

What Causes Myocardial Ischemia?

Myocardial ischemia occurs when myocardial oxygen demand exceeds oxygen delivery (Table 26-5) and is most commonly caused by coronary atherosclerosis. Ischemic heart disease is the leading cause of death and disability in the U.S.

What is Stable Angina, and What Causes it?

Stable angina refers to ischemic chest pain that is reliably provoked by stress or exertion and relieved by rest or nitroglycerin. Most patients have one or more focal narrowings in their coronary arteries caused by atherosclerotic plaques; blood supply may be adequate at rest, but not with the increased demand of exertion.

What Causes Unstable Angina and MI?

Atherosclerotic plaques may rupture. When this happens, platelets aggregate on the plaque causing subtotal or total occlusion. Subtotal occlusion of a coronary artery results in unstable angina; this term includes new onset of severe angina, increasing angina, and angina at rest. Total occlusion causes MI.

Table 26-5

Conditions That Exacerbate Cardiac Ischemia

	Decreased Oxygen Supply	Increased Oxygen Demand
Cardiac	Coronary atherosclerosis	Cardiac hypertrophy
	Coronary artery spasm	Tachyarrhythmia
		AS
Noncardiac	Anemia	Exercise
	Hypoxemia	Sinus tachycardia
	Hypovolemia	Hyperadrenergic states (e.g.,
	Hemoglobinopathy (e.g., sickle	anxiety, cocaine)
	cell anemia)	Hyperthyroidism
	Hyperviscosity	Fever
		Uncontrolled hypertension

Cardiology

Cardiology

DIAGNOSIS

How do I Diagnose Stable Angina?

The history and physical are the most important components of the initial evaluation of patients with chest pain. The history should focus on a thorough description of the chest pain and a review of the patient's CAD risk factors. The likelihood of ischemia increases with patient age, number of typical chest pain characteristics, and number of CAD risk factors (Table 26-6 and Box 26-1). The physical exam should detect signs of vascular disease, such as arterial bruits, and exacerbating factors (see Table 26-5). On completing your history and physical, make a rough estimate of the likelihood that your patient's symptoms are caused by CAD (Table 26-7). For example, a 60-year-old man with a history of hypertension and hyperlipidemia who complains of aching substernal chest discomfort that reliably begins about 20 minutes into his daily jog and clears within 5 minutes after he stops exercising has typical angina and a high likelihood of CAD. A 50-year-old man with a history of tobacco use who experiences sharp chest pain primarily when he uses his upper extremities has atypical chest pain and an intermediate likelihood of CAD as the cause of his symptoms.

When is a Stress Test Indicated?

In patients with an intermediate likelihood of CAD, an ETT may aid diagnosis (Table 26-8). False-positive and false-negative tests are possible, so it is important to use clinical judgment in interpreting the results. ETT has little impact on your diagnostic certainty in patients

Table 26-6

Chest Pain Characteristics Predictive of Cardiac Ischemia

	Ischemia More Likely	Ischemia Less Likely
Quality	Squeezing	Sharp
	Aching	Stabbing
	Pressure	Knifelike
	Heaviness	
	Tightness	
Location	Poorly localized	Sharply demarcated
	Substernal	
	Radiates to neck, jaw, teeth, shoulders, arms	
Duration	Minutes	Seconds only
		Hours to days
Provocation	Exertion	Position
	Emotional stress	
Relief	Rest	Change in position
	Nitroglycerin	

BOX 26-1

CORONARY ARTERY DISEASE RISK FACTORS

◆ Smoking
◆ Hypertension
◆ Hyperlipidemia
◆ Diabetes mellitus
◆ Family history of early CAD*

---
*First-degree male relative with MI before age 55 years or first-degree female relative with MI before age 65 years.

Table 26-7

Classification of Chest Pain

Typical	Pain of typical quality, location, and duration
	Provoked by stress or exercise
	Relieved by rest or nitroglycerin
Atypical	Meets 2 of the 3 criteria for typical chest pain
Noncardiac	Meets 0–1 of the 3 criteria for typical chest pain

Table 26-8

Predictive Ability of Exercise Treadmill Testing

Pre-ETT likelihood of CAD*	Post-ETT† likelihood of CAD	
	Positive Test	**Negative Test**
Low (<25%)	21%	3%
Intermediate (25%–75%)	83%	36%
High (>75%)	98%	83%

*Based on history.
†Assuming 50% sensitivity and 90% specificity.

with a high pretest likelihood of CAD. In these patients, the ETT serves a different function to separate patients who have a good prognosis from patients at higher risk for progressing from stable angina to unstable angina or acute MI.

How do I Diagnose Unstable Angina?

Unstable angina (1) is severe and new onset, (2) is of increasing severity, (3) occurs at rest, or (4) occurs post-MI or postrevascularization. The physical exam, ECG, and cardiac enzyme levels may be normal in this setting and do not rule out unstable angina. When abnormal,

Cardiology

however, they may alert you to patients who are at higher risk for progressing to MI or sudden cardiac death (Table 26-9).

How do I Diagnose Acute MI?

Diagnose acute MI rapidly to optimize patient outcome. Obtain an ECG without delay in any patient with suspected MI. Most patients with acute MI present with chest pain; when chest pain radiates to the arms or shoulders and is associated with diaphoresis, MI is more likely. Thirty percent of patients with acute MI do not have chest pain at the time of presentation, however. These patients are more likely to be older, female, or diabetic and instead may present with less typical symptoms, such as nausea, dyspnea or palpitations. Other patients with acute MI have no symptoms at all and do not present for evaluation at the time of their MI. In these patients, MI may be diagnosed months to years later based on ECG findings. In the acute setting, the ECG is less sensitive than cardiac enzyme measurements for the detection of myocardial injury. Because of its virtually immediate availability, however, early treatment decisions depend on the ECG findings. Patients with new ST segment elevations, new Q waves, or a new conduction defect (e.g., left bundle branch block) in the setting of acute ischemic symptoms are assumed to have acute MI. When the initial ECG has normal or nonspecific findings, and the patient has ongoing symptoms, repeat the ECG at 5- to 10-minute intervals. This may reveal evolving abnormalities that would allow the diagnosis of MI before cardiac enzyme levels become available.

Cardiology

Table 26-9

Risk Stratification of Patients with Unstable Angina

	Low Risk	Intermediate Risk	High Risk
History	New-onset angina, mild No ongoing pain Few risk factors	New-onset angina, severe Rest pain, now resolved	Prolonged, accelerating, or ongoing angina >3 risk factors
Exam	Normal	Hemodynamically stable	Hemodynamic instability, CHF
ECG	Normal or unchanged	T wave changes, but no ST segment deviation	ST segment deviation New bundle branch block
Lab	Normal cardiac enzymes	Normal or minimally elevated cardiac enzymes	Elevated cardiac enzymes
Age	Younger		Older (>65)
MI Risk	3%–6%	9%	18%
Death Risk	0%	1.5%	6%

What Cardiac Enzyme Tests should be Ordered?

Cardiac enzyme levels should be measured in all patients with acute coronary syndromes or nonspecific symptoms or ECG changes. CK and troponin I serum levels begin to increase 4–6 hours after the onset of symptoms and initially may be normal in patients who seek care promptly. Serial measurements allow the detection of the increase and decrease of these enzymes, which follow a typical time course (Table 26-10).

TREATMENT

What are the Goals of Therapy for Patients with Stable Angina?

The goals of therapy are to reduce symptoms, improve quality of life, and prevent future MI and death. Patients who achieve high levels of exercise without angina or evidence of ischemia during exercise tolerance testing have a good prognosis: <1% die of their CAD within the next year.

Who can be Treated Medically for Angina, and what Medicines can I Use?

Patients with stable angina and good exercise tolerance can be managed with lifestyle modification and medications. First-line therapies are aspirin or, if aspirin is contraindicated, clopidogrel to prevent platelet aggregation and a beta blocker to decrease myocardial oxygen demand. Rapid-acting nitroglycerin is used for episodes of angina that occur despite this therapy. Long-acting calcium channel blockers and nitrates can be added to or substituted for beta blockers in patients who do not completely respond, who are intolerant, or who have contraindications to beta blocker therapy. It is important to address each patient's CAD risk factors. Smoking cessation and treatment of hypertension and hyperlipidemia reduce the patient's risk for progressing to unstable angina or MI. Although drug therapy is frequently required, a healthy diet and regular exercise are important adjuncts in the treatment of hypertension and hyperlipidemia.

Which Patients with Stable Angina need Referral to Cardiology, and what Happens to Them?

Patients with angina or ECG abnormalities at low exercise intensity on ETT have a poorer prognosis: ≥5% of these patients die as a result of

Cardiology

Table 26-10

Time Course for Cardiac Enzyme Elevations in Acute Myocardial Infarction

	Onset	Peak	Duration
Troponin	4–6 h	18–24 h	Up to 10 d
CK	4–6 h	18–24 h	36–48 h

CAD in the next year. This group of patients should be referred to a cardiologist for further evaluation, which may include coronary catheterization and possibly revascularization by angioplasty, stenting, or CABG.

How do I Treat Patients with Unstable Angina?

The goals of initial management are to (1) relieve chest pain rapidly, (2) maintain stable hemodynamics, and (3) assess and reduce risk for acute MI and cardiac death. Admit patients with unstable angina to the hospital for continuous monitoring because hemodynamic instability can result from ischemia and its treatment. Initial treatment includes oxygen, sublingual nitroglycerin, and morphine to relieve pain; aspirin and heparin to reduce mortality and risk for progression to MI, possibly by preventing further clot development at the site of plaque rupture; and intravenous nitrates and beta blockers to reduce myocardial oxygen demand and improve coronary blood flow. When the patient is pain-free and hemodynamically stable, assess the patient's risk of dying or having a nonfatal MI (see Table 26-9). Generally, patients at intermediate to high risk for progression to MI are started on a platelet glycoprotein IIb/IIIa antagonist and referred for coronary catheterization. Patients at low risk are started on clopidogrel and observed. ETT is used to guide therapy in this low-risk group. Patients who do well on ETT may be managed medically, whereas patients who do poorly are referred for coronary catheterization. Smoking cessation and intensive control of lipids and BP reduce the patient's risk for MI and death due to cardiovascular disease after hospital discharge.

How do I Treat Patients with Acute MI?

The goals of treatment for patients with MI are listed in Table 26-11. As for patients with unstable angina, aspirin, nitrates, and beta blockers are the mainstays of early treatment. Attempts to reopen the occluded artery should begin as soon as possible; thrombolytic medications and angioplasty (with or without stenting) are effective. The decision about which modality to employ depends on patient characteristics and the availability of a cardiac catheterization facility. Depending on the technique used to re-establish perfusion in the affected artery, heparin or antiplatelet agents or both may be helpful in maintaining vessel patency. Patients who have received drug-eluting stents must receive a minimum of 12 months of clopidogrel after the stent placement to reduce the risk

Table 26-11

Goals for Management of Acute Myocardial Infarction

Immediate	Subacute	Long-term
Relieve pain	Identify patients with recurrent	Stop smoking
Restore hemodynamic stability	or ongoing ischemia	Control BP
Initiate reperfusion within 30 min	Monitor for complications	Lower lipids
Prevent recurrent thrombosis		
Detect and treat arrhythmia		

of early thrombosis. ACEIs improve survival after acute MI, but may cause hypotension and should be used with caution.

What are the Complications of Acute MI?

Patients should be monitored for complications of acute MI, which include atrial and ventricular arrhythmias, CHF, papillary muscle rupture leading to acute mitral regurgitation, and ventricular rupture. Patients with large anterior wall MI may develop clot in the LV.

When is the Patient Ready for Discharge?

Patients who have an uncomplicated post-MI course with no evidence of recurrent ischemia can undergo a low-level ETT within a few days of their MI. If the ETT is negative, they can be safely discharged from the hospital on medical management.

What Should I Prescribe When the Patient is Ready to Leave the Hospital?

First-line therapies for patients after MI are similar to therapies for patients with stable and unstable angina. Lifestyle changes include smoking cessation, healthy diet, and regular exercise. Unless there are specific contraindications to their use, aspirin and a beta blocker should be prescribed for all patients. Consider ACEIs, especially in patients with diabetes, hypertension, or depressed left ventricular function. Lipid-lowering therapy reduces the risk for recurrent MI; the target goal for low-density lipoprotein for patients with CAD is substantially <100 mg/dL, so medication is recommended when low-density lipoprotein levels are >100 mg/dL. The strongest data for survival are with the use of statins. All of these interventions offer a survival advantage.

Case 26-5

A 52-year-old man complains of the new onset of occasional exertional chest discomfort, which is dull, occurs on the left side, and resolves with rest. He smokes one pack of cigarettes daily and is otherwise healthy. On exam, his BP is 142/85 mm Hg. Heart and lung exams are normal. Distal pulses are present and equal bilaterally, and he has no bruits in his neck, abdomen, or groin. A resting ECG is normal. You refer him for ETT, and he exercises for 9 minutes. His heart rate increases from 84 to 160 beats/min at peak exercise and his BP increases from 137/80 to 190/100 mm Hg. He develops mild chest discomfort at peak exercise, and ECG shows 1-mm ST segment depressions, which return to baseline 3 minutes after he stops exercising.

   A. How would you classify his chest pain—typical, atypical, or noncardiac? Stable or unstable?
   B. What is your estimate of his pretest likelihood of CAD? How do his ETT results affect the likelihood that his symptoms are caused by CAD?

C. Should he be referred for catheterization or managed medically?
D. What medications would improve symptoms and reduce his risk for MI?

Case 26-6

A 66-year-old woman is brought into the emergency department by ambulance because of chest pressure that began 2 hours ago and has not gone away. Past medical history is significant for obesity, type 2 diabetes mellitus, hypertension, and hyperlipidemia. She takes aspirin, metformin, lisinopril, and lovastatin. On exam, she looks ill and is pale and sweaty. BP is 105/50 mm Hg, and heart rate is 55 beats/min. Lungs are clear, and heart is regular with no murmur or gallop heard. A chest radiograph is read as normal.

A. What is your differential diagnosis for her symptoms?
B. What additional tests will you order?
   Her ECG shows ST elevation in V_4–V_6. Baseline ECG from 2 years ago was normal.
C. What is your diagnosis?
D. What initial treatment do you prescribe?

Answers appear on pages 255–256.

VALVULAR HEART DISEASE

ETIOLOGY

Are all Murmurs Pathologic?

No. Many murmurs are flow murmurs without valvular pathology. These are benign, systolic, short murmurs heard in early systole, which are 1–2/6 in intensity, are loudest at the left upper sternal border, do not radiate, and do not cause symptoms. Children, teenagers, athletes, and patients with high output states such as anemia, fever, or hyperthyroidism often have flow murmurs. Systolic murmurs are more likely pathologic if the intensity is greater than 2/6, if they radiate, particularly to the carotids, are present in people >50 years old or are accompanied by cardiac or pulmonary symptoms. A diastolic murmur, in contrast, is always pathologic.

What are Common Causes of Systolic Murmurs?

Flow murmurs, AS and MR are common causes of systolic murmurs (Box 26-2). AS is most commonly due to calcification of a congenital bicuspid aortic valve in adults <60 years old and degenerative valve change in adults >60 years old. AS secondary to rheumatic heart disease most often occurs in adults 30–60 years old, but can occur in younger patients who have had repeated bouts of rheumatic fever. Aortic sclerosis is calcification

BOX 26-2

COMMON CAUSES OF MURMURS

Systolic Murmurs

Aortic sterosis (AS)
  Congenital bicuspid valve (age <60)
  Degenerative valvular disease (age >60)
Flow murmur
  Normal turbulence
  Anemia, fever, hyperthyroidism
Hypertrophic cardiomyopathy (HCM)
Mitral regurgitation (MR)
  Rheumatic heart disease
  Mitral prolapse
  Ischemic papillary muscle dysfunction

Diastolic Murmurs

Aortic regurgitation (AR)
  Congenital bicuspid valve
  Rheumatic heart disease
  Endocarditis
Aortic root dissection
  Marfan's syndrome
  Aortitis of syphilis or vasculitis
Mitral stenosis (MS)
  Rheumatic heart disease

of the aortic valve that can evolve into AS over time. Aortic sclerosis generally causes an early peaking systolic murmur, whereas significant AS is late peaking and harsh. Causes of MR are listed in Box 26-2. A third cause of a systolic murmur is HCM, also called subaortic stenosis. This is an inherited disorder that can cause ventricular hypertrophy, ventricular arrhythmias, exertional chest pain, dyspnea, syncope, or sudden death. The systolic murmur of HCM is created by obstruction to left ventricular outflow in systole owing to a thickened interventricular septum and abnormal motion of the mitral valve leaflets into the outflow tract. HCM is the most common identified cause of sudden death in athletes.

What are the Key Causes of Diastolic Murmurs?

AR and mitral stenosis are the most common causes of diastolic murmurs. AR can occur with congenital bicuspid valves, rheumatic heart disease, endocarditis, calcific aortic valve disease, ankylosing spondylitis, RA, and aortic root dilation or dissection (as with Marfan syndrome, vasculitis, or syphilitic aortitis). The predominant cause of mitral stenosis is rheumatic heart disease. The processes that cause regurgitation frequently cause stenosis as well (bicuspid aortic valve, rheumatic heart disease), so systolic and diastolic murmurs may be heard.

Cardiology

Cardiology

EVALUATION

My Patient has a Murmur. How should I Proceed?

Place the murmur in systole or diastole by palpating pulse; grade the murmur on a scale of 1–6 (Table 26-12); and describe pitch, location, and sites of radiation (carotids, chest wall sites). AR is frequently described as an early diastolic, 2/6, high-pitched decrescendo murmur heard best in the second right intercostal space radiating down the left sternal border.

How do I Differentiate Between the Systolic Murmurs of AS and MR?

Specific valvular abnormalities are often identifiable by the location and character of the murmur (Table 26-13; Figures 26-9 and 26-10). AS is crescendo-decrescendo (diamond-shaped), is heard best at the right upper sternal border, and radiates to the carotids. MR is holosystolic, is heard at the apex, and radiates to the axilla. Severe AS dampens

Table 26-12

Grading Cardiac Murmurs

Grade	Description
1	Cannot hear at first
2	Hear right away, not too loud
3	Loud, but no palpable thrill
4	Loud and associated with palpable thrill
5	Heard with stethoscope angled on chest
6	Heard with stethoscope off chest

Table 26-13

Characteristics of Common Valvular Abnormalities

Lesion	Timing	Loudest Location	Radiation
AS	Systolic crescendo-decrescendo	Second intercostal space	Carotid
MR	Pansystolic	Apex	Axilla, back
AR	Early diastole	Left sternal border	None
MS	Opening snap in early diastole, murmur in mid-diastole, with crescendo in late diastole	Apex, best to listen with bell in left lateral decubitus position	None

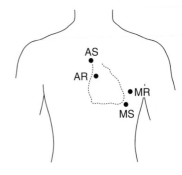

FIGURE 26-9 Location of murmurs from common valvular disorders.

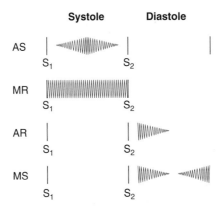

FIGURE 26-10 Visual representation of the sounds produced by common murmurs.

and delays the carotid pulse (pulsus parvus et tardus). To differentiate the murmur of AS from HCM, auscultate the heart while the patient abruptly stands from squatting or sitting, which decreases venous return. With this maneuver, an AS murmur *decreases* as decreased stroke volume decreases the amount of blood passing through the aortic valve. In HCM, the murmur intensity *increases* as the thickened ventricular walls are brought closer together with decreased stroke volume, creating greater obstruction to flow.

How do the Clinical Presentations of the Systolic Murmur Conditions Differ?

For AS and MR, a long asymptomatic period may precede the onset of symptoms. AS increases afterload and causes a compensatory hypertrophy. Symptoms include chest pain, dyspnea, exertional syncope, and decreased exercise tolerance. Chest pain is due to oxygen supply/

demand mismatch in a hypertrophied ventricle with impaired coronary perfusion. Hypertrophy results in increased left ventricular end-diastolic pressures causing dyspnea. The relatively fixed orifice of AS does not allow increase in cardiac output when needed, causing exertional syncope. MR is a volume load on the ventricle and causes left ventricular enlargement. Patients with MR also experience dyspnea and exercise intolerance and less frequently chest pain. MR may present acutely if MI causes a ruptured papillary muscle or if there is chordal rupture in patients with myxomatous valve disease. HCM often occurs in younger patients with a family history of an autosomal dominant inheritance pattern of early cardiac problems, particularly sudden cardiac death. For many patients, initial presentation of HCM is sudden cardiac death. When symptoms occur, they are similar to those of AS. Subtle declines in exercise tolerance represent symptomatic valve disease that requires therapy. This history may be difficult to elicit without careful, focused questioning because patients often attribute the subtle decline to being out of shape or aging.

How can I Differentiate Between the Diastolic Murmurs of AR and Mitral Stenosis?

The early diastolic high-pitched decrescendo murmur of AR is heard maximally in the second right intercostal space with radiation down the left sternal border. It almost mimics a breath sound. A wide pulse pressure often accompanies a pulse with a rapid rise and fall. To hear AR best, use the stethoscope diaphragm, and have the patient lean forward with his or her breath held. In contrast, the mitral stenosis murmur is low-pitched and loudest at the apex. An early diastolic accentuation may occur as blood rushes into the ventricle. In addition, a presystolic crescendo is often heard as the atrial kick sends blood across the stenotic mitral valve. Use a lightly placed bell over the apex or in the axilla, and ask the patient to lie in the left lateral decubitus position to hear the murmur of mitral stenosis best.

How do the Clinical Presentations of the Diastolic Murmur Conditions Differ?

AR and mitral stenosis can have long asymptomatic periods. AR creates a volume load on the ventricle and can result in left heart failure. Symptoms include exercise intolerance, dyspnea, and heart failure. Mitral stenosis obstructs blood flow into the LV, increasing left atrial pressures. This causes left atrial enlargement, pulmonary congestion, atrial fibrillation, and right heart failure. Rarely, patients with mitral stenosis present with hemoptysis.

Which Patients with Murmurs Need an Echocardiogram or ECG?

Obtain both tests for murmurs with pathologic features: systolic murmur grade *3/6 or greater*, age >55 years, any diastolic murmur, or concurrent cardiopulmonary symptoms.

TREATMENT

How should I Manage a Patient with Pathologic Valvular Disease?

All patients with pathologic valvular disease need close follow-up to detect the onset of symptoms. Definitive therapy is surgical, and the onset of symptoms is an indication for valve replacement. Review cardiopulmonary symptoms and exam at least annually. American College of Cardiology and American Heart Association recommendations regarding the frequency of echocardiography vary by severity of the valve disease and ventricular function, ranging from every 6 months to every 4 years. More severe disease or patients nearing criteria for valve replacement require echocardiograms more frequently. Patients with AR may benefit from afterload-reducing agents (ACEIs, nifedipine, or hydralazine). These drugs may delay surgery in asymptomatic patients with severe regurgitation. Atrial fibrillation is a common complication of atrial enlargement from mitral stenosis or MR. Atrial fibrillation requires anticoagulation (warfarin), cardioversion, or heart rate control (beta blocker, calcium channel blocker, or digoxin). Asymptomatic patients should be considered for valve replacement when there are signs of left ventricular decompensation. Criteria for left ventricular size and EF vary by the type of valve disease. With MR, valve replacement is recommended if EF is <60% or left ventricular end-systolic measurement is >45 mm. With AR, valve replacement is recommended when EF is <55%, left ventricular end-systolic diameter is >55 mm, or left ventricular end-diastolic diameter is >70 mm. All symptomatic patients should be considered for valve replacement. Acute AR and MR resulting from aortic dissection (AR), endocarditis (AR and MR), and MI (MR) require urgent valve replacement.

Are there any Special Issues in Managing Patients with AS?

In patients with severe AS, there is an inability to increase cardiac output when needed, and afterload reduction with ACEIs or hydralazine should be avoided. Preload-reducing agents, such as nitrates and diuretics, also should be avoided. Any patient with symptomatic severe AS should be referred for valve replacement. The management of severe AS (peak pressure gradient >64 mm Hg, valve area <0.7 cm^2) in asymptomatic patients with normal ventricular function is controversial.

Are there any Special Issues in Managing Patients with Mitral Stenosis?

Diuretics can reduce pulmonary congestion. Increased diastolic filling time improves flow across the stenotic valve. Treating tachycardia is important. In patients with atrial fibrillation, rate control or cardioversion or both markedly decrease symptoms. Systemic emboli are a complication of mitral stenosis, and lifelong warfarin is begun after any episode of atrial fibrillation. Consider valve replacement or valvuloplasty for dyspnea, uncontrollable pulmonary edema, recurrent

Cardiology

systemic emboli on anticoagulation, and severe pulmonary hypertension with right ventricular hypertrophy and hemoptysis. Percutaneous balloon valvuloplasty can be considered for nonregurgitant valves, but regurgitant or heavily calcified valves require replacement.

How can I Prevent Endocarditis?

Give high-risk patients (patients with prosthetic valves or previous endocarditis) a single 2-g oral dose of amoxicillin before dental, or respiratory tract procedures (when biopsy occurs).

Case 26-7

A 25-year-old woman comes in to establish care. On exam, she is very tall, wears glasses, and is quite flexible, with a positive thumb sign and positive wrist sign. She has a 2/6 early diastolic murmur heard at the right upper sternal border and left lower sternal border. She is a basketball player and has noticed she's been more out of shape over the last year.

    A. What valvular lesion is present?
    B. What is the underlying disease process?
    C. What diagnostic studies should you obtain?
    D. Outline your management of the valvular lesion.

Case 26-8

A 58-year-old man is seen for exertional dyspnea. He has a 3/6 systolic murmur on examination, loudest at the right upper sternal border and radiating to the carotids. You suspect AS.

    A. List as many physical exam features of severe AS as you can.
    B. Your assistant schedules an echocardiogram in 2 weeks. His blood pressure is 145/80 mm Hg. Do you initiate antihypertensive therapy today?

Answers appear on pages 256–257.

KEY POINTS – COMMON CARDIAC ARRHYTHMIAS

◆ When reading ECGs, look systematically at the rate, QRS width, RR interval, P waves, and PR intervals to determine the rhythm.

◆ An "irregularly irregular" rhythm is usually atrial fibrillation.

◆ Electrically cardiovert any patient who has an unstable arrhythmia.

◆ Assume any wide complex tachycardia is ventricular in origin and treat as VT.

◆ Do not treat patients with Wolff-Parkinson-White syndrome and atrial fibrillation with beta blockers, calcium channel blockers, or digoxin.

KEY POINTS – HEART FAILURE

◆ Patients presenting with heart failure should be classified by type of heart dysfunction and by functional class to guide treatment strategies.

◆ All patients with systolic dysfunction should be treated with ACEIs unless contraindicated.

◆ Treat volume overload with diuretics.

◆ Beta blockers should be considered for all patients, especially patients with ischemic heart failure.

◆ ACEIs, beta blockers, and aldosterone antagonists reduce mortality in patients with heart failure secondary to systolic dysfunction

KEY POINTS – ISCHEMIC HEART DISEASE

◆ Myocardial ischemia occurs when myocardial oxygen consumption exceeds delivery.

◆ Atypical symptoms are common, particularly in women, elderly individuals, and diabetics.

◆ Refer high-risk patients for catheterization; manage low-risk patients with medications.

◆ Time to reperfusion is critical to outcome in acute MI, so make a diagnosis and begin treatment as quickly as possible.

◆ Aggressive management of CAD risk factors decreases the likelihood of disease progression in patients with CAD.

◆ Post-MI medications that offer a survival advantage include aspirin, beta blockers, ACEIs, and HMG CoA reductase inhibitors.

Cardiology

KEY POINTS – VALVULAR HEART DISEASE

◆ All diastolic murmurs are pathologic.

◆ Monitor significant valvular disease by serial echocardiograms, and refer for valve replacement with symptoms or signs of left ventricular dysfunction.

◆ Acute valvular regurgitation, such as MR with papillary muscle or chordal rupture and AR with endocarditis, requires urgent intervention.

Case Answers

26-1 A-C. *Learning objectives:* **Recognize atrial fibrillation, state causes, and appropriately treat it.** This patient's rhythm strip shows atrial fibrillation with rapid ventricular response, a common arrhythmia that is "irregularly irregular." Atrial fibrillation should be confirmed with an ECG. Possible causes include pulmonary embolism, cardiac ischemia or failure, hypoxia (e.g., from aspiration pneumonia), alcohol withdrawal, electrolyte abnormalities, and thyroid abnormalities. The patient's rapid ventricular rate should be treated with a beta blocker or calcium channel blocker if there are no contraindications. Treatment of an underlying condition would help to treat the atrial fibrillation. Work-up should include assessment of electrolytes, cardiac enzymes, CXR, and additional studies to evaluate for pulmonary embolism. If these are unrevealing, consider echocardiogram to assess for structural heart disease, and check TSH.

26-2 A. *Learning objective:* **Recognize and treat VT.** This patient's rhythm strip shows a fast rhythm with a wide QRS indicating VT.

26-2 B. *Learning objective:* **Describe VT and treatment.** VT is a potentially lethal rhythm and should be treated with immediate cardioversion, particularly in this patient who has associated chest pain and is clinically unstable with a low BP.

26-2 C. *Learning objective:* **Outline cause of VT.** VT occurs most often with cardiac ischemia, but also may be secondary to drugs such as fluoroquinolones or TCA or electrolyte abnormalities.

26-3 A. *Learning objective:* **Recognize diastolic heart failure.** Diastolic heart failure commonly occurs in elderly patients with long-standing hypertension. Patients usually do not have a dilated left ventricle and may not present with typical volume overload.

26-3 B. *Learning objective:* **State the findings on ECG and echocardiogram in patients with diastolic HF.** This patient is likely to have LVH on ECG and a thickened ventricle on echocardiogram with a normal EF, but decreased end diastolic volume.

26-3 C.   *Learning objective:* **Choose appropriate first-line therapy in diastolic dysfunction.** Good BP control is key for patients with diastolic dysfunction, with an agent that does not decrease preload
too much, so avoid the nitrates and dihydropyridine calcium channel blockers. Beta blockers and verapamil are good choices because
they slow the heart rate and lengthen the PR interval, increasing
ventricular filling time. With either choice, the patient should be
monitored clinically for increasing pulmonary edema.

26-4 A.   *Learning objective:* **Recognize factors that contribute to worsening HF.** In this case, the patient's alcohol intake has increased
significantly, and he may be taking more ibuprofen, which can
worsen HF. His symptoms of difficulty sleeping and not seeing his
friends and his wife's report that he is different may indicate
depression, which is common in patients with HF.

26-4 B.   *Learning objective:* **Counsel patients about lifestyle issues as
part of HF management.** You should discuss that alcohol
depresses cardiac function, and that NSAIDs cause fluid retention
and precipitate worsening renal and cardiac function. You also
should discuss the importance of compliance with medications.
Patients with HF can become discouraged or depressed and stop
taking medications. They also may not understand the reasons
the medications are needed or that they need to take them
"forever."

26-4 C.   *Learning objective:* **Understand the principles of treating HF
exacerbations.** Because he is volume overloaded (JVP, S_3, lung
and peripheral edema), you should increase the furosemide dose
and maximize the ACEI, while monitoring creatinine and potassium. This may be a good time to add an aldosterone antagonist
(spironolactone or eplerenone). Although a beta blocker may help
in the long run, you would have to normalize his volume status
before adding one. Finally, as previously, you should discuss lifestyle
issues to maximize his care.

26-5 A.   *Learning objective:* **Be able to classify chest pain.** The patient's
chest pain is consistent with typical angina because of its quality
(dull, left-sided), and because it is provoked by exercise and relieved
by rest. Although it is of recent onset, it does not seem severe in
that it comes on only with exercise and is described as occasional.
Severe new-onset angina typically limits a person's usual activities
and is frequent.

26-5 B.   *Learning objective:* **Understand how the ETT result affects diagnostic thinking.** His pretest likelihood for CAD is high (>75%)
because of the typical quality of his chest pain and the presence
of cardiac risk factors (smoking and possibly hypertension). His
post-test likelihood for CAD approaches 100%. In this case, the
ETT has little impact on diagnostic certainty.

Cardiology

26-5 C. *Learning objective:* **Understand how to use ETT results to make decisions about management.** The patient had a normal hemodynamic response to exercise (HR and BP increased), and he was able to achieve a high intensity of exercise (HR 160 beats/min) before he developed symptoms (angina) and signs (ST segment depression) of ischemia. Symptoms and signs then resolved rapidly. This portends a relatively good prognosis and suggests that he should start with a trial of medication management. By comparison, someone whose BP didn't increase with exercise or who developed pain or ECG changes after just a few minutes of low-intensity exercise would have a higher risk and would need referral for further testing.

26-5 D. *Learning objective:* **Know how to treat stable angina.** Medications should include aspirin (or clopidogrel if he has a contraindication to aspirin), a beta blocker, and sublingual nitroglycerin for symptom control. He should have a fasting lipid profile and start a statin medication if low-density lipoprotein is >100 mg/dL. If BP remains elevated on a beta blocker, consider additional treatment to decrease BP to <130/80 mm Hg. Smoking cessation is crucial for reducing his risk for progressive CAD and MI.

26-6 A. *Learning objective:* **Recognize symptoms of MI.** The patient's age, symptoms, and cardiac risk factors all point to acute MI as the most likely diagnosis. Other "wouldn't want to miss" diagnoses to consider are aortic dissection and pulmonary embolism.

26-6 B. *Learning objective:* **Know to get an ECG immediately whenever MI is suspected.** The most important initial test in anyone with suspected MI is an ECG. This should be obtained immediately. Cardiac enzymes can then be drawn. Other important tests include CBC, electrolytes, creatinine, and coagulation studies. Abnormalities in these tests may influence treatment decisions. Someone with a severe anemia might not be a candidate for thrombolytic therapy, particularly if the cause of the anemia is GI bleeding.

26-6 C. *Learning objective:* **Know criteria for diagnosis of acute MI and recognize left bundle branch block.** The ECG shows a new left bundle branch block. This, in the setting of symptoms that are consistent with MI, is adequate for the diagnosis.

26-6 D. *Learning objective:* **Know what treatment to initiate for acute MI.** Initial treatment in the emergency department should include aspirin (chewed, not swallowed whole); a beta blocker, which in this case needs to be used with great caution given her bradycardia and new conduction abnormalities, and morphine and nitrates to relieve chest pain.

26-7 A. *Learning objective:* **Identify aortic insufficiency.**

26–7 B. *Learning objective:* **Recognize clinical presentation of Marfan syndrome.** The noncardiac exam is most suggestive of Marfan syndrome with aortic root and annular dilation leading to aortic insufficiency. A bicuspid aortic valve is less likely based on the non-cardiac exam suggestive of Marfan syndrome.

26-7 C.   *Learning objective:* **List initial studies in possible aortic insuffi-ciency.** Echocardiogram is the most important initial study. Also consider ECG and CXR as baseline studies.

26-7 D.   *Learning objective:* **Outline management of aortic insufficiency.** This patient's presentation as "out of shape" suggests symptomatic valve disease. If the echocardiogram confirms severe aortic insuffi-ciency, aortic valve replacement is indicated because of the pres-ence of symptoms. If the patient were asymptomatic, and the LV has not met criteria for aortic valve replacement, continued fol-low-up with serial echocardiograms is warranted. Concurrent after-load reduction is controversial, but can be considered in an effort to delay aortic valve replacement.

26-8 A.   *Learning objective:* **Identify key physical exam findings of aortic stenosis.** Findings include pulsus parvus et tardus, single S_2, and late peaking systolic ejection murmur.

26-8 B.   *Learning objective:* **Recognize that afterload reduction in severe AS can be dangerous.** Based on dyspnea and exam, this patient likely has severe AS. Because afterload reduction can precipitate hypotension, it is better to understand the underlying lesion before starting medication.

Cardiology

REFERENCES

Common Cardiac Arrhythmias

Blomström-Lundqvist C, Scheinman MM, Aliot EM, et al: ACC/AHA/ESC guide-lines for the management of patients with supraventricular arrhythmias—exec-utive summary. J Am Coll Cardiol 2003;42:1493.

Fuster V, Ryden LE, Asinger RW, et al: ACC/AHA/ESC guidelines for the manage-ment of patients with atrial fibrillation—executive summary. J Am Coll Cardiol 2001;38:1231.

Van Gelder IC: A comparison of rate control and rhythm control in patients with recurrent persistent atrial fibrillation. N Engl J Med 2002;347:1834.

Wyse DG: A comparison of rate control and rhythm control in patients with atrial fibrillation: The Atrial Fibrillation Follow-up Investigation of Rhythm Manage-ment (AFFIRM) investigators. N Engl J Med 2002;347:1825.

Heart Failure

Badgett RG, Lucey CR, Mulrow CD: Can the clinical examination diagnose left-sided heart failure in adults? JAMA 1997;277:1712.

Hunt SA, American College of Cardiology; American Heart Association Task Force on Practice Guidelines (Writing Committee to Update the 2001 Guide-lines for the Evaluation and Management of Heart Failure): ACC/AHA 2005 guideline update for the diagnosis and management of chronic heart failure in the adult. J Am Coll Cardiol 2005;46:e1.

Cardiology

Ischemic Heart Disease

Antman EM, Anbe DT, Armstrong PW, et al: ACC/AHA guidelines for the management of patients with ST-elevation myocardial infarction. J Am Coll Cardiol 2004;44:671.

Braunwald E: Application of current guidelines to the management of unstable angina and non-ST-elevation myocardial infarction. Circulation 2003;108 (suppl 3), 28.

Gibbons RJ, Abrams J, Chatterjee K, et al: ACC/AHA 2002 guideline update for the management of patients with chronic stable angina. J Am Coll Cardiol 2003;41:159.

Valvular Heart Disease

Bonow K, Carabello B, de Leon AC, et al; ACC/AHA Task Force Report: ACC/AHA guidelines for the management of patients with valvular heart disease. J Am Coll Cardiol 1998;32:1486.

Freeman RV, Otto CM: Spectrum of calcific aortic valve disease: Pathogenesis, disease progression, and treatment strategies. Circulation 2005;111:3316.

Otto CM: Evaluation and management of chronic mitral regurgitation. N Engl J Med 2001;354:740.

USEFUL WEB SITES

Heart Failure

ACC/AHA guidelines for the evaluation and management of chronic heart failure in the adult. http://www.americanheart.org/presenter.jhtml?identifier=11841

Ischemic Heart Disease

American College of Cardiology site includes several recent cardiology guidelines. www.acc.org

Valvular Heart Disease

http://www.acc.org/clinical/guidelines/valvular/exeIndex.htm

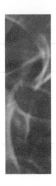

27

Dermatology

BARAK GASTER

 PRURITUS

ETIOLOGY

What are Common Causes of Pruritus?

Xerosis (dry skin), eczema, and scabies are common causes of itching (pruritus). Less common causes include systemic diseases such as renal failure, cholestasis, polycythemia vera, and lymphoma.

EVALUATION

How can I Determine What is Causing Itching?

Xerosis usually causes diffuse pruritus and is common in the elderly and in patients who bathe frequently. The skin appears dry and may be cracked, although there is usually no erythema. *Eczema* is focal scaling skin, particularly on the hands and flexor surfaces such as the popliteal and antecubital fossae. *Scabies* may be associated with burrows in the interdigital web spaces and a papular rash, especially in the axillae, around the waistline, on the male genitals, or on the buttocks. Red, itchy papules or nodules on the penis are pathognomonic for scabies infection. Sometimes a tiny scabies mite may be seen by looking at burrow scrapings under a microscope. Scabies burrows appear as white lines on the skin typically 1 mm wide and <½ inch long. Patients with scabies may have affected family members and almost always have intense pruritus, often worse at night. If a therapeutic trial for xerosis fails, and scabies is not identified, consider a workup for a systemic illness with a CBC, renal tests, and LFTs to screen for renal failure, cholestatic liver disease, and polycythemia vera.

TREATMENT

What Treatments are Useful?

For dry skin, use moisturizers, minimize bathing, and avoid hot water and deodorant soaps. Use moisturizing soap sparingly and in essential areas only. Treat scabies with permethrin or lindane cream overnight to the whole body below the neck. Prescribe enough for the simultaneous treatment of all intimate contacts (don't use lindane in children), even if they are asymptomatic. Persistent egg capsules beneath the skin may cause itching to endure a week past the treatment of the infection. Repeated applications beyond once or twice may worsen skin irritation and pruritus owing to irritation from the medication. In the morning, patients should wash their bedding and any clothes worn the previous 2 days. Itching may occur for 1–2 weeks after treatment, but does not indicate treatment failure. A short course of prednisone may be indicated if the itching is very severe.

MACULOPAPULAR RASHES

ETIOLOGY

What are the Most Common Causes of Erythematous Macules or Papules In Adults?

Drug reactions and viral infections cause diffuse maculopapular rashes. A rash caused by a viral infection is referred to as a "viral exanthem." Scabies causes more localized papular eruptions, but may cause diffuse pruritus.

EVALUATION

How can I Distinguish Viral from Drug-Related Rashes?

Because drug reactions and viral exanthems cause a diffuse, truncal rash, the history best delineates the likely cause. If a new medication was recently started, particularly a sulfa antibiotic or penicillin, a drug reaction is likely. If viral symptoms are present, a viral exanthem is more likely. Scabies also may cause papules, often intensely pruritic and crusted because of scratching. Although occasionally scabies is widespread, it is usually localized to the wrists, axillae, waist, or male genitals.

TREATMENT

What is the Treatment for Maculopapular Rashes?

Viral exanthems resolve spontaneously. Drug reactions resolve with removal of the offending agent. See previous section for treatment of scabies.

SCALING RASHES

ETIOLOGY

What are the Most Common Scaling Rashes In Adults?

Psoriasis, eczema, seborrheic dermatitis, pityriasis rosea, and tinea infection are common causes of scaling rashes.

Dermatology

EVALUATION

How can I Tell these Conditions Apart?

The pattern of body sites involved is helpful (Figure 27-1). Besides distribution, the appearance of the border and the presence of scale are useful. Psoriasis causes well-circumscribed, raised, salmon-colored plaques with adherent silvery scales. Eczema is often pruritic and frequently occurs in "atopic" individuals who are prone to allergies and asthma. Eczema rashes are often symmetric, are erythematous, and may contain small vesicles or pustules. If eczema is long-standing, scaling and thickening (lichenification) can occur. Seborrhea is nonpruritic and has indistinct margins with fine, greasy, yellowish scales and mild erythema. Pityriasis rosea is a mysterious, self-limited rash with distinct, oval-shaped, hyperpigmented lesions, each with an inner scaling ring. These lesions are distributed in an evergreen tree pattern over the trunk. Tinea corporis causes distinct erythematous lesions with scaly borders, which usually are not symmetric. Tinea versicolor usually occurs on the chest, back, and arms. The lesions are pink to coffee-colored patches in patients who have had little sun exposure and hypopigmented spots in individuals who are tan or of darker skin tone. Hyphae on a KOH preparation of skin scrapings are diagnostic of tinea conditions.

TREATMENT

What Treatments are Useful for Scaling Rashes?

Scaling rashes are generally treated with topical steroids, antifungals, or both (Table 27-1). For eczema, further preventive measures include the following: avoid skin irritants such as wool, newspaper ink, citrus peels, strong soaps, and household chemicals; minimize scratching with antihistamines and keeping fingernails short; prevent skin dryness with

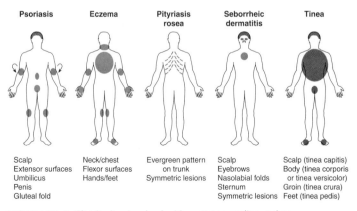

Psoriasis	Eczema	Pityriasis rosea	Seborrheic dermatitis	Tinea
Scalp	Neck/chest	Evergreen pattern on trunk	Scalp	Scalp (tinea capitis)
Extensor surfaces	Flexor surfaces	Symmetric lesions	Eyebrows	Body (tinea corporis or tinea versicolor)
Umbilicus	Hands/feet		Nasolabial folds	Groin (tinea crura)
Penis			Sternum	Feet (tinea pedis)
Gluteal fold			Symmetric lesions	

FIGURE 27-1 Classic sites involved with common scaling rashes.

Dermatology

Table 27-1	
Treatments for Scaling Rashes	
Cause of Scaling Rash	**Treatment**
Psoriasis	Coal tar lotion or shampoo, topical steroids (high to very high potency), sun exposure, UV light, methotrexate
Pityriasis rosea	Resolves without treatment after 2–8 weeks, antihistamines decrease itching
Seborrheic dermatitis	Selenium sulfide shampoo, steroid lotion (scalp), ketoconazole shampoo
Eczema	Topical steroids, moisturizer, irritant avoidance
Tinea	Antifungal cream

nonlanolin moisturizers, decreased bathing, and hot water avoidance. If eczema is secondarily infected with bacteria (e.g., impetigo), treat with antibiotics.

SKIN CANCERS

ETIOLOGY

What are the Main Types of Skin Cancer?

Melanoma is the most aggressive skin cancer. Associated with prior history of sunburns, it grows rapidly, metastasizes early, and can be deadly. Tissue depth of melanoma at the time of diagnosis determines prognosis. *Basal* and *squamous cell skin cancers* are slow-growing tumors associated with cumulative sun exposure, regardless of whether patients experienced actual sunburns. Although these skin cancers generally do not metastasize, they can invade and destroy local tissues if left untreated. *Actinic keratoses* are areas of mild atypia of the epidermis from chronic sun damage. They eventually can progress to squamous cell carcinoma, but the overall risk of progression is very small—<0.1% per year.

EVALUATION

How do I Recognize Skin Cancers?

Features that are concerning for melanoma are listed in Box 27-1. Basal cell carcinomas appear as shiny pink or pearly papules with telangiectasias. Squamous cell carcinoma is an indurated, yellowish plaque, often with scaling, erosions, or ulcerations. Actinic keratoses are usually more easily felt than seen, as a small patch of rough, adherent scale. Although melanoma can occur anywhere, the other three types of lesions generally occur on sun-exposed areas, especially the upper cheeks, below the eyes, on the ears, and around the nose.

Dermatology

BOX 27-1

FEATURES CONCERNING FOR MALIGNANT MELANOMA

A—asymmetry, especially a notched border
B—border irregularity, bleeding
C—color variation
D—diameter growing or >6 mm
E—elevation irregularity (e.g., a raised area within a macule)
F—feeling changes (e.g., new itching or burning)

How should a Suspicious Mole be Evaluated?

If there is a low suspicion for melanoma, small lesions can be removed with a punch biopsy. If there is concern for melanoma, excisional biopsy is indicated. Never perform a shave biopsy on a pigmented lesion because the depth of the lesion is crucial to prognosis if the lesion is a melanoma.

TREATMENT

Freeze actinic keratoses with liquid nitrogen. The lesions are so superficial that a single 10-second freeze is usually sufficient. Refer to dermatology for wider excision of malignant lesions.

VESICULAR LESIONS

ETIOLOGY

What are Common Causes of Vesicles?

Herpes zoster viruses reactivating as shingles, herpes simplex infection, and contact dermatitis are common causes of vesicles.

EVALUATION

How do I Distinguish Shingles from Herpes Simplex?

Shingles (or "zoster") is reactivation of dormant varicella zoster virus (the virus that causes chickenpox). Its dermatomal distribution, which typically does not cross the midline, clinches the diagnosis. Symptoms usually begin with painful burning along a single dermatome, followed by an outbreak of vesicles on an erythematous base in the same dermatome. Shingles occurs much more frequently in patients who are elderly or immunocompromised and is especially common in patients with HIV. Herpes simplex is usually sexually transmitted and causes vesicles and ulceration on the lips, in the mouth, or on the genitals; occasionally, herpes affects the fingers with weepy ulcerations, called herpetic

Dermatology

whitlow. To confirm the diagnosis of herpes simplex, obtain a sample of cells for viral culture from the base of an unroofed vesicle (rub firmly for an adequate sample).

What is PHN?

Post Herpetic Neuralgia (PHN) is pain occurring after shingles resolves. It may last a few weeks to 1 or 2 years in severe cases. The incidence and duration of PHN increase with age.

TREATMENT

How do I Treat Herpes Zoster and PHN?

Treat with 7 days of acyclovir (800 mg five times daily), famciclovir (500 mg three times daily), or valacyclovir (1 g three times daily). All are equally effective if taken in the correct dose. Valacyclovir and famciclovir are much more convenient to take, but more costly. Ideally, treatment for zoster should be started within 72 hours of symptom onset. These drugs shorten the time to healing and the duration of PHN, but they do not affect the incidence of PHN. Prednisone may decrease the acute pain, but has little to no effect on PHN and so should be used only when the acute rash is severe. All patients with active zoster should avoid coming into contact with pregnant women and individuals who do not have a history of chickenpox or varicella vaccination. Patients who have lesions on the forehead, on the nose, or around the eye and patients who have ocular symptoms should have urgent ophthalmologic evaluation to rule out corneal involvement. The pain of PHN may respond to TCAs, opioids, topical lidocaine, capsaicin cream, or gabapentin.

How do I Treat Herpes Simplex?

Outbreaks are self–limited, but may be shortened by 7 days of acyclovir (400 mg four times daily). Patients with frequent severe attacks can be given prophylactic acyclovir (400 mg twice daily). Lessen the risk of transmission by avoiding intimate contact with the involved area during outbreaks. Viral shedding occurs even without sores present, and daily suppressive therapy has been shown to reduce the risk of transmission.

KEY POINTS

◆ Scabies causes pruritic papules on the wrists, axillae, waist, and genitalia.

◆ Scaling rashes respond to either steroids or antifungals, depending on the cause.

◆ Pityriasis rosea is a benign, self-limited rash that has a characteristic evergreen tree pattern.

Dermatology

- Seborrhea is a common scaling rash on the face, which responds to low-potency steroids or antifungals.
- Psoriasis often responds to steroids, but, if severe, may require referral for nontopical therapy.
- Eczema management consists primarily of skin moisturizing and topical steroids.
- Zoster should be treated with antivirals to speed healing and shorten the course of PHN.
- Basal and squamous cell carcinomas almost never metastasize; excision halts local spread.

Case 27-1

A 28-year-old woman with allergic rhinitis and a history of childhood asthma reports an itchy rash on the flexor surfaces of her arms for 4 weeks. On exam, she has symmetric erythema on both antecubital fossae with significant excoriation and one area of associated yellowish crust.

    A. What is the most likely diagnosis?
    B. What do you make of the yellowish crusting?
    C. What would you recommend for treatment?

Case 27-2

A 62-year-old man has acute onset of facial pain followed by appearance of a rash on his forehead. His vision is normal. On exam, he has small red vesicles on his left forehead.

    A. What is the most likely diagnosis?
    B. What would you recommend for acute treatment?
    C. Is any other evaluation needed?

Case 27-3

A 52-year-old woman comes to the clinic because her husband has noticed a mole on her back that has grown recently. On exam, there is a 5-mm pigmented macular lesion just below the right scapula with a slightly irregular border.

    A. What other history and physical features should be noted?
    B. What is the main diagnostic concern?
    C. What is the next diagnostic step?

Dermatology

Case 27-4

An otherwise healthy, 25-year-old woman comes to the office with a pruritic rash that started on her lower extremities and is now diffuse. She began amoxicillin treatment 9 days ago for a sinus infection and still has 5 days left to complete the course. This patient has never been treated with a penicillin drug before. On physical exam, her vital signs are normal, and she has a diffuse macular and papular eruption

    A. What is the most likely cause of this eruption?
    B. What should you do to treat this patient?

Case Answers

27-1 A. *Learning objective:* **Recognize conditions associated with eczema and its typical distribution pattern.** This is a typical presentation of eczema. Some clues include young age, history of another "atopic" condition, and distribution of the rash on the flexor surfaces of the arms.

27-1 B. *Learning objective:* **Recognize the potential for secondary bacterial infection of an excoriated rash.** The yellow crusting is concerning for secondary bacterial infection. The appearance is similar to the "honey-crusting" seen with impetigo. Impetigo is usually caused by common skin flora, such as staphylococcal or streptococcal species.

27-1 C. *Learning objective:* **Design treatment for eczema with secondary bacterial infection.** The patient should first receive an antibiotic with activity against skin flora, such as cephalexin. Antihistamines may be added, especially at night, to minimize scratching. Keep fingernails short. When the infection has cleared, treat with a medium-potency topical steroid with liberal application of a lanolin-free moisturizer.

27-2 A. *Learning objective:* **Recognize the typical presentation of herpes zoster.** This is a typical presentation of herpes zoster. Clues are the patient's older age, the painful prodrome of the rash, and the rash's characteristic dermatomal distribution.

27-2 B. *Learning objective:* **Recognize the efficacy of antiviral therapy in the acute treatment of zoster.** Start immediate antiviral therapy with either oral acyclovir or valacyclovir to speed healing of the rash and to shorten the course of PHN, should it occur. Antivirals are more effective the sooner they are given. Efficacy is unclear if given >72 hours after the onset of symptoms.

27-2 C. *Learning objective:* **Recognize the risk of corneal involvement in facial zoster and the seriousness of this condition.** Because the patient has lesions on his forehead, he should be evaluated urgently by an ophthalmologist to rule out corneal involvement. If there are early signs of corneal lesions on careful exam, the patient should be given immediate high-dose intravenous acyclovir to prevent corneal scarring and possible blindness. Topical steroid drops and cycloplegics may be required if there is an associated uveitis.

27-3 A. *Learning objective:* **State the features of a suspicious mole.** In addition to noting the lesion's asymmetry, flatness, and size, ask whether the lesion has been itching or bleeding, and note whether it has any color variation. A complete exam also should include examination of the rest of the skin and whether regional lymph nodes are enlarged.

27-3 B. *Learning objective:* **Recognize a mole that is highly suspicious for melanoma.** The primary concern is for malignant melanoma. Whenever a patient notes that a pigmented lesion has been growing, especially if the borders are asymmetric, the suspicion for melanoma should be high.

27-3 C. *Learning objective:* **Design appropriate diagnostic evaluation of a highly suspicious mole.** Given the high clinical suspicion for melanoma, the most appropriate initial procedure should be definitive excision.

27-4 A. *Learning objective:* **Recognize a drug eruption.** This patient presents with a classic morbilliform rash and recent new drug exposure making this likely a drug-related eruption. When an individual has an initial exposure to a drug, it often takes 1–2 weeks before symptoms occur (the time necessary to develop a type IV hypersensitivity). The classic rapid response occurs only when a patient has been previously exposed to a drug.

27-4 B. *Learning objective:* **Be able to treat a drug eruption.** The most important treatment for a drug eruption is to stop the offending drug. This is often difficult in cases of polypharmacy, and a systematic approach should be used. Other treatments, including histamine blockers, topical antipuritics, and steroids, can be used for symptomatic relief.

Dermatology

USEFUL WEB SITE

Indiana University interactive site, where you can solve cases, and there are interesting cases with dermatology findings. http://erl.pathology.iupui.edu/cases/dermcases/dermcases.cfm

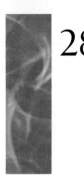

28

Endocrinology

TIMOTHY C. EVANS, DAWN E. DEWITT, KIM O'CONNOR, BRADLEY D. ANAWALT, and ANNE EACKER

 ADRENAL DISORDERS

ETIOLOGY

What Causes Adrenal Insufficiency?

The most critical adrenal insufficiency state results from cortisol loss. Adrenocortical insufficiency has three forms—primary, secondary, and tertiary. *Primary insufficiency*, also known as Addison's disease, is most often due to autoimmune destruction, sometimes in association with other glandular autoimmune disease—affecting thyroid, pancreatic islets, and ovaries. Adrenocortical destruction also may result from infections (tuberculosis, HIV, and several species of fungi) or hemorrhage (anticoagulants or meningococcemia). *Secondary adrenal insufficiency* is caused by decreased ACTH production secondary to disruption of pituitary function, most often in association with other pituitary hormone deficiencies.

What is Tertiary Adrenal Insufficiency?

The most common cause of adrenocortical insufficiency in the U.S. is *tertiary insufficiency* from exogenous glucocorticoid use, which suppresses hypothalamic-pituitary-adrenal function, but does not destroy those tissues. Prolonged suppression of endogenous cortisol production can result from 20 mg of predisone (or its equivalent) per day for several weeks. Prolonged corticosteroid treatment should be tapered slowly, rather than abruptly discontinued, and return of appropriate adrenal cortisol production should be documented before discontinuation. Clinical insufficiency also can occur in a patient taking corticosteroids despite the patient's usual steroid dose if there is great stress, and the suppressed adrenals are unable to respond. A 65-year-old woman on long-term, moderate-dose corticosteroids for RA who develops

268

BOX 28-1

CAUSES OF ADRENAL INSUFFICIENCY

Common Causes

Autoimmune disease
Steroid use*
Tuberculosis

Uncommon Causes

Bilateral adrenal hemorrhage
Fungal infection
CMV adrenalitis (AIDS patients)
Lymphoma
Metastatic cancer
Pituitary failure[†]

---

*Tertiary adrenal insufficiency.
[†]Secondary adrenal insufficiency.

pneumonia may present with hypotension and tachycardia when her adrenals are unable to respond to the need for greater cortisol production. Although she may be septic, this is also a common presentation for adrenal insufficiency. Causes of adrenocortical insufficiency are listed in Box 28-1.

What Types of Adrenal Excess are There?

All of the adrenal cortical and medullary hormones can be inappropriately excessive and result in specific clinical syndromes. Cushing's syndrome is a state of chronic glucocorticoid excess from any source. Long-term exogenous glucocorticoid use is the most common cause. Cushing's disease is caused by a pituitary adenoma secreting ACTH and is the second most common cause of adrenal excess. Less common are adrenal hyperplasia, adrenal adenoma, and ectopic ACTH production, usually from small cell lung cancer. Excess aldosterone may result from primary adrenal overproduction (adenoma or bilateral hyperplasia) or may be secondary to high renin states. Excess adrenal androgen production may result from adrenal carcinoma or congenital adrenal hyperplasia syndromes. Pheochromocytoma is an adrenal medullary tumor that overproduces the catecholamines epinephrine and norepinephrine.

EVALUATION

How does a Patient with Adrenal Insufficiency Present?

Except for the unusual instance of sudden adrenal destruction (e.g., bilateral hemorrhage), the onset of adrenal insufficiency symptoms is usually precipitated by the stress of another acute condition. In the ambulatory setting, a patient with chronic adrenal insufficiency presents with nonspecific chronic complaints, particularly fatigue, anorexia, vague abdominal complaints, arthralgias, myalgias, and episodes of volume depletion or hypotension. Think of this diagnosis in patients who make recurrent emergency department visits for abdominal pain and volume depletion. Patients feel much better after receiving intravenous saline. Acute adrenal insufficiency, or adrenal crisis, manifests with cardiovascular collapse mimicking sepsis (Table 28-1). With chronic primary adrenal failure, the compensating pituitary overproduces ACTH and a by-product, MSH, which results in diffuse hyperpigmentation accentuated in the palmar creases and gums. Patients with secondary or tertiary adrenal insufficiency resulting from pituitary failure or suppression usually present with similar fatigue, arthralgias, and myalgias,

Table 28-1

Presenting Signs and Symptoms of Adrenal Insufficiency and Cortisol Excess

	Adrenal Insufficiency	**Cortisol Excess (Cushing's Syndrome)**
Symptoms	Weakness and fatigue	Weakness and fatigue
	GI symptoms—anorexia, nausea, vomiting, abdominal pain, diarrhea	Psychiatric symptoms
		Easy bruising
	Dizziness	Amenorrhea
	Fever	Impotence
	Myalgias, arthralgias	
	Amenorrhea	
	Anxiety, irritability, confusion, depression, psychosis	
Signs	Hypotension/orthostasis*	Central obesity with thin extremities
	Weight loss	Facial plethora, moon face
	Hyperpigmentation*	Hypertension
		Hirsutism
		Acne
		Abdominal striae
		Edema
		Osteoporosis
Lab Test Results	Hyperkalemia*	Hypokalemia
	Nongap metabolic acidosis	Metabolic alkalosis
	Hyponatremia	Hyperglycemia
	Hypoglycemia	Leukocytosis, lymphocytopenia
	Eosinophilia, lymphocytosis, neutropenia	

*Occur with primary adrenal insufficiency, not in secondary or tertiary adrenal insufficiency, where mineralocorticoid levels are preserved and ACTH and MSH are suppressed.

Endocrinology

but the abdominal symptoms and hypotension are less prominent because mineralocorticoid production is preserved. Hypothyroidism and hypogonadism also may be present if there is panhypopituitarism. In that case, hyperpigmentation does not occur because the pituitary is producing neither ACTH nor MSH. Lab abnormalities are listed in Table 28-1.

How do I Diagnose Adrenal Insufficiency?

When there is a question of adrenal insufficiency, stimulation tests are combined with random cortisol to determine the adrenal reserve (unless a random cortisol is already known to be >20 μg/dL [>550 nmol/L]). After a basal cortisol blood draw, supraphysiologic synthetic ACTH (e.g., Cortrosyn, 0.25 mg intravenously) is administered, and a second serum cortisol is measured after 30–60 minutes. A serum cortisol >20 μg/dL (>550 nmol/L) at baseline or after stimulation rules out primary adrenal insufficiency. This test is less sensitive in patients with acute adrenal insufficiency (<1–2 weeks' duration) and patients with partial ACTH deficiency. For such patients, the low-dose (1 μg) ACTH stimulation test may be helpful. A serum ACTH level also may help to distinguish primary (high ACTH) from secondary (low ACTH) adrenal insufficiency. When established, the etiology of adrenal insufficiency may be pursued with visualization of adrenals and pituitary and skin tests. In suspected adrenal crisis, treatment should not be withheld while waiting for the cortisol results. Synthetic glucocorticoids, such as prednisone (but not dexamethasone), cross-react in the cortisol assay.

When should I Suspect Adrenal Excess?

Poorly controlled hypertension can arise from excess cortisol, aldosterone, or catecholamines. Screen for adrenal excess with careful history, physical, and electrolytes in young hypertensive patients, older patients with new-onset hypertension, and patients with difficult-to-control hypertension. Hypokalemia and metabolic alkalosis can occur with elevated cortisol or aldosterone. Additional clues to excess cortisol include a cushingoid appearance with central obesity, moon facies, purple striae, hirsutism, and proximal muscle wasting. Patients with Cushing's syndrome also may have glucose intolerance, osteoporosis, and psychiatric symptoms. Pheochromocytoma classically causes episodic severe hypertension, with associated sweating, tachycardia, and headaches. Pheochromocytomas occasionally are part of several familial MEN-2 syndromes.

How do I Diagnose Cushing's Syndrome?

Because the most common cause of Cushing's syndrome is administration of high-dose glucocorticoid, a thorough history is essential. Screening for endogenous cortisol excess is best accomplished by a 24-hour urine free cortisol (normal <100 μg/24 h [<275 nmol/24 h]). Levels >250 μg/day (>688 nmol/L) diagnose Cushing's syndrome; intermediate levels should be interpreted cautiously. Physiologically elevated cortisol or "false-positive" tests may occur in any state of stress, including any significant illness, depression, obesity, or alcoholism. Before searching for causes of Cushing's syndrome, it is crucial first to establish that there is unexplained inappropriate hypercortisolism. When endogenous hypercortisolism is established, the work-up turns to distinguishing pituitary ACTH, primary adrenal, or ectopic ACTH causes.

How do I Investigate for Hyperaldosteronism or Pheochromocytoma?

In patients with hypertension and hypokalemia or difficult-to-control hypertension, a serum aldosterone-to-renin ratio is used to screen for hyperaldosteronism. A high aldosterone in the setting of low renin strongly suggests primary hyperaldosteronism. If aldosterone and renin are elevated, renal artery stenosis may be the cause and warrants further evaluation. Screen for pheochromocytoma by 24-hour urine catecholamines, metanephrines, and vanillylmandelic acid. Subsequent evaluation of hyperaldosteronism or pheochromocytoma includes visualization studies.

TREATMENT

How do I Treat Adrenal Insufficiency?

In patients with suspected primary adrenal insufficiency and hemodynamic instability, give intravenous fluids and dexamethasone 4 mg intravenously immediately, which would not interfere with subsequent cortisol testing, or hydrocortisone 100 mg intravenously every 6–8 hours. Search for precipitating infection or other physical sources of stress. Maintenance therapy for chronic adrenal insufficiency is with hydrocortisone 15–20 mg in the morning and 5–10 mg in the late afternoon. For patients with primary adrenal insufficiency, mineralocorticoid also is replaced with fludrocortisone 0.1 mg daily. For minor illnesses, patients can be educated to take two to three times their maintenance glucocorticoid dose for 2–3 days and then return to maintenance. More serious illnesses may require higher stress doses up to maximal stress dose hydrocortisone, 100 mg intravenously every 6–8 hours, which is tapered as the patient stabilizes.

How do I Treat Adrenal Excess Syndromes?

When cortisol, aldosterone, or catecholamine excess is due to an adrenal tumor, surgical removal is indicated. This must be done carefully with pheochromocytoma; prepare preoperatively with alpha and beta blockade to block catecholamine bolus effects. Aldosterone excess secondary to bilateral adrenal hyperplasia can be treated with spironolactone therapy. Cushing's disease secondary to pituitary or ectopic ACTH production requires surgical removal of the source of ACTH.

Endocrinology

Case 28-1

A previously well 35-year-old man presents with muscle weakness and cough. He has a round face, purple abdominal striae, and thin arms and legs. His BP is 150/96 mm Hg, and fasting glucose is 119 mg/dL (6.6 mmol/L). He has gained 18 lb since his last clinic visit 1 year earlier.

A. What is a likely cause of his difficulty?
B. What is the screening test for this diagnosis?
C. What causes this problem?

Case 28-2

A 40-year-old woman has long-standing Hashimoto's thyroiditis treated with levothyroxine 0.112 mg daily. She presents with fever, weakness, anorexia, increased pigmentation of palmar creases, and BP of 98/64 mm Hg. Her TSH is 1.24 mU/L. CXR shows a right middle lobe infiltrate.

A. What diagnosis do you consider likely?
B. What is the screening test for this diagnosis?
C. What treatment would you administer?

Case 28-3

A 56-year-old man has long-standing hypertension, which has never been well controlled despite four antihypertensive agents. His BP is 160/102 mm Hg, and pulse is 76 beats/min. His exam is otherwise normal. Electrolytes are significant for potassium of 2.4 mEq/L.

A. What diagnosis would you consider?
B. How would you screen for this disorder?
C. What would be the treatment?

Answers appear on page 303.

DIABETES

ETIOLOGY

What is the Difference Between Type 1 and Type 2 Diabetes?

Diabetes is defined by insulin deficiency caused by inadequate production or insulin resistance. Inadequate insulin action results in high blood glucose. Type 1 diabetes results from a combination of genetic predisposition and an environmental trigger (e.g., viral infection), which causes autoimmune destruction of pancreatic islet beta cells. These patients are generally young and slender. In type 2 diabetes mellitus, insulin secretion is insufficient to overcome insulin resistance. Patients are usually obese and >30 years old. More cases are occurring in adolescents and young adults as the younger population becomes more obese.

What are the Risk Factors for Diabetes?

The major risk factor for type 1 diabetes mellitus is an affected identical twin. Risk factors for type 2 diabetes mellitus include prior gestational diabetes or newborn weight >9 lb, overweight, inactivity, race (Native American, Hispanic, African American, Asian American, or Pacific Islander), hypertension, family history (of type 2 diabetes mellitus), dyslipidemia, polycystic ovary syndrome (PCOS), and previous glucose intolerance. Many drugs increase insulin resistance, including steroids, thiazide diuretics, niacin, protease inhibitors, glucosamine, beta blockers, and atypical antipsychotics.

What is Diabetic Ketoacidosis (DKA)?

DKA occurs in type 1 diabetes mellitus when absolute insulin absence and lack of glucose usage causes accelerated starvation that forces the body to make ketones for fuel. Clinical features include hyperglycemia, elevated ketones, and anion-gap acidosis. Common precipitants include infection (50%) and lack of insulin.

What is Hyperosmolar Hyperglycemic Nonketotic Coma (HHNC)?

When patients with type 2 diabetes mellitus get extremely hyperglycemic, they become hyperosmolar. Ketoacidosis is uncommon because patients have enough insulin to prevent ketone production. High glucose draws free water out of cells and creates an osmotic diuresis, leading to dehydration and altered mental status. Many patients with HHNC are elderly and unable to drink enough fluids to compensate. Coma occurs in 10%; mortality is 10%-17%. Common precipitants include infection, heart attack, stroke, uremia, pancreatitis, and parenteral nutrition.

EVALUATION

How do I Diagnose Diabetes?

Diagnose diabetes by a single plasma glucose $\geq$200 mg/dL ($\geq$11.1 mmol/L) with symptoms (e.g., polydipsia, polyuria, polyphagia, or weight loss) or a fasting plasma glucose $\geq$126 mg/dL ($\geq$7 mmol/L) with confirmation by repeat testing. Glycosylated hemoglobin (hemoglobin A_{1c}) is not a criterion because it is insensitive and may be falsely low. Oral glucose tolerance testing is mainly used to screen for gestational diabetes.

Who should be Screened for Diabetes?

Patients often have impaired glucose tolerance and prediabetes for 10-12 years before diagnosis. The American Diabetes Association recommends screening individuals with one or more risk factors beginning

Endocrinology

at age 30. Screening includes risk factor evaluation and fasting plasma glucose. The ADA recommends checking a fasting glucose every 3 years in patients after the age of 45.

What is Prediabetes?

A fasting glucose 100–126 mg/dL is termed "impaired fasting glucose." Patients with impaired fasting glucose are at higher risk for development of diabetes. It should be viewed as a risk factor more than as a distinct disease entity.

How do Patients with Diabetes Present?

Patients <20 years old with type 1 diabetes mellitus may present abruptly with DKA precipitated by an acute stressor, such as a bacterial infection. Ketoacidosis may be accompanied by coma (in 10%), Kussmaul breathing (rapid deep breaths in response to acidosis), fruity breath from elevated acetone, dehydration, hypotension, and tachycardia. Many patients with type 1 diabetes mellitus present with more gradual onset of malaise, weight loss, polydipsia, polyuria, or blurred vision. Patients with type 2 diabetes mellitus commonly present either without obvious symptoms or with weeks to months of polyuria, polydipsia, weight loss, or symptoms of end-organ complications, such as altered vision (retinopathy), peripheral edema (nephropathy), or sensory changes in the distal extremities (neuropathy). Diabetes also can manifest with recurrent infections, such as boils, carbuncles, and vaginal yeast infections in women. Elderly patients with new-onset type 2 diabetes mellitus may present with life-threatening hyperosmolar coma.

After I have Made the Diagnosis, What Other Evaluation is Important?

At diagnosis, 10%-15% of patients with type 2 diabetes mellitus have neuropathy, 37% have retinopathy, and 50% have CAD. Pertinent history and physical (Table 28-2) and monitoring should be aimed at detecting complications (Table 28-3). Hemoglobin A_{1c} estimates average blood glucose over the prior 3 months. Obtain a baseline hemoglobin A_{1c}, and repeat every 6 months in patients who are stable at target and every 3 months in patients above target or who are changing therapy. Because patients with type 1 diabetes mellitus may have autoimmune destruction of other endocrine glands, check TSH.

What Tests are Appropriate for Patients with DKA or Hyperosmolar Coma?

Obtain electrolytes, renal function, ABG, CBC, and urinalysis. Look for a precipitating infection with blood and urine cultures and a CXR, even if the patient is afebrile. Elevated WBC (12,000–15,000), glucose >250 mg/dL (>14 mmol/L), elevated potassium owing to cellular shifts, and anion-gap acidosis with compensatory respiratory alkalosis are expected. Serum osmolarity >330 mOsm/kg can cause altered mental

Table 28-2

Pertinent History and Physical Findings in Patients with Diabetes

	History	Physical

New Diagnosis of Diabetes	Duration of symptoms
	Polyuria, polydipsia
	Current diet and exercise pattern
	Cardiovascular symptoms
	Cardiovascular risk factors
	Cigarette use
	  Cholesterol
	  Hypertension
	  Family history of cardiovascular disease
	  Family history of diabetes
	Vision disturbance
	Sensory changes in extremities
	Medications
		BP (assess cardiovascular risk)
		Weight and height for BMI
		Funduscopic exam (for retinopathy)
		Thyroid exam (concurrent autoimmune disease)
		Carotid, femoral, abdominal renal artery bruits (for atherosclerotic disease)
		Sensory exam with monofilament (neuropathy)
		Extremities for edema, ulcers
		Skin (fungal infections may provide portal of entry for cellulitis)
		Acanthosis nigricans

Periodic Follow-up	Hyperglycemia or hypoglycemia symptoms Glucose monitoring results Changes in vision Changes in foot sensation Daily self-exam of feet Medication tolerance Diet and exercise habits	Same as above

status. If the serum osmolarity is <330 mOsm/kg with altered mental status, or if mental status does not reverse after several hours of treatment, consider head CT and LP.

TREATMENT

What are the Goals of Treatment?

In the Diabetes Control and Complications Trial (DCCT), patients with type 1 diabetes mellitus treated with intensive therapy were 50%-75% less likely to have progression of retinopathy, nephropathy, and neuropathy than patients receiving conventional therapy. The goal of intensive treatment for type 1 diabetes is hemoglobin A_{1c} $\leq$6.5% (normal 4%-6%), with fasting glucose <110 mg/dL (<6.1 mmol/L) and 2-hour postprandial glucose <140 mg/dL (<7.8 mmol/L). A goal of hemoglobin A_{1c} <7% is now recommended for all patients. The best view of the guidelines is to get the hemoglobin A_{1c} as low as safely possible.

Table 28-3

Screening and Treatment for Complications of Diabetes

	Screening Test	Recommendation	Treatment
Retinopathy	Ophthalmology referral	Type 1: yearly beginning 5 y after diagnosis; at diagnosis if age >30 Type 2: yearly starting at diagnosis	Laser therapy
Nephropathy	Urine protein-to-creatinine ratio or 24-h urine (microalbuminuria = 30–300 mg/24 h)	Type 1: yearly beginning 5 y after diagnosis Type 2: yearly	ACEI Angiotensin receptor blocker BP control
Neuropathy	Foot exam: deformity, lesions, and sensory testing with 5.0 monofilament	Daily patient self-checks Foot exam at every visit Yearly sensory testing	TCAs Gabapentin Carbamazepine Capsaicin cream
Heart disease	ECG at diagnosis in patients with type 2; pursue cardiac testing if chest or respiratory complaints	Type 1: fasting lipids at diagnosis, then follow lipid screening guidelines Type 2: fasting lipids yearly	Lower lipids with statin to LDL <100 mg/dL (<2.6 mmol/L) Beta blockers post-MI
Gastroparesis	Ask about symptoms of early satiety, nausea, emesis	Upper GI series or nuclear medicine gastric emptying study	Metoclopramide Erythromycin

How do I Start Treatment in Patients with Newly Diagnosed Diabetes?

Diet, exercise, and self monitoring blood glucose (SMBG) are the foundation of treatment. Aggressively lower CAD risk with smoking cessation and treatment for elevated BP and hyperlipidemia. Glucose is best checked two to four times daily, before meals or before bed. Increased frequency of glucose monitoring is appropriate in patients with unstable readings. Patients with frequent hypoglycemia or severe hyperglycemia benefit from more frequent monitoring. Continuous glucose sensing monitors are available and can be an invaluable aid in tight glucose control. Type 1 patients require insulin. Type 2 patients may require oral medications or insulin. Educate patients about sweating, shaking, hunger, or confusion as signs of hypoglycemia and averting a reaction with candy (seven jelly beans) or other food. Careful glucose monitoring should accompany any change in regimen.

How do I Choose a Starting Dose of Insulin?

Patients with type 1 diabetes mellitus need multiple daily subcutaneous insulin injections: *rapid-acting* to cover meals (prandial) and *long-acting* for basal requirements. Numerous preparations are available (Table 28-4). Estimate total daily insulin dose by weight, starting at 0.5–1 U/kg/d. Type 1 patients and patients who have type 2 diabetes mellitus with little insulin resistance need less insulin. Basal (glargine and detemir) and prandial (lispro or aspart or glulisine) combination regimens give half of insulin as basal and the other half before meals based on premeal glucose level and anticipated intake. For less intensive therapy with two shots per day, many patients do well with premixed insulins (e.g., aspart 70/30 mix), although some patients need an additional injection of rapid insulin at lunch. If nighttime hypoglycemia is a problem, give NPH at bedtime and rapid insulin with dinner so that the peak effect coincides with the morning growth hormone and cortisol peaks that naturally increase blood glucose. Alternatively, insulin glargine, a 24-hour peakless basal insulin, causes less hypoglycemia than NPH.

Table 28-4				
Selected Human Insulin Formulations and Pharmacokinetics				
Insulin	**Action**	**Onset** **(= lag time*)**	**Peak (h)**	**Duration (h)**
Lispro (Humalog); Aspart (NovoLog)	Immediate	5–15 min	0.5–1.5	≤5
Regular (Humulin R)	Rapid	30–60 min	1–5	5–7
NPH (Humulin N)	Intermediate	3–4 h	6–12	18–28
70/30 premix (NovoLog Mix 70/30); 75/25 premix (Humalog mix 75/25)	70%/30% mix of intermediate and rapid	30–60 min rapid; 3–4 h intermediate	6–15	22–28
Glargine (Lantus)	Prolonged	2 h	No peak	24

*Lag time refers to the amount of time between an insulin injection and when a patient should eat. Lag time is approximately equal to onset of action (e.g., 30 minutes for regular insulin; little or no lag time with lispro or aspart).

When are Medications Necessary in Patients with Type 2 Diabetes?

Asymptomatic patients near ideal body weight, with no complications and hemoglobin A_{1c} <7% can be managed with diet and exercise. Patients who are symptomatic, have complications, and have a fasting glucose >300 mg/dL (>16.6 mmol/L) or hemoglobin A_{1c} >9%, diet and oral agents are usually not enough, so insulin is appropriate initial therapy. Most patients with type 2 diabetes mellitus require diet and an oral agent. Most type 2 diabetes mellitus patients need insulin after 8–10 years of diabetes.

Which Oral Agent Should I Use?

Multiple oral agents are available (Table 28-5). Nonobese patients who need more than dietary treatment should start with a sulfonylurea to stimulate pancreatic insulin secretion and decrease insulin resistance. Patients who are overweight or have high TG do well on metformin, which lowers lipids and doesn't cause the weight gain common with sulfonylureas and insulin. Metformin is absolutely or relatively contra-indicated in patients >80 years old, with CHF, with liver disease, with excessive alcohol use, and with increased creatinine (>1.4 mg/dL [>125 mmol/L] in women and >1.5 mg/dL [>133 mmol/L] in men) because of the risk of lactic acidosis. Metformin must be stopped temporarily in patients with sepsis, hypoxia, or dehydration and in patients undergoing surgery or procedures requiring intravenous contrast dye. Increase doses of oral medications weekly as needed. Oral agents lower hemoglobin A_{1c} 1%-2% except acarbose (0.5% reduction).

What Should I do if One Oral Agent is not Enough?

Many patients require combination therapy, either a sulfonylurea plus met-formin or an oral agent plus insulin. The combination of metformin and glyburide lowers hemoglobin A_{1c} about 3%. Thioglitazones (rosiglitazone and pioglitazone) also are available for combination use. They should be avoided in patients with CHF or with CAD. They also should not be used in patients with renal insufficiency. There is evidence for increased cardio-vascular events in patients who have received rosiglitazone. The major side effect of this class is the development of severe edema. If hemoglobin A_{1c} remains >7%, start 0.1 U/kg of NPH or insulin glargine at bedtime. Bedtime insulin decreases fasting glucose and causes less weight gain. Acute illness or medications such as prednisone can exacerbate hypergly-cemia, necessitating short-term insulin use. Bedtime insulin can be increased 2–4 U every 3 days until fasting glucose is consistently 80–110 mg/dL (4.5–6.2 mmol/L). Inhaled insulin is an option for patients who do not wish to use injectable insulin. Inhaled insulin is short-acting and is used at mealtime.

How can I Prevent Nephropathy and Renal Failure?

Slow the progression of nephropathy by controlling hypertension aggres-sively to BP <130/80 mm Hg. Use an ACEI when urine microalbumin is >30 mg/L (or per gram of creatinine or per 24 hours). Angiotensin

Table 28-5

Common Oral Agents Used to Treat Patients with Type 2 Diabetes

Drug (Example)	Primary Action	Major Side Effects	Can Be Used in Combination	Dose
Sulfonylureas (glyburide)	Increase pancreatic insulin secretion	Hypoglycemia, weight gain	Metformin, insulin	1.25–20 mg/d
Biguanides (metformin)	Decrease gluconeogenesis	GI intolerance, lactic acidosis	Sulfonylurea	1000–2550 mg/d; divide bid-tid
Meglitinides* (repaglinide)	Increase pancreatic insulin secretion	Hypoglycemia, weight gain	Metformin	0.5–4 mg before each meal
Thiazolidinediones (pioglitazone, rosiglitazone)	Increase uptake at the muscle	Edema, weight gain, CHF, possibly liver toxicity	Sulfonylurea, metformin, insulin	15–45 mg/d (pioglitazone); 2–8 mg/d (rosiglitazone)
Alpha glucosidase inhibitors (acarbose)	Slows down absorption	Intestinal gas, abdominal pain	Sulfonylurea, metformin	50–100 mg tid

*Repaglinide has shorter half-life, can be given with meals, and skipped when meals are skipped. Possibly less hypoglycemia, but more expensive than sulfonylureas.

receptor blockers are an appropriate option in patients who can't tolerate ACEIs. ACEIs cannot be used in pregnancy, or when they cause hyperkalemia or angioedema. Elevated creatinine alone should not prevent ACEI use because even patients with creatinine values of 3–4 may benefit. Patients with higher creatinine values are at increased risk for hyperkalemia. Monitor electrolytes and keep patients volume replete. Ensure that patients do not take potassium supplements. Beta blockers and thiazide diuretics are preferred choices for hypertension despite mild adverse effects on glycemic control and lipids, and patients with CAD gain greater benefit than harm from beta blockers.

How do I Adjust Therapy when Patients can't Eat?

When patients are ill or fasting for a procedure, adjust therapy to avoid hypoglycemia. Patients with type 2 diabetes mellitus can hold or decrease sulfonylurea doses and monitor glucose. Patients on metformin must stop this medication before procedures or surgery because of the small risk of lactic acidosis; restart after 48 hours if creatinine is stable. Patients with type 1 diabetes mellitus always need insulin, regardless of food intake, to prevent ketoacidosis. Because hepatic production accounts for about half of the serum glucose, give patients half their total 24-hour insulin dose in long-acting form (or half of one dose if taking twice-daily NPH), and monitor frequently. Alternatively, you may use an insulin drip.

How do I Treat Hypoglycemia?

Hypoglycemia is the most common endocrine emergency. Intensive therapy and decreased renal clearance of insulin or sulfonylureas are risk factors. Low serum glucose alters mental status and induces a catecholamine response (sweating, shakiness, weakness, nausea, and anxiety). Beta blockers blunt hypoglycemic symptoms except for sweating. Give oral glucose to conscious patients and intravenous glucose or glucagon to unconscious patients. Hospitalize the patient if he or she doesn't respond rapidly or if decreased renal clearance may cause recurrent symptoms.

When do I Need to Hospitalize Patients with Diabetes?

DKA, hyperosmolar coma, severe infections, severe nausea and vomiting, and cardiac ischemia are common reasons to hospitalize patients with diabetes. Cellulitis and foot ulcers often require intravenous antibiotics. Malignant otitis externa is an uncommon but life-threatening pseudomonal infection of the external ear canal that requires intravenous antibiotics. Other life-threatening infections seen with diabetes include rhinocerebral mucormycosis, emphysematous cholecystitis (*Escherichia coli* or *Clostridium*), emphysematous pyelonephritis (*E. coli* or other gram-negative rods), and necrotizing fasciitis (mixed anaerobes and aerobes).

A Patient with Diabetes is Hospitalized for Cellulitis. How Should I Manage the Glucose?

Good control in the hospital (<180 mg/dL [<10 mmol/L]) decreases hospital length of stay and mortality. Patients can be given their usual regimen if glucose remains controlled. "Supplemental" insulin (additional rapid insulin before meals for high glucose measurements) may be appropriate. "Sliding scale" insulin given for a high glucose level without anticipating caloric intake is unacceptable because of the risk of hypoglycemia. If the patient's glucose cannot be easily controlled by insulin injections, use an insulin drip, and give intravenous glucose if the patient is not eating.

How do I Treat Patients with DKA?

Patients with DKA usually require intensive care for aggressive hydration with normal saline, intravenous insulin, and electrolyte monitoring and replacement. Give regular or rapid insulin, bolus of 0.1 U/kg, followed by an insulin drip for at least 12–24 hours, with hourly monitoring and adjustments. Check potassium and phosphate because these are often depleted. Serum potassium levels may not reflect total body depletion because acidosis causes shift from cells to plasma. When the serum glucose is <180 mg/dL (<10 mmol/L), intravenous fluid can be changed to 5% dextrose in ½ normal saline to prevent hypoglycemia and provide calories and free water. Subcutaneous insulin can be resumed when bicarbonate normalizes, and the patient is eating. Continue the insulin drip at least 1 hour after the first subcutaneous injection to prevent recurrent ketone production. DVT prophylaxis and diagnosis and treatment of infections are important.

How do I Treat Patients with Hyperosmolar Coma?

Hydration with isotonic saline is the mainstay of therapy. Insulin may be needed in lower doses than for DKA (5–10 U bolus and 0.1 U/kg/h). As with DKA, look for and treat any precipitating infection.

Case 28-4

A 52-year-old man is referred to you for care of his type 2 diabetes. He was diagnosed 6 months ago after presenting with a random glucose of 220 mg/dL (12.3 mmol/L) and increased thirst, polyuria, and weight loss. He was started on glyburide and metformin, but has not had significant improvement in his symptoms. He has a daughter with type 1 diabetes. He has been well except for a long history of excessive alcohol intake and two hospitalizations for pancreatitis. On review of symptoms, he reports frequent, greasy stools. His exam is notable for a BMI of 19 and is otherwise normal except for mild epigastric tenderness. Glucose today is 300 mg/dL (16.6 mmol/L) and hemoglobin A$_{1c}$ is 10%.

   A. What type of diabetes is most likely in this patient?
   B. What tests would help you confirm an alternate diagnosis?
   C. How should you treat him now?

Case 28-5

A 42-year-old woman with type 2 diabetes diagnosed 10 years ago returns for care after a 2-year absence. She has not previously had complications documented, but is concerned about her feet feeling like they are "going to sleep." She does not smoke and has not had hypertension. Today, BMI is 29, and BP is 135/90 mm Hg. Rapid hemoglobin A_{1c} in the office is 9% on glyburide and metformin at maximum doses. Rapid test for microalbumin is positive.

    A. What other screening does this patient need for complications?
    B. What should be done about her microalbuminuria and BP?
    C. How would you address her elevated hemoglobin A_{1c} (poor control)?

HYPERLIPIDEMIA

ETIOLOGY

Why are Lipids Important?

Hyperlipidemia is associated with an increased risk for CAD, the leading cause of morbidity and mortality in the U.S. In particular, treating high levels of low-density lipoprotein (LDL) has been shown to reduce the risk of future CAD events. Depressed high-density lipoprotein (HDL) and elevated TG levels also are independently associated with increased risk of CAD events, although treatment of these isolated conditions has not been shown definitively to decrease the risk of future events. Very high TG levels (>1000 mg/dL [>11.3 mmol/L]) also can cause life-threatening pancreatitis.

What Causes Hyperlipidemia?

Although some lipid abnormalities are caused by known inborn errors of lipid metabolism, most lipid disorders arise from a combination of dietary factors, lack of exercise, and some degree of genetic susceptibility. Coexisting conditions and medications (Box 28-2) also may affect lipid levels.

EVALUATION

Whom should I Test for Hyperlipidemia?

Anyone with known CAD or CAD equivalents (diabetes, peripheral artery disease, abdominal aortic aneurysm, carotid disease) should be tested for hyperlipidemia. Controversy exists about when to screen individuals without known cardiovascular disease or CAD equivalents. The National Cholesterol Education Program (NCEP) currently recommends screening every 5 years in all adults >20 years old. The U.S. Preventive Services Task Force, which uses stricter requirements for the evidence on which they base their guidelines, recommends screening

BOX 28-2

SECONDARY CAUSES OF HYPERLIPIDEMIA

Chronic renal failure
Diabetes mellitus, uncontrolled
Drugs
    Corticosteroids, anabolic steroids
    Hormones—progestins, testosterone
    Atypical antipsychotics
    Protease inhibitors
    Thiazide diuretics, selective beta blockers
    Retinoic acid derivatives
    Immunosuppressives—cyclosporine
Hypothyroidism
Nephrotic syndrome
Obstructive liver disease
Obesity
PCOS
Smoking

men 35–65 years old and women 45–65 years old. A reasonable approach would be to begin screening at age 35 and earlier only if the patient has significant cardiovascular risk factors (Box 28-3) or a family history of hyperlipidemia. Screening is appropriate in adults >65 years old who have never been screened and have risk factors for CAD. Testing at an older age in low-risk individuals may be less important because lipid levels are less likely to increase after age 65, and there is no known benefit of primary prevention in the elderly.

BOX 28-3

**CARDIOVASCULAR RISK FACTORS BESIDES ELEVATED
LOW-DENSITY LIPOPROTEIN CHOLESTEROL***

Age (men ≥45 years old or women ≥55 years old)
Cigarette smoking
Diabetes mellitus
Family history of premature CAD
    CAD event in a first-degree male relative <55 years old
    CAD event in a first-degree female relative <65 years old
HDL <40 mg/dL[†]
Hypertension (BP ≥140/90 mm Hg or on medication)

---

*National Cholesterol Education Program guidelines.
[†]Note: HDL ≥60mg/dL counts as a negative risk factor.

What Tests are Available?

A complete lipid panel provides direct measurement of total cholesterol (TC), HDL, and TG and is measured after a 9- to12-hour fast, usually in the morning before breakfast. LDL is calculated based on the formula: LDL = TC − HDL − TG/5. You also may order isolated TC, TG, or HDL levels.

What Test Should I Use?

For screening purposes, measure nonfasting levels of TC and HDL for convenience and decreased expense. If the TC is ≥200 mg/dL (≥5.2 mmol/L) or the HDL is <40 mg/dL (<1.03 mmol/L), a complete fasting lipid panel is indicated. Obtain a fasting lipid panel to guide therapeutic decisions in any patient in whom treatment is possible or currently under way. When looking for causes of pancreatitis, an isolated TG level may be useful. In patients with elevated TG or elevated LDL, check a TSH and glucose before starting treatment for hyperlipidemia. Hypothyroidism and diabetes can increase lipid levels.

What Happens When the Lab Can't Calculate the LDL Level?

If the patient's TG level is >400 mg/dL (>4.5 mmol/L), the LDL cannot be accurately calculated. This is problematic because treatment guidelines are generally based on LDL levels. To circumvent this problem, you can assume the TG to be 400 mg/dL (4.5 mmol/L). This provides a conservative (high) estimate of LDL (LDL = TC − HDL − 400/5—i.e., 80) because TG level >400 mg/dL (>4.5 mmol/L) would subtract more from the LDL figure.

TREATMENT

How do I Decide Whom to Treat?

Treatment decisions are usually based on an estimation of the patient's overall risk of future CAD events and on the patient's LDL. Aggressive treatment is indicated for anyone with known CAD or CAD equivalents. The NCEP extends these guidelines to anyone with a calculated 10-year risk of CAD events ≥20%. For patients with less risk, treatment is less aggressive (Table 28-6). The 10-year risk of events can be calculated using a point system or computerized risk model. One example of such a risk calculator, based on the Framingham study, is provided on the National Heart, Lung, and Blood Institute web site (see web site reference at the end of the chapter). These risk assessment tools should be used for all patients with two or more risk factors.

Are Diet, Exercise, and Other Lifestyle Modifications Helpful?

A regular exercise program can lower LDL and TG levels and increase HDL levels. Eating a diet low in total fat (25%-35% of total calories) and saturated fats (<7% of total calories) and high in soluble fiber and plant stanols and sterols can decrease LDL levels by 5%-15%. Cohort

Table 28-6

National Cholesterol Education Program Guidelines (Simplified) for Treatment of Hypercholesterolemia

Patient's Cardiovascular Risk Factor Profile	Goal LDL (by Diet or Drugs)	Threshold LDL for Starting Drug Therapy
High risk: CAD, other atherosclerotic disease, diabetes mellitus, or 10-y risk >20%	<100 mg/dL (optional goal <70 mg/dL)	≥100 mg/dL
Moderately high risk: ≥2 risk factors and 10-y risk 10%-20%	<130 mg/dL	≥130 mg/dL
Moderate risk: ≥2 risk factors and 10-y risk <10%	<130 mg/dL	≥160 mg/dL
Lower risk: 0–1 risk factors	<160 mg/dL	≥190 mg/dL

studies suggest that numerous dietary modifications reduce cardiovascular risk; diet and exercise are recommended in all individuals with hyperlipidemia. Before starting medications, a 6- to 12-week trial of lifestyle modification, with or without referral to a dietitian, is often appropriate and can be sufficient to treat mild hyperlipidemia. Diet, exercise, weight loss, and alcohol restriction are first-line therapy for hypertriglyceridemia. A lipid-lowering medication should be started at the same time in high-risk patients with high LDL levels. If significant lifestyle changes are made, the need for long-term drug therapy can be reconsidered.

What Medications are used to Treat Hyperlipidemia?

Primary prevention studies have shown that cholesterol-lowering drug treatment for 5–7 years decreases risk of CAD by 30% in patients with high total cholesterol or average cholesterol and low HDL. Decreasing the risk of future cardiovascular events has been most clearly documented with HMG CoA reductase inhibitors (statins), and these should be considered first-line therapy in patients with known CAD, CAD equivalents, and elevated LDL. Some consideration may be given to cost, differing effects on the lipid profile, and side effects (Table 28-7) when choosing between other available agents; however, treatment is focused on reducing LDL levels, and this is done most efficiently with statins. The lowest cost statins are simvastatin, pravastatin and lovastatin. Side effects of statins include rare myopathy and generally insignificant liver enzyme elevations. The most common and frequently limiting side effect of statins is myalgias. For patients without known CAD who have high LDL and low HDL levels, niacin is a low-cost alternative. The flushing and headache associated with niacin can be attenuated by pretreatment with aspirin, slow upward dose titration, or use of extended-release formulations. Older extended-release niacin preparations were associated with hepatotoxicity; newer preparations seem to be safer.

Table 28-7

Lipid-Lowering Medications

Drug	Cost	Action	Side Effects
HMG CoA reductase inhibitors (statins)	$–$$$	LDL ↓↓ TG ↓ HDL ↑	Myalgias Elevated liver enzymes GI distress Headache, insomnia
Nicotinic acid (niacin)	$	LDL ↓ TG ↓↓ HDL ↑	Flushing, headache, tachycardia, pruritus Hyperuricemia Hyperglycemia Hepatotoxicity
Fibric acid (gemfibrozil) Fenofibrate	$ $$	LDL ↓ TG ↓↓ HDL ↑↑	Myopathy, small increased risk with statins, greatly increased risk with cyclosporine, erythromycin, and ketoconazole Gallstones Hepatotoxicity GI malignancy Nausea
Bile-acid sequestrants (colestipol, cholestyramine)	$$	LDL ↓ TG ↑ HDL —	Decreased absorption of many other medications GI distress, constipation
Cholesterol absorption inhibitors (ezetimibe)	$$$	LDL ↓↓ TG ↓ HDL ↓ LDL ↓↓↓ (in combination with statin)	Elevated liver enzymes when combined with statin Myalgias

In some patients who have extremely elevated TG or low HDL levels in the absence of elevated LDL, a fibric acid derivative, such as gemfibrozil, may be indicated. A fibric acid derivative is especially important in patients with TG >500 mg/dL (>5.6 mmol/L) because the short-term risk of pancreatitis from elevated triglycerides is high. Bile acid sequestrants also may be used, usually in combination with another agent, to lower LDL levels further. Both of these agents commonly cause some GI upset and may interfere with statin absorption. The newer agent, ezetimibe, a cholesterol absorption inhibitor, can be used as first-line therapy for patients who cannot tolerate statins. The addition of ezetimibe to a statin results in greater LDL reduction than with either agent alone. Studies on cardiovascular outcomes with ezetimibe are not yet available.

Are Treatment Goals the Same in Women?

Lipid-modifying drugs offer benefits to women comparable to the benefits seen in men. In women, HDL and TG levels are better predictors of CAD risk, however, than LDL or total cholesterol. Treatment regimens may need to extend beyond reaching LDL goals.

Is HRT a Reasonable Alternative for Treatment of Hyperlipidemia in Postmenopausal Women?

Although estrogen has been shown to decrease LDL and TG levels and to increase HDL levels, evidence from The Women's Health Initiative provides evidence that hormone replacement therapy (HRT) does not decrease the risk of cardiovascular events and can increase risk of cardiovascular and thromboembolic events. Estrogen (with or without progestin) should not be used for the treatment of hyperlipidemia. At this time, the only indication for HRT is severe hot flashes not controlled by other treatment modalities.

Are there Other Alternatives to Cholesterol-Lowering Medications?

Increasing dietary omega-3 fatty acids by consuming fish and fish oil (3 g/d or two fish meals weekly) has been shown to reduce total cholesterol, reduce TG, increase HDL, and decrease mortality. Soluble dietary fiber (found in legumes, oat bran, fruit, and psyllium) also has been associated with significant lowering of cholesterol levels. Mild-to-moderate consumption of alcohol (<1 oz/d = 2 oz whiskey, 8 oz wine, or 24 oz beer) is associated with increased HDL levels and reduced incidence of CAD. The potential harmful effects of excess alcohol ingestion preclude routine recommendations for its use in preventing CAD, however.

Are there any Other Ways to Decrease the Risk of Future CAD Events?

Assess and treat any other cardiovascular risk factors. Counsel patients to quit smoking, and aggressively treat hypertension and diabetes mellitus. These are well-established, effective ways of preventing CAD events.

Case 28-6

For each of the following cases, decide whether to test for hyperlipidemia, and which test you would order.

A. A 36-year-old man with no medical problems told by his wife to get a physical exam.

B. A 40-year-old woman with tobacco use and diabetes mellitus.

C. A 29-year-old healthy woman whose mother had a heart attack at age 60.

D. A 70-year-old healthy man with no history of tobacco use, CAD, diabetes, or peripheral vascular disease. He has never had cholesterol checked before.

E. A 30-year-old obese woman whom you follow in clinic for irregular periods and acne.

F. A 19-year-old athletic man here for a sports physical.

Case 28-7

A 58-year-old man has type 2 diabetes mellitus and hypertension. His fasting lipid and glucose panel is as follows: total cholesterol 265 mg/dL, TG 505 mg/dL, HDL 40 mg/dL, LDL "cannot be calculated." Glucose is 300 mg/dL (16.5 mmol/L). BP is 150/88 mm Hg.

    A. Calculate the LDL level assuming the TG level is 400 mg/dL (3.3 mmol/L). Is the actual LDL level higher or lower than this estimate?

    B. What is his target LDL?

    C. What therapy, if any would you recommend at this time?

Case 28-8

A 57-year-old overweight, postmenopausal woman with hypertension taking a hydrochlorothiazide diuretic, hypothyroidism, and occasional tobacco use is in the clinic for a preventive health visit. She does not exercise regularly. Fasting lipid panel is as follows: total cholesterol 212 mg/dL (5.5 mmol/dL), TG 220 mg/dL (2.5 mmol.L) (high), LDL 145 mg/dL (3.75 mmol/dL), HDL 39 mg/dL (1 mmol/L), TSH 3.2 (normal). BP is 122/70 mm Hg.

    A. She heard that hormones can help her cholesterol levels, and she wants to know if she should be on HRT?

    B. What is her target LDL, and would you start treatment?

    C. Modification of which risk factor would have the most impact on her CAD risk?

Answers appear on page 307.

MALE HYPOGONADISM

ETIOLOGY

What is Male Hypogonadism?

Male hypogonadism is a *syndrome* of low serum androgen levels associated with symptoms and signs of androgen deficiency, including sexual dysfunction, loss of sense of well-being, weakness, tender gynecomastia, sarcopenia (loss of muscle mass), and osteoporosis. Sometimes, hypogonadism is diagnosed in men whose serum testosterone levels are in the low-normal range at the time of diagnosis. These men may benefit from treatment because their serum testosterone level is below their normal baseline level. The male gonad has two important functions: production of sex steroid hormones and spermatogenesis. Men with deficient testosterone production inevitably have decreased or absent spermatogenesis and diminished fertility. Technically, an isolated defect in spermatogenesis is a form of male hypogonadism, but the term "hypogonadism" is normally used to denote testosterone deficiency.

Endocrinology

What are the Types of Male Hypogonadism?

Primary hypogonadism is defined as testosterone deficiency caused by a testicular defect. Secondary hypogonadism describes pituitary or hypothalamic dysfunction that results in decreased secretion of the gonadotropins, FSH, and LH; gonadotropin deficiency leads to defects in testosterone and sperm production.

What Causes Hypogonadism?

The most common cause of primary hypogonadism is Klinefelter's syndrome (1 in 800 live male births), a syndrome associated with very small testes and an XXY karyotype. Other causes of primary hypogonadism include postpubertal orchitis (mumps), bilateral orchiectomy, and testicular trauma (Table 28-8). Common causes of secondary hypogonadism include large pituitary tumors (macroadenomas), hyperprolactinemia, and hemochromatosis; hypogonadism is often the sole or first sign of these diseases. Supraphysiologic levels of glucocorticoids (either from endogenous hypersecretion or from exogenous administration) also suppress gonadotropin secretion and cause secondary hypogonadism. A rare congenital cause (1 in 10,000 male births) of secondary hypogonadism is Kallmann's syndrome, which is associated with inadequate secretion of gonadotropin-releasing hormone from the hypothalamus to the pituitary. Any severe chronic systemic illness, such as uremia and HIV disease, also may cause secondary hypogonadism, and many of these patients may benefit from androgen replacement therapy. Men who are hospitalized with any severe acute disease commonly have transient suppression of circulating gonadotropins and testosterone levels that normalize with resolution of the acute disease. Older men (>60 years old) often have low or low-normal serum testosterone levels. It is controversial whether these men have hypogonadism that would benefit from androgen replacement therapy.

Table 28-8

Common Causes of Primary and Secondary Hypogonadism

Cause	Distinguishing Features
Primary Hypogonadism	**Elevated gonadotropins**
Klinefelter's syndrome	Very small testes, XXY karyotype
Postpubertal mumps orchitis	History of postpubertal orchitis
Orchiectomy	No testes
Trauma	History of trauma
Secondary Hypogonadism	**Low or normal gonadotropins**
Hyperprolactinemia	May be due to medications
Pituitary macroadenoma	Headaches, visual complaints
Hemochromatosis	Early: arthralgias, hyperpigmented skin
	Late: liver failure, diabetes mellitus, heart failure
Cushing's syndrome	Easy bruisability; proximal muscle weakness

DIAGNOSIS

When should I Suspect Male Hypogonadism?

Male hypogonadism is a common disorder that is often undiagnosed for years after the onset because the symptoms and signs are often vague and nonspecific (Box 28-4). Hypogonadism should be suspected in men who complain of sexual dysfunction, weakness, or gynecomastia. Sexual dysfunction resulting from hypogonadism usually manifests as decreased libido and sexual pleasure; hypogonadism is seldom the sole cause of erectile dysfunction. All men with osteopenia or osteoporosis should be evaluated for hypogonadism. Hypogonadism also should be considered in men with unexplained hypoproliferative anemia.

What Tests should I Order to Make the Diagnosis of Hypogonadism?

When male hypogonadism is suspected, order serum total or calculated free and weakly bound testosterone levels plus serum FSH and LH levels. Testosterone is found in three circulating forms: free (unbound), weakly bound to albumin, and avidly bound to sex hormone–binding globulin (SHBG). Testosterone that is bound to albumin is thought to be bioavailable to tissues, but testosterone bound to SHBG is not thought to be bioavailable. Although there are commercial platform assays for free bioactive serum testosterone, these assays tend to under-estimate the true free testosterone levels and should not be used. Some laboratories offer an assay known as the "calculated free and weakly bound testosterone assay." This assay estimates serum free (unbound) and weakly bound (bound to albumin) testosterone levels based on a formula that uses the measured serum total testosterone, SHBG, and albumin levels. The calculated free and weakly bound testosterone assay

---

BOX 28-4

COMMON MANIFESTATIONS OF MALE HYPOGONADISM

Symptoms

Decreased sexual function (diminished libido)
Decreased energy
Diminished sense of well-being
Weakness
Tender gynecomastia
Infertility

Signs

Decreased rate of facial hair growth
Gynecomastia extending beyond areola
Small or soft testes (<3.5 cm in longest axis)
Atraumatic/osteoporotic fracture

has been shown to correlate well with "gold standard" assays (equilibrium dialysis and ammonium precipitation), and calculated free and weakly bound testosterone levels can be useful in the diagnosis of men with borderline low-normal testosterone levels or suspected abnormal SHBG levels (e.g., higher SHBG levels with aging or lower SHBG levels with diabetes and obesity). Serum FSH and LH levels are helpful in determining the etiology of the hypogonadism and can confirm hypogonadism in men with low-normal serum testosterone levels. In primary hypogonadism, serum FSH and LH levels are elevated even in men with low-normal serum testosterone levels. No further evaluation is necessary in primary hypogonadism, although a serum karyotype may be useful to confirm Klinefelter's syndrome. In secondary hypogonadism, serum testosterone levels are decreased, and serum FSH and LH levels are inappropriately normal or low. Measure serum prolactin in all patients with secondary hypogonadism; if elevated, investigate for causes of hyperprolactinemia. In all young men (<50 years old) with secondary hypogonadism and patients with extremely low testosterone levels and secondary hypogonadism, order a pituitary imaging study (CT or MRI) to exclude a pituitary macroadenoma. In patients with secondary hypogonadism, it also is reasonable to measure serum iron saturation or ferritin to exclude hemochromatosis. A careful history and physical exam for evidence of thin skin (easy bruisability and violaceous striae) and proximal muscle weakness is generally an adequate evaluation for Cushing's syndrome as the cause of secondary hypogonadism.

TREATMENT

How do I Treat Male Hypogonadism?

Treatment should address androgen replacement and fertility restoration. Androgen replacement should be considered for all hypogonadal men, but therapy to restore fertility is expensive and should be reserved for men with secondary hypogonadism who are attempting to conceive within the next 1–2 years. Men with primary hypogonadism are generally infertile and do not respond to medical therapy to improve fertility. Men with secondary hypogonadism might have improved fertility after normalization of FSH and LH levels by appropriate treatment with gonadotropin-releasing hormone or gonadotropin replacement therapy.

What Options are Available for Androgen Replacement Therapy?

Androgen replacement therapy may be safely and effectively accomplished with transdermal testosterone (a patch system or a gel), a buccal testosterone system, or intramuscular testosterone ester injections (Table 28-9). After intramuscular administration of testosterone, serum testosterone levels peak at 24–48 hours and gradually decrease until the next dose. Occasionally, men have difficulty with cyclic acne and moodiness around the time of the peak level after intramuscular testosterone injection.

Table 28-9

Forms of Androgen Replacement Therapy Available in the United States

Route	Frequency	Advantages	Disadvantages
Transdermal patch	Daily	Provides physiologic testosterone levels	Expensive Often causes a dermatitis Difficult to adjust dosage May not provide enough testosterone
Transdermal gel	Daily	Provides physiologic testosterone levels Easy to adjust dosage	Very expensive May rub off on to intimate contacts
Buccal testosterone	Twice daily	Provides variable testosterone levels Difficult to adjust dosage	May irritate gums Twice-daily administration inconvenient
Intramuscular testosterone enanthate or cypionate injection	Every 7–14 d	Inexpensive if self-injected (or injected by friend) Relatively easy to adjust dosage	Supraphysiologic testosterone levels for 2–3 d postinjection Requires injections

What are the Risks and Benefits of Androgen Replacement Therapy?

Androgen replacement therapy has been shown to improve sexual function and sense of well-being and increase strength and bone mass in hypogonadal men. The most common side effect of androgen replacement therapy is erythrocytosis, and a hematocrit must be checked after initiation of therapy, an increase in dosage, and periodically thereafter (at least annually). Overall, the data suggest that there is a neutral effect or a small benefit to cardiovascular risk factors, such as LDL, visceral adiposity, and coronary endothelial function, when hypogonadal men take androgen replacement therapy. There is no evidence that androgen replacement therapy increases the risk of prostate disease, but hypogonadal men >45–50 years old should be offered counseling and screening for prostate disease. Most experts recommend an annual serum PSA in all men >50 years old who are taking testosterone therapy.

Case 28-9

A 32-year-old man reports painful, enlarged breast tissue. He and his wife have had difficulty conceiving. His physical examination is unremarkable except that he has tender gynecomastia that extends beyond both areolae, and he has small testes. His serum testosterone level is low, and his serum gonadotropins are elevated.

    A. What type of hypogonadism does he have?
    B. What it the most likely diagnosis?
    C. What is the treatment?

Case 28-10

A 42-year-old man reports fatigue, decreased energy, and diminished sex drive. He has recently started taking a beta blocker for treatment of hypertension. His serum testosterone level is low, and his gonadotropin levels are normal.

    A. What is the differential diagnosis?
    B. What further diagnostic studies should be done?

Answers appear on page 307.

THYROID DISEASE

ETIOLOGY

What are the Most Likely Causes of Hypothyroidism?

In >95% of patients, hypothyroidism is due to thyroid gland failure or removal. *Iatrogenic hypothyroidism* from ablation, irradiation, or removal of the thyroid gland is the most common cause in developed nations. *Iodine deficiency* is the most common cause worldwide. If iodine is plentiful and the thyroid intact, *autoimmune (Hashimoto's) thyroiditis* can develop with antithyroid antibodies. It may coexist with other autoimmune disorders, such as type 1 diabetes, pernicious anemia, vitiligo, and polyendocrine failure syndromes. The drugs *amiodarone, lithium,* and *interferon* can cause hypothyroidism. Less than 5% of hypothyroidism is secondary, usually due to *pituitary failure.* This diagnosis is important to make because giving thyroid hormone without cortisol replacement can precipitate fatal adrenal crisis.

What are the Most Likely Causes of Hyperthyroidism?

Sixty percent to 80% of hyperthyroidism is due to *Graves' disease,* from an antibody that stimulates the TSH receptor. *Excessive thyroid hormone replacement* commonly causes hyperthyroidism. Occasionally, patients take thyroid hormone surreptitiously to lose weight and present with hyperthyroidism. *Toxic multinodular goiter* accounts for 5% of cases and is typically seen in patients >50 years old. Two types of thyroiditis, *subacute (granulomatous) thyroiditis* and *lymphocytic thyroiditis,* may have periods of transient hyperthyroidism and hypothyroidism. *Subacute thyroiditis* is likely viral and characterized by pain, fever, and elevated ESR; *lymphocytic thyroiditis* is likely a variant of autoimmune thyroiditis and occurs often in the postpartum period. Less common causes include *iodinated contrast material* or *excess iodine in the diet,* especially if the patient is iodine deficient or has pre-existing multinodular goiter.

What Causes Thyroid Nodules?

Although thyroid nodules can be palpated in only 5% of patients, autopsies show 50% prevalence. Of clinically recognized nodules, 80% are due to colloid nodules, cysts, and thyroiditis. Fifteen percent are due to benign follicular neoplasms. About 5% of solitary thyroid nodules are malignant, >90% from papillary or follicular carcinoma—well-differentiated, slow-growing, and curable when found early. Of thyroid cancers, 5% are due to medullary thyroid carcinoma, which is usually sporadic, but may be inherited, sometimes as part of MEN-2. Lymphoma occasionally complicates Hashimoto's thyroiditis. Anaplastic thyroid carcinoma is rare, but particularly aggressive with average survival of 3–7 months. Risk factors for thyroid malignancy are listed in Box 28-5.

EVALUATION

What Questions are Pertinent if I Suspect Hyperthyroidism?

Symptoms of hyperthyroidism are due to action of excess thyroid hormone in the cell and enhanced beta-adrenergic activity. Ask about

---

BOX 28-5

RISK FACTORS FOR THYROID MALIGNANCY IN PATIENT WITH SOLITARY THYROID NODULE

History

Family history of medullary thyroid carcinoma or MEN-2
History of head and neck irradiation

Physical

Very firm nodule
Nodule >4 cm in size
Fixation of nodule
Associated lymphadenopathy
Hoarseness

weight loss despite a healthy appetite, nervousness, anxiety, excessive sweating, palpitations, heat intolerance, and altered menses (although amenorrhea is rare). Elderly patients may have a less obvious presentation and complain of "apathetic" symptoms, such as anorexia, weakness, and slowed mentation. In older patients, heart failure, angina, or arrhythmias may be precipitated or worsened by thyroid disease, so obtain a good cardiopulmonary review of systems (Box 28–6).

What should I Look for on Exam When I Suspect Hyperthyroidism?

Clinical findings almost always include tachycardia; warm, moist, "velvety" skin from excess sweating; an enlarged thyroid; and a fine tremor. Palpation of the thyroid may reveal diffuse enlargement in Graves' disease; multiple nodules in multinodular goiter; or a tender, firm gland in viral thyroiditis. With auscultation, a bruit may be heard over the thyroid gland. Check for signs of sympathetic overstimulation, including tachycardia, arrhythmias, hyperreflexia, lid retraction causing stare, and *lid lag* on oculomotor testing (white sclera visible above the iris with downward gaze); these all reverse with treatment. Findings specific to Graves' disease include *exophthalmos* (protrusion of the eyeballs or extraocular muscle impairment) owing to retro-orbital infiltration and inflammation of eye muscles, which does not reverse with antithyroid

---

BOX 28-6

SYMPTOMS AND SIGNS OF HYPERTHYROIDISM

Symptoms

Diarrhea, frequent stools
Fatigue, insomnia
Menstrual irregularities
Nervousness, irritability
Palpitations
Sweating, heat intolerance
Tremor
Weakness
Weight loss

Signs

Abnormal thyroid gland exam
Cardiac findings—tachycardia, atrial fibrillation, CHF, hypertension
Lid lag (all causes)
Pretibial myxedema (Graves' disease only)
Proptosis (Graves' disease only)
Proximal muscle weakness

therapy, and *pretibial myxedema* (localized indurated nonpitting edema) seen on the anterior shins.

What History and Physical Findings Suggest Hypothyroidism?

Onset is usually insidious in primary hypothyroidism, so patients and physicians may overlook symptoms. Hypothyroid patients often are fatigued, but most fatigued patients do not have hypothyroidism. Slowing of metabolic processes may cause cold intolerance, altered menses, constipation, or weight gain. Dry skin, hoarseness, and hair changes may be due to accumulation of glycosaminoglycans. Infiltration of glycosaminoglycans into the muscle can cause muscle pain and stiffness. Patients with multiple new symptoms of recent onset are much more likely to have hypothyroidism. It is likely that there would be no abnormalities on exam, especially early in the course of hypothyroidism. Look for hypothermia; bradycardia; pale, cool, doughy skin; pitting edema in the lower extremities; periorbital edema; macroglossia; decreased breath sounds suggesting pleural effusion; or distant heart sounds suggesting pericardial effusion. Neurologic manifestations include impaired mentation, dementia, ataxia, psychosis, carpal tunnel syndrome, "hung-up" reflexes with a delayed relaxation phase, or bradykinesia (Box 28-7). (See "When should I Hospitalize a Patient for Thyroid Disease?")

BOX 28-7

SYMPTOMS AND SIGNS OF HYPOTHYROIDISM

Symptoms

Coarse hair
Cold intolerance
Constipation
Dry skin
Fatigue, hypersomnolence
Hoarseness
Impaired mentation, depressed mood
Menstrual irregularities
Peripheral and periorbital edema
Weakness, myalgias, muscle cramps
Weight gain

Signs

Altered mental status, coma, depression, psychosis
Bradycardia, hypotension, CHF
Edema
Pericardial effusion
Pleural effusion
Reflexes with a delayed relaxation phase

What Studies do I Order if I Suspect Hypothyroidism or Hyperthyroidism?

Order a TSH. If the TSH is abnormal, repeat the TSH, and check a free T_4. Hypothyroidism or hyperthyroidism may be associated with numerous other lab abnormalities, but no other lab studies are necessary initially. In hypothyroid patients, you may find normocytic anemia, hypercholesterolemia, elevated CK, or hyponatremia. In hyperthyroidism, there may be mildly elevated transaminases or elevated calcium from increased bone turnover. ECG may show bradycardia with hypothyroidism or tachyarrhythmia (often atrial fibrillation) with hyperthyroidism.

What does it Mean if My Patient has an Elevated TSH?

TSH cannot be interpreted alone. The most common cause of an elevated TSH is an underactive thyroid gland (primary hypothyroidism). A reduced free T_4 confirms this. If free T_4 is in the normal range, and the patient is asymptomatic, subclinical hypothyroidism is present. TSH is sensitive to small changes in T_4, and it increases before a decrease in T_4 is detected. In rare cases, free T_4 and TSH are elevated, implicating a TSH-producing pituitary or gynecologic tumor and associated hyperthyroidism (secondary).

Does a Reduced TSH Imply Primary Hyperthyroidism?

A reduced TSH usually implies primary hyperthyroidism, and this is confirmed by the clinical picture and a high free T_4. If the TSH is low, but the free T_4 is in the normal range, subclinical hyperthyroidism is likely present. In hospitalized patients, a suppressed TSH may reflect the *euthyroid sick syndrome*. Unless there are signs and symptoms of hyperthyroidism or an elevated free T_4, the abnormalities should be rechecked after hospitalization rather than treated. In the rare instance where TSH and free T_4 are reduced, and hypothyroid symptoms are present, secondary hypothyroidism from pituitary failure owing to adenoma, surgery, or radiation is likely.

When do I need to Check a Free T_3?

T_4 is the inactive form of hormone produced in the thyroid, which is converted to active T_3 in the periphery. If TSH is low in the setting of hyperthyroid symptoms, but free T_4 is normal or low, obtain free T_3 to look for *T_3 toxicosis*, which occurs only rarely.

When do I need to Check Antithyroid Antibodies?

In general, it is unnecessary to check antithyroid antibodies. Most Hashimoto's and many Graves' disease patients have thyroid peroxidase (TPO) or antithyroglobulin antibodies or both. Patients with Graves' disease also may have thyroid receptor antibodies. Usually the diagnosis can be made without these measures. There are a couple of situations in which specific antibody testing might be useful. In subclinical hypothyroidism (asymptomatic patient with elevated TSH, normal free T_4), the presence of TPO antibodies greatly increases the likelihood of progression to overt hypothyroidism, and in postpartum thyroiditis, TPO antibodies increase the likelihood of persistent hypothyroidism. These patients are often treated with levothyroxine. Patients with Graves' disease may present with ophthalmopathy (exophthalmos) without overt hyperthyroidism. The presence of thyroid-receptor (thyroid-stimulating immunoglobulin) antibodies obviates the need for further work-up for retro-orbital mass or vascular lesion.

How do I tell the Difference Between a Malignant and Benign Thyroid Nodule?

FNA is the initial evaluation of choice for any patient with a clinically palpable nodule. It yields a benign diagnosis in 70%-80% of patients and a malignant diagnosis in 5%. The remaining 10%-20% of biopsy specimens are nondiagnostic. In 10% of them, the TSH is suppressed, and surgery can be avoided if a radioactive iodine scan shows a "hot" nodule (takes up radiolabeled iodine) because this is unlikely to be malignant. In the remaining nondiagnostic biopsy specimens, surgical exploration of the thyroid is usually necessary because 2 of 10 would be malignant.

TREATMENT

What are the Options for Treatment of Hyperthyroid Patients?

Initial medications for symptom management include *propranolol* to block sympathetic stimulation and decrease tremor, palpitations, and tachycardia. In Graves' disease or toxic multinodular goiter, antithyroid medications *PTU* and *methimazole* decrease thyroid hormone production and release. Methimazole is used most frequently because it works more quickly and is dosed once daily, but PTU is considered to be safest in pregnancy. Although most patients achieve a euthyroid state after 6 weeks with one of these agents, 35%-40% with Graves' disease relapse eventually when the medication is stopped. Both agents can cause agranulocytosis, so patients should be evaluated urgently if any fever or pharyngitis symptoms arise.

Radioiodine ablation is effective for Graves' disease and is the treatment of choice for multinodular goiter and solitary adenoma, but leads to iatrogenic hypothyroidism in most patients. It is contraindicated in pregnancy. Check TSH periodically after ablation, and treat if indicated. If the patient has significant exophthalmos, preradiation steroids and ophthalmology referral should be considered because radiation may irreversibly worsen the condition.

Surgical removal of the thyroid gland is reserved for severe local compressive symptoms, failure of or contraindication to other therapies (pregnancy and radioactive iodine), retrosternal extension of an enlarged thyroid gland, or possible malignancy. In acute thyroiditis, NSAIDs are first-line therapy. *Glucocorticoids* shorten the course and decrease thyroid pain, but are rarely needed. Consider bone density testing in patients with prolonged hyperthyroidism, particularly if iatrogenic, to assess for bone loss.

How do I Treat Hypothyroid Patients?

Start clearly hypothyroid patients (elevated TSH, reduced free T_4) on oral thyroxine at around 100 µg/d. Titrate dose up slowly from 25 µg/d if the patient is elderly or has known cardiovascular disease to prevent precipitation of angina or MI. Asymptomatic patients with subclinical hypothyroidism (normal free T_4 and mildly elevated TSH) can be followed without therapy, although patients may feel better if treated with low-dose thyroxine. Thyroid hormone should not be taken at the same time as vitamins, calcium, or iron because all of these can bind the thyroid hormone and make it not be absorbed. TSH takes 4–6 weeks to reflect changes in thyroid hormone replacement. Aim for a TSH in the middle of the normal range.

When should I Hospitalize a Patient for Thyroid Disease?

Hypothyroid myxedema coma is an endocrine emergency with high mortality even with intensive therapy. Patients present with stupor and possibly coma, hypothermia, bradycardia, heart failure, or hypoventilation. It may develop insidiously or be precipitated by infection, sedative drugs, or failure to take thyroid replacement. There may be associated coagulopathy, hyponatremia (from SIADH), or adrenal insufficiency. This is the only indication for parenteral levothyroxine, along with high-dose glucocorticoids to prevent adrenal crisis, and intensive supportive therapy, particularly vigilance for infection. Life-threatening hyperthyroidism, or thyroid storm, also requires hospitalization for supportive therapy and initiation of antithyroid drugs, including iodine to inhibit hormone release, beta blockers to decrease adrenergic effects and block peripheral conversion of T_4 to T_3, and possibly glucocorticoids. Iopanoic acid or ipodate (radiographic contrast agents) can be added to block hormone release and decrease peripheral T_4 to T_3 conversion.

Case 28-11

A 45-year-old woman reports fatigue and weight gain. Her menstrual cycles are with increased flow, but less regular than when she was younger. She reports a family history of "thyroid problems." On exam, her vital signs are normal except she is mildly overweight; thyroid is nonpalpable.

A. What is your differential diagnosis for her fatigue?
B. Her TSH is 7.1. On repeat testing, her TSH is 6.2, and her free T_4 is normal at 1. What thyroid condition is present?
C. Are there any further tests that might be useful to you?
D. What is your management plan?

Endocrinology

Case 28-12

A 60-year-old man presents for his annual exam. He has no significant past medical history. On exam, there is a firm, 1-cm nodule in the right lobe of his thyroid, which you have not noted previously.

A. What further history is important to obtain?
B. What is the appropriate management?
C. Evaluation reveals no concerning findings. At his annual exam 1 year later, he asks if additional testing is necessary. When you examine his neck, there has been no interval change. What do you recommend?

Case 28-13

A 20-year-old woman presents to establish care, reporting increased anxiety. She has had difficulty sleeping for the last several weeks. She is most concerned about irrational thoughts that the police are following her. She has no significant past medical or family history. On exam, her pulse is 105 beats/min, and BP is normal. Her extraocular muscles are intact, but the sclera are visible above and below her iris when she looks at you. Her thyroid seems enlarged diffusely, but nontender. Cardiac exam is regular, but with tachycardia. Extension of her arms reveals a fine tremor.

A. What is your differential diagnosis for her paranoia?
B. Her TSH is undetectable, and her free T_4 is 2.1. What is the diagnosis?
C. What is the likely cause? What exam findings are specific for this diagnosis?
D. What are the next steps in her management?
E. Are there any other lab tests that might be abnormal?

Answers appear on page 309.

Answers appear on page 309.

KEY POINTS – ADRENAL DISORDERS

◆ Adrenal insufficiency is most commonly the tertiary form, resulting from glucocorticoid use.

◆ Patients who look septic might have adrenal insufficiency.

◆ Think of adrenal insufficiency in patients with recurrent episodes of abdominal pain and volume depletion.

◆ If you suspect adrenal crisis, do not wait for test results—give hydrocortisone or dexamethasone immediately.

◆ Hyperpigmentation, hypotension, and hyperkalemia occur with primary, but not secondary or tertiary, adrenal insufficiency.

(continued)

♦ Consider hyperaldosteronism, Cushing's syndrome, and pheochromocytoma in patients with poorly controlled hypertension.

♦ Suspect cortisol excess in patients with hypertension, diabetes, central obesity, hypokalemia, and characteristic physical findings.

KEY POINTS – DIABETES

♦ Type 1 diabetes mellitus is caused by autoimmune-induced absolute insulin deficiency.

♦ Type 2 diabetes mellitus is caused by relative insulin deficiency and insulin resistance.

♦ Diagnose diabetes by two fasting glucose values >126 mg/dL (>7 mmol/L), or a random glucose >200 mg/dL (>11.1 mmol/L) plus symptoms.

♦ Patients with type 1 diabetes mellitus require insulin to avoid DKA; intensive therapy reduces complications.

♦ Therapy for type 2 diabetes mellitus begins with diet and exercise; oral agents and insulin are often required to optimize glucose levels and prevent complications.

KEY POINTS – HYPERLIPIDEMIA

♦ Screen otherwise healthy patients with nonfasting total cholesterol and HDL.

♦ Recognize CAD equivalents.

♦ Treatment goals should be commensurate with estimated future risk of CAD events.

♦ Statins prevent death and cardiovascular events in patients with known CAD.

KEY POINTS – MALE HYPOGONADISM

♦ Hypogonadism should be excluded in all men with sexual dysfunction, osteoporosis, unexplained weakness, unexplained anemia, or symptomatic gynecomastia.

Endocrinology

◆ It is important to distinguish between primary hypogonadism (with elevated serum gonadotropins) and secondary hypogonadism (with low or inappropriately normal serum gonadotropins).

◆ Hyperprolactinemia, pituitary macroadenoma, hemochromatosis, and Cushing's syndrome are the most common causes of secondary hypogonadism.

KEY POINTS – THYROID DISEASE

◆ When TSH and free T_4 are abnormal in opposite directions, there is a primary thyroid problem.

◆ TSH is very sensitive—small changes in T_4 cause large changes in TSH.

◆ TSH levels lag behind dosage changes by about 4–6 weeks.

◆ In the elderly or in patients with coronary artery disease, start with low-dose replacement.

◆ The procedure of choice for the initial work-up of a thyroid nodule is FNA.

Case Answers

28-1 A. *Learning objective:* **Recognize the clinical presentation of Cushing's syndrome.** This patient has a classic clinical presentation of Cushing's syndrome. The most common manifestations of Cushing's syndrome are centripetal obesity with purple abdominal striae, facial plethora, glucose intolerance or overt diabetes, weakness, hypertension, psychological changes, and easy bruising.

28-1 B. *Learning objective:* **Choose the correct screening test for Cushing's syndrome.** The best screening test is the 24-hour urine free cortisol. An alternative for patients unable to collect a 24-hour urine sample accurately is the 1-mg overnight dexamethasone suppression test, in which 1 mg of dexamethasone is given between 11 pm and midnight. Serum cortisol is checked the next morning at 8 am and should be suppressed to <5 g/dL (<138 nmol/L). Whatever test is used, remember that any acute illness or stress leads to an appropriate increase in cortisol. Elevation of the urine or serum cortisol must be evaluated in the context of the clinical situation.

28-1 C. *Learning objective:* **Distinguish exogenous and endogenous Cushing's syndrome, and identify causes of the latter.** Most Cushing's syndrome is a result of exogenous glucocorticoid administration. In the absence of that history, the most common cause of endogenous Cushing's syndrome is pituitary ACTH-producing adenoma. Less common are primary adrenal overproduction or ectopic ACTH production.

28-2 A. *Learning objective:* **Recognize the clinical presentation of adrenal insufficiency.** This presentation suggests adrenal insufficiency. It is likely to be primary insufficiency because of the hypotension and increased pigmentation, the latter resulting from increased MSH associated with increased pituitary ACTH production. The etiology in this case is probably autoimmune adrenalitis considering the patient's associated autoimmune thyroiditis. The clinical syndrome was probably precipitated by pneumonia because she needs increased stress levels of cortisol in this circumstance. Although the CXR is not suggestive, consider TB as a possible cause of the adrenal insufficiency.

28-2 B. *Learning objective:* **Identify the screening test for adrenal insufficiency.** In the setting of acute illness, such as pneumonia, the adrenal should normally produce stress levels of cortisol resulting in a serum level >20 μg/dL (>550 nmol/L). The random cortisol should be followed by a second serum cortisol level drawn 30–60 minutes after ACTH administration, 0.25 mg intravenously, to confirm adequate adrenal reserve in the event the baseline was not >20 μg/dL (>550 nmol/L).

28-2 C. *Learning objective:* **Describe acute and long-term replacement of adrenocortical steroids.** For acutely ill, hypotensive patients with adrenocortical insufficiency, intravenous fluids and full stress doses of glucocorticoid should be administered: hydrocortisone, 100 mg intravenously every 6-8 hours. This can be tapered to maintenance dose as the patient is stabilized, and the acute problem resolves. Maintenance-dose glucocorticoid is hydrocortisone, 15-20 mg orally in the mornings and 5-10 mg orally in the late afternoons. Patients with primary adrenal insufficiency also need mineralocorticoid replacement with fludrocortisone, 0.1 mg orally each day.

28-3 A. *Learning objective:* **Recognize the clinical setting of hyperaldosteronism.** Secondary causes of hypertension should be considered in young patients, older patients with new-onset hypertension, and patients with difficult-to-treat hypertension. Hypokalemia in a patient with hypertension is most often associated with diuretics used in treatment. Hypokalemia, even when associated with diuretics, also raises the possibility of hyperaldosteronism. Primary hyperaldosteronism may result from an adrenal aldosterone-producing tumor or from bilateral hyperplasia. Hyperaldosterone secondary to high renin results from causes of renal artery stenosis.

28-3 B. *Learning objective:* **Describe the screening test for hyperaldosteronism.** Screen for hyperaldosteronism with an aldosterone-to-renin ratio. The primary stimuli of aldosterone secretion are the renin-angiotensin system and hyperkalemia. When aldosterone is high despite a low renin, primary hyperaldosteronism is suggested.

When aldosterone and renin are elevated in a well-hydrated recumbent individual, hyperaldosteronism secondary to high renin states, such as renal artery stenosis, should be considered.

28-3 C.   *Learning objective:* **Understand aldosterone receptor blockade.** An aldosterone-producing adenoma is usually removed surgically. When this is impossible, or when the cause of primary hyperaldosteronism is bilateral hyperplasia, spironolactone is used specifically to block the renal aldosterone receptor. Likewise, spironolactone can be used to block aldosterone effect in secondary hyperaldosteronism.

28-4 A.   *Learning objective:* **Recognize causes of diabetes in adults other than type 2 diabetes.** This patient was presumed to have type 2 diabetes because of his age at diagnosis. Given his BMI and family history, however, it is much more likely that he has either latent autoimmune diabetes of adults or type 1 diabetes. Additionally, his history of pancreatitis and alcohol use with steatorrhea suggests possible insulin deficiency based on beta cell destruction secondary to chronic pancreatitis.

28-4 B.   *Learning objective:* **Understand how to differentiate between type 1 diabetes, type 2 diabetes, and chronic pancreatitis diabetes using available tests.** Although insulin antibodies are not as sensitive in adults as in children, about 10% of adults classified as having type 2 diabetes actually have type 1 diabetes, and in one series 76% of suspected late-onset patients had GAD antibodies. It is worth considering ordering IA-2, ICA, and GAD antibodies; if elevated, it is more likely the patient has autoimmune type 1 diabetes. A low C-peptide or lack of response to glucagon may be helpful because this confirms lack of insulin production. Most helpful in this case may be an abdominal x-ray. If the pancreas shows calcifications, chronic pancreatitis may be most likely (seen in this case).

28-4 C.   *Learning objective:* **Understand when to initiate insulin.** This patient is on two oral agents with a hemoglobin A_{1c} of 10% (defined as poor control). In addition, he is highly likely to be insulin deficient. At this time, it would be most appropriate to stop his oral sulfonylurea because it is probably of little benefit (stimulates pancreatic release of stored insulin). Because he is so insulin deficient, adding twice-daily insulin, either NPH or premix convenience insulin such as aspart 70/30 mix, would be the treatment of choice. Continuing his metformin is debatable because he is unlikely to be significantly resistant, but is a matter of clinical judgment, unless he is found to have type 1 (autoimmune) diabetes, in which case it is contraindicated because of risk of compounding ketoacidosis with lactic acidosis.

28-5 A.   *Learning objective:* **Appropriately screen for complications of diabetes.** This patient should be scheduled for a dilated eye exam or equivalent (some centers do nondilated retinal exams using special equipment). She also should have a foot exam with documentation of foot deformities, lesions, and sensitivity to a 10-g monofilament (e.g., using the modified Michigan score for risk).

28-5 B. *Learning objective:* **Start appropriate treatment for microalbuminuria and hypertension in type 2 diabetes mellitus.** Very poor glucose control can falsely elevate urinary protein excretion, but given her paresthesias, she is likely to have nephropathy and neuropathy, and this is likely to be a true positive. Spot urinary microalbumin could be confirmed with a protein-to-creatinine ratio or a 24-hour urine, but the clinical diagnosis and outcome are unlikely to be different. She should be counseled and started on an ACEI regardless of her BP (which is above the recommended BP for patients with diabetes, but would need to be confirmed at three visits to generate a diagnosis of hypertension).

28-5 C. *Learning objective:* **Know when to start insulin in type 2 diabetes mellitus.** This patient has poor control despite maximal oral therapy. In this case, it is best to start NPH insulin or insulin glargine at bedtime. A good starting dose is 0.1–0.2 U/kg with dose escalation of 2–4 U every 3 days until fasting capillary blood glucose levels are approximately 110–126 mg/dL (6.2–7 mmol/L).

28-6 A-F. *Learning objective:* **Know whom to screen, and how to screen for hyperlipidemia.**

28-6 A. **Nonfasting cholesterol.** No cardiovascular risk factors are present. Recommendations for screening differ among organizations. NCEP recommends starting at age 20 in all adults. U.S. Preventive Services Task Force recommendations are to start screening at age 35 in low-risk men and age 45 in low-risk women. Earlier screening is recommended if patients have risk factors for CAD. If total cholesterol is >200 mg/dL (>5.2 mmol/L) or HDL is <40 mg/dL (<1.03 mmol/L), proceed to fasting lipid panel.

28-6 B. **Fasting lipid panel.** Diabetes is considered a CAD equivalent. Tobacco use is an additional risk factor. You need to know the patient's LDL to determine if therapy is indicated or to tailor therapy.

28-6 C. **Nonfasting cholesterol.** Although she is young and healthy the fact that her mother had a heart attack before age 65 is a risk factor. Proceed to fasting cholesterol if TC is high or HDL is low.

28-6 D. **None.** He has no CAD risk factors or CAD equivalent illnesses (diabetes, peripheral arterial disease, abdominal aortic aneurysm, or carotid disease). Lipid levels are less likely to increase after age 65, and at this time there is no known benefit of primary prevention in the elderly. If he develops CAD risk factors in the future, screening could be considered.

28-6 E.   **Nonfasting or fasting lipid panel.** The combination of obesity, acne, and irregular menses suggests PCOS, which is associated with insulin resistance and dyslipidemia. Generally, choose fasting levels if you think medical therapy is likely.

28-6 F.   **None.** He is <20 years old with no cardiovascular risk factors.

28-7 A.   *Learning objective:* **Be able to calculate LDL, or use an estimate of LDL when TG levels are high.** Use the formula LDL = TC − HDL − TG/5. Substitute the number 400 in this formula for TG levels to estimate LDL when TG >400 mg/dL (>4.5 mmol/L). His estimated LDL is 145 mg/dL (3.75 mmol/L). This approach overestimates LDL, but allows treatment decisions to be made based on estimated LDL.

28-7 B.   *Learning objective:* **Recognize CAD equivalents and targets for treatment.** CAD equivalents include diabetes, peripheral arterial disease, abdominal aortic aneurysm, and carotid disease. Target LDL for known CAD and CAD equivalents is <100mg/dL (<2.6 mmol/L). More aggressive lipid lowering to <70 mg/dL (<1.8 mmol/L) may be appropriate in some patients.

28-7 C.   *Learning objective:* **Recognize the need for immediate treatment of hypertriglyceridemia when TG >500 mg/dL (>5.6 mmol/L).** Address LDL treatment goals after TG treated to <500 mg/dL (<5.6 mmol/L). Treatment should encompass diet (<15% calories from fat), physical activity, and weight loss. He also needs aggressive diabetes and BP management because his glucose is 300 mg/dL, and BP >130/85 mm Hg is too high in a diabetic. LDL is always the primary focus of therapy *except* when TG >500 mg/dL (>5.6 mmol/L) because the short-term risk of pancreatitis from hypertriglyceridemia is high in this setting and needs to be addressed. Start a fibrate to treat high TG. When TG <500 mg/dL (<5.6 mmol/L), reassess LDL. If >100 mg/dL (>2.6 mmol/L), start a statin.

28-8 A.   *Learning objective:* **HRT should not be used to treat hyperlipidemia.** Although estrogen has been shown to decrease LDL and TG levels and to increase HDL levels, evidence from the Women's Health Initiative shows that HRT does not decrease the risk of cardiovascular events and can increase risk of cardiovascular and thromboembolic events. At this time, the only indication for HRT is severe hot flashes not controlled by other treatment modalities.

28-8 B.   *Learning objective:* **Recognize the need to use NCEP guidelines and Framingham data risk assessment calculator to determine LDL goals.** The decision to treat dyslipidemia is based on absolute risk of an event over the next 10 years and the severity of dyslipidemia. Known CAD, CAD equivalents, or 10-year risk of >20% warrant immediate medical therapy. Her risk factors for CAD include age (>55 years old), low HDL, hypertension, and occasional tobacco use. NCEP advises using the Framingham data risk calculator for intermediate-risk patients with two or more risk factors for CAD. The risk calculator is less important in patients who fall in low-risk or high-risk categories. Almost all patients who fall in the low-risk category (no or one risk factor) have a 10-year risk <10%. In patients with known CAD or CAD equivalents, their 10-year risk is already >20%. See the web site http://hin.nhlbi.nih .gov/atpiii/calculator.asp?usertype=prof to determine this patient's 10-year risk. Based on the NCEP table, she falls in the moderate-risk category with two or more risk factors. Her calculated risk over 10 years is 8%. This makes her target LDL <130 mg/dL with recommendation for drug therapy to start if LDL >160 mg/dL. If her calculated risk is 13%, her target LDL would still be <130 mg/dL, but drug therapy is recommended if LDL >130 mg/dL.

28-8 C.   *Learning objective:* **Emphasize the importance of risk factor modification and the use of the risk assessment calculator as a teaching tool for patients.** Smoking cessation would have the biggest impact on risk reduction in this patient. By using the Framingham risk calculator, notice that her 10-year risk of CHD decreases from 8% to 3% if she becomes a nonsmoker. Showing her the dramatic decrease in her risk may help influence her to quit.

28-9 A.   *Learning objective:* **Distinguish between primary and secondary hypogonadism.** Elevated gonadotropins indicate primary hypogonadism (testicular failure).

28-9 B.   *Learning objective:* **Identify the most common causes of primary hypogonadism.** Klinefelter's syndrome (XXY karyotype) is the most common cause of primary hypogonadism. Klinefelter's syndrome is associated with small testes. Other common causes of primary hypogonadism include trauma, bilateral orchiectomy, and postpubertal mumps orchitis.

28-9 C.   *Learning objective:* **Understand the goals of therapy in primary and secondary hypogonadism.** Androgen replacement therapy should be considered for all men with hypogonadism. Men with primary hypogonadism are generally infertile, although occasionally a man with primary hypogonadism might conceive with assisted reproductive techniques. Men with secondary hypogonadism may be fertile with appropriate hormonal therapy (gonadotropin-releasing hormone or gonadotropin therapy). Androgen replacement therapy is much cheaper than hormone therapy for fertility.

28-10 A. *Learning objective:* **Recognize the presentation of male hypogonadism.** The differential diagnosis of these vague symptoms includes depression, CHF, adverse drug effect (beta blocker), and hypogonadism.

28-10 B. *Learning objective:* **Understand the evaluation of secondary hypogonadism.** Order a pituitary MRI to exclude a macroadenoma and iron studies to exclude hemochromatosis. Perform a careful history and physical to look for Cushing's syndrome.

28-11 A. *Learning objective:* **Outline a reasonable differential diagnosis for her fatigue.** The differential diagnosis of fatigue is broad because it is a common and nonspecific symptom. Given her age and gender and family history, hypothyroidism is possible. Psychological diagnoses, including depression, anxiety, or an adjustment disorder, are common in the outpatient setting. Anemia is always on the differential diagnosis in a woman who is menstruating. Other potential diagnoses include a sleep disorder, type 2 diabetes mellitus, or hepatitis C.

28-11 B. *Learning objective:* **Recognize subclinical hypothyroidism.** Because her free thyroxine is in the normal range, and her TSH is only mildly elevated, her hypothyroidism is said to be "subclinical," rather than "overt." It's difficult to say whether her fatigue and weight gain can be attributed to her mildly elevated TSH.

28-11 C. *Learning objective:* **State role of thyroid antibodies.** No additional tests are necessary to confirm the diagnosis of subclinical hypothyroidism, but if antithyroid microsomal (antithyroid peroxidase) antibodies are positive, they are predictive of progression to overt hypothyroidism over time.

28-11 D. *Learning objective:* **Outline possible management strategies for subclinical hypothyroidism.** There are two options for managing a patient with subclinical hypothyroidism: initiating treatment now or following her laboratory studies closely. It would be reasonable to treat this patient with levothyroxine at 1.6 µg/kg/d, which is usually 100–112 µg/d, to see if her symptoms can be improved. Levothyroxine dosing can be adjusted based on repeat TSH testing after at least 1 month has elapsed. Alternatively, she could be followed with TSH testing every 6 months to 1 year and treated when she develops overt hypothyroidism.

28-12 A. *Learning objective:* **Identify key historical points in patients with a thyroid nodule.** Although <10% of thyroid nodules are malignant, it is important to assess for risk factors and symptoms related to thyroid malignancy. Possible symptoms include dysphagia, dysphonia, hoarseness, and cough, all suggestive of compression. Risk factors include family history of medullary thyroid carcinoma or personal history of head and neck irradiation.

28-12 B. *Learning objective:* **Outline the first steps in the work-up of a thyroid nodule.** With a thyroid nodule, always check TSH first because this guides the diagnostic work-up. Most patients also require an FNA to rule out malignancy, unless TSH is suppressed below the normal range. If the TSH is suppressed, the patient may have a "toxic nodule," which would be confirmed by thyroid uptake scan. If the FNA is indeterminate to rule out malignancy, the patient may need repeat FNA and possibly partial or complete thyroidectomy.

28-12 C. *Learning objective:* **Identify appropriate management for a stable nodule with prior negative evaluation.** If an adequate sample was obtained on FNA, with benign pathology, and the nodule is unchanged on exam, no further testing is indicated. The patient should continue to have yearly physical exams of his thyroid.

28-13 A. *Learning objective:* **Outline a brief differential for paranoia.** A primary psychiatric disorder, such as schizophrenia, mania, or psychotic depression, is possible. Stimulant abuse, such as cocaine or methamphetamines, is also a concern. The exam findings of stare, tachycardia, and tremor suggest hyperthyroidism.

28-13 B. *Learning objective:* **Recognize the lab test results and exam findings of hyperthyroidism.** This patient has overt hyperthyroidism given her symptoms of anxiety, insomnia, and psychiatric disturbance; exam findings of tachycardia, stare, thyroid goiter, and tremor; and lab abnormalities of suppressed TSH and elevated free thyroxine. No other laboratory studies are necessary.

28-13 C. *Learning objective:* **Identify Graves' disease as the most likely cause of her hyperthyroidism.** Given her age, gender, and the diffusely enlarged thyroid, Graves' disease is most likely as the cause of her hyperthyroidism. An exam finding specific for Graves' disease is proptosis, with protrusion of the globe of the eye, resulting in part from inflammation from the autoimmune process in the retro-orbital area. Lid lag and stare can be found in hyperthyroidism of any cause and are not specific for Graves' disease.

28-13 D. *Learning objective:* **State initial management for Graves' disease and hyperthyroidism.** Initial management includes a beta blocker to treat her tachycardia, anxiety, and tremor and antithyroid medication, such as propylthiouracil or methimazole, to normalize her lab abnormalities and treat her other symptoms. Given her psychiatric symptoms, she may require inpatient hospitalization.

REFERENCES

Adrenal Disorders
Boscaro M, Barzon L, Fallo F, et al: Cushing's syndrome. Lancet 2001;357:783.
Oelkers W: Adrenal insufficiency. N Engl J Med 1996;335:1206.

Diabetes
Expert Committee on the Diagnosis and Classification of Diabetes Mellitus: Report of the Expert Committee on the Diagnosis and Classification of Diabetes Mellitus. Diabetes Care 2005;28:S37.

Hyperlipidemia
Executive Summary of the Third Report of the National Cholesterol Education Program (NCEP) Expert Panel on Detection, Evaluation, and Treatment of High Blood Cholesterol in Adults (Adult Treatment Panel III). JAMA 2001;285:2486.
Grundy SM, Cleeman JI, Merz CN, et al: Implications of recent clinical trials for the National Cholesterol Education Program Adult Treatment Panel III guidelines. Circulation 2004;110:227.
U.S. Preventive Services Task Force. Screening and treating adults for lipid disorders: Recommendations and rationale. Am J Prev Med 2001;20:73.

Endocrinology

Male Hypogonadism

Darby E, Anawalt BD: Male hypogonadism: An update on diagnosis and treatment. Treat Endocrinol 2005;4:293.

Thyroid Disease

Castro MR, Gharib H: Continuing controversies in the management of thyroid nodules. Ann Intern Med 2005;142:926.
Cooper DS: Antithyroid drugs. N Engl J Med 2005;352:905.
Pearce EN, Farwell AP, Braverman LE: Thyroiditis. N Engl J Med 2003;348:2646.
Roberts CG, Ladenson PW: Hypothyroidism. Lancet 2004;363:793.
Sherman SI: Thyroid carcinoma. Lancet 2003;361:501.

USEFUL WEB SITES

Diabetes

American Diabetes Association web site: http://www.diabetes.org/main/application/commercewf

Hyperlipidemia

National Heart Lung and Blood Institute web site risk calculator: http://hin.nhlbi.nih.gov/atpiii/calculator.asp?usertype=prof

Endocrinology

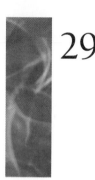

29

Gastroenterology

LISANNE R. BURKHOLDER and
CHRISTOPHER KNIGHT

 BILIARY TRACT DISEASE

ETIOLOGY

What are Cholelithiasis and Choledocholithiasis?

Cholelithiasis occurs when gallstones are present in the gallbladder without causing symptoms. Choledocholithiasis occurs when gallstones are present in the common bile duct and is usually accompanied by the symptoms of cholangitis—fever, jaundice, and RUQ pain.

What are Cholecystitis and Cholangitis?

Blockage of the bile ducts leads to inflammation and infection and presents as cholecystitis or cholangitis. Blockage is usually due to gallstones, but rarely caused by cholangiocarcinoma, Primary Sclerosing Cholangitis (PSC), or extrinsic compression by tumor or adenopathy. Cholecystitis is inflammation or infection of the gallbladder from obstruction of the cystic duct, usually by a gallstone. Cholangitis is a deadly infection arising in the common bile duct owing to ductal obstruction; the gallbladder is usually uninvolved. The organisms causing biliary infections are usually enteric gram-negative rods, anaerobes, or enterococcus, which have ascended the biliary tree from the gut. Cholangitis can be a complication of instrumentation of the biliary tree during ERCP. PSC causes bile duct inflammation and scarring from unclear cause. PSC leaves the biliary ducts thickened and irregularly narrowed and eventually causes cirrhosis and hepatic failure. Patients with ulcerative colitis are at risk for PSC.

EVALUATION

What is a Pertinent History?

The classic patient with gallstones is "fat, fertile, forty and female," a derogatory but accurate characterization of the risk factors. Cystic

312

duct occlusion presents as postprandial RUQ pain, worse with fatty food ingestion, 3–4 hours after eating. It commonly occurs at night (between 10 PM and 2 AM). It can be intermittent or progressive. If blockage persists, pain becomes steady, often radiating to the right shoulder. High fever is rare. In contrast, cholangitis is a GI emergency, presenting in 50–75% of cases with a triad of high spiking fevers with rigors, jaundice, and RUQ pain; elderly or immunosuppressed patients may present only with confusion, hypotension, or sepsis, without the classic triad. If tumor is obstructing the common bile duct, painless jaundice may develop gradually over weeks before onset of infection. When bile flow to the intestine is completely obstructed, urine is dark (bilirubinuria), and stools are light. More than 30% of patients with cholangitis have concomitant pancreatitis, with pain radiating to the back. With PSC, patients have intermittent flares of jaundice, pruritus, RUQ pain, and sometimes frank cholangitis.

What do I Look for on Physical Exam?

Fever, tachycardia, hypotension, and RUQ pain and guarding can occur with cholecystitis and cholangitis. Peritoneal signs are usually absent. Jaundice is a feature of cholangitis, but is absent in cholecystitis. Fifty percent of patients with cholecystitis have a palpably enlarged gallbladder. The classic exam finding is Murphy's sign: Palpate the liver edge deeply at the midclavicular line and ask the patient to inhale. When the inflamed gallbladder meets the hand, the patient abruptly stops breathing in. Sensitivity and specificity are low for this maneuver.

What Lab Tests and Studies should I Order?

When cholecystitis or cholangitis is suspected, order CBC, blood cultures, LFTs, amylase, and an imaging study. The hallmarks of cystic or common duct blockage are elevated alkaline phosphatase and GGT; in cholangitis, bilirubin also is elevated. A thickened, edematous gallbladder wall on ultrasound or CT suggests cholecystitis; common bile duct dilation >1 cm suggests cholangitis, even if stones are not seen, which is often the case. Magnetic resonance cholangiopancreatography also is available now for imaging the biliary tree in patients without a clear diagnosis. ERCP should not be delayed when cholangitis is likely, however, and can diagnose and treat cholangitis. If cholecystitis is suspected, but ultrasound is normal, a HIDA nuclear medicine scan can radiolabel bile and confirm cholecystitis by absence of tracer uptake in the gallbladder. ERCP confirms PSC by the beaded appearance of the bile ducts or cholangiocarcinoma by brush biopsy of the bile duct.

TREATMENT

What Treatment Steps are Appropriate for Patients with Cholecystitis or Cholangitis?

For cholecystitis or cholangitis, start broad-spectrum intravenous antibiotics to cover gram-negative enteric, gram-positive (*Clostridium, Enterococcus*), and anaerobic (*Bacteroides*) organisms; ampicillin plus gentamicin plus metronidazole are often used in combination in the sickest patients. Levofloxacin or imipenem can be substituted if there is concurrent renal failure. Employ volume resuscitation as needed. Cholecystis may respond to antibiotics alone and warrants eventual elective cholecystectomy; asymptomatic gallstones do not require removal. Worsening fever or leukocytosis warrants urgent cholecystectomy. For cholangitis, consult a gastroenterologist immediately for emergent ERCP with sphincterotomy to decompress the pus in the common bile duct.

Do Most Patients Recover from Cholecystitis and Cholangitis?

Cholecystitis requires urgent surgery 25% of the time. Complications of cholecystitis include empyema, gangrene, and gallbladder perforation and carry a 30% mortality. Cholangitis is fatal if untreated. Suspect coexisting pancreatitis with pleural effusion and pain left of the midline or radiating to the back.

Case 29-1

A 49-year-old woman reports recurrent episodes of RUQ pain lasting 1–2 hours, usually occurring after eating at her favorite fast-food restaurant. She has come to an after-hours clinic today because her pain has persisted longer than usual and is now radiating to her midback; she also is vomiting and feeling quite unwell. Temperature is 38.8° C, pulse is 120 beats/min, BP is 100/80 mm Hg, and respirations are 28. She is jaundiced, and her abdomen is obese with RUQ tenderness.

A. What could be causing her symptoms?
B. Can she be treated at home?
C. What management steps are warranted?

Answers appear on page 327.

 LIVER DISEASE

ETIOLOGY

How is Liver Disease Categorized?

Liver disease is categorized by whether it affects the biliary tree or the parenchymal cells. Biliary tree disorders elevate alkaline phosphatase and bilirubin primarily. Hepatocellular injury elevates liver transaminases (ALT, AST) more dramatically than bilirubin or alkaline phosphatase. This section focuses on causes of hepatocellular and parenchymal injury.

What are the Causes of Elevated Transaminases?

Transaminases >2000 mg/dL are caused by viral hepatitis, drug-induced hepatitis, or ischemic hepatitis such as occurs with shock. More modest transaminase elevations may be caused by viral or drug-induced hepatitis; other causes include alcohol, passive liver congestion from right-sided heart failure, autoimmune disorders, inherited storage disorders, tumors, and nonalcoholic steatohepatitis.

What Epidemiologic Features Distinguish the Major Causes of Viral Hepatitis?

The epidemiology of viral hepatitis is summarized in Table 29-1. Hepatitis A and E are passed by the fecal-oral route, whereas hepatitis B, C, and D are acquired parenterally, usually through sexual contact, transfusion, or injection drug use. *Hepatitis A virus* is endemic in developing countries, where it causes approximately 35% of cases of acute viral hepatitis. Infection with HBV is often asymptomatic. Less than 5% of individuals who are infected as adults develop chronic infection; by contrast, 90% of perinatally acquired HBV infections become chronic. HCV is the most common chronic blood-borne infection in the U.S., with 60% of transmission due to injection drug use. In contrast to HBV, in HCV, sexual transmission is rare, and chronic infection is much more common. The course of infection is insidious, and most patients do not notice any symptoms during the first 2 decades of infection. *Hepatitis D virus* requires coinfection with HBV to replicate. Seroprevalence is low in the U.S. except in injection drug users and recipients of multiple transfusions. *Hepatitis E virus* infection is usually inconsequential and self-limited, although mortality rates >30% have been seen in

Table 29-1

Epidemiologic Features of Viral Hepatitis

Virus	Transmission	Risk Factors	% Who Become Chronic Carriers	Incubation Period (Days)
A	Fecal-oral	Travel in developing countries	None	15–60
B	Parenteral	IVDU, male-male sex, health care worker, unprotected sex, tattoos	10% (90% if perinatal)	45–160
C	Parenteral	Same as HBV, intranasal cocaine use	55%–85%	14–180
D	Parenteral	IVDU, coinfection with HBV, unprotected sex	2%–70%	42–180
E	Fecal-oral	No cases seen in U.S.	None*	15–60

*Hepatitis E infection carries 30% mortality if acquired in the third trimester of pregnancy.

women infected during the third trimester of pregnancy. Vaccines are available for hepatitis A and B.

What are the Most Important Causes of Chronic Liver Disease?

Chronic liver disease is any condition that causes hepatic inflammation for >6 months. Chronic liver disease from all causes is the 10th leading cause of death among U.S. adults. The most common causes of chronic liver disease include alcohol and chronic viral hepatitis from HBV and HCV. Other causes include autoimmune disease, hemochromatosis, Wilson's disease, and alpha-1-antitrypsin deficiency. Alcohol also is a common cocontributor to cirrhosis in the other conditions, particularly HCV.

How does Alcohol Cause Liver Damage?

The pathogenesis is unknown. The spectrum of disease includes fatty liver infiltration, alcoholic hepatitis, and cirrhosis. Cirrhosis occurs more frequently in individuals who have a history of alcoholic hepatitis and continue to drink.

What Drugs Cause Hepatocellular Injury?

Numerous medications can cause drug-induced hepatitis. Some of the most notorious are antilipid agents (statins and fibrates), acetaminophen, trazodone, phenytoin, nitrofurantoin, isoniazid, valproic acid, methyldopa, and sulfonamides. Natural products, such as chaparral, coltsfoot, kava, and comfrey, also can cause hepatitis.

What are Autoimmune Hepatitis and Primary Biliary Cirrhosis?

Autoimmune hepatitis causes liver inflammation. Although autoantibodies are often found, they do not directly cause the hepatitis. Type 1 is responsible for 80% of adult cases in the U.S. Both types occur predominantly in younger women, although type 1 sometimes affects older age groups, whereas type 2 is almost always seen in young women and girls. Primary biliary cirrhosis also is an autoimmune liver disease that predominantly affects women—95% of patients are female. In contrast to the other diseases described in this chapter, primary biliary cirrhosis affects intrahepatic bile ducts more than hepatocytes.

What are Some of the Inherited Causes of Liver Disease?

Autosomal recessive causes of liver disease include hemochromatosis, Wilson's disease, and alpha-1-antitrypsin deficiency. Hemochromatosis results from abnormally increased intestinal iron absorption and iron deposition in a variety of organs, including the liver, heart, pancreas, and pituitary. In Wilson's disease, impaired copper excretion into the bile results in accumulation of copper in the liver and other tissues resulting in cirrhosis or neuropsychiatric abnormalities or both. A new diagnosis of Wilson's disease is extremely rare in patients >35 years old. Alpha-1-antitrypsin deficiency causes emphysema, chronic hepatitis, and eventual cirrhosis.

EVALUATION

When should I Suspect Liver Disease?

Acute hepatitis is often obvious; patients present with RUQ pain and jaundice. Nausea, anorexia, and malaise also are often present. If hepatic failure has occurred, encephalopathy and coagulopathy are likely as well. Chronic hepatitis is often insidious and nonspecific with fatigue, anorexia, or pruritus; use the history and physical to detect risk factors and subtle signs (see later).

What Components of the Clinical History are Pertinent?

Assess risk factors for viral hepatitis (e.g., intravenous drug use, prior transfusion, tattoos, cocaine use, occupational exposures, sexual behavior, travel history, or birthplace in an endemic area). Ask about toxin exposure, including alcohol and medications. Family history of liver or autoimmune disease also is pertinent.

What Clues to Liver Disease Should I Look for on Physical Exam?

Scleral icterus is often visible when bilirubin level is >2.5–3 mg/dL. Most patients with chronic liver disease remain anicteric until acute exacerbation or end-stage disease occurs. Other signs of chronic liver disease include spider angiomata, palmar erythema, Terry's nails (dark red distal nail, pale proximal nail), gynecomastia, and jaundice. Portal hypertension can develop in advanced cirrhosis, resulting in spleno-megaly and, beyond a critical threshold, ascites. The most specific phys-ical exam test for ascites is the *fluid wave*. To test for a fluid wave, you tap quickly on one side of the abdomen and feel for the impulse on the opposite side. Because the wave can be transmitted by subcutaneous tissue and fluid, you must have the patient or an assistant hold pressure with the edge of the hand in the midline to prevent the wave from prop-agating through the abdominal wall. Other manifestations of portal hypertension include caput medusae (engorged vessels around the umbilicus), bleeding esophageal varices, severe hemorrhoids, muscle wasting, encephalopathy, and peripheral edema. Patients with hemo-chromatosis may be bronze in color. Patients with alcohol-induced liver disease or hemochromatosis may have testicular atrophy. Patients with Wilson's disease may have Kayser-Fleischer rings (brownish rings at the periphery of the corneas). Patients with alpha-1-antitrypsin defi-ciency may present with early emphysema in the lung bases.

What Laboratory Tests should I Order When I Suspect Liver Disease?

Liver enzymes (also called liver transaminases or aminotransferases) are sensitive indicators of active liver injury and include ALT and AST. The ALT is more specific for liver injury, whereas the AST may be elevated as a result of skeletal, cardiac, and liver muscle injury or injury to the brain and kidney. Transaminases are elevated with all causes of hepatitis. The degree of elevation is usually higher in acute than in chronic injury and correlates with the severity of liver injury only in acute, but not chronic, hepatitis. Acute viral hepatitis can cause transaminase elevations 100 times normal. In contrast, alcohol-induced hepatitis usually elevates transaminases to about two to three times normal, with a characteristic AST-to-ALT ratio of 2:1. In advanced cirrhosis, enzymes may be normal despite ongoing damage because nearly all the normal hepatocytes have been destroyed.

When you detect liver disease, look first for alcohol, medications, or toxins (including natural products and wild mushrooms) that could be causing liver injury. If no cause is found, continue the work-up with viral hepatitis antibody screening. If viral serologies are negative, look further for storage or autoimmune disorders (see later). For patients with minimal alcohol use or who deny a previously applied diagnosis of alcohol-induced liver disease, have a low threshold for ruling out other treatable causes of liver disease.

What Lab Tests can I Use to Assess the Severity of Liver Disease?

In contrast to acute hepatitis, transaminase levels do not correlate well with the degree of accumulated injury in patients with chronic hepatitis. Albumin and PT are more sensitive markers of hepatic biosynthetic function in patients with chronic liver disease. Albumin <3 g/dL or an increased PT >11–16 seconds indicates significantly reduced hepatic synthetic function. Hyperbilirubinemia is common in acute and chronic liver disease.

What is a MELD Score, and How is it Helpful?

In advanced liver disease, the Model for End-stage Liver Disease (MELD) score can be computed using the patient's bilirubin, PT (expressed using the INR), and creatinine. The MELD score is a powerful predictor of mortality: Patients with a MELD score <10 have a 3-month mortality of <10%, whereas patients with a MELD score ≥30 have a 3-month mortality >70%. Because of its predictive power, the MELD score has been adopted as the primary eligibility criterion for liver transplantation.

How do I Interpret Hepatitis Serologic Profiles?

Some general rules are helpful. Antigen is present with active acute or chronic infection; IgM antibodies signal early response to acute infection, and IgG antibodies develop later in infection and persist with chronic infection or resolution (Table 29-2). In HCV infection, the likelihood of becoming a chronic carrier is so high that positive antibody tests are usually presumed to indicate chronic infection. Active HCV infection can be confirmed by testing for HCV RNA by PCR.

Table 29-2

Interpretation of Serologic Tests for Viral Hepatitis

Test	Interpretation
Hepatitis A	
IgM antibody	Acute infection
IgG antibody	Past infection
Hepatitis B	
Surface antigen (HBsAg)	Acute or chronic infection
Envelope antigen (HBeAg)	Correlates with higher infectivity
IgM antibody against core protein (HBcIgM)	Acute infection
IgG antibody against core protein (HBcIgG)	Prior infection or vaccination
IgG antibody against surface protein (HBsAg)	Long-term immunity after vaccination or prior infection
Hepatitis C	
IgG antibody	Infection, likely chronic
Viral load (HCV RNA)	Active infection

When should I Test for Hemochromatosis?

Test all first-degree relatives of affected patients for iron overload with serum iron, ferritin, and transferrin saturation, and consider testing for the hemochromatosis gene (if present in the affected relative). Also test patients with chronic liver disease and negative viral serologies. Elevated ferritin and a transferrin saturation >55% are suggestive, but not specific for hemochromatosis; liver biopsy or genetic testing is required to confirm the diagnosis. Other causes of chronic liver disease also may cause elevations in ferritin and transferrin saturation and iron deposition in the liver, making interpretation of iron studies challenging. Screening the general population for hemochromatosis is controversial; repeated phlebotomy is a safe and effective therapy, but it is unclear whether or not all individuals with mild iron overload or the hemochromatosis genotype, or both, require therapeutic phlebotomy.

What Lab Test Results Suggest Autoimmune Hepatitis?

Type 1 autoimmune hepatitis is characterized by hypergammaglobulinemia, ANA, and anti–smooth muscle antibody. Type 2 is characterized by antibody to liver/kidney microsome type 1 without ANA and anti–smooth muscle antibody. Either type may be accompanied by other autoimmune diseases, although this is more common with type 2.

What Lab Test Results Suggest Primary Biliary Cirrhosis?

Primary biliary cirrhosis affects intrahepatic bile ducts and often shows striking elevations in alkaline phosphatase. The most specific serologic marker is antimitochondrial antibody, present in 95% of cases.

What Lab Tests do I Use to Diagnose Wilson's Disease?

Wilson's disease decreases the serum ceruloplasmin to <20 mg/dL and increases urinary copper excretion. Twenty percent of patients with Wilson's disease have a normal ceruloplasmin; an elevated 24-hour urine copper excretion suggests the diagnosis, and liver biopsy with quantitative copper measurement confirms the diagnosis. Kayser-Fleischer rings, single brownish lines on the outer edge of the corneas seen by slit-lamp exam, are pathognomonic, but not always present.

What Complications of Cirrhosis should I Recognize?

Cirrhosis leads to fibrosis of the liver parenchyma with increased vascular resistance in the hepatic sinusoids resulting in increased resistance to portal blood flow. This is referred to as portal hypertension. Clinical features associated with portal hypertension include esophageal varices as blood detours around the liver through small vessels in the esophagus, massive GI bleeding if these varices rupture, and ascites owing to leakage of fluid from the portal system with risk of associated SBP. Cirrhosis also may result in hepatic encephalopathy, hepatorenal syndrome, and hepatocellular cancer.

Should I Screen for Hepatocellular Carcinoma in Patients with Chronic Liver Disease?

Serum AFP and imaging studies (ultrasound or CT) are used to detect hepatocellular carcinoma. There is no evidence, however, that screening increases the rate of detecting potentially curable tumors, despite the fact that cirrhosis of any etiology is associated with the development of hepatocellular carcinoma. In areas where HBV is endemic, half of patients with hepatocellular carcinoma are HBsAg positive. A similar risk pattern is seen with HCV infection.

When should a Patient be Referred for Liver Biopsy?

Obtain a liver biopsy specimen to confirm hemochromatosis, Wilson's disease, autoimmune hepatitis, and primary biliary cirrhosis. Biopsy is useful to determine eligibility for antiviral therapy in hepatitis B or C. Biopsy also is a prognostic tool: Patients with evidence of portal or mild periportal hepatitis tend to have a benign course; patients with bridging or multilobular necrosis or cirrhosis are at high risk for progressive disease.

TREATMENT

What Treatments are Available for Chronic Viral Hepatitis?

The treatment of chronic viral hepatitis is a rapidly evolving field. The goals of therapy for hepatitis B and C differ. HBV treatment is directed at halting viral replication and sustaining seroconversion as evidenced by the development of anti-HBeAg antibody. HCV treatment is directed at eliminating the virus. Alpha-interferon is approved by the Food and Drug Administration for the treatment of hepatitis B and C. This treatment is expensive and has multiple side effects, including flulike symptoms, fatigue, bone marrow suppression, and neuropsychiatric effects. With HBV, treatment is reserved for patients with active viral replication and elevated aminotransferases. Of treated individuals, 30%-40% respond to therapy as evidenced by loss of HBeAg and a return of the serum ALT to normal. Lamivudine is an alternative therapy for chronic HBV infection with fewer side effects, but half the overall sustained virologic response owing to development of viral resistance to the drug. In patients treated with lamivudine, long-term maintenance therapy may be required to prevent viral recurrence and return of hepatic inflammation. Combining interferon and lamivudine in chronic HBV remains experimental, but shows some promise. The nucleotide analog adefovir is another treatment option for patients with chronic hepatitis B. Interferon is recommended for chronic HCV in patients at the greatest risk for the progression to cirrhosis, as evidenced by elevated ALT levels, detectable HCV RNA, and liver biopsy findings of portal or bridging fibrosis. Most patients receive combination therapy with peginterferon (a long-acting depot form of interferon) and ribavirin. Patients with high viral loads or genotype 1 disease have lower clearance rates and are often treated with an extended course of therapy (48 weeks instead of 24 weeks). Advise patients with chronic hepatitis of any type to abstain from all alcohol ingestion to prevent accelerated progression to cirrhosis.

What Treatments are Available for Drug-Induced Hepatitis?

Stop the drug, and watch to ensure that LFTs and clinical symptoms improve. Certain drugs have specific antidotes that are effective if administered early; the most important is N-acetyl cysteine, a specific antidote for acetaminophen toxicity that should be administered orally or intravenously in patients with severe acetaminophen overdose.

What Treatments are Available for Autoimmune Hepatitis and Primary Biliary Cirrhosis?

Although both diseases have autoantibodies, the treatments are quite different. Autoimmune hepatitis often responds well to immunosuppressant drugs, such as glucocorticoids and azathioprine. Primary biliary cirrhosis is notoriously unresponsive to these drugs; the only drug of convincing (if modest) value in primary biliary cirrhosis is ursodeoxycholic acid (ursodiol). Either disease can lead to liver transplant if the disease progresses despite therapy.

What is the Treatment for Alcoholic Liver Disease?

For acute alcoholic hepatitis, some patients are helped by corticosteroids. Severity is defined by the discriminant function [4.6 × (patient PT − control PT in seconds) + bilirubin]. Patients with a discriminant function >32 or evidence of encephalopathy should be treated with prednisolone. For patients with chronic alcoholic liver disease, there may be improvement with abstinence, even in patients with advanced cirrhosis. Many transplant centers require a period of abstinence (often ≥6 months) before a patient is eligible for transplant.

How do I Treat the Complications of Cirrhosis?

Treat *ascites* with sodium restriction to <2 g/d. A loop diuretic such as furosemide or an aldosterone antagonist such as spironolactone or both can be added. Use large-volume paracentesis for tense ascites in symptomatic patients in whom diuretics fail or are contraindicated. The use of albumin infusions with large-volume paracentesis (to reduce the risk of hepatorenal syndrome) is controversial, but is often considered when paracentesis volumes exceed 3–4 L. *Esophageal variceal hemorrhage* is treated with endoscopic variceal banding (preferred) or sclerotherapy. TIPS decompresses portal hypertension and reduces recurrent variceal bleeding or refractory ascites, but does not reduce overall mortality and may increase encephalopathy. Beta blockers, with or without oral nitrates, are effective at reducing first-time esophageal hemorrhage and recurrent esophageal hemorrhage. The mainstay of treatment for *hepatic encephalopathy* is lactulose, which facilitates the removal of ammonium ion. Rifaximin is an oral antibiotic that is effective therapy for hepatic encephalopathy. It is a good option for patients who do not tolerate lactulose. *Hepatorenal syndrome* with oliguria and poor renal perfusion causing a renal sodium concentration <10 mEq/L is a grave prognostic sign. There is no treatment other than temporizing with dialysis while awaiting liver transplantation. *Hepatocellular tumors* can be resected if surgically feasible or may be treated with liver transplantation if overall prognosis is favorable, and there is no evidence of distant metastasis. Otherwise, elective palliative therapy involves angiographic embolization or radiofrequency ablation of affected areas.

How do I Treat Hemochromatosis?

Treat hemochromatosis with phlebotomy, removing 500 mL one to two times a month to a goal hemoglobin <11 g/dL and ferritin <100 ng/mL. This prevents iron overload and cirrhosis.

What Patients should be Referred for Liver Transplantation?

Patients with end-stage liver disease or fulminant hepatic failure should be referred early to transplant centers for consideration of liver transplantation. Waiting lists are long, and patients must fulfill specific criteria, including mental stability, psychosocial support, probability that they will survive the operation, and funding. Contraindications are based on outcome data and include alcohol intake over the preceding 6 months, other substance abuse, active infection outside the hepatobiliary system that would make immunosuppression an unacceptable risk, and incurable extrahepatic malignancy. Prioritization for transplant is by the MELD score (see earlier), with higher scores having higher priority.

How can I Prevent Hepatitis?

Vaccines are available for hepatitis A and B. The hepatitis A vaccine is given in two doses 6 to 12 months apart and is recommended for travelers to endemic areas, military personnel, individuals with chronic liver disease, and individuals engaging in high-risk sexual activity. HBV vaccine is given in three doses, spaced by 1 and 6 months. It is recommended in infants, individuals at occupational risk, sexually active young adults, injection drug users, inmates of correctional facilities, hemodialysis patients, international travelers, and residents of areas where HBV is endemic.

Case 29-2

A 70-year-old man comes to the clinic 10 days after hospital discharge, concerned that he has been looking yellow for the last week. He reports feeling quite tired and is particularly bothered by generalized itching. His stool is light in color, and he thinks that his urine looks brown. He hasn't been eating because of loss of appetite.

A. What is your differential diagnosis?
B. What laboratory tests would be useful in determining the etiology of his illness?
C. What other information would be useful?

Case 29-3

A 50-year-old man is diagnosed with HCV. He believes that he initially was infected on his 40th birthday when he injected intravenous drugs for the first and only time. He has had no subsequent care and is referred to a hepatologist for further evaluation.

A. Which diagnostic studies would be useful in determining the extent of his disease?
B. What factors would lead you to treat him?
C. What advice would you offer to prevent accelerated progression to cirrhosis?

Answers appear on pages 327–328.

 PANCREATITIS

ETIOLOGY

What are Causes of Acute and Chronic Pancreatitis?

Causes of acute pancreatitis are listed in Table 29-3; no cause is identified in 15%-20% of cases. Pancreatitis can become chronic if the underlying cause is not treated. Excess alcohol use is the most common cause of chronic pancreatitis.

Table 29-3

Causes of Acute Pancreatitis

Common	Uncommon
Alcohol	Drugs (didanosine, zalcitabine, stavudine, sulfonamides, tetracycline, thiazides, pentamidine, azathioprine, estrogen, valproate)
Gallstones	Viral
	TG >1000
	Idiopathic
	Trauma
	Hypercalcemia

EVALUATION

How do Patients with Pancreatitis Present?

Patients with acute or chronic pancreatitis report severe steady epigastric pain, often radiating to the back, worse with lying down, and relieved by sitting up. Nausea and vomiting are common and exacerbated by eating. If pancreatic edema or gallstones occlude the common bile duct, jaundice ensues.

What do I Look for on Physical Exam?

In patients with acute presentations, look for tachycardia, hypotension, volume depletion owing to third spacing of fluids, or low-grade fever secondary to inflammation or infection. The abdomen is usually diffusely tender. Retroperitoneal pancreatic hemorrhage may manifest as bruising around the umbilicus (Cullen's sign) or flank (Turner's sign), although both of these signs are rarely seen.

What Tests should I Order?

Order CBC, amylase or lipase, chemistry panel, calcium, LFTs, LDH, glucose, TG, and x-rays of the abdomen and chest. Pancreatic calcifications on x-ray are pathognomonic of chronic pancreatitis. CXR may show pleural effusion. Abdominal CT scan may show necrotic pancreatic tissue, an indication for antibiotic prophylaxis. If patients are refractory to therapy, repeat abdominal CT scan may show developing complications, such as pancreatic pseudocyst or abscess. Follow CBC, calcium, BUN, Pao_2, and base deficit (from ABG) to assess for worsening prognosis by Ranson criteria (Box 29-1), one of many available scoring systems; APACHE (Acute Physiology, Age, and Chronic Health Evaluation) score may predict disease severity more accurately.

TREATMENT

What is the Treatment for Pancreatitis?

Treatment is mostly supportive, to allow inflammation to subside and monitor for complications. Rest the bowel by keeping the patient

BOX 29-1

RANSON CRITERIA PREDICT MORTALITY RATES

Mortality is 2% with 0–2 criteria, 40% with 5–6 criteria, nearly 100% with >7 criteria.

Initial Evaluation

Age >55
WBC >16,000
AST >250 u/L
LDH >350 u/L
Glucose >200 mg/dL

Changes in the First 48 Hours

Hematocrit decrease >10%
BUN increase >5 mg/dL
Ca <8 mg/dL
Pao_2 <60 mm Hg
Base deficit >4

---

without food, and suction gastric secretions with an NG tube if significant vomiting persists. Resuscitate with intravenous saline as needed and then maintenance (5% dextrose in ¼ normal saline). Parenteral nutrition may be required if the pancreatitis is prolonged by more than 1–2 days. ERCP relieves an obstructing gallstone, but may worsen pancreatic inflammation. Manage pain with patient-controlled intravenous narcotics. Watch for complications of pseudocyst, abscess, sepsis, and ARDS. Severely ill patients and patients with necrotic pancreatic tissue on CT scan may benefit from prophylaxis with a broad-spectrum antibiotic, such as imipenem. Follow daily amylase, LFTs, and CBC until they return to normal to track resolution of inflammation. Refer for elective cholecystectomy when the pancreatitis resolves if stones were the cause. Mortality is 10% overall in patients hospitalized with pancreatitis.

Case 29-4

A 45-year-old man reports several hours of severe midepigastric pain radiating to the back associated with emesis worsened by eating. He takes saquinivir/ritonavir, lamivudine, and didanosine for HIV infection diagnosed 1 year ago, with a nadir CD4 count of 50. He also smokes a pack of cigarettes and drinks two to six beers daily. Pulse is 110 beats/min, BP is 100/60 mm Hg, temperature is 38.3° C, and respirations are 24. His upper midabdomen is very tender, and you cannot find any costovertebral angle or point tenderness on his back.

   A. What could be causing this man's abdominal pain?

B. What tests do you want to order to confirm your diagnosis and assess his prognosis?
C. Read the answer to part B for test results, and list your management for this patient.

KEY POINTS – BILIARY TRACT DISEASE

◆ RUQ pain, high fever, and jaundice is cholangitis until proven otherwise.

◆ Cholangitis is a GI emergency and warrants urgent imaging and a GI consult.

KEY POINTS – LIVER DISEASE

◆ The most common presenting symptoms of chronic liver disease are fatigue, anorexia, and pruritus.

◆ HBV rarely progresses to chronic infection and cirrhosis unless acquired perinatally.

◆ HCV is the most common chronic blood-borne infection in the U.S. with most patients unaware that they are infected.

◆ Patients with severe alcoholic hepatitis (discriminant function >32) benefit from corticosteroids.

◆ The MELD score is a useful tool for assessing severity and determining prognosis and priority for transplant in patients with advanced liver disease.

KEY POINTS – PANCREATITIS

◆ Pancreatitis radiates to the back, whereas cholecystitis radiates to the right shoulder.

◆ Gallstone disease and alcohol abuse are the two main causes of pancreatitis.

◆ Treat pancreatitis with bowel rest, intravenous hydration, and parenteral nutrition; consider antibiotics, and monitor for complications.

Case Answers

29-1 A. *Learning objective:* **Recognize biliary colic leading to cholangitis accompanied by pancreatitis.** The patient's preceding RUQ pain episodes are most likely biliary colic from gallstones lodging in the cystic duct and spontaneously resolving. Now, she sounds as though she could have developed cholangitis with the classic triad of fever, jaundice, and RUQ pain. The midabdominal pain radiating to the back also suggests concurrent pancreatitis. Patients with other causes of biliary obstruction, such as lymphadenopathy or tumor, usually present with painless jaundice of gradual onset. Perforated duodenal ulcer is possible because it can cause RUQ pain and pain radiating to the back, although it would not explain her jaundice. Other pains that might radiate to the back include discitis and abdominal aortic dissection, although neither of these would explain all her presenting findings.

29-1 B. *Learning objective:* **Recognize the severity of infection when cholangitis is suspected, and hospitalize for further treatment.** Cholangitis is potentially life-threatening, as is pancreatitis. She needs treatment in the hospital.

29-1 C. *Learning objective:* **Design a management plan for patients with suspected cholangitis.** First, confirm your diagnosis with blood testing and abdominal imaging, either ultrasound or CT scan. Elevated WBC, bilirubin, GGT, and alkaline phosphatase in the setting of a dilated common bile duct with the presence of stones in the gallbladder suggest cholangitis caused by choledocholithiasis (the biliary duct stones are rarely seen). Elevated amylase suggests concurrent pancreatitis, and the pancreas also may look edematous on CT scan. The patient needs intravenous antibiotics, such as ampicillin plus gentamicin plus metronidazole, and urgent ERCP to decompress the bile ducts. Treatment of concurrent pancreatits may require bowel rest and appropriate supportive care, including parenteral nutrition.

29-2 A. *Learning objective:* **State the differential diagnosis for jaundice.** The differential includes viral, alcoholic, autoimmune, and drug-induced hepatitis. Biliary obstruction owing to gallstone or neoplasm also is possible. Hereditary causes of liver disease are unlikely in this patient because of the acute onset and the patient's older age, although hemochromatosis occasionally occurs later in women because of the phlebotomy-like effect of menses.

29-2 B. *Learning objective:* **Order appropriate laboratory studies in a jaundiced patient.** Given jaundice, order a broad panel, including ALT, AST, bilirubin, albumin, PTT, PT INR, and alkaline phosphatase. If transaminases are elevated to a greater degree than bilirubin and alkaline phosphatase, order hepatitis A, B, and C serologies. If bilirubin and alkaline phosphatase are more elevated, order RUQ ultrasound to rule out biliary obstruction.

29-2 C. *Learning objective:* **Obtain a thorough history to look for potential exposures as the cause of an acute hepatitis.** Quantitate alcohol intake. Ask about potential toxic exposures and medications, especially in elderly patients or in the setting of ongoing heavy alcohol use; include over-the-counter remedies, particularly acetaminophen. This patient had elevated aminotransferases in the 1000 range and a bilirubin of 10.2. Hepatitis serology studies were normal except for a positive hepatitis A virus IgG antibody indicating old infection. A careful review of his medical history revealed that he had been recently hospitalized with MI and had been discharged on trazodone to help with sleep, a possible cause of drug-induced hepatitis. Withdrawal of trazodone resulted in resolution of his symptoms and normalization of bilirubin and aminotransferases.

29-3 A. *Learning objective:* **Identify appropriate diagnostic studies in the evaluation of HCV.** HCV RNA tests, viral load, and liver biopsy are useful diagnostic studies for determining the extent of disease. The alanine aminotransferase level is an inexpensive and useful test that is best for monitoring HCV infection and the efficacy of therapy in the intervals between molecular testing. HCV genotype is useful for planning the duration of potential treatment because it is advisable to treat patients infected with genotype 1 for 48 weeks and patients infected with genotypes 2 and 3 for 24 weeks.

29-3 B. *Learning objective:* **Identify factors that would influence treatment of HCV.** HCV treatment is appropriate for patients who are at the highest risk for progression of their disease. This includes patients with detectable levels of HCV RNA who have persistently elevated ALT levels and liver biopsy results showing moderate necrosis and inflammation.

29-3 C. *Learning objective:* **Recognize the main factor that accelerates progression to cirrhosis.** Advise patients with any form of chronic hepatitis to abstain from alcohol ingestion to prevent acceleration and progression to cirrhosis of the liver.

29-4 A. *Learning objective:* **Recognize pancreatitis, and list potential causes relevant to the patient's presentation.** This sounds like pancreatitis with abdominal pain radiating to the back, in a patient with some risk factors, including alcohol use and medications that themselves can cause pancreatitis (didanosine) or that can increase TG (protease inhibitors such as saquinivir and ritonavir). Patients with CD4 counts <50 also are at risk for external compression of the biliary tree from MAC-induced lymphadenopathy, which would be a rare cause of pancreatitis. Primary HIV infection and other viral infections (mumps, HBV, coxsackievirus, HSV, herpes zoster virus, CMV) may cause pancreatitis. *Toxoplasma, Cryptosporidium, Pneumocystis carinii,* and MAC infections can rarely cause pancreatitis, although these infections would be expected at lower CD4 counts. The patient also could have gallstones because this is still one of the most common causes of pancreatitis. Other, less likely causes of abdominal pain radiating to the back include lower lobe pneumonia, peptic ulcer, aortic dissection, thoracic radiculopathy, discitis, or vertebral osteomyelitis.

29-4 B. *Learning objective:* **Order appropriate investigations in patients with abdominal pain and probable pancreatits.** Order amylase or lipase, CBC, triglycerides, LFTs, chemistry panel, calcium, LDH, and glucose, and if hypoxic, consider an ABG. Order chest and abdominal films, looking for pancreatic calcifications (chronic alcohol-induced pancreatitis), free air under the diaphragm (perforated ulcer), pulmonary infiltrate (lower lobe pneumonia), pleural effusion, or early ARDS. Abdominal CT may confirm pancreatitis and may help in making a decision about whether to use antibiotics. This man had an amylase of 890 U/L, triglycerides 4500 mg/dL (50 nmol/L), WBC 18,000/m^2, hematocrit 30%, AST 320 U/L, glucose 220 mg/dL (12.1 mmol/L), pleural effusion on CXR, and chronic calcifications in the pancreas on abdominal films, giving him three Ransom criteria with his pancreatitis. He could have alcohol-induced, medication-induced, or hypertriglyceridemia-induced pancreatitis.

29-4 C. *Learning objective:* **Appropriately manage patients with pancreatitis.** Start with intravenous normal saline volume resuscitation and bowel rest, and consider placing an NG tube, starting antibiotics, and parenteral nutrition. Retest blood for follow-up assessment of Ranson criteria. Elevated TG can be a complication or cause of pancreatitis. If the TG remain >500 mg/dL (>5.6 mmol/L) after he is better, the patient may need treatment of TG or a change of his HIV regimen to one without a protease inhibitor.

REFERENCES

Biliary Tract Disease
Kalloo AN: Gallstones and biliary disease. Prim Care 2001;28:591.
Lee YM, Kaplan M: Medical progress: Primary sclerosing cholangitis. N Engl J Med 1995;332:924.

Liver Disease
Giboney PT: Mildly elevated liver transaminase levels in the asymptomatic patient. Am Fam Physician 2005;71:1105.
Kamath PS, Wiesner RH, Malinchoc M, et al: A model to predict survival in patients with end-stage liver disease. Hepatology 2001;33:464.
Kim AI, Saab S: Treatment of hepatitis C. Am J Med 2005;118:808.
Menon KV, Gores GJ, Shah VH: Pathogenesis, diagnosis, and treatment of alcoholic liver disease. Mayo Clin Proc 2001;76:1021.
Schmitt B, Golub RM, Green R: Screening primary care patients for hereditary hemochromatosis with transferrin saturation and serum ferritin level: Systematic review for the American College of Physicians. Ann Intern Med 2005;143:522.

Gastroenterology

Pancreatitis
Acute pancreatitis. Hosp Med 2000;61:382.

USEFUL WEB SITE

Liver Disease
United Network for Organ Sharing site has information on transplants and includes a MELD calculator under Resources. www.unos.org

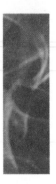

30

Geriatrics

JEFFREY I. WALLACE

BENIGN PROSTATIC HYPERPLASIA

ETIOLOGY

What Causes BPH?

BPH, a nonmalignant enlargement of the prostate, is due to excessive cellular growth of glandular and stromal elements of the prostate. BPH pathophysiology is characterized by increased adrenergic tone (dynamic component) leading to smooth muscle contraction and prostate growth owing to androgenic stimulation (static component).

EVALUATION

How do I Make the Diagnosis of BPH?

The diagnosis of BPH is suggested by symptoms that reflect bladder irritation (urinary frequency, urgency, nocturia) and obstruction (hesitancy, straining, weak stream, dribbling, retention). Rule out other conditions causing these symptoms (e.g., prostatitis, urethral stricture, infection, prostate or bladder cancer) by history, urinalysis, and rectal exam. On rectal exam, prostatitis results in a tender, tense prostate; a nodule suggests possible malignancy.

How can I Gauge the Severity of BPH?

The American Urological Association (AUA) Symptom Index is a valid and reliable indicator of symptom severity using seven questions regarding specific symptoms (Table 30-1). Peak urine flow (normal >15 mL/sec) and PVR (normal <100 mL) are useful to gauge disease severity. Prostate size does not correlate well with symptom severity or degree of obstruction.

Table 30-1

American Urological Association Symptom Index for Patients with Benign Prostatic Hyperplasia

Questions: Over the past month, how often have you . . .	Answer Score
1. Had the sensation of not emptying your bladder completely?	0 = not at all
2. Had to urinate again within 2 hours of last void (frequency)?	1 = <1 time in 5
3. Stopped and started again several times while urinating?	2 = less than half the time
4. Found it difficult to postpone urination (urge)?	3 = half the time
5. Had a weak urinary stream?	4 = more than half the time
6. Had to push or strain to begin urination?	5 = almost always
7. Had to get up to urinate after going to bed?	Number times: 0, 1, 2, 3, 4, >5
BPH Symptom Score (Sum of Answers)	
Mild	= 0–7
Moderate	= 8–19
Severe	= 20–35

Besides Symptoms, are there any Other Serious Problems Associated with BPH?

Long-standing BPH can infrequently cause urinary retention, renal insufficiency, UTI, gross hematuria, and bladder stones. If these occur, surgery is generally indicated.

TREATMENT

How do I Decide When and How to Treat BPH?

BPH is a disease that primarily affects quality of life. Patient perception of symptom severity (AUA Symptom Score) is a major determinant in making treatment decisions. Treatment options range from watchful waiting to surgery (Figure 30-1).

What Medications are Used to Manage BPH?

Two classes of medication and one herbal remedy improve BPH symptoms. *Alpha-1-adrenergic antagonists,* such as doxazosin, terazosin, alfuzosin, and tamsulosin, work fairly rapidly (within several weeks) by blocking alpha-1-adrenergic receptors in the bladder neck and prostate that constrict outflow. Side effects, which occur in 5%-10% of patients, include orthostatic hypotension and weakness. Tamsulosin and alfuzosin selectively block prostatic alpha-1 receptors and cause less asthenia, dizziness, and hypotension, but can cause more retrograde ejaculation. The second class of medications, 5-alpha-reductase inhibitors (*finasteride*

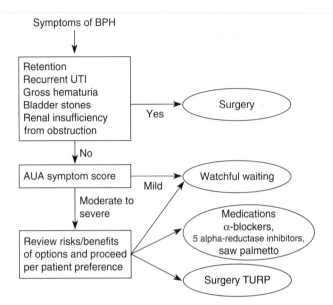

FIGURE 30-1 Treatment algorithm for BPH. AUA, American Urological Association.

and *dutasteride*), work by decreasing prostatic DHT (the chief intracellular androgen) and shrinking prostate size by about 20%. Over 6–12 months, these agents reduce urinary retention symptoms and need for surgery. 5-alpha-reductase inhibitors have fewer side effects (decreased libido, impotence in 3%-4%) than alpha-1 blockers, but take much longer to work and are generally second-line therapy. The herbal product *saw palmetto* seems to be effective in relieving the symptoms of prostate obstruction with minimal side effects. The mechanism of action of saw palmetto is unclear, but may include antiandrogen, anti-inflammatory, and antiproliferative effects. (A well-crafted year-long study showed no benefit from saw palmetto. These results are counter to prior findings and should be substantiated.) *Invasive or surgical interventions* offer benefit for patients in whom medical therapy fails, but risks include impotence, incontinence, blood loss requiring transfusion, and infection. The most common surgical procedure is TURP (transurethral resection of the prostate).

DEMENTIA

ETIOLOGY

What are the Three Most Common Causes of Dementia In Older Adults?

Alzheimer's disease accounts for about two thirds of dementia cases. Traditionally, multi-infarct dementia is cited as the next most common cause of dementia (15%-25%). More recent studies suggest that vascular dementia may be overdiagnosed, however, and that a previously under-diagnosed entity, Lewy body dementia, may account for 10%-20% of cases. Alcohol, at 10%, is the third most common cause of dementia in some case series.

What are the Most Common Causes of "Reversible Dementia"?

Drugs and depression ("pseudodementia") are the most common reversible causes. After drugs and depression, only 5% of remaining cases are potentially treatable; $\leq 1\%$ are truly fully reversible. The most common potentially reversible causes of cognitive impairment are vitamin B_{12} deficiency, hypothyroidism, and normal pressure hydrocephalus. Dementia is often only partially reversed with treatment of these conditions (perhaps because they often coexist with Alzheimer's disease).

EVALUATION

How does One Establish the Diagnosis of Dementia?

Although a hallmark sign, memory deficits alone are insufficient to diagnose dementia. Impairments must exist in at least one other cognitive area (e.g., language, motor skills, personality), at a level severe enough to interfere with usual function. The mini-mental state examination (MMSE) is a useful 30-item instrument to measure and document cognitive impairment objectively.

What is the Appropriate Work-Up for a Patient Suspected to have Dementia?

Perform a thorough history and exam with focus on neurologic and mental status evaluations. Obtain CBC, electrolytes, BUN, creatinine, LFTs, vitamin B_{12}, thyroid screen, and syphilis serology. Most experts recommend a noncontrast head CT scan to rule out tumor, subdural hematoma, or hydrocephalus. Brain imaging is absolutely indicated for patients with focal neurologic signs, headache, or other atypical features. LP and EEG are not routinely required.

What "Red Flags" Increase the Likelihood of a Diagnosis Other than Alzheimer's Disease?

Sudden onset or onset at a younger age (especially <60 years old), a history of rapid cognitive decline over weeks to months rather than years, or the presence of focal neurologic signs or symptoms increases the chance of a diagnosis other than Alzheimer's disease.

TREATMENT

What are the Basic Management Approaches to Patients with Dementia?

Review and discontinue drugs likely to impair cognition. Depression often coexists with dementia (especially early in the course of disease),

Geriatrics

so carefully assess for depression, and consider a trial of therapy, usually with a selective serotonin reuptake inhibitor. Similarly, diagnose and treat other coexisting medical conditions that, although not the cause of cognitive impairment, can affect mood, comfort, and function. Use nonpharmacologic approaches to improve patient function and behavior, along with caregiver education, support, and respite.

What Pharmacologic Treatments are Available to Prevent or Treat Alzheimer's Dementia?

Three cholinesterase inhibitors (donepezil, rivastigmine, and galantamine) and memantine (an N-methyl-D-aspartate receptor antagonist) are currently available to treat Alzheimer's disease. These agents can improve cognition, behavior, and overall function, but their main effect is mostly to slow rates of decline, and, on average, changes in these parameters are small. Vitamin E and ginkgo biloba also may slow the rate of decline in Alzheimer's disease, but data on these agents have not been strong or consistent. Although estrogen, anti-inflammatory agents, and statin lipid-lowering drugs have been associated with lower prevalence rates of Alzheimer's disease, to date, trials show that estrogen and anti-inflammatories have failed to prevent or slow progression of Alzheimer's disease. Further study is needed before these drugs should be considered for prevention or treatment of Alzheimer's disease.

How about Managing Common Behavioral Problems, such as Agitation and Sleep Problems?

Nonpharmacologic strategies work as well, if not better, than medications. Seek out and address medication side effects, infection, injury or pain, exacerbation of pre-existing illness, or inconsistency in the environment that may be causing agitation or sleep disturbances. Increased physical activity can help behavior and sleep problems. Low-dose neuroleptics (e.g., haloperidol 0.5–1 mg, risperidone 0.5–2 mg, olanzapine 2.5–5 mg) may be helpful for severe agitation, persistent hallucinations, or delusions. None of these agents are approved by the Food and Drug Administration for the treatment of dementia-related behavioral disturbances, however, and antipsychotic agents have been associated with an increased risk of mortality in this patient population.

Geriatrics

Case 30-1

An 83-year-old man with history of hypertension, type 2 diabetes, and hyperlipidemia is brought in by his daughter for a gradual worsening of confusion over the past several years. His daughter describes that he has had several angry outbursts and is more irritable. He also has had memory changes, such as forgetting the names of his grandchildren. Although he used to walk daily to the nearby park alone, recently he has been getting lost. For this reason, he also has stopped driving. In the clinic, BP is 150/90 mm Hg. There is a right facial droop and positive Babinski's sign. The rest of the physical exam is normal. On MMSE, the patient scores 18/30. CT scan of the head shows small, old subcortical ischemic infarcts, but no hemorrhage or mass.

A. Does this patient have dementia?
B. What is your management for this patient?
C. What are some complications secondary to his mental status?

POLYPHARMACY

ETIOLOGY

Why do Older Adults have More Adverse Drug Effects than Younger Patients?

Most studies on the efficacy and safety of medications exclude the very old (patients >75 years old) and patients with multiple medical problems. As a result, the benefits, risks, and dosages of drugs in younger, healthier populations may not apply to older patients. Older adults are at higher risk for adverse effects because they take more medications (30% take at least four drugs) and have more underlying disease. Older adults also have altered pharmacokinetics (e.g., reduced renal clearance not accurately reflected by serum creatinine) and pharmacodynamics (e.g., more sensitive to warfarin and psychoactive drugs). Finally, polypharmacy decreases compliance, with its own adverse effects.

EVALUATION

When should I Suspect an Adverse Effect from Drugs or Polypharmacy?

Always suspect drugs as a cause of new symptoms. Adverse consequences are often nonspecific, such as dizziness, falls, confusion, or altered bowel and bladder function. Particularly scrutinize hospitalized patients because 25% of admissions of older adults are for drug-related problems—most often resulting from adverse effects, rather than patient errors or noncompliance.

Are Particular Medications More Commonly Associated with Adverse Effects in Elderly Patients?

Problematic drugs include antihypertensives, NSAIDs, H_2 blockers, digoxin, narcotics, and sedatives. These agents are often clearly medically indicated; they are mentioned here to increase vigilance, rather than prohibit their use. The Beers list is a well-known expert panel consensus compilation of drugs that may be inappropriate for use in elderly patients and includes propoxyphene, muscle relaxants, long-acting benzodiazepines, TCAs, and diphenhydramine.

TREATMENT

How can I best Avoid Polypharmacy and Adverse Drug Events in Elderly Patients?

Regardless of age, the risk for adverse reactions increases with each added medication. Be particularly judicious when initiating drugs in elderly patients. Try to limit patients to at most four drugs, which is often very difficult in patients with multiple chronic conditions. Start at the lowest recommended dose. Carefully assess for drug interactions and for dosage changes necessitated by altered metabolism. Calculate creatinine clearance, rather than relying on serum creatinine to assess renal function. Use Medisets (a box with compartments for each day to hold pills), simple regimens, and patient education to reduce patient errors. Review over-the-counter agent use as well.

How can I Safely Withdraw Medications in Elderly Patients?

Although some drugs require slow tapering to avoid physiologic withdrawal (i.e., steroids or drugs that interact with receptors such as beta blockers, benzodiazepines, and antidepressants), do not be reluctant to withdraw drugs carefully whenever problematic polypharmacy is suspected. In one study of drug reduction among older adults, about one in four medications was stopped, and 74% of drug discontinuations occurred without incident; no deaths were associated with the infrequent disease exacerbations that did occur when medications were stopped.

URINARY INCONTINENCE

ETIOLOGY

What are the Basic Categories of Urinary Incontinence?

Keeping in mind that mixed etiologies are common, there are four basic categories, each with characteristic symptoms and risk factors (Table 30-2): overflow, stress, urge, and functional.

What are Common Causes of Acute Incontinence?

Remember reversible causes with the mnemonic "DRIP" (Box 30-1). These often present suddenly and are usually reversible. Frequently implicated drugs include diuretics, anticholinergic agents that impair bladder contractility, and narcotics. Isolated nocturnal incontinence is often from volume overload states (CHF, lower extremity edema) secondary to the diuresis that occurs with recumbence.

Geriatrics

Geriatrics

Table 30-2

Mechanisms, Symptoms, and Treatment of the Four Types of Urinary Incontinence

Incontinence Type	Mechanisms and Risk Factors	Characteristic Symptoms	Treatment
Overflow	Outlet obstruction BPH, stricture Decreased bladder contractility Diabetic neuropathy	Hesitancy, dribbling Small-volume leakage	Avoid anticholinergic agents For BPH Alpha blockers 5-alpha-reductase inhibitor Saw palmetto TURP For stricture Urethral dilation
Stress	Weak sphincter Altered pelvic muscle strength Multiple childbirths Vaginal atrophy	Exacerbated by cough, laugh, bending Small-volume leakage	Pelvic muscle exercises Pessary Periurethral collagen injections Surgery Alpha agonists Topical estrogen
Urge	Detrusor Hyperreflexia Decreased CNS inhibition Parkinson's disease, stroke Detrusor Overactivity Increased bladder contraction UTI, renal stone Outlet obstruction	Sudden urge Large-volume leakage	Avoid irritants (caffeine, alcohol) Scheduled voiding Anticholinergic agents— oxybutynin, tolterodine
Functional	Physical or cognitive impairment	Inability to get to toilet Large-volume leakage	Adapt environment Commode, urinal Scheduled voiding

BOX 30-1

COMMON REVERSIBLE CAUSES OF ACUTE INCONTINENCE

D—Drugs, delirium
R—Restricted mobility, retention
I —Infection, fecal impaction
P—Polyuric states (e.g., CHF, diabetes)

EVALUATION

What is the Best Way to Discern the Cause of a Patient's Incontinence?

Inquire about timing and volume of urine loss and about specific symptoms related to urge or stress incontinence, outlet obstruction, and functional problems. If incontinence is new or suddenly worse, consider DRIP causes. Because the bladder control reflex arc is located at S2–4, focus the examination on relevant neurologic evaluation of sacral dermatomes and lower extremity function. Also perform a rectal exam (evaluate prostate, sphincter tone, anal wink, and for fecal impaction) and pelvic exam (atrophy, vaginitis, prolapse). Assess for a volume overload state, cognitive impairment, and physical impairment. Send urinalysis, glucose, BUN/creatinine, and calcium. Obtain PVR; >100 mL is likely overflow incontinence, whereas <100 mL is likely urge or stress incontinence.

TREATMENT

What are Common Treatment Approaches to Incontinence?

Greater than 50% of patients are cured and most others are markedly improved with standard therapies. Nonpharmacologic interventions are often the most effective and include scheduled voids, bladder training (including Kegel exercises to strengthen pelvic muscles and biofeedback and techniques to decrease urges), addressing mobility issues, and adult protective garments. Medications and surgical options are guided by etiology (Figure 30-2; see Table 30-2). For urge incontinence, agents with antimuscarinic effects can decrease urgency, but anticholinergic side effects (dry mouth, constipation, confusion) may limit their use, especially in the elderly. No medications help overflow incontinence; avoid anticholinergic medications that may decrease bladder tone and worsen obstruction. Refer to urology for hematuria, PVR >100 mL, prostate nodule, prolapse, or if diagnosis is unclear after initial evaluation or empiric therapy fails.

Geriatrics

Geriatrics

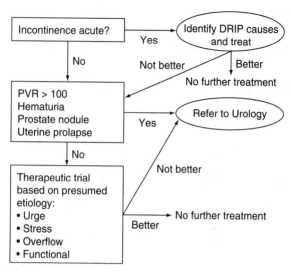

FIGURE 30-2 Algorithm for the management of urinary incontinence.

Case 30-2

A 69-year-old woman presents with a new onset of urinary incontinence, worsening over the past month. She also describes difficulty walking over the past 3 months and has required the use of a walker. Her son, who is her primary caregiver, reports that the patient has memory impairment. He reports that she has difficulty recalling recent events, and he has observed changes in his mother's behavior. Her past medical history is significant for a head injury resulting in a subdural hemorrhage 8 months ago. There have been no recent changes to her medications. Vital signs are normal.

A. What is your differential diagnosis?
B. What is the most likely diagnosis and management?

KEY POINTS – BENIGN PROSTATIC HYPERPLASIA

◆ Use history and directed evaluations to detect and assess severity of BPH.

◆ Patient symptoms and preferences should guide interventions for BPH.

KEY POINTS – DEMENTIA

◆ Most dementia is not reversible; Alzheimer's disease is the most common cause.

◆ Drugs and depression are the most common potentially reversible causes of dementia.

◆ Function and behavior are optimized through excellent general medical care, nonpharmacologic interventions, and the judicious use of drugs.

KEY POINTS – POLYPHARMACY

◆ The biggest risk factor for adverse drug events is number of medications prescribed.

◆ Compliance decreases as the number of drugs and complexity of the regimen increase.

◆ With careful monitoring, many medications can be safely stopped in older adults.

KEY POINTS – URINARY INCONTINENCE

◆ Most urinary incontinence can be cured or markedly improved using combined nonpharmacologic and pharmacologic interventions.

◆ History and directed exam are the key to determining the causes of incontinence.

Case Answers

30-1 A. *Learning objective:* **Identify key features necessary to diagnose dementia.** This patient has memory deficits along with impairment in other cognitive areas—motor skills, language, or personality. The MMSE is a good objective measurement of cognitive impairment, but is not a tool to diagnose dementia. The patient likely has multi-infarct dementia, one of the most common causes of dementia after Alzheimer's dementia. This is due to an accumulation of defects secondary to multiple cerebral infarcts. Patients often present with a stepwise progression of dementia.

30-1 B.   *Learning objective:* **Outline treatment plan for multi-infarct dementia.** Treatment for patients with multi-infarct dementia involves addressing risk factors for vascular events, in particular, aggressive control of hypertension and treatment of high cholesterol levels to reduce the risk of further infarctions. Nonpharmacologic approaches (distraction, physical activity, day centers) should be the first step to manage problem behaviors, but if such efforts fail, and behavior is impairing care, distressing to the patient, or causing safety problems, treatment with small doses of neuroleptics is appropriate.

30-1 C.   *Learning objective:* **Recognize complications associated with dementia.** Complications of multi-infarct dementia include urinary incontinence, aspiration pneumonia, and, in more severe cases, seizure disorders secondary to the infarcted area serving as a seizure focus.

30-2 A.   *Learning objective:* **Recognize acute causes of urinary incontinence and cases that may report urinary incontinence as an associated symptom.** Common causes of acute incontinence include the "DRIP" mnemonic—drugs, delirium; restricted mobility, retention; infection, fecal impaction; polyuric state (CHF or diabetes). Urinary incontinence also can be a presenting symptom with other findings. This patient also has behavior changes and memory impairment and describes gait disturbances. The differential in this case also should include UTI, subcortical dementia, stroke, hemorrhage, neoplasm, or hydrocephalus.

30-2 B.   *Learning objective:* **Understand the manifestations of normal pressure communicating hydrocephalus.** This patient has the triad of normal pressure communicating hydrocephalus, which includes: urinary incontinence, dementia, and gait ataxia. Normal pressure hydrocephalus can be idiopathic or follow a head injury, meningitis, or SAH. CT or MRI showing enlarged lateral ventricles is consistent with a diagnosis of normal pressure hydrocephalus, but ultimately this diagnosis is made on clinical grounds. Treatment is a lumbar-peritoneal or ventriculoperitoneal shunt.

USEFUL WEB SITE

Urinary Incontinence
American Geriatrics Society web site, which has many cross-references to clinical guidelines and updates regarding health problems of older adults. http://www.americangeriatrics.org/

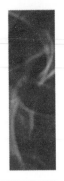

31

Hematology and Oncology

KEITH D. EATON, HEIDI S. POWELL, and ALEXANDER D. SCHAFIR

 BLEEDING DISORDERS

ETIOLOGY

What General Processes Cause Abnormal Hemostasis?

Hemostasis requires a dynamic balance between factors that promote clot formation and factors that promote anticoagulation. The tendency to bleed or to clot can be inherited or acquired. The types of bleeding problems you encounter in the outpatient setting are likely to be quite different from the bleeding problems you might see in hospitalized patients.

What are the Most Common Causes of Abnormal Bleeding?

Common causes are summarized in Table 31-1. Von Willibrand's disease (vWD) is the most likely inherited cause; it is due to a lack of the protein that links platelets to damaged endothelium. The most common acquired cause is **NSAIDs and aspirin**, with bleeding in 10% of patients taking these agents. Idiopathic thrombocytopenic purpura (ITP) is an acquired disease caused by autoantibodies that bind to the surface of platelets and shorten their life span. These antibodies may be associated with a variety of systemic illnesses, including SLE, HIV infection, and lymphoproliferative disorders. ITP is usually an outpatient diagnosis. Hospitalized patients with thrombocytopenia should be evaluated for alternative causes.

What are the Most Likely Causes of Bleeding in a Hospitalized Patient?

The leading diagnosis depends on how sick your patient is and what underlying medical problems are present. In the ICU, Disseminated Intravascular Coagulation (DIC) is a common cause of abnormal

Table 31-1

Prevalence of Common Inherited and Acquired Bleeding Disorders

Bleeding Disorder	Prevalence	Factors Involved
Inherited Disorders		
vWD	1/100	von Willebrand factor deficiency
Hemophilia A	1/5000–10,000*	VIII deficiency
Hemophilia B	1/30,000–50,000*	IX deficiency (Christmas disease)
Acquired Disorders		
NSAIDs	1/10	Platelet dysfunction
ITP	1/10,000	Platelet antibodies
DIC	—	Platelet and factor consumption
End-stage liver disease	—	Vitamin K–dependent factor deficiency (II, VII, IX, X)
Warfarin	2/100/y	Vitamin K–dependent factor deficiency (II, VII, IX, X)

*Prevalence among live male births only because these are X-linked conditions.

bleeding. This is a final common pathway of many conditions, including sepsis, massive trauma and transfusion, acute head injury, acute promyelocytic leukemia, and adenocarcinoma. **Liver disease** (acute or chronic) with its associated vitamin K–dependent factor deficiencies (II, VII, IX, X) is common in patients who are bleeding briskly enough to be hospitalized. Overanticoagulation is a common cause of bleeding necessitating hospitalization. Of the several million patients in the U.S. taking **warfarin** for CHF or atrial fibrillation, about 2% per year have significant bleeding complications.

What is Hemophilia?

Hemophilia A and B are X-linked deficiencies of factors VIII and IX (see Table 31-1). Although we expect a pedigree similar to that of the royal families of Victorian Europe, about 30% of hemophiliacs have a spontaneous, de novo mutation.

EVALUATION

How do I Gauge if Prior Bleeding is Excessive?

Although prior excessive bleeding is your clue to a true bleeding disorder, it is often over-reported. Quantify the blood loss. Did epistaxis require cautery, packing, or transfusion? Was transfusion required after a minor surgical procedure (dental extraction, tonsillectomy, circumcision)? Have menses been heavy for >3 days or prolonged for >6–7 days? Has there been anemia or iron therapy in the past, especially in men (who do not have menses or pregnancy to blame)?

How do I Distinguish Between Hereditary and Acquired Disorders?

A careful history reveals helpful clues. Ask about lifelong problems with hemostasis to uncover inherited problems: at birth, circumcision, tonsillectomy, tooth extractions (requiring wound packing or suturing), postpartum, nosebleeds. The one exception to this rule is vWD because severity varies and may worsen later in life. Ask about medications, especially the recent addition of an anti-inflammatory drug or anticoagulant, which might suggest an acquired cause. Acute bleeding in a hospitalized patient who has a history of excellent hemostasis is almost always from an acquired condition.

Does the Type of Bleeding Help me Generate a Differential Diagnosis?

Yes; Table 31-2 summarizes differential diagnoses. Hematochezia, melena, hematemesis, hemoptysis, and hematuria are almost never due to a bleeding disorder, so evaluate these patients for an anatomic cause of blood loss.

What Lab Tests do I Order if I Suspect a Bleeding Problem?

Common tests ordered are listed in Table 31-3. CBC determines if bleeding has caused anemia. Platelet count identifies altered platelet numbers, but tells you nothing about platelet function. PT assesses activity of the extrinsic and common pathways in the coagulation

Table 31-2

Type of Bleeding Suggested by Particular History and Physical Clues

Clinical Symptom	Likely Bleeding Problem
Bruising	Connective tissue disorder (Ehlers-Danlos syndrome, scurvy), vitamin K deficiency (liver failure)
Bruises on extremity extensor surfaces	Physical abuse
Delayed (hours-days) postsurgical bleeding	Hemophilia, vitamin K deficiency, factor deficiency (secondary hemostasis problem)
Joint or deep muscle bleed	Hemophilia
Oozing catheter sites in hospitalized patient	DIC
Palpable purpura	Vasculitis, cryoglobulinemia, endocarditis
Petechiae, mucosal hemorrhage, bruises from minor trauma	Decreased or dysfunctional platelets (primary hemostasis problem)

Table 31-3

Key Features of Lab Abnormalities Seen with Specific Bleeding Disorders

Condition	BT	Plts	PT	PTT	TT	FDP	F	Other Tests
ASA or NSAIDs	↑↑							
vWD	↑	↓ in IIB						Platelet aggregation decreased only with ristocetin
Hemophilia A or B				↑				Factor levels*
Warfarin			↑↑↑	↑↑				LFT
Liver disease	↓		↑↑	↑↑	↑			Exam, LFT
DIC	↑↑	↓↓	↑	↑	↑↑	↑↑↑	↓↓	

BT, bleeding time; F, fibrinogen; FDP, fibrin degradation products; Plts, platelets; TT, thrombin time.

*Factor VIII levels may be low in vWD and hemophilia A because von Willebrand factor complexes with factor VIII and prolongs its half-life in the circulation.

cascade and is elevated with warfarin, vitamin K deficiency, liver disease, and DIC. PTT measures intrinsic pathway activity and is prolonged with DIC and heparin use (but not LMWH). Prolonged PTT also can occur with deficiency of a clotting factor or presence of a lupus inhibitor. To tell which is true, mix some normal serum in with the patient's sample (a "1:1 mix"), and repeat the assay; factor deficiencies correct, whereas inhibitors continue to prolong the PTT. Fibrin degradation products (D-dimer) appear with thromboembolism or DIC.

Case 31-1

A 37-year-old woman with a history of RA presents with a new rash around her ankles and multiple dime- to quarter-sized bruises on her arms after working in her garden. She denies any recent illness or problems with bleeding or bruising in the past and takes no medications. On exam, there are palatal petechiae. There are several purpuric lesions on each of her forearms, all <1.5 cm in diameter and most <1 week old (i.e., little change in color to green or yellow). There is no adenopathy or organomegaly. The rash around her ankles consists of nearly confluent, nonblanching, pinpoint erythematous lesions.

A. What is the most likely diagnosis, and how is her history of RA relevant?
B. What lab studies would you order to investigate this?
C. What do you recommend for therapy?

TREATMENT

How do I Use Blood Products?

Supply the missing components needed for adequate hemostasis (Table 31-4). If the problem is DIC, the key to the patient's survival is to correct the underlying disorder quickly. Mortality in DIC attributed to shock and sepsis is >50%.

If the Diagnosis is Most Likely ITP, do I Give Platelets?

No, because transfused platelets would likely be destroyed about as fast as they were infused. Use high-dose prednisone (1 mg/kg/d) to block the immune process responsible for destroying platelets for 2–7 days, or until the platelet count increases to >30,000/μL. Taper prednisone slowly over 3–4 weeks. If bleeding is severe, or if the initial platelet count is <10,000/μL, IVIG may be considered. The response to IVIG is quicker than the response to prednisone, such that the platelet count usually increases within 24 hours. Many patients with chronic ITP require splenectomy. Immunize these patients with the *Haemophilus*, polyvalent pneumococcal, and meningococcal vaccines several weeks before splenectomy. Platelet count >30,000/μL in ITP is sufficient for adequate hemostasis.

Table 31-4

Use of Blood and Other Products for Bleeding Disorders

Product	Contents	When to use
FFP	All clotting factors, no platelets	Multifactor deficiency, vitamin K deficiency, warfarin excess, liver disease with bleeding
Vitamin K		Same as for FFP
Cryoprecipitate (from FFP)	Fibrinogen, VIII, von Willebrand factor, XIII	PTT prolonged, heparin excess, severe vWD, fibrinogen depletion, DIC, factor VIII deficiency
Protamine sulfate		PTT prolonged from regular heparin (not LMWH)
Platelets		Bleeding time prolonged, NSAIDs, aspirin, massive bleeding or transfusion
Rho (D) immunoglobulin		ITP in Rh-positive patients
Specific factor concentrates	VIII or IX	Hemophilia long-term maintenance
DDAVP*		Preoperatively for mild vWD

FFP, fresh frozen plasma.
*Do not use desmopressin in patients with type IIB vWD because it exacerbates associated thrombocytopenia and may worsen hemostasis.

CLOTTING DISORDERS

What are Heritable Causes of Hypercoagulability?

The list of possible heritable causes of hypercoagulability is growing steadily; all of the causes mentioned here are autosomal dominant. Deficiencies of the physiologic anticoagulant proteins C and S and antithrombin III are detected in 5%-15% of patients <45 years old with DVT. Activated protein C resistance (also called factor V Leiden mutation) may be diagnosed in 50% of patients with recurrent DVT. This is common in women who develop blood clots while taking oral contraceptives. The prevalence of this mutation is estimated at 3%-6% in whites, although it is much less common in Asians and African Americans. A prothrombin (G20210A) polymorphism has been identified more recently as associated with an increased risk of thromboembolism and MI in young patients (2% prevalence in whites). Hyperhomocysteinemia is associated with arterial and venous clots. Thromboembolism remains idiopathic in most cases.

What are the Risk Factors for Thrombosis?

Risk factors for arterial thrombosis (MI, stroke) include hypertension, hyperlipidemia, elevated Lp(a) lipoprotein, diabetes, smoking, and vasculitis. Risk factors for venous clotting include immobilization, anesthesia, surgery, pregnancy, estrogen use, malignancy (especially adenocarcinomas), nephrotic syndrome, CHF, age >50, and prior thrombosis.

What are Antiphospholipid Antibodies?

Antiphospholipid antibodies are acquired IgG or IgM antibodies that come in two classes—anticardiolipin antibodies and lupus anticoagulants. Lupus anticoagulants artifactually prolong the PTT assay. In this setting, the PTT time is not corrected by the addition of plasma, as would be the case for a factor deficiency. The term "lupus anticoagulant" is a misnomer because these antibodies generally are not associated with lupus, and they cause clotting, rather than bleeding. Presence of a lupus anticoagulant and thrombosis, low platelets, or recurrent fetal loss is referred to as APAS—an acquired hypercoagulable state associated with lupus and other autoimmune disorders. It is typically seen in young women. Thirty-five percent of patients with APAS have venous or arterial thromboembolism (or both); the risk of thrombosis approaches 70% with APAS and concurrent lupus, and patients are often given long-term anticoagulation.

Whom do I Screen for the Presence of an Underlying Hypercoagulable State?

The British Society for Hematology has recommended screening in the following situations:

- Thrombosis in a patient <45 years old without risk factors (even with the first event)
- Recurrent thrombosis or thrombosis at an unusual site (cerebral or visceral vein thrombosis)
- Arterial thrombosis in a patient <30 years old
- Family history of venous thrombosis
- Stillbirth *or* three or more unexplained spontaneous abortions

How do I Screen for a Hypercoagulable State?

Obtain protein C and S levels before starting warfarin; remember these may be artifactually low because of consumption of factors in the acute thrombosis. Obtain an antithrombin III level before starting heparin. Activated protein C resistance (by PCR), the presence of antiphospholipid antibodies, and homocysteine levels can be assayed while patients are on anticoagulant therapy. Factor V Leiden and prothrombin G20210A polymorphisms can be detected using PCR-based tests from DNA.

TREATMENT

How do I Anticoagulate a Patient with a DVT?

Patients with an acute DVT need to be treated initially with either standard (unfractionated) heparin or low molecular weight heparin (LMWH). Standard heparin is less expensive and requires frequent monitoring of the PTT and dose adjustments to achieve a therapeutic anticoagulation. The advantage is that it is short-lived and can be reversed more easily than LMWH. Once- or twice-daily subcutaneous LMWH can be given instead. Although LMWH is more expensive per dose, costs are less because of less monitoring and the ability to administer therapy outside of the hospital. LMWH does not alter PTT, and monitoring is not done routinely. For obese (>300 lb) patients and patients with abnormal renal function, the anti-Xa assay can be used to assess the degree of anticoagulation. Oral warfarin can begin soon after the therapeutic anticoagulation levels have been achieved. Physicians vary widely in how aggressively they "load" the warfarin therapy, starting with 5–10 mg for the first few days, then adjusting based on the PT and INR. Heparin is continued until PT is therapeutic on warfarin (INR 2–3). Some hematologists continue heparin 2 days beyond the time a therapeutic INR has been reached to prevent warfarin-associated skin necrosis, which is especially a risk in patients with protein C or S deficiency. Warfarin necrosis occurs as a result of rapid loss of short half-life clotting factors during the initiation of warfarin, causing a transient imbalance in the clotting cascade toward thromboembolism.

My Patient has a Postsurgical DVT. His PT has been Therapeutic on Heparin for 5 Days, but his Platelet Count is Decreasing, and by Duplex Ultrasound his DVT is Enlarging. What's Going on?

Your patient is one of the approximately 2% of patients who develop Heparin-induced thrombocytopenia (HIT). HIT is suspected when platelets decrease below normal or decline >50% from baseline. Extension of the DVT despite adequate anticoagulation means your patient is also one of the 0.2%-0.6% who develop Heparin-induced thrombosis (HITT). A heparin-dependent antibody (usually IgG) that activates platelet aggregation causes HITT. The clotting events associated with HITT may be venous or arterial and are life-threatening. *Stop* all heparin, including catheter flushes. Remove all heparin-bonded catheters. Post a sign above the patient's bed explicitly stating, "*No* heparin flushes." Because this is an antibody-mediated phenomenon, it may occur after the heparin already has been discontinued. Call a hematologist to assist with options for replacing heparin, such as the direct thrombin inhibitors hirudin and argatroban. HIT and HITT are the reason careful platelet monitoring must accompany all heparin use.

How Long do I Continue Warfarin Therapy?

Warfarin is usually given for 3–12 months after an initial event when a reversible cause was present, such as pregnancy, surgery or trauma. Consider indefinite warfarin therapy if the hypercoagulable state is a persistent risk (APAS, CHF, paroxysmal nocturnal hemoglobinuria, nephrotic syndrome, active malignancy). Lifelong anticoagulation also is recommended in patients with a history of multiple events, multiple genetic risk factors, a strong family history, or an initial event in an unusual site. Although it is tempting to base the length of warfarin therapy on the severity of the initial event, this has no real bearing on the patient's subsequent risk for recurrence. Of patients who develop a diagnosed lower extremity DVT, 40%-50% have a pulmonary embolism. Overall, the risk of a significant bleeding complication owing to warfarin therapy is about 2% per year, but is significantly higher for patients >70 years old. Avoid warfarin in women planning pregnancy and through the first trimester.

When should I Consider Prophylactic Anticoagulation?

Give prophylactic subcutaneous heparin during immobility (e.g., postoperatively) to any patient with a prior clot (i.e., with surgery) or with an identified genetic risk, even in the absence of a personal history of thrombosis. Women with factor V Leiden mutation who become pregnant are at a much greater risk for DVT (odds ratio 16.3; 95% confidence interval 4.8–54.9), but there is no evidence supporting prophylaxis in this population, unless there is a personal prior history of DVT.

Is there a Role for Aspirin in a Hypercoagulable Patient?

Aspirin and NSAIDs are antiplatelet agents and are useful in preventing arterial thrombosis (e.g., MI and stroke). A patient with APAS who has a history of predominantly arterial thromboses is often treated with the combination of warfarin and aspirin, with close monitoring of the INR and clinical status. In all other patients taking warfarin for venous thrombosis, aspirin and NSAIDs are discouraged because the risk of bleeding complications increases with the use of these agents.

Case 31-2

A 27-year-old woman of Irish descent is admitted to the medical floor with a left iliofemoral DVT 4 weeks postpartum. She is gravida 4, para 3, aborta 1 (four pregnancies, three live births, and one spontaneous abortion). She denies any prior thrombosis. Her family history is significant for a maternal grandmother who died of a pulmonary embolism at age 63 and a maternal uncle who developed a DVT after a flight to London from Seattle.

A. What are the two most likely diagnoses?
B. What laboratory studies would you perform, and how would anticoagulation therapy affect the accuracy of the evaluation?
C. What do you recommend for therapy?
D. How would you approach diagnostic screening of the extended family?

BREAST CANCER

See section on Breast Health in Chapter 40 for a discussion of breast cancer.

COLON CANCER

ETIOLOGY

Who gets Colon Cancer?

In the U.S., 56,000 people die from colon cancer each year, making it the second deadliest malignancy after lung cancer. Similar to breast cancer, most patients have no risk factors other than age. Lifetime incidence of colon cancer is 5% overall. Lack of physical activity, consumption of red meat, obesity, and alcohol and cigarette use are associated with higher rates of colon cancer. Certain uncommon conditions impart a particularly high risk. A family history of colon cancer in a first-degree relative increases risk approximately twofold. Ulcerative colitis increases risk 10-fold after 10 years of active disease. Hereditary nonpolyposis colorectal cancer (HNPCC), an autosomal dominant condition, accounts for 2%-5% of colon cancer, with early onset of cancer of the colon and other organs and multiple affected relatives. Patients with HNPCC have a 70%-90% chance of developing colon cancer. Familial Adenomatous Polyposis (FAP), also autosomal dominant, accounts for <1% of colon cancer. The colon becomes studded with polyps at an early age, with a colon cancer diagnosis on average by age 16, and nearly all FAP patients who do not undergo prophylactic colectomy are diagnosed with colon cancer by age 50. HNPCC and FAP should be considered in families with early-onset colon cancer, other associated malignancies, and multiple affected relatives.

EVALUATION

What Screening is Recommended?

Starting at age 50, screen for polyps with colonoscopy every decade or, alternatively, with sigmoidoscopy every 3–5 years and annual stool occult blood testing. Individuals at higher risk need earlier and more frequent screening. For patients with a first-degree relative with colon cancer, begin screening at 10 years younger than when the relative developed the disease. Digital rectal exams may detect rectal cancers, but have not been shown to improve outcomes.

What Symptoms Might my Patient with Colon Cancer Develop?

Distal colon cancers tend to obstruct, producing cramping, thin stools, bloating, or perforation. Stool in the proximal colon is more liquid, so cancers there cause symptoms by ulcerating and bleeding. Every adult with unexplained iron deficiency anemia needs a colonoscopy. Dyspnea may be the chief complaint of a patient with a cecal carcinoma and a low hematocrit. Approximately one in five patients presents with metastatic disease, usually in the liver, although the chest and brain also can be sites of metastasis.

How do I Stage Colon Cancer?

The more recent TNM classification categorizes colon cancers into stages I-IV and roughly parallels the older Dukes' classification scheme, which divided cancers into stages A-D. Both systems have been used to decide on appropriate treatment and to estimate prognosis (Table 31-5). Staging work-up includes full examination, including a look for nodal, neurologic, chest, and liver involvement. CXR and CT scan of the abdomen and pelvis are warranted to stage patients appropriately before surgery.

Table 31-5

TNM Classification of Colon Cancer

Stage*	Definition	Treatment	5-Year Survival (%)
I	Limited to mucosa and submucosa	Excision	95
II	Local extension to subserosa or beyond	Excision	75
III	Regional lymph node involvement	Excision, plus adjuvant chemotherapy	50
IV	Metastases (liver > lung > bone > CNS)	Chemotherapy or irradiation, excision of 1–3 liver metastases	5

*Dukes' classification A = TNM I, B = TNM II, C = TNM III, and D = TNM IV.

TREATMENT

How do I Treat Colon Cancer?

Surgery is the primary treatment for stage I-III colon cancer. Adjuvant chemotherapy after surgery is recommended for patients with stage III disease and in selected patients with high-risk stage II disease. Adjuvant chemotherapy agents include 5-fluorouracil with leucovorin with or without oxaliplatin; these reduce recurrence rates and mortality by 30%. In patients with resectable liver metastases as the only metastatic site, resection for cure is sometimes possible. For metastatic disease, treatment with palliative chemotherapy has been shown to prolong survival by many months. Many newer and investigational agents are available, and patients should be treated by an oncology specialist to receive the most up-to-date advice and to participate in treatment trials. Chemotherapy for elderly patients is controversial.

How do I Detect Recurrences Early?

Perform regular exams, blood tests, and colonoscopy. Measure CEA level before excision; a persistently elevated or rising level predicts recurrence.

LEUKEMIA

ETIOLOGY

What Causes Leukemia?

Leukemias are the neoplastic, clonal proliferation of blood cells or their precursors. Leukemias are classified according to the stage of maturation (blast or mature-appearing cells) and type of cell involved (lymphoid or myeloid). There are four common leukemias: CLL, CML, ALL, and acute myeloid leukemia (AML). CLL and AML are diseases of the elderly, with average presentation at age 60 for CLL and 65 for AML. CML is a disease of middle age, with an average age of 42 at presentation. Almost all patients with CML have a translocation between chromosomes 9 and 22, called the Philadelphia chromosome. ALL incidence peaks in young children, but also is seen in adults. AML can arise from the myelodysplastic syndrome. Certain genetic conditions and exposure to radiation, benzene, and chemotherapy all are associated with the development of acute leukemias, but most cases have no identifiable risk factors.

EVALUATION

What are Common Symptoms of Leukemia?

Infiltration of normal bone marrow causes pancytopenia (neutropenia, anemia, and thrombocytopenia), resulting in infection, dyspnea, fatigue, bleeding (especially from the nose or gums), and bruising. Patients may describe fatigue, night sweats, or fever. Infiltration of tissues may result in enlarged nodes, liver, and spleen or masses in the gingiva, skin (leukemia cutis), or soft tissue (chloroma). When the WBC is >150,000, vascular sludging, or leukostasis, may result in stroke, headache, tinnitus, blindness, priapism, or myocardial injury.

What will I See on a Peripheral Blood Smear?

If you see >10,000 mature lymphocytes in the blood of an elderly patient, he or she likely has CLL. In CML, there are 30,000–300,000 WBC, mostly myeloid cells in later stages of maturation with <5% blast forms. When blast forms are >20%, the CML has progressed to a more acute blast phase. Leukemoid reactions or reactive elevations of WBC caused by certain infections may look similar. Leukemoid reactions can be differentiated from CML by testing for a *BCR/ABL* gene rearrangement using PCR. Pancytopenia is the hallmark of acute leukemia, usually with circulating blasts of either myeloid (AML) or lymphoid (ALL) lineage. Leukemia can manifest with a low, high, or numerically normal WBC. Auer rods are pathognomonic for AML—these look like red cigars in the myeloid blast cell cytoplasm.

What Other Tests are Used to Diagnose Leukemias?

Bone marrow biopsy and aspiration are helpful: >30% mature B lymphocytes are present in CLL; mature cells predominate in CML; blasts predominate in AML and ALL. Flow cytometry of bone marrow aspirate specimens identifies membrane antigens that differentiate the blast forms seen with acute leukemias. Cytogenetics can be performed on bone marrow or peripheral blood specimens to identify genetic rearrangements in malignant cells, which provide diagnostic and prognostic information and aid in choosing therapy. One specific translocation between chromosome 9 and 22 is the Philadelphia chromosome and is pathognomonic for CML.

What Special Complications should I Watch Out for?

In CLL, clonal lymphocytes can produce monoclonal immunoglobulins and depress the synthesis of normal immunoglobulins. The resulting hypogammaglobulinemia impairs humoral immunity, causing infections by *Staphylococcus aureus, Streptococcus pneumoniae,* and *Haemophilus influenzae.* Fifteen percent of patients have antibodies against erythrocytes or platelets, conditions known as autoimmune hemolytic anemia or thrombocytopenia. In AML/ALL, bone marrow failure at presentation is the rule, often with sepsis, DIC, or renal failure. Cranial nerve palsies and leukemic meningitis are seen in ALL, especially in children.

TREATMENT

Do I need to Treat the Chronic Leukemias?

Neither CLL nor CML requires urgent treatment in their chronic, asymptomatic phases. CLL may not cause symptoms for many years, and it typically affects older patients who often die of other diseases

Hematology and Oncology

first. Indications for treatment include worsening fatigue, anemia, thrombocytopenia, or worsening lymphadenopathy. Chemotherapy with chlorambucil or fludarabine can be used to help palliate symptoms of CLL. Newer treatments combining chemotherapy with antibodies against CLL cell antigens are now commonly used. Associated autoimmune hemolytic anemia or thrombocytopenia may require prednisone or splenectomy. For CML, hydroxyurea can be used to decrease the WBC. Emergent leukapheresis can reduce cell counts rapidly when sludging causes end-organ damage. Imatinib (Gleevec), specifically inhibits the tyrosine kinase up-regulated by the *bcr/abl* oncogene of CML and seems to give excellent control of the disease for several years with few serious side effects or toxicity. For patients with CML, allogeneic bone marrow transplant is offered to patients <60 years old—this is most successful early in the chronic phase of disease and is the only curative therapy. After several years, patients with CML develop a blast crisis (similar to AML) that responds poorly to chemotherapy or transplantation and is usually lethal.

How do I Treat the Acute Leukemias?

ALL and AML are treated with combination chemotherapy (two or more drugs) in stages—induction, consolidation, and maintenance. Induction chemotherapy is the initial, often successful, attempt to induce a complete remission. Recurrence within 1 year is the rule, unless monthly consolidation chemotherapy is given. The agents used depend on the leukemia cell type and patient age, but may include antimetabolites such as cytarabine or 6-thioguanine, anthracyclines such as daunorubicin or idarubicin, or etoposide. Patients with ALL also require CNS therapy (radiation, intrathecal chemotherapy, or systemic delivery of drugs that penetrate the blood-brain barrier) to prevent CNS relapse. Patients with ALL also may require years of low-dose maintenance therapy. Autologous or allogeneic bone marrow transplants are sometimes used, especially for patients with poor response to chemotherapy or poor prognosis as predicted by cytogenetics. Long-term disease-free survival in adults is 15%-20% for AML and 40% for ALL.

What is the Role of Bone Marrow Transplant?

Hematopoietic cell transplantation is used to treat a variety of hematologic malignancies, including AML, ALL, and CML. Otherwise lethal doses of chemotherapy and radiation are given, and the patient is "rescued" by an infusion of his or her own (autologous) or a donor's (allogeneic) stem cells. In the case of allogeneic transplantation, an immunologic "graft versus leukemia" effect helps to control the underlying malignant clone. Because of the high degree of toxicity associated with transplantation, these therapies traditionally have been used in patients <60 years old. More recently, nonmyeloablative transplantation has come into clinical use, in which lower doses of chemotherapy are given along with immunosuppressants to allow for engraftment of donor stem cells. This approach is tolerated in older patients and offers potentially curative therapy based on the graft versus leukemia effect.

What are Potential Complications of Treatments for Leukemia?

Hydroxyurea can cause bone marrow suppression. Imatinib can cause capillary leakage (pulmonary edema, ascites, pleural effusions, edema), GI symptoms, and cytopenias, and can be hepatotoxic, but is generally well tolerated. Bone marrow transplantation purposefully ablates native bone marrow, leaving patients transiently susceptible to many serious infections and dependent on RBC and platelet transfusions until the transplant repopulates the bone marrow. Treatment that rapidly lyses large numbers of tumor cells, such as induction chemotherapy for acute leukemia, can precipitate renal failure secondary to the tumor lysis syndrome, in which purine metabolites released from leukemic cells increase uric acid and potassium. Cytarabine and etoposide cause alopecia, mucositis, nausea, vomiting, neuropathy, and bone marrow suppression with a nadir around 14 days after administration. Anthracyclines such as daunorubicin are known to cause arrhythmias, heart failure (even years after administration), secondary leukemias, and infertility in addition to the usual myelosuppression, GI effects, and alopecia seen with other chemotherapy agents.

█ LUNG CANCER

ETIOLOGY

Who gets Lung Cancer?

Lung cancer is the leading cause of cancer deaths in the U.S., accounting for >160,000 deaths annually—more than the next three most common cancers combined. Because of increasing smoking rates among women, lung cancer mortality has far surpassed that of breast cancer among women in the U.S. Approximately 85% of patients who die of lung cancer are current or former smokers, and many of the nonsmokers affected die from passive exposure. Workers exposed to asbestos (plumbers, shipbuilders) have four times the risk of nonsmokers. Smoking is synergistic with asbestos, and together they increase the risk of lung cancer 100 times. Although in theory screening for such a common, fatal disease makes sense, trials of screening with sputum cytology or CXR or both have not been shown to decrease mortality, and these screening methods are not recommended. Screening with chest CT has a higher sensitivity for smaller and more potentially curable lesions. Many noncancerous lesions are discovered, however, which must be investigated, exposing the patient to potential harm and cost. At this time, there are no data from randomized clinical trials indicating decreased mortality with this procedure.

What Types of Lung Cancer are There?

Multiple histologic types of lung cancer are classified into one of two groups based on natural history and response to therapy (Table 31-6). Squamous cell carcinoma, adenocarcinoma, and large cell carcinoma

Table 31-6

Classification of Lung Cancers

Stage	Involvement	Treatment	5-Year Survival (%)
SCLC			
Limited	Disease site can be encompassed in a radiation port in one hemithorax	Chemotherapy and radiotherapy with or without prophylactic cranial irradiation	12
Extensive	More than "limited"	Chemotherapy with or without prophylactic cranial irradiation	<1
NSCLC			
1	No nodes or metastases	Surgical resection and adjuvant chemotherapy for selected patients	60–70
2	Ipsilateral bronchial or hilar nodes only	Surgical resection and adjuvant chemotherapy	40–50
3	Distal nodes or local extension	Chemotherapy, surgery, or radiotherapy or some combination	15–25
4	Distant metastases	Palliative radiotherapy or chemotherapy	2

are lumped together as non small cell lung cancer (NSCLC). This subset accounts for >80% of lung cancer and is treated with combinations of surgery, radiation, and chemotherapy depending on the stage of disease and the underlying health of the patient. Small cell lung cancer (SCLC) is a less common histologic subtype and is seen in about 15%-20% of lung cancer patients. It is a systemic disease—with rapid spread to the mediastinum, nodes, liver, bone, and CNS. Chemotherapy often produces dramatic responses in patients with SCLC and can extend life expectancy significantly and palliate symptoms.

EVALUATION

How might a Patient with Lung Cancer Present?

The most common presenting symptom is cough, and the second most common is dyspnea. A lung mass may bleed or obstruct an airway, producing hemoptysis, dyspnea, or postobstructive pneumonia. Local extension to the mediastinum, pleura, and chest wall may result in chest pain, pleural and pericardial effusions, compression of the superior vena cava, or paralysis of mediastinal nerves. Patients with lung cancer may present with signs of distant metastases before ever having any pulmonary symptoms, including bone pain, liver inflammation, adrenal insufficiency, or neurologic symptoms. Many paraneoplastic syndromes are associated with particular lung cancers. SIADH occurs in about 10% of patients with SCLC and causes hyponatremia. SCLC also can release ACTH and cause Cushing's syndrome. Humorally mediated hypercalcemia is common in squamous cell carcinoma. These tumors increase serum calcium by secreting parathyroid hormone analogues—bone metastases are rarely a cause of hypercalcemia in lung cancer.

How do I Evaluate a Single Nodule on a CXR?

Many diseases may cause nodules, such as benign tumors (hamartomas, lipomas), arteriovenous malformations, infections (TB, abscesses, fungal diseases), rheumatologic disease (Wegener's granulomatosis, RA), infarction, hemorrhage, primary lung cancers, or metastatic cancers. A complete history and physical is important. Certain features of the nodule suggest cancer, including irregular borders and eccentric calcification. Nodules that are unchanged after 2 years are unlikely to be cancer, so old CXR may be helpful. CT and PET scanning can aid in the evaluation of a concerning chest radiograph, but ultimately, suspicious lesions require biopsy.

What Tests are Required to Stage Lung Cancer?

Patients suspected to have lung cancer should have a thorough history and physical, looking for signs of metastasis to nodes, bone, brain, or liver. Blood tests should include CBC, electrolytes, creatinine, calcium, liver panel, and alkaline phosphatase. Chest CT should be obtained to look for extent of disease. Abnormal findings should guide the ordering of further testing. In patients with NSCLC, if CT suggests stage IIIB (extensive invasion of local structures, contralateral lung involvement) or stage IV (distant metastasis) disease, and biopsy confirms this, surgical resection is not an option. PET may help identify suspicious lymph nodes in the hilar area or mediastinum that require biopsy by bronchoscopy, mediastinoscopy, or thoracoscopy. Sometimes staging is not completed until after surgical resection has occurred. Patients with SCLC require brain imaging, bone scan, and chest and abdominal imaging to differentiate limited from extensive stage disease. Of patients with SCLC, 40% have CNS metastasis.

TREATMENT

What is the Approach to Treatment?

For advanced lung cancers (stage IIIb/IV NSCLC or extensive SCLC), treatment is palliative with chemotherapy or radiation to shrink, but not eliminate, bulky tumor masses impinging on crucial structures. Earlier stages of NSCLC (I-IIIA) are surgically resected, and most patients also receive adjuvant chemotherapy with agents such as cisplatin and vinorelbine. SCLC is sensitive to combined chemoradiotherapy, but relapse after treatment is the general rule. Etoposide and cisplatin have traditionally been used, although many other regimens exist in this rapidly developing field. One third of patients with SCLC have disease limited to a hemithorax, and although 80%-90% respond initially, average survival is <20 months. Patients with extensive stage disease have average survival of <13 months. Patients with SCLC CNS metastasis can be offered radiation therapy (see Table 31-6).

 NON-HODGKIN'S LYMPHOMA

ETIOLOGY

What Causes NHL?

NHL comprises a diverse group of lymphoid tumors of unknown etiology. NHL causes about 19,000 deaths each year, mostly in middle-aged patients. NHL can be a complication of HIV infection. Other associations include HTLV infection, *Helicobacter pylori* infection, prior chemotherapy or radiation therapy, and autoimmune disease. Because of the relatively low prevalence, screening is not recommended.

What are the Different Types of NHL?

Most lymphomas are due to clonal proliferation of B lymphocytes residing in lymph nodes. Primary CNS lymphomas are usually seen in patients with immunocompromise, such as HIV infection. GI lymphomas have been associated with *H. pylori* infection, Crohn's disease, and celiac sprue. T cell lymphomas are less common and may manifest as cutaneous malignancy (mycosis fungoides) or in association with HTLV infection (seen predominantly in Southern Japan, parts of Africa and the Caribbean, and in IVDU in the U.S.). Lymphomas also are classified as indolent, aggressive, and highly aggressive based on their rapidity of progression.

EVALUATION

How do Patients with NHL Present?

About two thirds of patients present with enlarged nodes. **Indolent** lymphomas may exist for years before the patient notices waxing and waning painless adenopathy. Sometimes, patients report abdominal fullness or early satiety secondary to hepatosplenomegaly. **Aggressive** lymphomas may act like acute leukemias, with rapid, progressive enlargement of lymph nodes. Any lymphoma may manifest with generalized "B" symptoms: fever, night sweats, and ≥10% weight loss over the previous 6 months. B symptoms more often accompany aggressive lymphomas and portend a worse prognosis. Patients also may report fatigue, pruritus, or GI symptoms. Physical exam should focus on presence of lymph nodes (including in the neck, axillae, groin, and tonsils); abdominal exam for organomegaly; and testicular, neurologic, and skin exams.

What Work-up is Necessary?

Lymphomas can involve any lymphoid tissue and the CNS, so a complete history and physical are critical, with special focus as noted in the previous question. You also would want a lymph node biopsy of an entire node to evaluate nodal architecture and adequately diagnose the type of lymphoma. When lymphoma has been suggested by node biopsy, you would need bone marrow biopsy, LP, and head and body imaging for staging the tumor. Basic blood tests should be drawn to identify complications, including CBC, renal function, electrolytes, calcium, uric acid, and LFTs. Serum beta-2-microglobulin and LDH may reflect prognosis and disease activity in patients with NHL and help monitor response to therapy. SPEP may reveal circulating paraproteins or hypogammaglobinemia. Cytogenetics and cell surface immunophenotyping (flow cytometry) and immunohistocytochemistry may characterize the malignant cells further for diagnostic and treatment decisions.

What Defines the Stages of NHL?

The stages are I-IV, as follows: I, single nodal area; II, several nodal areas on the same side of the diaphragm; III, several nodal areas on both sides of the diaphragm; and IV, disseminated disease. Each stage is subclassified as "B" for presence of B symptoms, as described previously.

TREATMENT

Which Patients with NHL Require Treatment, and How Effective is Therapy?

In general, indolent lymphomas are not curable, so asymptomatic indolent lymphomas are not treated. If symptoms occur, these may be improved with chemotherapy. Aggressive and highly aggressive lymphomas are potentially curable, are often responsive to treatment, and are rapidly fatal if not treated. For symptomatic or more aggressive tumors, various combinations of radiation and chemotherapy are used, depending on the histology of the tumor and extent of disease. Overall, 5-year survival is about 50%, but that does not tell the whole story. Patients with low-grade lymphomas live many years, but are rarely cured, whereas patients with aggressive lymphomas are cured about 50% of the time.

PROSTATE CANCER

ETIOLOGY

How Many Men have Prostate Cancer?

Prostate cancer is the most common newly diagnosed cancer in men (i.e., it has the highest incidence). About 30,000 men die of this disease each year in the U.S. It is unique in its high prevalence of "latent" disease: 70% of men in their 80s who die from other causes have microscopic foci of prostate cancer. In contrast, only 3% of prostate cancers lead to death. The incidence is highest in blacks, less in whites, and least in Asians. Mortality per case is higher in African Americans. Family history is a risk factor.

EVALUATION

Should I Screen My Patient for Prostate Cancer?

There is currently insufficient evidence to recommend for or against screening. Digital rectal exams, PSA, and transrectal ultrasound can detect tumors that would never cause symptoms or are already incurable. Additionally, treatments may cause incontinence and impotence with unclear benefit. You must help your patient make a personal decision in the face of uncertainty.

What Symptoms Suggest Prostate Cancer?

Early cancers often produce no symptoms, and most cases are detected by screening. Some men report symptoms of dysuria, hematuria, or trouble voiding, but this is uncommon. The first symptom may be metastatic bone pain. Sorting out the few men with treatable prostate cancer from the millions with symptomatic BPH is a clinical dilemma.

How is Prostate Cancer Classified?

Prostate cancer is staged clinically by how far the cancer has extended (Table 31-7). Pelvic CT scan is not sensitive enough to detect extracapsular extension and pelvic node or seminal vesicle involvement; some cancers are fully staged only at the time of surgery. Each cancer also is assigned a Gleason grade based on histologic features. Tumors are graded 1–5 on two accounts: primarily on the level of differentiation and secondarily on structural architecture. These two scores are added, with the most well-differentiated tumors having the best prognosis and scoring 2–4, moderately differentiated tumors scoring 5–7, and poorly differentiated tumors having the worst prognosis and scoring 8–10. Stage and grade assist with treatment decisions and prognosis.

When and Where should I Look for Metastatic Prostate Cancer?

Bone is the most common distant site, usually involving the pelvic girdle and vertebrae. Some physicians obtain radionuclide bone scan in all patients with a prostate cancer diagnosis, although others are more selective, ordering the test only when PSA is >10, Gleason score is

Table 31-7

Staging of Prostate Cancer

Stage	Criteria
T1	Microscopic, not palpable on rectal exam
T2	Palpable, confined to prostate gland
T3	Protrudes beyond prostate capsule or into seminal vesicles
T4	Tumor fixed, extends locally well beyond gland
Metastatic	Tumor spread to pelvic nodes or bone

>5, or there is palpable extension of tumor on rectal exam. Lung and liver are rarely sites of distant metastasis.

TREATMENT

What are the Treatment Options for Men with Prostate Cancer?

Treatment options include observation, radiation, surgery, and hormonal therapy. For disease limited to the prostate, the decision to treat is usually based on Gleason score. Nonaggressive tumors are candidates for watchful waiting. More aggressive cancer limited to the prostate may be cured with radical prostatectomy or radiation therapy, although there is controversy among experts whether benefits outweigh risks of side effects. The treatment for tumor extending through the capsule is another area of controversy. When lymph nodes, bone, lung, or liver is involved, the cancer cannot be cured; in contrast to breast and colon cancer, even a single positive lymph node makes recurrence nearly certain. Consequences of surgical or radiation therapy include urinary incontinence and impotence for many patients. Radiation also can cause chronic proctitis. Long-term survivors of radiation therapy may have an increased risk of bladder and rectal cancers.

Is there a Role for Palliative Therapy in Patients with Metastatic Prostate Cancer?

Palliative treatment is the rule for symptomatic metastatic disease. Because this tumor is responsive to androgens, the use of antiandrogens, orchiectomy, estrogens, or LHRH analogues reduces androgen synthesis and decreases symptoms. Bone pain resulting from metastases also responds well to anti-inflammatory agents, but may require use of opioid analgesics. Chemotherapy has been shown to decrease pain and prolong palliation and has been shown more recently to confer a modest improvement in survival.

How Long will my Patient Live?

Five-year survival for local disease is >90%. Five-year survival decreases to 80% for locally invasive disease and 30% for metastatic disease (better than for most other metastatic cancers). All of these rates are lower for African Americans, who may have more aggressive tumors or may get less timely or less aggressive treatment.

TUMORS IN YOUNGER ADULTS

What Cancers of Younger Adults should I Look Out For?

Hodgkin's disease is a tumor of lymphoid tissue, commonly manifesting with painless, rubbery nodes, which is highly curable with radiation or chemotherapy or both. **Testicular cancer** is the most common cancer in men 15–35 years old. It also is highly curable; owing to the ignorance and embarrassment of patients and physicians, the diagnosis is often delayed. It is more common in whites and in men with undescended testes. The patient may present with a painless testicular mass or supraclavicular nodes. Treatment modalities include surgery, radiation, and chemotherapy, depending on stage and pathologic subtype. Overall cure rates are 95%. In contrast to most solid tumors, patients with advanced disease have excellent cure rates of 80%. Early stages of **ovarian cancer** are asymptomatic. Ovarian cancer manifests late, often with ascites or pain from peritoneal spread. Most patients die (16,000/y in the U.S.), and there is no effective screening. Deaths from **cervical cancer** have declined to <4000/y in the U.S., and many of these could be prevented with regular Pap smears. The major risk factor is infection with HPV, and the disease is particularly aggressive in patients with HIV.

Case 31-3

A 61-year-old, 80-pack-year smoker presents with neck and upper back pain. CXR shows hyperinflation, flattened diaphragms, bullae, and a 2-cm right upper lobe nodule. Calcium is 10.5 mg/dL.

 A. What is your diagnostic plan?
 B. What are the characteristics of a lung nodule that suggest malignancy?
 C. What are possible explanations for his abnormal calcium level?

Case 31-4

A 50-year-old woman reports feeling very tired. She used to play soccer with her daughters, but now she gets out of breath just unloading the car. She had a prolonged nosebleed yesterday for the first time in years.

 A. What are diagnoses to consider, and what questions should you ask?
 B. What would you look for on exam? Would this pin down the diagnosis?
 C. What complications might occur?

Case 31-5

A 40-year-old man reports chills for the last few days. He has smoked 2 packs per day since age 15 and "coughs all the time, but I think it is getting worse." His 43-year-old brother had a bleeding adenoma removed from his colon last year. You see that he is tired and thin, and you find a clump of nodes in the left supraclavicular fossa. CXR shows left hilar enlargement.

 A. What is a Virchow's node?
 B. What tests do you order?
 C. If he is cured by chemotherapy, would there be long-lasting effects?

Case 31-6

A 58-year-old woman elects to have a screening colonoscopy because her neighbor just died of colon cancer. You find a 2-cm ulcerating adenocarcinoma in her ascending colon. LFTs, a CT scan of the abdomen, and CXR are normal. She undergoes hemicolectomy, and tumor is found in two regional lymph nodes.

   A. Should she have been screened earlier? If so, why and how?
   B. What stage of colon cancer does she have?
   C. Do you recommend any further treatment?

Case 31-7

A 70-year-old man comes to you for a routine physical exam. On rectal exam, you find that his prostate is mildly irregular and firm in one area. He tells you that his father had prostate cancer at age 57.

   A. What evaluation do you suggest?
   B. How can you help him decide on treatment?
   C. He is concerned about his 35-year-old son and 92-year-old uncle, and he hopes that you will see them for screening, too. What do you say?

Hematology and Oncology

KEY POINTS – BLEEDING DISORDERS

◆ Ask about prior dental procedures, surgeries, and menses to uncover excessive bleeding.

◆ Mucosal and catheter site oozing in hospitalized patients suggests DIC; petechiae suggest a platelet problem; palpable purpura suggests vasculitis or immune complex deposition; delayed bleeding suggests factor deficiency.

◆ Bleeding from the bowel, bladder, or lungs is generally not due to a bleeding disorder and requires rapid evaluation to find the cause.

◆ Give FFP to stop bleeding in patients with liver disease or warfarin excess.

◆ Give prednisone or IVIG, not platelets, to patients with ITP.

KEY POINTS – CLOTTING DISORDERS

◆ Overlap heparin and warfarin use in patients with DVT to prevent warfarin-induced clotting.

◆ Screen for hypercoagulable state in patients with recurrent thromboses, recurrent fetal loss, unusual or arterial sites of clotting, or a family history of frequent blood clots and patients <45 years old with DVT and no risk factors.

◆ Monitor platelets in patients before and during heparin use to look for HIT.

KEY POINTS – COLON CANCER

◆ Common risk factors for colon cancer are age >50 years, family history, and ulcerative colitis.

◆ Screen individuals >50 years old, or earlier if there are risk factors.

◆ Patients with iron deficiency anemia need endoscopic evaluation to assess for colon cancer.

KEY POINTS – LEUKEMIA

◆ Symptoms of leukemia are caused by cytopenias, infiltration of organs and bone marrow, alterations in immunity, and the large burden of clonal cells in the blood.

◆ Leukemia is diagnosed by peripheral smear, bone marrow biopsy, immunologic markers (flow cytometry), and cytogenetics.

◆ CLL may never need treatment; CML always becomes acute over time, and early transplant is the only cure.

◆ Acute leukemias are treated urgently with combination chemotherapy.

KEY POINTS – LUNG CANCER

◆ Screening asymptomatic individuals for lung cancer is not currently recommended.

◆ SCLC is treated with chemotherapy for extensive disease. Limited stage disease is treated with chemotherapy and radiation.

◆ NSCLC is best treated by surgery, but you must look carefully to prove that the tumor is resectable.

◆ Talk to smokers about quitting every time you see them.

Hematology and Oncology

(Continued)

◆ Hyponatremia resulting from SIADH and hypercortisolism resulting from tumor ACTH release can occur with SCLC.

KEY POINTS – NON-HODGKIN'S LYMPHOMA

◆ Suspect NHL when diffuse or persistent lymphadenopathy is present.

◆ NHL is a common complication of HIV infection.

◆ Treatment decisions depend on subtype, stage, and age and condition of the patient.

KEY POINTS – PROSTATE CANCER

◆ It is unknown whether screening for prostate cancer is beneficial or harmful.

◆ Treatment is with surgery and radiation, but some patients may be better off without treatment.

◆ Metastatic disease cannot be cured, but antiandrogen therapies and anti-inflammatory medications may reduce bone pain symptoms.

Case Answers

31-1 A.   *Learning objective:* **Suspect ITP when petechiae appear in the setting of autoimmune disease.** The most likely diagnosis is ITP. The patient's autoimmune history puts her at a slightly higher risk of acquiring additional autoimmune complications such as ITP. The combination of ITP and autoimmune hemolytic anemia is known as Evans' syndrome and is seen in patients with underlying autoimmune disorders such as lupus and RA.

31-1 B.   *Learning objective:* **Order appropriate lab tests for the work-up of low platelets.** CBC would yield the most pertinent information for acute management. Typical platelet counts with an initial diagnosis of ITP are <50,000 and can be 1000–5000. Evaluating for the presence of antiplatelet antibodies is not helpful because they do not correlate with the presence of ITP or with disease activity in patients with chronic ITP.

31-1 C.   *Learning objective:* **Treat ITP appropriately with steroids; add IVIG only if acute bleeding is present.** The highest risk for life-threatening bleeding associated with ITP is in the first month with a platelet count of <20,000. She has evidence of a primary hemostasis problem (petechiae, purpura), but no acute bleeding at present. She can be treated with prednisone for 2–7 days, followed by a slow taper over ≥1 month. If she had evidence of acute bleeding (which she does not), IVIG (1 g/kg/d × 2 days) would be indicated because the onset of action of IVIG is hours rather than days.

31-2 A. *Learning objective:* **Develop a differential diagnosis for DVT in young patients.** Statistically, the two most likely diagnoses are an inherited factor V Leiden mutation (activated protein C resistance; genetic frequency of approximately 5%) or the prothrombin G20210A mutation (genetic frequency of approximately 3%).

31-2 B. *Learning objective:* **List appropriate diagnostic tests in the work-up of hypercoagulable state.** The most important studies to perform, in terms of probability, would be DNA/PCR screening for factor V Leiden and the prothrombin mutation. These are not affected by anticoagulation therapy. Blood should be drawn, however, to test for other autosomal dominant hypercoagulable disorders, such as protein C, protein S, and antithrombin III deficiencies, with careful consideration of how heparin (antithrombin III) or warfarin (proteins C and S) would affect the results. In the setting of acute thrombosis, the measured levels of protein C, protein S, and antithrombin III may be falsely decreased.

31-2 C. *Learning objective:* **Order appropriate anticoagulant therapy.** Anticoagulation therapy should be initiated with heparin, followed by warfarin for at least 6 months. Prophylaxis in future situations with risk of thrombosis (surgery, trauma, immobilization) is recommended. It is not recommended, however, during pregnancy.

31-2 D. *Learning objective:* **Recognize the heritable nature of many coagulation disorders, and know the appropriate approach to family members.** The family history strongly suggests a heritable disorder. Screening of family members with a history of thrombophilia is indicated if it has not already been done. First-degree relatives of patients with one or more abnormal test results should be examined to determine whether they should receive primary prophylaxis (e.g., anticoagulation during elective surgery). Whether to screen all potential carriers who have not been affected is more controversial. In all of medicine, the issue of genetic susceptibility on the basis of specific testing is becoming a management issue. In general, any genetic testing in an otherwise healthy individual should be performed in conjunction with the help of a genetic counselor who is able to describe clearly the relative risks and benefits of obtaining such information. Concerns about discrimination involving third-party insurance carriers and potential employers must be considered. If a family history indicates that the genetic vulnerability poses a risk only as an adult, testing is usually deferred until the family member is 18 years old.

31-3 A. *Learning objective:* **Design appropriate work-up for a solitary pulmonary nodule.** Perform a complete history and physical to identify other causes of this nodule besides lung cancer (e.g., aspergilloma, metastatic gastric cancer). Review old CXR to establish the history of the lesion. Characterize the lesion by chest CT, and look for enlarged chest nodes. Bone scan may reveal bony metastases causing back pain. Chance of cancer is high; an early-stage NSCLC that might be cured by excision is the best possible tumor you could find.

31-3 B. *Learning objective:* **List CXR features of pulmonary nodules that suggest malignancy.** Malignant nodules are more likely to double in volume (not diameter) between 7–465 days. Nodules unchanged for 2 years are unlikely to be cancer. Eccentric or stippled calcifications, irregular shape, and poorly defined borders all suggest malignancy. The "pretest probability" also is important—a nodule in a 25-year-old nonsmoker is unlikely to be lung cancer.

31-3 C. *Learning objective:* **List potential causes of hypercalcemia in a man with a pulmonary nodule.** A squamous cell lung cancer might produce parathyroid-like hormones or, less likely, bony metastases (remember his sore back) causing elevated calcium. Other potential causes unrelated to lung cancer include hyperparathyroidism, immobility, and multiple myeloma. CXR showed an eccentrically calcified nodule; work-up for nodes and metastases was negative; FEV_1 was high enough to allow lobectomy that showed adenocarcinoma with negative regional nodes. Elevated calcium persisted, and eventually a parathyroid adenoma was removed ("you can have fleas *and* lice"). He knew it was a close call, and this helped him to quit smoking.

31-4 A. *Learning objective:* **Think of leukemia when someone has dyspnea, fatigue, and bleeding.** Common causes of "low energy," such as depression and CHF, don't cause bleeding. The nosebleed may be coincidental; consider other diagnoses, such as pneumonia, TB, anemia, and lung cancer. History of other bleeding helps distinguish incidental from worrisome cause; the patient reports bleeding from her gums, too.

31-4 B. *Learning objective:* **Learn how to diagnose acute leukemia.** Look for gum infiltration, adenopathy, petechiae, lung consolidation, meningitis, and focal neurologic deficits. Peripheral smear with blasts is a strong hint, but a bone marrow biopsy specimen showing >30% blasts defines leukemia. Auer rods—"red cigars" in the cytoplasm—clinch the diagnosis of AML. Next, you need the hematopathologist to subtype the AML by identifying characteristic membrane antigens using flow cytometry.

31-4 C. *Learning objective:* **Anticipate the common complications of AML.** Look for sepsis (fever, tachycardia, hypotension), and check coagulation studies to rule out DIC. If the WBC is >150,000, consider sludging and tumor lysis with renal failure. CNS involvement is uncommon in adults. If she develops a cranial nerve VII palsy, however, she needs head CT and LP.

31-5 A. *Learning objective:* **List cancers that can cause nodes in the supraclavicular fossa.** Virchow's node is a left supraclavicular node from metastatic intestinal cancers (stomach, colon). The patient is at risk for colon cancer because of his brother's colon cancer. Testicular cancers can present in the neck, but he is a bit old. Perform a testicular exam to be sure. His 50 pack-years of smoking increases lung cancer risk. Fever could be due to postobstructive pneumonia, a "B" symptom of lymphoma, sarcoidosis, or TB.

31-5 B. *Learning objective:* **Describe the work-up for chest lymphadenopathy.** Although node biopsy is tempting, further imaging first helps you decide between a needle biopsy (to look for lung cancer or intestinal cancer) or excisional biopsy (needed for lymphomas). Chest and abdominal CT scans show no lung mass, but there is diffuse adenopathy and splenomegaly you and your attending missed on exam. The biopsy shows an intermediate-grade lymphoma, which is stage IIIB.

31-5 C. *Learning objective:* **Learn the long-term effects of some cancer treatments.** He undergoes intensive chemotherapy with CHOP (cyclophosphamide, hydroxydaunomycin, Oncovin [vincristine], prednisone). He is alive at 5 years, but is sterile and has an increased risk for a second primary cancer at any site.

31-6 A. *Learning objective:* **Understand the principles and methods of screening for colon cancer.** Almost all colon cancers could be prevented if their antecedent polyps were discovered and removed. Current recommendations are for screening to start at age 50, or earlier if there is a family history or other risk factors. Colonoscopy is the most effective method. Compared with flexible sigmoidoscopy plus fecal occult blood testing, colonoscopy has greater immediate costs, inconvenience, and a modestly increased chance of complications.

31-6 B. *Learning objective:* **Understand Dukes' classification and the necessary work-up.** See Table 31-5. The normal CT scan, CXR, and LFT suggest that there are no metastases. Regardless of the depth of invasion of the original cancer, the involvement of regional lymph nodes defines Dukes' stage C. Before surgery, you would have ordered a CEA level to help you prognosticate later.

31-6 C. *Learning objective:* **Understand the role of adjuvant chemotherapy in the treatment of colon cancer.** For her stage C tumor, you would recommend fluorouracil and leucovorin for 6 months. Less advanced tumors are simply excised. Treatment for metastatic disease varies, but may include resection of isolated metastases, chemotherapy, or comfort care.

31-7 A. *Learning objective:* **Understand the evaluation of a prostate nodule.** Most palpable prostate nodules are benign and result from calcification, scarring, or other processes. Suspicious nodules may be evaluated by measuring the PSA, transrectal ultrasound, and often biopsy. In this case, the PSA was "high-normal," and a biopsy specimen showed a tiny focus of intermediate grade. (The exam findings were coincidental.) The grade, or Gleason score, is based on histologic appearance and may predict the aggressiveness of the tumor.

31-7 B. *Learning objective:* **Counsel patients about difficult treatment decisions.** Your patient faces a potentially difficult decision because he is 70 years old, his tumor is very small, the benefits of treatment are uncertain, and the morbidity of treatment is substantial. Help your patient make a list of questions that he should have answered to decide about treatment: What might happen if he does nothing? What are the common complications of treatment? Guide your patient through a discussion that defines his particular values, fears, and goals. Does he value most the chance to live a long time, or is he particularly fearful of the incontinence and impotence that may occur after therapy?

31-7 C. *Learning objective:* **Understand how screening decisions for prostate cancer are influenced by individual patient characteristics.** Screening is not appropriate for the son or the uncle, even with their family history and elevated risk for prostate cancer. Because prostate cancer is so rare at age 35, the son's PSA would be either normal or perhaps falsely elevated. The chances for a true positive are tiny. The 92-year-old uncle has a high chance of having prostate cancer, but no treatment would be indicated unless he had symptoms, so there is no reason to screen.

REFERENCES

Bleeding Disorders
Cobas M: Preoperative assessment of coagulation disorders. Int Anesthesiol Clin 2001;39:1.

Clotting Disorders
Thomas RH: Hypercoagulability syndromes. Arch Intern Med 2001;161:2433.
Whiteman T, Hassouna HI: Hypercoagulable states. Hematol Oncol Clin N Am 2000;14:355.

USEFUL WEB SITES

Clotting Disorders
American Society of Hematology Education Book. www.asheducationbook.org

Prostate Cancer
National Cancer Institute. http://www.cancer.gov/cancer_information/
The American Cancer Society. http://www.cancer.org
The National Comprehensive Cancer Network. http://www.nccn.org

Hematology and Oncology

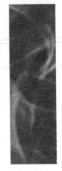

32

Infectious Diseases

HENRY ROSEN, DOUGLAS S. PAAUW, MELISSA M. HAGMAN, MARY B. MIGEON, and LISANNE R. BURKHOLDER

 BIOTERRORISM

ETIOLOGY

What is Bioterrorism?

Bioterrorism is the dissemination of potentially lethal biologic agents—bacteria, viruses, and toxins—with the intent of generating illness, death, and panic in a population. The degree of fear \and anxiety generated may be disproportionate to the number of the individuals afflicted.

Why is it Appropriate to include a Review of Bioterrorism Agents in the Medical Curriculum?

Dissemination of anthrax spores by U.S. mail in fall 2001 infected 20–30 individuals, killed 5, and produced a high level of anxiety among >200 million U.S. citizens. Despite the fact that very few practitioners encountered a case of anthrax, many or most had to deal with personal, patient, and community anxieties about the threat. They also needed to be able to recognize an instance of cutaneous or inhalational anthrax had it appeared before them. Although it seems impractical to know the details of each otherwise rare agent, it seems appropriate to be aware of general principles relevant to the recognition and management of the most likely agents of bioterrorism.

What are the Likely Agents of Bioterrorism?

Potential agents of bioterrorism are limited only by the imagination of the bioterrorist. Features that might be sought in a bioterrorism agent include the following:

- Easy dissemination
- Ugly manifestations

- Bleeding
- Skin discoloration
- Disfigurement
- Intense pain
- Deranged behaviors
- Infectious by aerosol route
- Civilian populations susceptible
- High rates of morbidity and mortality
- Person-to-person transmission
- Unfamiliar to physicians—difficult to diagnose and treat
- High capacity to cause panic and social disruption
- Prior development for biologic warfare by governmental entities

The agents that are deemed to best fit the above-listed criteria have been designated "category A" agents and are listed in Box 32-1. A second and third tier of potential bioterrorism agents, designated "category B" and "category C," are listed in the Centers for Disease Control and Prevention (CDC) web site provided at the end of this chapter. We discuss only anthrax, other agents of ulceroglandular fevers, and smallpox in this chapter.

What makes Anthrax a Category A Bioterrorism Agent?

Special features that favor use of anthrax as a bioterrorism agent include the following. The initial presentation of inhalational anthrax is difficult for physicians to diagnose because it is a vague illness that is similar to a mild upper respiratory illness. By the time fulminant symptoms have developed, antibiotics are ineffective, so morbidity and mortality of undiagnosed exposure are high. Anthrax exists in a spore (hibernating) form that is long-lived in the environment and withstands conditions that 32 would kill growing bacteria. As to dissemination, mechanisms have been developed to disperse the spores finely, substantially reducing the inhaled dose required to cause infection. This has been termed

---

BOX 32-1

LIKELY CLASS A AGENTS FOR BIOTERRORISM*

Anthrax
Other ulceroglandular fevers
    Plague
    Tularemia
Smallpox
Hemorrhagic fever viruses
    Ebola
    Marburg
Botulinum toxin

---

*For class B and class C agents, refer to http://www.bt.cdc.gov/

"weaponizing." In the natural form, anthrax also can be aerosolized, but this is less effective as a bioterrorism agent because the spores tend to cluster and stick to environmental surfaces.

How Deadly is Smallpox, and is Vaccine Effective at Preventing Disease?

Smallpox is a viral disease that affects only humans and that can be prevented by vaccination. As a consequence of a vigorous worldwide vaccination and isolation campaign, natural smallpox was eradicated in 1977. In the U.S., vaccinations were no longer administered after 1972. The CDC continues to hold a small supply of the virus, and concern remains that bioterrorists may choose to use this poxvirus as a weapon. Smallpox is a devastating disfiguring disease that is associated with a mortality rate of approximately 30% in nonimmune populations. There is probably significant, but incomplete, immunity among individuals who have been vaccinated decades (50 years) before exposure. Although smallpox is contagious by the aerosol route, infectivity does not emerge until the diagnostic features of the disease are evident, making quarantine of individuals with symptoms an effective strategy to diminish person-to-person spread of disease.

EVALUATION

What are the Clinical Features of Ulceroglandular Fevers?

Ulceroglandular fevers have in common the following features. They are acquired by inoculation of bacteria into the skin usually by microtrauma or by the bite of an arthropod vector. Local replication of the bacteria produces local inflammation and, later, tissue necrosis resulting in an ulcer—often with a black scar at the center. Lymph nodes that drain the affected area become swollen—hence the glandular component of the disease. The principal agents of ulceroglandular fevers are plague (*Pasteurella [Yersinia] pestis*), tularemia (*Francisella tularensis*), and anthrax (*Bacillus anthracis*). Each of the agents of the ulceroglandular fevers has a natural life cycle in animals and is endemic, albeit at low levels, in the U.S. All of these agents are treatable with common antimicrobials when given early in the course of the disease. Each of the agents rarely can be acquired by an aerosol route, producing a much more difficult to diagnose and more deadly infection.

How does a Patient with Anthrax Present?

The clinical presentation of **cutaneous anthrax** is an ulceroglandular fever syndrome that, in approximately 80% of cases, resolves without specific treatment. Antimicrobials are effective for the remaining 20% of individuals. A special feature of anthrax skin lesions is the remarkable degree of brawny edema at the margins of ulcers. The edema reaction is thought to be mediated by a particular toxin, edema toxin. **Inhalation anthrax** is characterized early by an upper respiratory illness with sore throat, mild fever, and myalgias, followed by mediastinal lymphadanopathy with lymph nodes growing so large as to produce pain, respiratory distress, and stridor. Large pleural effusions also are a prominent characteristic. Although naturally acquired inhalation disease rarely leads to pneumonia, inhalation anthrax associated with bioterrorism agents has resulted in pneumonias in about half of the cases. When inhalation disease is evident, blood cultures for gram-positive rod bacteria are usually positive. Death is usually associated with overwhelming sepsis and, often, with bacillary meningitis.

How does a Patient with Smallpox Present?

Usually patients become severely ill with fever, headache, backache, and vomiting 2–3 days before onset of a rash. When the rash begins, the patient becomes infectious. The rash begins on the face, hands, and forearms (different from the *truncal* predominance in chickenpox) and involves the palms and soles, in contrast to most other viral exanthems. Oropharyngeal virus is aerosolized through coughing. Symptoms suggestive of smallpox should prompt early communication with local health authorities and rapid quarantine to prevent spread of disease.

TREATMENT

How do I Treat Anthrax?

Doxycycline and quinolones are effective if given early in the course of the disease. Ciprofloxacin is the only drug with a specific Food and Drug Administration–approved treatment indication for anthrax.

How do I Treat Smallpox?

For close contacts of a smallpox patient, treat by vaccination, which is effective if given within a few days of exposure. No specific antimicrobials are available.

What is the Role of the Practitioner in Coping with Bioterrorism Agents?

It's impossible to know all about these ordinarily rare disorders. Rapid self-education through local CME resources and reliable web sites such as the one maintained by the CDC is appropriate. The goals of self-education are to be able to recognize the more classic manifestations of an agent when it is identified. A key role of the practitioner is to communicate medical events of concern to local health authorities. Such events would include an increase in individuals ill with a similar or unusual syndrome, an increase in unexplained diseases or deaths, a single case of a disease due to an uncommon agent, an unexpected seasonal or geographic distribution of a disease, an unusual age distribution (e.g., varicella or measles in adults), or acquisition of a disease by an unusual route of transmission. Box 32-2 summarizes the practitioner's role in coping with bioterrorism agents.

Infectious Diseases

BOX 32-2

ROLE OF THE PRACTITIONER IN COPING WITH BIOTERRORISM— THE 5 R'S

- ◆ Rapid self-education
- ◆ Recognition of syndromes
- ◆ Reporting to public health agencies
- ◆ Rx of patients
- ◆ Realistic reassurance of worried well

How do I Provide Psychological Care to the Worried Well?

The first issue is to become knowledgeable about the bioterrorism agent of immediate concern and to gain a reasonable view of the epidemiologic risks associated with that agent. If you personally can honestly be reassured and can speak with your patients in an informed manner, this may help significantly in providing truthful reassurance. Real risks should not be negated. For individuals who manifest extreme anxiety, anxiolytic drugs may be beneficial. Prophylaxis or empiric treatment in the form of vaccines, antiserum, or prophylactic antibiotics should be restricted to circumstances set out in guidelines developed by public health authorities. Risks of vaccination or widespread prophylactic antibiotic therapy need to be balanced against the potential benefits. Public health guidance is crucial in making these decisions.

ENCEPHALITIS

ETIOLOGY

What is Encephalitis, and What Causes It?

Encephalitis is inflammation of the brain tissue. Viral causes predominate, but fungus, rickettsial infection, toxoplasmosis, and TB also are important etiologies. Without question, the most important cause of acute encephalitis in the U.S. is the herpesvirus, especially HSV type 1. HSV is an important cause of viral meningitis as well. HSV 2 can cause meningitis and encephalitis. It should be considered in the differential diagnosis if the patient has sexual risk factors. Rare eastern equine encephalitis, St. Louis encephalitis, and rabies cases are reported each year. West Nile virus has been reported in all states in the U.S. Only 1 in 150 people infected with West Nile virus has clinical symptoms. Symptoms of encephalitis secondary to West Nile virus are more common in the elderly. *Toxoplasma* encephalitis is common in HIV-infected patients with low CD4 counts (see sections on HIV). The mortality rate of untreated HSV encephalitis is 70%.

EVALUATION

What are the Typical Clinical Features of Herpes Encephalitis?

The clinical features of herpes encephalitis include fever, nausea, vomiting, headache, and alterations in level of consciousness with lethargy and confusion. HSV can involve the temporal lobe, causing personality change, temporal lobe seizures, and odd behavior. Other symptoms include speech disturbances, ataxia, cranial nerve defects, and visual field loss. Patients who present with coma or in whom the diagnosis is missed have a high likelihood of death, and neurologic sequelae are common in survivors.

When Should I Suspect West Nile Virus?

West Nile virus (and other arboviruses) should be strongly considered in patients who have onset of unexplained febrile illness, encephalitis or meningitis or both, or flaccid paralysis in summer or early fall. Other clinical signs seen with West Nile virus include weakness, a maculopapular rash (50%), and visual symptoms.

What Testing Should be Done to Evaluate Suspected Encephalitis?

CSF in patients with HSV encephalitis usually shows a pleocytosis with lymphocytes and PMN. PMN may predominate early in infection. RBC are frequently present in the CSF. CT, MRI, or EEG can localize the area of brain involvement. In the past, definitive diagnosis was made by brain biopsy because culture of HSV from CSF is difficult. HSV DNA PCR performed on CSF is replacing brain biopsy for diagnosis because it is rapidly performed and highly sensitive and specific. Testing for West Nile virus and other arboviral infections is through serologic and CSF testing for IgM antibody.

TREATMENT

How do I Treat HSV Encephalitis?

Treat with high-dose intravenous acyclovir. Because of high mortality rates, begin therapy as soon as you consider the diagnosis. No treatment is effective for other viral encephalitides.

ENDOCARDITIS

ETIOLOGY

What Causes Endocarditis?

Endocarditis is an infection of heart valves. Endocarditis typically begins with a pre-existing valve abnormality that is seeded during a period of transient bacteremia. Native valve disease is usually due to

Infectious Diseases

Staphylococcus aureus in IVDU and to streptococcal species in other patients. Prosthetic valve disease within 2 months of valve replacement is likely nosocomial and due to *Staphylococcus epidermidis, S. aureus,* or gram-negative organisms. Disease that occurs >2 months after valve replacement follows the native valve pathogen profile. *Streptococcus bovis* endocarditis is associated with colon cancer and should prompt a colonoscopy.

DIAGNOSIS

How do I Recognize the Clinical Presentation of Endocarditis?

Most patients with endocarditis have fever and systemic toxicity. Endocarditis also can be subtle, however, causing nonspecific symptoms such as fatigue, weight loss, arthralgias, and abdominal or back pain. Some patients present with complications, including CHF, stroke, arrhythmia, vertebral osteomyelitis, or lung abscess. Ask about risk factors, such as injection drug use, prior valve abnormality, or recent invasive procedures (dental, GI, genitourinary, gynecologic) likely to cause transient bacteremia. On exam, assess dentition for source of infection. Look for evidence of emboli, including conjunctival hemorrhages, splinter hemorrhages in nail beds, and red nontender Janeway lesions on the palms and soles. Evaluate for immunologic phenomena of the fundi (Roth's spots) and the palms and soles (tender red Osler's nodes). Listen for a new heart murmur or abnormal lung sounds. Document a thorough neurologic exam as a baseline in case of future embolic events.

How do I Diagnose Endocarditis?

Clinical criteria for diagnosis are shown in Box 32-3. Before starting antibiotics, obtain at least three sets of blood cultures drawn 1 hour apart. Do not withhold antibiotics in acutely ill patients, however. Echocardiography is necessary in almost all suspected cases of endocarditis. Transthoracic echo (TTE) is a reasonable first test, but it cannot rule out endocarditis because sensitivity is only 55%-65%. Transesophageal echo (TEE) is more sensitive and is recommended for suspected prosthetic valve endocarditis, myocardial abscess, or valve perforation. TEE should be obtained despite normal TTE if suspicion of endocarditis remains high. CXR may show evidence of septic emboli in right-sided endocarditis or CHF in left-sided endocarditis. An ECG showing new PR interval prolongation may indicate perivalvular abscess. Hematuria on urinalysis suggests glomerulonephritis.

TREATMENT

What Antibiotics are Appropriate for Endocarditis?

Treat with empiric bactericidal antibiotics based on the presentation. For native valve infections, start nafcillin and gentamicin. Consider adding ampicillin to improve enterococcal coverage. Substitute vancomycin for nafcillin if the patient is penicillin allergic, uses intravenous drugs, or resides in an area with a high incidence of methicillin-resistant

---

BOX 32-3

MODIFIED DUKE CRITERIA FOR DIAGNOSIS OF ENDOCARDITIS

Major Criteria

1. Two separate positive blood cultures with a typical microorganism
2. Persistently positive blood cultures with any microorganism
3. Positive serologic test or single positive blood culture for *Coxiella burnetti* (Q fever)
4. New regurgitant murmur or characteristic echocardiography findings—vegetation, myocardial abscess, new dehiscence of a prosthetic valve

Minor Criteria

1. Presence of a predisposing heart condition or injection drug use
2. Fever >38° C
3. Vascular or embolic phenomena—mycotic aneurysm, intracranial hemorrhage, stroke, splenic/pulmonary infarct
4. Immunologic phenomena—glomerulonephritis, Osler's nodes, Roth's spots, positive rheumatoid factor
5. Serologic evidence of infection or positive blood cultures not meeting major criteria

Definite Diagnosis (with High Sensitivity and Specificity):

2 major criteria *or*
1 major criterion plus 3 minor criteria *or*
5 minor criteria

Possible Diagnosis

1 major criterion plus 1 minor criterion *or*
3 minor criteria

S. aureus. Prosthetic valve infections should be treated empirically with vancomycin, gentamicin, and rifampin. When culture results are available, narrow antibiotic coverage and treat for 4–6 weeks. Uncomplicated tricuspid valve *S. aureus* endocarditis can be treated with 2 weeks of nafcillin and an aminoglycoside. Surgical management should be considered in patients with new CHF, perivalvular extension of infection, persistently positive blood cultures despite appropriate antibiotics, or emboli with a large residual mobile vegetation.

GENITAL INFECTIONS

ETIOLOGY

What are Common Causes of Genital Discharge?

In women, vaginal discharge is often normal and varies in amount and quality through the hormonal cycle. In men, penile discharge aside from

Table 32-1

Pathologic Causes and Location of Genital Discharge

Women	Cervicitis	Vaginitis
	Gonorrhea	*Candida*
	Chlamydia	*Trichomonas*
	Polymicrobial GNR,	Bacterial Vaginosis
	Streptococcus species	Atrophic vaginitis of low estrogen

Men	Urethritis
	Gonorrhea
	Chlamydia
	Reiter's syndrome (rare)

GNR, gram-negative rods.

ejaculation warrants further evaluation. Pathologic causes of discharge in women include inflammation or infection of the cervix or vagina (**cervicitis** and **vaginitis**) and in men **urethritis** (Table 32-1). In men and women, discharge may be absent despite infection. In particular, chlamydia is often clinically silent; untreated chlamydia may cause infertility in women.

What is Bacterial Vaginosis (BV)?

BV is an overgrowth of normal vaginal flora. There is no infection or inflammation—hence the term *vaginosis* rather than *vaginitis*. Seventy-five percent of women are asymptomatic. This condition waxes and wanes, is not dangerous or sexually transmitted, but may cause increased discharge and postcoital fishy odor that may be bothersome to patients and, if so, merits treatment. In pregnancy, BV may be associated with preterm labor and so should be treated.

What Causes Genital Ulcers?

HSV is the most common cause of superficial, painful, often recurring genital ulcers. Particularly with primary infection, patients may have accompanying fevers and myalgias. Much less commonly, painful ulcers occur with chancroid, caused by *Haemophilus ducreyi*, although these are usually deep, friable, and undermined at the edges. Chancroid is endemic in Southeast Asia and Africa. Painless, deep, and indurated ulcers are seen with primary syphilis. Toxic epidermal necrolysis is a rare, potentially fatal, drug reaction that can cause painful genital and oral ulcers.

What Causes Genital Growths?

Human papilloma virus (HPV) causes genital warts or condylomata acuminata, which are broad-based and verrucous. These can appear at any location in the perineum, including perirectally. Condom use does not prevent transmission of this virus, which is easily spread from skin-to-skin contact. More than half of the general population has serologic evidence of exposure; most infections clear spontaneously within 2 years. Certain subtypes of HPV (16, 18, and others) play a causative role in cervical and other genital cancers. Genital growths also may be skin tags, molluscum contagiosum, and skin cancer.

My Patient Reports Pelvic Pain. What are Common Genitourinary Causes?

In women, UTI, menstrual pain, ovarian cyst rupture, ectopic pregnancy, endometriosis, and pelvic inflammatory disease (PID) all can cause pain. PID is a polymicrobial infection of the upper genital tract in women, usually caused by some combination of *Chlamydia*, gonorrhea, enteric gram-negative rods, and streptococci. Chronic pelvic pain is closely associated with a history of sexual abuse. In men, deep pelvic or perineal pain can be due to prostatitis or UTI.

EVALUATION

What Historical Points are Important in Evaluating Genital Infections?

Ask about new sexual partners, previous infections, and unprotected or high-risk sex. Also, inquire into last menstrual period, irregular vaginal bleeding, new discharge, pain with intercourse, fevers, or new skin or genital lesions. In women with vaginal discharge, history alone is unreliable for diagnosis. Vaginal itching, which is often thought to represent vaginal yeast infection, may be due to BV, condylomata, or HSV and is not predictive of *Candida*.

What Examination is Necessary for Patients Reporting Genital Symptoms?

Examine the external genitalia for dermal or mucosal ulceration, redness, discharge, or new lesions. Include testicular and prostate exams in men, pelvic speculum and bimanual exams in women, and inguinal lymph node exam in both sexes. For women with discharge or pain on exam, obtain CBC and urine pregnancy test, and perform a wet prep and KOH microscopic exam on vaginal secretions from the vaginal wall and a Gram stain on any cervical discharge. For both sexes, order urinalysis and gonorrhea and *Chlamydia* testing. This can be performed by urethral (men) or cervical (women) swab for culture or nucleic acid amplification testing (NAAT), a DNA-based test that is extremely sensitive and specific. The specimen can be from a swab of the urethra (men) or cervix (women). A less invasive method is to run the NAAT on the first 15 mL of urine ("dirty catch"). This collection technique is different from the clean-catch midstream sample most patients are accustomed to obtaining, so instruct patients carefully because samples are not processed if sent to the lab with >20 mL in the cup. Further testing to consider includes syphilis testing with RPR and HIV testing in patients with genital symptoms or any other sexually transmitted disease diagnosis, including *Trichomonas*, HSV, genital warts, gonorrhea, and *Chlamydia* infections.

How do I Perform a Microscopic Exam of Vaginal Discharge?

In a woman with new or symptomatic discharge, studies show that routine office speculum and bimanual pelvic exams are not adequate to determine the cause. Further sampling is required. Using a cotton swab, obtain fluid from the vaginal wall, and place in a small amount of saline. The swab must stay moist because even a few seconds of drying can decrease sensitivity for *Trichomonas*. Use this swab to prepare saline and KOH slides. The saline slide may reveal WBC suggesting inflammation of any cause; clue cells suggesting BV (grainy-appearing squamous cells coated with bacteria); or trichomonads, which are motile and slightly larger than WBC. The KOH slide may show candidal hyphae after the normal cells have lysed. WBC also should be seen on the saline slide to confirm the diagnosis of candidal vaginitis because nonpathologic yeast colonization is common. pH testing is useful; vaginal pH is normally 4.5 and can be tested directly using pH paper along the vaginal wall. pH is above normal with BV, *Trichomonas*, and estrogen-deficient states.

How do I Diagnose PID?

Diagnosis of PID can be tricky because of a range of presenting symptoms from subtle to severe. Tubo-ovarian abscess, tubal infection and inflammation, and endometritis all are forms of PID. Minimal criteria for diagnosis include pelvic pain or cervical motion tenderness; presence of fever >38.3° C, cervical discharge, elevated ESR or C-reactive protein, and positive cervical or endometrial cultures enhance diagnostic specificity. Less than half of women with PID have an elevated WBC. Endometrial biopsy, imaging, or laparoscopy also can make the diagnosis of PID more definitively. Because none of these tests have adequate sensitivity and specificity, however, the recommendation now is to have a low threshold to treat in a clinical presentation consistent with PID.

Should I Perform Routine Screening for Any of These Infections?

Chlamydia screening is indicated in high-risk populations of women <25 years old and women with two or more new sexual partners per year. HPV, BV, and gonorrhea are not routinely screened. Annual pap smear is indicated for women with new partners in the prior several years to screen for cervical atypia that may arise in the setting of HPV infection, whereas women in a single long-term, monogamous relationship with three prior normal annual paps can safely undergo pap screening every 3 years.

TREATMENT

What are Current Therapies for Genital Infections?

See Table 32-2 for pathogens, diagnosis, and treatment of common genital infections. Gonorrhea, *Chlamydia,* and *Trichomonas* are reportable conditions in most states, and partners require evaluation and treatment. BV requires treatment only if the patient is pregnant or is bothered by her symptoms. One third of cases of symptomatic BV resolve

Table 32-2

Pathogens, Diagnosis, and Treatment in Genital Infections

Pathogen	Diagnosis	Treatment*
Cervix, Endometrium, Urethra		
Chlamydia	NAAT or culture	Azithromycin 1000 mg × 1
Gonorrhea	NAAT or culture	Ceftriaxone 125 mg IM × 1, *or* Cefixime 400 mg × 1
PID—polymicrobial, including gonorrhea, *Chlamydia*, *Streptococcus* species, GNR, anaerobes	Pelvic pain, fever; cervical motion tenderness; elevated ESR, C-reactive protein; cervical cultures or urine NAAT; imaging, laparoscopy; endometrial biopsy	*Outpatient:* Ofloxacin 400 mg bid × 14 d *and* Metronidazole 500 mg bid × 14 d, *or* Ceftriaxone 250 mg IM × 1 *and* Doxycycline 100 mg bid × 14 d *Inpatient:* Cefoxitin 2 g IV q6h, *or* Cefotetan IV 2 g q12h *and* Doxycycline 100 mg bid × 14 d
Vagina		
Candida	Hyphae, WBC on KOH; pH <4.5	Fluconazole 150 mg × 1, may repeat × 1, *and/or* Topical antifungal
Trichomonas	Flagellates on wet mount; pH >4.5	Metronidazole 2 g × 1
BV	Clue cells, WBC on wet prep; pH >4.5; positive whiff test	Metronidazole 500 mg bid × 7 d *or* Metronidazole vaginal gel 0.75% bid × 5 d
Genital Mucosa		
HSV	Direct fluorescent antibody or culture of ulcer; serology†	*Suppressive:* Acyclovir 400 mg bid‡ *Acute:* Acyclovir 400 mg tid × 5–10 d
HPV	Exam; biopsy if needed	Cryotherapy Topical imiquimod or podophyllin

GNR, gram-negative rods.
*Oral unless otherwise noted.
†Does differentiate HSV type 1 from HSV type 2, but does not distinguish past infection from new infection and so is not diagnostic for a current lesion.
‡Valacyclovir and famciclovir also are effective, but are more expensive.

spontaneously; conversely, although treatment is effective, one third of cases relapse. HSV can be treated acutely to shorten duration of outbreaks or with daily suppressive therapy for severe or frequent outbreaks. Genital warts are easily removed with cryotherapy or topical podophyllin, although the underlying HPV infection cannot be eradicated. Topical treatment also comes in forms the patient may use at home. HPV vaccine is now available as a cervical cancer preventive in young women. For PID, treat empirically for even mildly suggested disease because testing can be insensitive, and because consequences of untreated infection are so severe. Partners need to be treated as well. PID is considered polymicrobial because definitive identification of a organism can be elusive. The treatment regimen should be broad, including coverage for *Chlamydia*, gonorrhea, *Streptococcus* species, and anaerobic bacteria. For stable patients, outpatient treatment is adequate with a follow-up exam in 3–5 days to verify there has been a reduction in symptoms and pain on exam. If not, further evaluation or perhaps admission is indicated.

What are the Potential Complications of PID Infection?

Even with treatment, 25% of women with PID experience repeat infections, chronic pelvic pain, dyspareunia, ectopic pregnancy, and infertility.

Can I Treat a Vaginal Yeast Infection Empirically?

Yes, but only if the patient has been on antibiotics recently. Otherwise, it is best to perform a full exam because several studies have shown inaccurate diagnoses by physicians and patients based on history and inspection alone. Microscopic exam is especially important in patients with recurrent symptoms because the diagnosis may be incorrect, or the yeast may be resistant to routine therapy. Send a vaginal swab for culture and sensitivity in these cases. Also, screen for elevated blood glucose and consider HIV testing in patients with recurrent yeast infections because diabetes and HIV infection are risk factors. Topical antifungal cream treatment may provide relief more rapidly than oral fluconazole therapy.

Case 32-1

A 23-year-old woman presents with recent lower pelvic pain including with intercourse. She feels well otherwise and has never had similar symptoms.

A. What is your differential diagnosis?
B. What tests would you obtain?
C. On exam, you find cervical motion tenderness, but no vaginal discharge or cervical changes. Her urine pregnancy test is negative. How would you proceed?

HIV INFECTION PRIMARY CARE

ETIOLOGY

What Terminology is Useful in Categorizing HIV Infection?

HIV infection is classified by numbers 1, 2, or 3 depending on the $CD4^+$ count, and by letters A, B, or C depending on the occurrence of specific

Table 32-3			
Classification of HIV Infection			
CD4⁺ Count per mm³	**A—Asymptomatic, or Persistent Generalized Lymphadenopathy**	**B*— Symptomatic, not Category C**	**C†—AIDS-Indicator Conditions**
>500	A1	B1	**C1**
200–499	A2	B2	**C2**
<200	**A3**	**B3**	**C3**

Boldface indicates diagnosis of AIDS
*Examples of category B conditions include bacillary angiomatosis, oral thrush, cervical dysplasia/carcinoma, oral hairy leukoplakia, herpes zoster (recurrent or multidermatomal), and ITP.
†Examples of category C conditions include PCP, cryptococcal meningitis, toxoplasmosis, CMV retinitis, AIDS dementia complex, TB, recurrent bacterial pneumonias, Kaposi's sarcoma, CNS lymphoma, and other NHL.

conditions (Table 32-3). AIDS is defined as category C disease or a CD4⁺ count <200 (A3, B3). Begin your oral presentation of any HIV-infected patient by giving the classification, last CD4⁺ count, and viral load.

Why are CD4⁺ Cell Counts and HIV Viral Load Important?

CD4⁺ count indicates the severity of immunosuppression and is used to determine (1) disease classification, (2) when to start or change antiretroviral therapy, (3) when certain opportunistic infections are likely (Figure 32-1), and (4) when to start opportunistic infection prophylaxis. Quantitative HIV viral load gives prognostic information beyond that provided by the CD4⁺ count. The higher the viral load, the more rapidly the patient is becoming immunosuppressed. In addition, viral load is used to assess efficacy of antiretroviral therapy within weeks of any change.

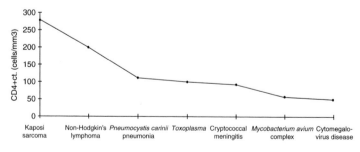

From the New England Journal of Medicine (324: 1332-B, 1992)

FIGURE 32-1 Occurrence of AIDS-indicating conditions in the natural history of HIV infection, according to mean CD4⁺ cell count. (From N Engl J Med 1998;324:1332–8.)

What is the Risk of Acquiring HIV Infection from a Needle-Stick Injury?

Fear of contracting HIV in the health care setting through needle-stick or mucosal splash accidents is a significant stress for all health care professionals. The risk of infection is low, estimated in a CDC study to be 0.5% for percutaneous exposure (3 in 860). Based on other data, the risk is probably less (approximately 0.2%) than that reported by the CDC. The risk for HIV transmission is greater if blood is seen on the needle, the needle stick is a deep wound from a hollow-bore needle, if gloves weren't worn, or if the source patient has advanced HIV disease.

EVALUATION

How do I Diagnose HIV Infection?

Screen for HIV infection with an enzyme-linked immunosorbent assay (ELISA) test. This test detects HIV antibodies with sensitivity and specificity of >99%. The PPV of the ELISA (i.e., the likelihood that a patient with a positive test actually has HIV infection) ranges from 20% in very low risk populations to >95% in patients with strong risk factors. Because the ELISA is not 100% specific, use a Western blot to confirm any positive ELISA. This test detects serum antibodies directed against specific HIV-1 proteins of various molecular weights and is defined as positive when two or more of the following antibody bands are present: p24, gp41, or gp120/160. Indeterminate Western blots are common; without p24, gp41, or gp 120/160 bands, the patient does not need further evaluation and does not have HIV infection.

What is the Window Period?

The window period is the period of time between acquiring infection and development of antibodies. Antibody-based tests remain negative in this window period. Greater than 90% of patients seroconvert within 4 weeks of infection. Three tests can detect HIV infection before the appearance of antibody: viral p24 antigen and viral load testing with nucleic acid polymerase chain reaction or branched-chain DNA assays. The p24 antigen is transiently positive and less sensitive for acute HIV infection than are the viral load tests (PCR or branched-chain DNA assay). Occasionally, when risk of acute infection is high, and a patient is still within the window period, viral load testing may be used for diagnosis instead of the usual antibody-based tests.

What Key Questions Should I Ask Patients with HIV Infection at Clinic Visits?

Your main goal is to assess the immune status of your patient. In patients with high $CD4^+$ counts, focus on skin or mouth symptoms, side effects from any medications, general health (weight loss, fatigue, itching, loss of appetite), and any patient concerns. In patients with low $CD4^+$ counts (<300), the risk of opportunistic infection is much

Table 32-4

History Questions to Ask HIV-Infected Patients at Routine Clinic Visits

	Diseases Concerned About
Patient with high CD4+ count (>300)	
Medication side effects	Pancreatitis—didanosine, stavudine, zalcitabine
	Neuropathy—didanosine, zalcitabine, stavudine
	Myositis—zidovudine
	Jaundice—atazanavir, indinavir
	Kidney stones—indinavir
	Diarrhea—nelfinavir, and other protease inhibitors (PIs)
	Hepatitis—all PI, nevirapine
Skin changes	Seborrheic dermatitis, generalized pruritus
General health (fatigue, weight change, anorexia)	Medication side effects, depression, TB
Patient with low CD4+ count (<300)	
Headache, seizure, weakness, general fever, weight loss, night sweats	MAC, AIDS wasting syndrome, toxoplasmosis, cryptococcus
Dysphagia	Candidal esophagitis (CMV or HSV esophagitis less commonly)
Diarrhea	C. difficile, cryptosporidia, MAC
Abdominal pain	MAC, lymphoma, acalculous cholecystitis, nephrolithiasis
Cough, dyspnea	Pneumonia, especially PCP
Visual changes	CMV

greater. Mean $CD4^+$ count is <100 for most common opportunistic infections. Ask these patients about diarrhea, dysphagia, thrush, headache, fever, or changes in vision (Table 32-4). It is important to ask patients about adherence to antiretroviral therapy at each visit. Even missing a few doses a week affects the possibility of suppressing the virus. Patients who take >95% of their doses have a >80% chance of suppressing the virus to nondetectable levels compared with only a 50% chance if they are taking 85% of the doses.

What are the Important Parts of the Physical Exam to Include in All Visits?

Perform skin and oral exams at each visit in all patients. Look for any of the three forms of candidiasis: Pseudomembranous candidiasis causes well-recognized thick, white plaques on the tongue and palate; atrophic candidiasis causes a painful, red, shiny tongue or hard palate; and angular cheilitis causes cracking and fissuring at the corners of the mouth. Look for hairy leukoplakia, aphthous ulcers, KS, and gingivitis. Perform a careful skin exam. Test for peripheral neuropathy in patients on didanosine, zalcitabine, and stavudine therapy. This can be done easily by breaking a cotton-tipped applicator and using the sharp broken end and the soft cotton end to distinguish sharp from light touch sensation. Examination of the anal and perineal area should be done annually in patients with a history of receptive anal intercourse. These patients are at an increased risk for anal cancer.

When should I Obtain HIV RNA Viral Load and CD4$^+$ Counts?

Current recommendations for obtaining quantitative measurement of HIV RNA are (1) before starting antiretroviral therapy, (2) 4 weeks after starting a new antiretroviral regimen, and (3) every 3–4 months during antiretroviral therapy to assess whether modifications are needed. Check CD4$^+$ counts every 6 months when CD4$^+$ is >500 and every 3 months when CD4$^+$ is <500.

What are the Indications for Resistance Testing?

Evidence of virologic failure (increasing viral loads) is the main reason to do resistance testing. If a patient's viral load increases suddenly, suspect that he or she has stopped the antiretroviral regimen. Resistance occurs over time, so a slow increase in viral loads is most consistent with development of resistance. Resistance testing should be done when patients are on their current antiretroviral regimen. The minimal viral load required for resistance testing is 1000 copies/mL.

TREATMENT

When should I Start Antiretroviral Therapy?

Patients who present with acute HIV infection should be enrolled in trials looking at the efficacy of aggressive antiretroviral therapy shortly after infection occurs. Some providers treat acute infection regardless of CD4$^+$ count and viral load with triple-drug combinations including PI, although we do not know long-term outcomes with this approach. In patients with CD4$^+$ counts >350 and an undetectable viral load, monitoring without antiretroviral therapy is appropriate. When the CD4$^+$ count is <350, antiretroviral therapy can be considered and should be encouraged if the viral load is high (>55,000). Watching closely without antiretroviral therapy is a reasonable approach in patients with CD4$^+$ counts >200, but with low or nondetectable viral loads. If the patient has symptomatic HIV disease or has a CD4$^+$ count <200, the patient should receive antiretroviral therapy. Antiretroviral therapy should be started only when patients can commit to making all follow-up visits and taking medications without missing doses so as to decrease the risk of developing viral resistance.

What Antiretroviral Drug should I Use?

Combination therapy is the rule. The most potent combination is two NRTI with a PI. Another excellent option is two NRTI with an NNRTI, either efavirenz or nevirapine (Table 32-5).

Table 32-5

Antiretroviral Medications, Dose, and Side Effects

Drugs	Typical Dose	Side Effects
NRTI		
Zidovudine	300 mg bid	Nausea, headache, myopathy, anemia, neutropenia
Didanosine	400 mg qd	Neuropathy, pancreatitis
Zalcitabine	0.75 mg tid	Neuropathy, pancreatitis, mucosal ulcer
Stavudine	40 mg bid	Neuropathy, pancreatitis
Lamivudine	300 mg qd	Minimal
Abacavir	300 mg bid	Life-threatening hypersensitivity
Tenofovir	300 mg qd	Nausea, asymptomatic increased CPK
Emtricitabine	200 mg qd	Minimal
NNRTI		
Nevirapine	200 mg bid	Rash, liver failure
Efavirenz	600 mg qd	Rash, agitation, confusion
PI		All PI can increase cholesterol, TG, transaminases
Indinavir	800 mg q8h	Kidney stones, elevated bilirubin
Nelfinavir	1250 mg bid	Diarrhea
Ritonavir	400 mg bid with saquinavir	Nausea, vomiting, perioral paresthesias
Saquinavir	400 mg bid with ritonavir	Nausea, diarrhea
Amprenavir	1200 mg bid	Nausea, diarrhea
Lopinavir-ritonavir (Kaletra)	400 mg/100 mg bid	Nausea, diarrhea
Atazanavir	400 mg qd	Nausea, diarrhea, elevated bilirubin
Fosamprenavir	1400 mg bid or 1400 mg qd with ritonavir 200 mg qd	Nausea, diarrhea
Tipranavir	500 mg bid with ritonavir 200 mg bid	Nausea, diarrhea Intracranial hemorrhage
Darunavir	600 mg bid with ritonavir 100 mg bid	Nausea, diarrhea
Fusion protein inhibitor		
Enfuvirtide	90 mg subq infection bid	Fatigue, diarrhea nausea

Can I Give Triple-Drug Therapy Once a Day?

Yes, many of the medications are available to be dosed once a day. Atazanavir, tenofovir, lamivudine, emtricitabine, didanosine, efavirenz, and fosamprenavir or amprenavir plus ritonavir all are available to be given once a day.

What are the Side Effects of Antiretroviral Agents?

Zidovudine can cause headaches, nausea, and vomiting when first started. Anemia and neutropenia occur with longer term use and are more common in patients who have lower CD4$^+$ counts. Patients on the drug for >6 months can develop myopathy. Didanosine, zalcitabine, and stavudine can cause peripheral neuropathy and pancreatitis. Zalcitabine also can cause mucosal ulceration. Stavudine causes more side effects than most other nucleosides. It has been linked to fat wasting (lipoatrophy) and is contraindicated in pregnancy. All nucleoside drugs have the potential to cause fatty liver with fatal lactic acidosis. This problem is most likely with stavudine and didanosine. Think about this possibility in patients on nucleosides who are losing weight and having abdominal pain and nausea. Abacavir can cause a life-threatening allergic reaction. The non-nucleoside drug nevirapine causes rash in 15% of patients and can rarely cause liver failure. The non-nucleoside drug efavirenz can cause insomnia, nightmares, and problems concentrating. All the PI (indinavir, ritonavir, nelfinavir, amprenavir, fosamprenavir, atazanavir, lopinavir, and saquinavir) can cause transaminase elevations. Indinavir is known for its propensity to cause kidney stones, so patients on this drug should be counseled to stay well hydrated. PI can increase TG and decrease high-density lipoprotein cholesterol levels and cause glucose intolerance, so lipids and glucose should be monitored regularly (see Table 32-5). Atazanavir seems to be the exception, rarely causing lipid or glucose problems. It can cause unconjugated hyperbilirubinemia.

What is Lipodystrophy?

Patients on PI or stavudine can develop changes in body fat distribution referred to as lipodystrophy. Typical features are temporal wasting and sunken cheeks, thin arms and thin legs with a protuberant abdomen ("protease paunch"). Veins on the arms and legs become prominent, and there is an increased incidence of paronychia. Metabolic abnormalities include increased glucose and TG and decreased high-density lipoprotein cholesterol.

When should I Start Prophylaxis Against PCP?

Patients who have any of the following conditions should receive PCP prophylaxis: CD4$^+$ count <200, previous PCP, or oral candidiasis. Trimethoprim-sulfamethoxazole is the most effective agent. It also provides prophylaxis against toxoplasmosis and may prevent bacterial sinusitis and bacterial pneumonias. For patients who cannot tolerate trimethoprim-sulfamethoxazole, dapsone is a reasonable option. Atovaquone and aerosolized pentamidine are third-line options, but are less effective than trimethoprim-sulfamethoxazole or dapsone. Because aerosolized pentamidine is not a systemic therapy, patients may develop *Pneumocystis* at sites other than their lungs. *Pneumocystis* prophylaxis can be stopped in patients on HAART who have CD4$^+$ counts >200 and nondetectable viral loads for at least 6 months.

When should Patients Receive MAC Prophylaxis?

Current recommendations start MAC prophylaxis when $CD4^+$ count is <50. Favored regimens are azithromycin 1200 mg weekly or clarithromycin 500 mg twice a day. MAC prophylaxis can be stopped in patients on HAART who have $CD4^+$ counts >100 and nondetectable viral loads for at least 6 months.

What do I do if I Get a Needle-Stick Injury from an HIV-Infected Patient?

First, try to prevent needle-stick injury by wearing gloves whenever you draw blood, manipulate intravenous lines, or examine a mucosal surface. Wear eye protection for any procedure (endoscopy, bronchoscopy, surgery). *Never* recap needles: This is the most common cause of needle-stick injury. Use of zidovudine after needle-stick injury seems to decrease the risk of transmission. Current practice is to give zidovudine plus lamivudine for lower risk exposures and to add a third drug (usually a PI) for high-risk exposures. If the source patient has known zidovudine resistance, substitute tenofovir, abacavir, or didanosine for the zidovudine in the prophylactic regimen. Nevirapine should never be used for postexposure prophylaxis because severe hepatitis can occur.

Case 32-2

A 27-year-old HIV-infected man with A2 HIV disease comes to establish primary care. He was diagnosed with HIV 3 years ago and believes he was infected about 6 years ago. His $CD4^+$ count done 2 months ago was 340 and viral load was 75,000. He reports no symptoms. He has had only sporadic, routine care in the past and was previously on zidovudine plus didanosine therapy for about 6 months.

A. Would you start antiretroviral therapy?
B. What tests should you obtain?

◼ COMPLICATIONS OF HIV INFECTION

ETIOLOGY

What Types of Skin Problems Affect Patients with HIV Infection?

Skin findings that occur at higher $CD4^+$ counts include seborrheic dermatitis, allergic reactions (medication, insect bites), and exacerbations of psoriasis. Later in the course of HIV infection, patients can develop KS and molluscum contagiosum. In patients with HIV infection, molluscum can cluster together to form giant molluscum 1–2 cm across; this is an indication of a markedly depleted immune system.

Patients with very low CD4$^+$ counts (<50) can develop large cutaneous ulcers, often in the perirectal region, which should be considered HSV until proved otherwise.

My Patient with HIV Infection has a Mouth Lesion. What Could This Be?

Possibilities include hairy leukoplakia, *Candida* infection, aphthous ulcers, gingivitis, and KS. Hairy leukoplakia appears as white plaques on the side of the tongue and is due to EBV. Hairy leukoplakia is specific for HIV infection and indicates a higher risk for disease progression to AIDS. In one study of CD4$^+$ count–matched patients, 22% of patients with hairy leukoplakia progressed to AIDS within 2 years compared with 9% of patients without hairy leukoplakia. Candidiasis ("thrush") occurs generally when the CD4$^+$ count is <300 and is a marker of immunodeficiency. Patients with oral candidiasis are at higher risk for developing other opportunistic infections and should receive *Pneumocystis* prophylaxis. Thirty percent of patients with KS have mouth involvement.

My Patient is Short of Breath. What Diseases do I Need to Consider?

Of cases of *P. carinii*, 95% occur with CD4$^+$ counts <200 and at a mean CD4$^+$ count <100. TB is more common in patients with HIV, especially in the presence of intravenous drug use, homelessness, or origin from an endemic area (Africa, Latin America, and Southeast Asia). With HIV infection and a positive PPD, the yearly risk of developing TB is 7%. This compares with a lifetime TB risk with positive PPD but no HIV infection of 10%. Bacterial pneumonia also is more common. It occurs at high CD4$^+$ counts and may be the first hint to the presence of HIV disease. *Streptococcus pneumoniae* and *Haemophilus influenzae* are the most common organisms involved. Estimated annual rates of pneumococcal pneumonia in HIV-infected patients are 10%. *Pseudomonas aeruginosa* is another important cause of community-acquired pneumonia when CD4$^+$ count is <50. Bacteremia and recurrent pneumonias are more likely in the setting of HIV infection. HIV infection also causes cardiomyopathy, which may manifest as dyspnea.

What Causes Headaches in HIV-Infected Patients?

Headache is common. If the CD4$^+$ count is >500, nonopportunistic infections are more likely (sinusitis, HIV meningitis). When the CD4$^+$ is <200, consider the three major opportunistic diseases—cryptococcus, toxoplasmosis, and lymphoma. Sinusitis, HIV meningitis, and tuberculous meningitis also can occur at these lower CD4$^+$ counts.

My Patient has Diarrhea. What Causes do I Need to Consider?

Approximately 50% of AIDS patients have GI problems, with diarrhea from enteric pathogens being the most common complaint. Common pathogens include CMV, *Cryptosporidium*, *Giardia*, MAC, and

Clostridium difficile. Cryptosporidium is a small noninvasive parasite of animals and was a rare cause of self-limited diarrhea in immunocompetent patients before the AIDS epidemic. Cryptosporidiosis is characterized by a persistent watery diarrhea, cramping abdominal pain, anorexia, and weight loss. *Giardia* is the most common nonopportunistic protozoan parasite in AIDS patients. It is seen in 15% of AIDS patients with symptomatic diarrhea. *C. difficile* is extremely common in patients with HIV disease because frequent hospitalizations results in colonization, and antibiotic use leads to overgrowth. HIV infection itself also can cause diarrhea, but is a diagnosis of exclusion. Many of the medications used to treat HIV disease cause diarrhea, especially protease inhibitors.

What are the Causes of Esophagitis?

Dysphagia (difficulty swallowing) and odynophagia (painful swallowing) are symptoms suggesting esophagitis in AIDS patients. These symptoms can significantly decrease food intake and worsen nutritional status. *Candida* esophagitis is the most frequent cause, especially when oral candidiasis is present. CMV, HSV, and the drug zalcitabine also can cause symptomatic esophageal ulcerations.

What Causes Fever in HIV-Infected Patients?

When $CD4^+$ count is >500, nonopportunistic causes are more common: bacterial pneumonia, pulmonary TB, or sinusitis, which is an almost universal problem in patients with HIV. In patients with lower $CD4^+$ counts (<200), opportunistic infections are more likely. With diarrhea, consider the enteric pathogens *C. difficile, Salmonella,* and MAC. For fever with pulmonary symptoms, consider bacterial pneumonia, TB, or PCP. If no focal signs accompany fever, think of cryptococcal meningitis because 10%-20% of patients do not have headache. Other poorly localized conditions causing fever in HIV-infected patients include lymphoma; extrapulmonary TB, common with low $CD4^+$ counts; MAC, which can cause night sweats and anemia; hepatitis, owing to HBV or HCV or toxin effect (e.g., from trimethoprim-sulfamethoxazole); CMV infection; and sinusitis. Don't forget the possibility of drug fever (especially due to trimethoprim-sulfamethoxazole). The drug abacavir can cause a life-threatening allergic reaction with fever.

EVALUATION

When should I Suspect Pneumonia in an HIV-Infected Patient?

The symptoms of bacterial pneumonia in HIV-infected patients are similar to symptoms in non–HIV-infected individuals, including dyspnea, productive cough, high fever, and fatigue. Tachycardia, tachypnea, and hypoxia may be present on exam, although lung exam may be unrevealing. In patients with *Pseudomonas* and $CD4^+$ counts <100, x-ray may show cavitary lesions.

Does TB Manifest Differently in HIV-Infected Patients?

Clinical manifestations of TB vary by the CD4$^+$ count. At CD4$^+$ counts >300, symptoms and x-ray findings are more typical, including weight loss; night sweats; fevers; productive cough; and upper lobe infiltrates, pleural effusions, or cavitary lesions on x-ray. At CD4$^+$ counts <200, clinical manifestations are less typical, extrapulmonary TB becomes common (two thirds of cases), and CXR findings are atypical with bilateral hilar adenopathy and lower lobe disease. Upper lobe infiltrates and pulmonary cavities are rare in patients with frank AIDS.

How does PCP Pneumonia Manifest?

Patients with PCP usually present with dry, nonproductive cough, low-grade fever, and progressive dyspnea and fatigue over 2–3 weeks. Exam is often unrevealing except for an increased respiratory rate. ABG often shows a decreased Po_2 and a widened A-a gradient. LDH is commonly elevated and is a prognostic factor for severity of illness. Bilateral interstitial infiltrates are typical on x-ray, but in severe cases alveolar/lobar infiltrates occur as well. In 20% of cases, CXR is normal. Spontaneous pneumothorax in a patient with HIV disease is usually a sign of underlying PCP.

What Tests are Warranted in Patients with Headache in the Setting of HIV Infection?

Work-up of patients with headache and low CD4$^+$ count (<200) consists of an imaging procedure (MRI or contrast CT scan) followed by LP. Characteristic CT findings are listed in Table 32-6. Send CSF for cell count, protein, glucose, Gram stain, cryptococcal antigen, and bacterial culture; strongly consider mycobacterial culture. Serum cryptococcal antigen is 99% sensitive for cryptococcal meningitis. Review if the patient has had *Toxoplasma* titers checked—if this was negative, toxoplasmosis is unlikely because >90% of patients with CNS toxoplasmosis have had a prior positive IgG with a reactivation of previous infection. CNS lymphoma requires brain biopsy for diagnosis, although it is usually diagnosed by exclusion after an unsuccessful trial of therapy for toxoplasmosis.

Table 32-6

Patterns Seen on Head CT Scan in HIV-Related CNS Disease

Disease	Pattern	Enhancement	Location
Toxoplasmosis	Ring mass	++	Basal ganglia
Lymphoma	Solid mass	+++	Periventricular
Progressive multifocal leukoencephalopathy	No mass	None	Subcortical white matter

How should I Evaluate an HIV-Infected Patient Who has a Fever?

Look for a focal process, and let history and physical guide your work-up. The $CD4^+$ count is the most important factor in determining risk of opportunistic infection. Obtain CBC with differential, CXR, blood cultures, urinalysis, and ALT/AST (HCV is common with intravenous drug use; HBV is common in patients with intravenous drug use or male-male sex). If no focal signs exist, consider additional tests, including blood cultures for mycobacteria and serum cryptococcal antigen. Other tests, such as head CT with contrast administration, LP, stool cultures, and sinus CT, should be based on symptoms suggesting focal abnormalities. If the patient has diarrhea, obtain stool *C. difficile* toxin and stool culture for enteric pathogens and atypical mycobacteria. Consider colonoscopy if the cause remains unclear. With pulmonary symptoms, obtain CXR, sputum Gram stain, and sputum cultures for TB. Pulmonary disease is usually one of three—bacterial pneumonia, TB, or PCP. PCP prophylaxis makes PCP unlikely, and fluconazole use makes cryptococcus unlikely.

My Patient has Persistent Dysphagia After 2 Weeks of Fluconazole. What should I do Next?

Obtain endoscopic biopsy with viral cultures to identify infection other than *Candida*. CMV appears on endoscopy as large shallow superficial ulcerations often involving most of the esophagus. Stop zalcitabine because this medication can cause esophageal ulceration.

TREATMENT

How do I Treat PCP Infection?

Treatment is with high-dose trimethoprim-sulfamethoxazole (first choice), pentamidine, trimethoprim-dapsone (for mild disease), atovaquone, or clindamycin-primaquine. These regimens all seem to have equivalent efficacy. Side effects are common, occurring in 50% of cases treated with trimethoprim-sulfamethoxazole or pentamidine. The major side effects with pentamidine are renal insufficiency; pancreatic islet cell destruction, which can cause transient hypoglycemia or permanent hyperglycemia; and hypotension. Early use of corticosteroids in patients with moderate-to-severe PCP can improve survival and decrease the occurrence of respiratory failure. Give steroids to patient with Po_2 <75 or an alveolar-arterial oxygen gradient >35.

What Treatments are used for the Various Causes of Diarrhea?

Ganciclovir decreases CMV-induced nausea and diarrhea. Treat *Giardia* and *C. difficile* with oral metronidazole. Common enteric bacteria respond to appropriate antibiotics with gram-negative coverage. *Cryptosporidium* is harder to eradicate (azithromycin and paromomycin are used); these patients may benefit from a hypomotility agent, such as loperamide or diphenoxylate/atropine.

Infectious Diseases

How do I Treat Esophagitis?

Patients with oral candidiasis and dysphagia can be given empiric keto-conazole, 200 mg daily, or fluconazole, 100–200 mg daily. Treat endo-scopically diagnosed CMV with ganciclovir, herpes with high-dose acyclovir, and documented *Candida* with fluconazole or ketoconazole.

How do I Treat Cryptococcal Meningitis?

Treat initially with intravenous amphotericin B, usually for 2 weeks. Follow with lifelong suppressive therapy using oral fluconazole.

Case 32-3

A 30-year-old man with C3 HIV disease (CD4$^+$ count 60) presents with severe headaches and confusion that have progressed over the past 2 weeks. He has had intermittent fevers for the past 3 weeks. His friends state he has been more forgetful, and on the day of admission he became belligerent and did not recognize his partner. He takes zidovudine, 200 mg three times daily; lamivudine, 150 mg twice daily; Atazanavir 400 mg QD every 8 hours; and dapsone, 100 mg once daily. Exam shows severe seborrheic dermatitis, molluscum contagiosum, oral hairy leukoplakia, and left lower extremity weakness with a left up-going toe. Lab values are HCT 31, WBC 2.0, Na 134, K 3.9, Cl 98, HCO$_3$ 26, creatinine 1.0, and BUN 18.

A. What does the seborrheic dermatitis tell you?
B. What is the importance of molluscum contagiosum and oral hairy leukoplakia in patients with HIV disease?
C. What is the differential diagnosis for this patient?
D. What work-up would you pursue?

MENINGITIS

ETIOLOGY

What is the Definition of Meningitis?

Meningitis is inflammation of the meninges from infectious (bacterial, viral, or fungal) or noninfectious causes (sarcoid, malignancy, drug reaction, or hemorrhage from vasculitis).

What are the Most Common Causes of Infectious Meningitis?

Viral meningitis is much more common than bacterial meningitis, with enteroviruses accounting for 70% of all cases of viral meningitis. Herpes simplex meningitis is usually associated with episodes of primary HSV 2 infection. Acute HIV infection can cause meningitis and is underdiag-nosed. In adults with bacterial meningitis, the most common etiologic

Table 32-7		
Causes of Bacterial Meningitis in Adults		
Common	**Uncommon**	**Special Circumstances**
Streptococcus pneumoniae	*Haemophilus influenzae*	Neurosurgical patients *Staphylococcus aureus* Gram-negative rods
Neisseria meningitidis		Alcoholics or immunosuppressed patients *Listeria*

agent is *S. pneumoniae,* occurring in 30%-50% of patients. *Neisseria meningitidis* (meningococcus) is the second most common cause, occurring in 10%-35% of adult patients with bacterial meningitis. *H. influenzae,* a common cause of bacterial meningitis in children before the onset of vaccination against *Haemophilus,* is rare in adults, causing only 1%-2% of adult meningitis cases (Table 32-7).

What are the Risk Factors for the Different Organisms Causing Bacterial Meningitis?

Pneumococcal meningitis may occur in the presence of pneumococcal pneumonia (15%-25% of cases), otitis media, or CSF leaks after trauma. Risk factors for pneumococcal meningitis, similar to pneumococcal pneumonia, include alcoholism, cirrhosis, sickle cell anemia, asplenism, multiple myeloma, and CLL. Neisserial meningitis usually occurs in young adults, is rare in adults >45 years old, and is the most common cause for epidemic bacterial meningitis. Also, complement deficiency increases the risk, particularly with deficient terminal components (C-5 through C-8). *Listeria monocytogenes* is a gram-positive rod, which is more prevalent in the setting of alcoholism, pregnancy, or hematologic malignancy. Of adults with *Listeria* infections, 20%-30% have no risk factors, however.

EVALUATION

What are the Typical Symptoms of Bacterial Meningitis?

Classic symptoms seen in adults include fever (77%), headache (87%), altered mental status (69%), and meningismus (83%). Less than half of patients have the classic triad of fever, stiff neck, and altered mental status. More nonspecific symptoms include nausea, vomiting, rigors, profuse sweats, weakness, myalgias, and photophobia. The presenting signs vary depending on the infecting organism and the underlying immune status of the patient. Presence of mental status change is the strongest indicator of bacterial meningitis.

What Signs should I Look for if I Suspect Meningitis?

Kernig's and Brudzinski's signs are present in 50% of bacterial meningitis cases. Perform these tests as follows. For Kernig's sign, attempt to

Infectious Diseases

extend the knee with the hip flexed. This is positive when radicular pain in the back or leg causes resistance to further extension. For Brudzinski's sign, flex the patient's neck. In a positive test, this maneuver produces flexion in the hip. Perform a careful skin exam because 66% of patients with meningococcus have a petechial rash.

Does Meningitis Present Differently in Elderly and Immunosuppressed Patients?

The usual signs of meningeal inflammation (nuchal rigidity, headache, Kernig's and Brudzinski's signs, fever) may not be present in elderly patients or patients with immune dysfunction, such as neutropenia or HIV disease. In elderly patients, confusion and mental status changes are the most reliable findings (80%-90%), although these are nonspecific because they occur with many other conditions.

What are the Typical Clinical Features of Viral Meningitis?

The clinical features of viral meningitis include a prodrome of headache, malaise, and fever with normal mental status. Viral meningitis is particularly common in individuals <40 years old. Exam is usually unrevealing; look for genital ulcers or blisters suggesting HSV 2, generalized adenopathy suggesting HIV, or parotitis suggesting mumps.

Should I Obtain a CNS Imaging Test Before LP?

The question frequently arises whether CNS imaging is required before LP. Obtain a CT scan or MRI before LP in any patient with a focal neurologic exam, papilledema or loss of venous pulsations on funduscopic exam, seizures, or HIV infection and $CD4^+$ count <200 or other severely immunosuppressed patients. HIV-infected patients more commonly have mass lesions secondary to toxoplasmosis, TB, or lymphoma. Look for evidence of midline shift, indicating CNS mass lesion and increased intracranial pressure; if present, risk for herniation and subsequent death with LP is approximately 6%.

What Tests should I Order on CSF?

Send CSF for glucose, protein, cell count with differential, bacterial culture, and Gram stain. In patients at high risk for TB or fungal meningitis, test for TB with an AFB smear and culture and for cryptococcal disease with cryptococcal antigen testing. Not all patients need AFB and fungal testing of the CSF.

What does the CSF Look Like in Patients with Bacterial Meningitis?

CSF in bacterial meningitis shows >500/mm^3 PMNs, markedly elevated protein >100 mm/dL (and often >250 mg/dL, with normal 23–38 mg/dL), and glucose <40% of serum glucose (Table 32-8). About 80% of patients have a positive Gram stain (*S. pneumoniae* 83%, *H. influenzae* 76%, *N. meningitidis* 66%).

Table 32-8

Cerebrospinal Fluid Findings with Meningitis of Various Causes

Etiology	WBC	WBC Differential	Protein (mg/dL)	Glucose* (mg/dL)	Gram Stain
Viral	5–500	>50% mono	0–150	Normal	No organisms
Bacterial	100–2000	>90% PMN	80–500	<35	80% gram positive
Cryptococcus	40–400†	>80% mono	40–150	Normal	>90% cryptococcal antigen
TB	100–1000	>80% mono	40–150	Normal or lower	AFB smear positive
Subdural or epidural abscess	50–300	Variable	75–300	Normal	No organisms

*Normal glucose is >40 mg/dL or >50% of simultaneous blood glucose; glucose may be decreased in viral, fungal, or parameningeal infections.
†Lower in immunocompromised patients with HIV.
mono, monocytes.

What Tests are Useful if I Suspect Bacterial Meningitis, But the Gram Stain and Culture are Negative?

CIE can detect the presence of capsular polysaccharide from *H. influenzae*, *S. pneumoniae*, and *N. meningitidis*. This is particularly useful for evaluating patients who have received antibiotics because the polysaccharide persists after bacterial lysis.

What does the CSF Test Look Like in a Patient with Viral Meningitis?

In contrast to the high PMN count of bacterial meningitis, the typical pattern of viral meningitis is a total cell count <500/mm^3 with a mononuclear predominance, protein moderately elevated but not usually >100 mm/dL (normal 22–38 mg/dL), and a normal glucose level. Early in the course of viral meningitis, PMNs may predominate. A repeat LP within 6–8 hours often shows a shift to mononuclear predominance.

TREATMENT

What Therapy should be Used for Suspected Bacterial Meningitis?

With the increase in pneumococcal resistance to penicillin, empiric therapy for meningitis must cover penicillin-resistant organisms.

Vancomycin plus a third-generation cephalosporin (ceftriaxone or cefotaxime) is recommended. If the patient has risk factors for *Listeria*, or if this organism is seen on Gram stain, add ampicillin as well. A third-generation cephalosporin alone is adequate when meningococcus is seen on Gram stain or in elderly patients with probable gram-negative meningitis by Gram stain. If *S. aureus* is suspected by history or Gram stain, use vancomycin plus a third-generation cephalosporin until sensitivities are available. Do not use cefoperazone or ceftazidime because they have poor anti-streptococcal effect. Narrow the spectrum of coverage after an organism is identified. If you need to obtain a CT scan before obtaining LP in a patient with a high suspicion for bacterial meningitis, obtain blood cultures first, then give antibiotics *before* sending the patient for the CT scan.

Case 32-4

A 73-year-old man is brought by his daughter to the emergency department with mental status changes over the past 24 hours. He reports no concerns or symptoms. Past medical history is significant for CAD, CHF, and BPH. Vital signs are BP 100/60 mm Hg, pulse 110 beats/min, and temperature 39.8° C. Exam shows there is no rash, chest is clear, there is no heart murmur, and abdomen is nontender. Lab results are HCT 38, WBC 23,000 with 90% PMN, Na 136, K 4.9, Cl 100, HCO_3 18, BUN 30, and creatinine 2.0.

A. What tests would you order?
B. What is the most likely diagnosis for this patient?

Case 32-5

A 37-year-old alcoholic presents with obtundation and fever. He was found seizing on a downtown sidewalk. His old chart shows multiple emergency department visits for alcohol intoxication, lacerations, and one episode of pancreatitis. Vital signs are BP 90/60 mm Hg, pulse 120 beats/min, and temperature 40.8° C. Exam shows skin is without rash, and neck is stiff with a positive Brudzinski's sign. Breath sounds are decreased at the right base; there is no heart murmur. He is sleepy with a symmetric neurologic exam, and toes are up-going bilaterally. Lab test results are Na 128, K 3.8, Cl 96, HCO_3 12, HCT 39, and WBC 2.9. CXR shows right lower lobe infiltrate.

A. What tests would you order?
B. What is your differential diagnosis?
C. What treatment would you start?

PNEUMONIA

ETIOLOGY

How Common and How Dangerous is Pneumonia?

Community-acquired pneumonia is common, with >4 million cases annually in the U.S. Most patients are treated as outpatients with a mortality rate of about 1%, although 20% of patients require hospitalization, where death rates are 25%. Pneumonia is the sixth leading cause of death overall.

How do People get Pneumonia?

Pneumonia is inflammation of lung parenchyma from infection. Organisms reach the lung by oropharyngeal aspiration, inhalation, or hematogenous spread. Defects in host defenses often contribute (i.e., impaired glottic reflex, insufficient cough, impaired ciliary function usually from smoking, or deficient immunity). Important risk factors for pneumonia are listed in Table 32-9.

Table 32-9

Organisms and Mechanisms Causing Pneumonia in Patients with Specific Risk Factors for Pneumonia

Risk Group	Specific Likely Organisms	Mechanisms of Acquiring Pneumonia
Alcoholism	*Streptococcus pneumoniae* Anaerobes *Haemophilus influenzae* *Klebsiella pneumoniae* *Mycobacterium tuberculosis*	Decreased glottic reflex Seizures Stupor Aspiration of oral and gastric flora Poor WBC function and humoral immunity
Injection drug use	*S. pneumoniae* Anaerobes *Staphylococcus aureus* Septic PE *(tricuspid endocarditis)* (often MRSA) *M. tuberculosis*	Aspiration during times of altered consciousness (heroin) or seizures (cocaine) HIV infection
Smoking-induced lung disease	*S. pneumoniae* *H. influenzae* *Moraxella catarrhalis* *Legionella*	Impaired mucociliary transport Colonized lower respiratory tract Resistance due to prior frequent antibiotics

(continued)

Table 32-9

Organisms and Mechanisms Causing Pneumonia in Patients with Specific Risk Factors for Pneumonia (Continued)

Risk Group	Specific Likely Organisms	Mechanisms of Acquiring Pneumonia
HIV infection	S. pneumoniae H. influenzae Pneumocystis carinii Pseudomonas aeruginosa	Impaired cellular immunity Prophylactic antibiotics and CD4$^+$ <100 make pseudomonal infection more likely
Nursing home residence	K. pneumoniae S. aureus (often MRSA) M. tuberculosis (reactivation or primary)	Lowered immunity Predisposing illness Institutional exposures Neurologic disease or medications cause altered cognition and aspiration Colonization with gram-negative rods
Postviral superinfection	S. pneumoniae S. aureus H. influenzae	Viral infections disrupt mucociliary function Viruses interfere with cell-mediated host defense mechanisms (influenza, CMV) Develops 7–19 d after viral infection

MRSA, methicillin-resistant *S. aureus.*

What Organisms Cause Community-Acquired Pneumonia?

Microbiologic confirmation of the cause is obtained only in about 50%-70% of cases at best, even using invasive studies. *S. pneumoniae* and *H. influenzae* are most common; both occur in patients with predisposing conditions (see Table 32-9), although these are not always present. *Mycoplasma pneumoniae* and *Chlamydophila* are probably the most common causes in young healthy adults. Anaerobic pneumonias occur with periodontal disease because anaerobes flourish amid rotting teeth and gums; edentulous patients rarely get anaerobic infections. Anaerobic infections also are more common with aspiration of mouth flora during periods of unconsciousness or with swallowing disorders. Aspiration is a common cause for pneumonias developing in IVDU (heroin decreases the gag reflex; cocaine can cause seizures) and alcoholics. Bacterial pneumonia can occur after viral upper respiratory infections, usually soon after symptoms of the viral infection begin to improve. *S. pneumoniae* and *S. aureus* are the most common causes of pneumonia after a preceding viral upper respiratory infection.

How is Hospital-Acquired Pneumonia Different from Community-Acquired Pneumonia?

Hospital-acquired pneumonia occurs in 10% of hospitalized patients. Common culprits are gram-negative rods (often resistant to multiple antibiotics) and *S. aureus* (including MRSA), followed by anaerobes and *S. pneumoniae*. Gram-negative pneumonias carry a high mortality (40%) because the organisms are aggressive, and concurrent underlying medical conditions complicate recovery. Mortality in patients with nosocomial pneumonias can be 50%, partially related to the presence and severity of comorbid conditions.

What are Some Uncommon Causes of Pneumonia?

Legionella occurs sporadically or as an epidemic; patients with underlying lung disease are at greatest risk. Consider psittacosis (*Chlamydophila psittaci*) with exposure to birds, especially in pet shop workers or bird keepers. *Chlamydophila* occurs in young adults. Q fever from inhalation of aerosolized *Coxiella burnetii* is seen in livestock handlers.

What causes Pleural Effusions in Patients with Pneumonia?

Exudative pleural effusion accompanies about 40% of pneumonias and is due to pleural inflammation. Most of these parapneumonic effusions are small, are sterile, and resolve with treatment of the pneumonia. Some become infected, creating a purulent empyema, which can cause persistent infection, sepsis, and permanent scarring if left untreated.

EVALUATION

What Questions should I ask when I Suspect Pneumonia?

Classic symptoms of bacterial pneumonia include cough producing bloody or purulent sputum, high fever often accompanied by rigors or chills, dyspnea, and pleuritic chest pain. Patients with pneumococcal pneumonia classically present with a single shaking chill at onset followed by high fever, pleuritic chest pain, and cough productive of bloody or "rusty" sputum. *Legionella* may cause myalgias, headache, confusion, and diarrhea. "Atypical" presentations are more subdued and suggest less inflammatory organisms, such as viruses, *Mycoplasma, Pneumocystis, Chlamydophila,* or uncommonly Q fever or psittacosis. For atypical presentations, cough (when present) is usually nonproductive, fevers are lower grade, and myalgias or severe headache may be present. Extrapulmonary manifestations may be prominent with *Mycoplasma,* such as meningitis, bullous myringitis (otitis media), cerebellar ataxia, and erythema multiforme. Hoarseness or sore throat suggests *Chlamydophila.* Ask about occupational or animal exposure, especially when symptoms are atypical, an organism cannot be found, or patients do not respond to empiric therapy for common organisms. Foul-smelling sputum suggests anaerobes. Prior TB exposure, weight loss, anorexia, and night sweats are clues to TB infection.

In what Situations Might Typical Pneumonias Manifest Atypically?

Elderly patients may have few symptoms referable to the chest, and the main finding is confusion, disorientation, or anorexia. Neutropenic patients rarely have productive cough because there are no WBC to produce sputum; the earliest and most pronounced symptom of pneumonia is isolated fever. Some lower lobe pneumonias may manifest with minimal chest symptoms and abdominal pain secondary to irritation of the diaphragm.

What Exam Findings Support a Diagnosis of Typical Lobar Pneumonia?

Tachypnea, tachycardia, and fever are common. With early lobar pneumonia, breath sounds may be decreased over the affected parenchyma, although occasionally breath sounds are louder as a result of better transmission of tracheal airway sounds through consolidated lung (called bronchial breath sounds). Always compare breath sounds from side to side to detect subtle asymmetry. Dullness to percussion can represent consolidation or pleural effusion. Rales may be heard over the affected lobe and are most prominent with resolving pneumonia as air passages begin to open up again. Other signs of lobar consolidation include whispered pectoriloquy and tactile fremitus. Whispered pectoriloquy is elicited by having the patient whisper something (try their phone number or social security number). Transmission of sound is good through consolidated lung, and you can easily hear the whispered words when your stethoscope is placed over the area. Elicit tactile fremitus by having the patient say "toy boat" while you place your hands symmetrically on the patient's chest; vibrations are increased over areas of consolidation and are decreased when fluid or air is present in the pleural space. Use this technique when dullness to percussion is present to differentiate effusion from infiltrate.

What Lab Tests are Warranted if I Suspect Pneumonia?

Check oxygen saturation, CBC, sputum Gram stain and culture, electrolytes, and kidney function. In typical bacterial presentations, WBC increases, often with a left shift (excess immature forms or bands). In contrast, WBC is often normal in viruses, *Mycoplasma,* or *Chlamydophila*. A decreased WBC in the presence of pneumonia is a poor prognostic sign. In particularly ill-appearing patients, consider blood cultures and ABG. Positive blood cultures occur in 25% of pneumococcal pneumonias and are associated with poorer prognosis (20%-40% mortality). ABG may reveal hypoxia and respiratory alkalosis. *Mycoplasma* is suggested by hemolytic anemia or cold agglutinins (seen in 50%). Confirm diagnosis by an increase in convalescent antibody titers. *Mycoplasma* and *Chlamydophila* are often treated empirically without confirming a diagnosis. *Legionella* causes hyponatremia and a sputum Gram stain with leukocytes, but no organisms. Diagnose *Legionella* by urinary antigen (type 1 only), DNA probe, direct fluorescent antibody, culture, or increase in convalescent antibody titer.

How do I Interpret Sputum Gram Stain and Cultures?

Sputum specimens are often contaminated with saliva and oral flora, as indicated by epithelial cells and multiple organisms on Gram stain: >25 epithelial cells per low-power field correlates with an inadequate specimen. An adequate specimen from deep in the chest, with <10 epithelial cells and >25 WBC per low-power field, and with one dominant organism (more the exception than the rule) can guide initial empiric therapy. Gram stain is most reliable for *S. pneumoniae* and least reliable for the difficult-to-see pleomorphic gram-negative rods of *H. influenzae*. If you see WBC with no organisms, consider *Legionella*, *Mycoplasma*, *Chlamydophila*, TB, or psittacosis. Sputum culture is less useful than stains because it is negative in 50% of patients with blood culture–positive pneumonia. Sputum culture is more useful in the diagnosis of TB because stains may miss this disease.

How can CXR Help with the Diagnosis of Pneumonia?

The causative organism cannot be accurately predicted by x-ray, but certain appearances are more typical of some organisms than others (Table 32-10).

Table 32-10

Likely Organisms as Suggested by Specific Chest Film Findings in Pneumonia

Chest Film Findings	Likely Organisms
Alveolar/airspace lobar infiltrate with air bronchograms,* silhouette sign†	*Pneumococcus, Haemophilus,* other typical organisms
Upper lobe infiltrates	TB, *Klebsiella*
Apical scarring	Prior TB
Bilateral lower lobe infiltrates	Anaerobes (aspiration)
Upper lobe posterior segment or lower lobe superior segment R > L	Anaerobes (aspiration) Right lung > left lung (right main stem bronchus more straight)
Patchy bilateral infiltrates	*Mycoplasma pneumoniae*
Patchy unilateral segmental infiltrates	*Chlamydia pneumoniae, M. pneumoniae*
Diffuse interstitial infiltrates	*Pneumocystis* and viral pneumonias
Cavitation‡	*Mycobacterium tuberculosis, Staphylococcus aureus,* or gram-negative rods

*Bronchus remains aerated and dark, whereas surrounding alveoli are fluid-filled and bright.
†Silhouette sign is the loss of a heart border or diaphragm shadow as a result of focal adjacent lung consolidation.
‡Appearance of a hollow round cavity owing to necrosis and liquefaction of lung parenchyma.

TREATMENT

How do I Choose Empiric Treatment for a Patient with Pneumonia?

Identify and target the most likely organism (Table 32-11). Severity of illness and local resistance patterns also guide empiric antibiotic choice and route of administration. Switch to a narrow spectrum antibiotic when or if sensitivities become available. For community-acquired pneumonia in a patient <45 years old who has no specific risk factors, use a macrolide (azithromycin, clarithromycin, or erythromycin) or doxycycline. For nosocomial pneumonia with gram-negative rods on sputum Gram stain, cover dually with an aminoglycoside and

Table 32-11

Empiric Antibiotic Treatment Options for Pneumonia by Risk Factor and Suspected Pathogens

Risk Factor	Empiric Therapy Options
COPD	Cefuroxime (oral) Ceftriaxone (IV) Amoxicillin-clavulanate Quinolone (levofloxacin, moxifloxacin)
Aspiration	Clindamycin Amoxicillin-clavulanate or ampicillin-sulbactam
Elderly	Amoxicillin-clavulanate or ampicillin-sulbactam
Nosocomial infection	Aminoglycoside plus antipseudomonal penicillin or third-generation cephalosporin or quinolone

Suspected Pathogen	
Pneumococcus or Haemophilus	Second- or third-generation cephalosporin Amoxicillin-clavulanate or ampicillin-sulbactam
Mycoplasma	Erythromycin (also clarithromycin or azithromycin)
Legionella	Erythromycin in high dose (1 g IV q6h) Quinolones
Staphylococcus	Vancomycin (if MRSA or culture unknown) Nafcillin or first-generation cephalosporin if MSSA
Anaerobes	Clindamycin Metronidazole Amoxicillin-clavulanate or ampicillin-sulbactam
Psittacosis	Tetracycline or doxycycline Erythromycin
Chlamydophila	Tetracycline
Q fever	Tetracycline Chloramphenicol

MRSA, methicillin-resistant *S. aureus;* MSSA, methicillin-sensitive *S. aureus.*

an extended spectrum antipseudomonal penicillin (ticarcillin, mezlocillin, piperacillin), an antipseudomonal third-generation cephalosporin (ceftazidime or cefoperazone), or a quinolone with activity against *S. pneumoniae* (levofloxacin, or moxifloxacin). With clusters of gram-positive cocci on Gram stain in a nosocomial pneumonia, cover empirically for *S. aureus* and gram-negative rods until culture results are back. Coverage for *S. aureus* should cover methicillin-resistant *S. aureus*.

What should I Know about Resistance to Antibiotics?

Most strains of pneumococcus are penicillin sensitive and low-dose penicillin (600,000–1,200,000 U/d) is effective when the diagnosis is made. Pneumococcal resistance to penicillin and cephalosporins is 30% in some areas. Pneumococcal resistance to penicillin is due to alterations in penicillin binding protein. Beta-lactamase production is not a factor in pneumococcal penicillin resistance, but is important in *S. aureus* and anaerobe resistance. Third-generation cephalosporins and advanced generation quinolones (levofloxacin, and moxifloxacin) have reasonable activity against pneumococcal strains with intermediate resistance to penicillins. Vancomycin is the most active antibiotic against penicillin-resistant pneumococcus. Methicillin resistance to *S. aureus* is common in community-acquired and hospital-acquired organisms.

How do I Manage a Parapneumonic Effusion?

Pleural tap is indicated to differentiate a sterile parapneumonic effusion from an infected empyema. Empyema must be drained expeditiously by chest tube or surgery to cure the infection, prevent sepsis, and avoid loculation, fibrosis, and permanent impairment of lung function. Treat for empyema if pleural fluid WBC and LDH are high, pH is <7.1, glucose is <40 mg/dL, or cultures of pleural fluid grow organisms. If parameters are borderline, do another pleural tap in 12 hours.

Can Pneumonia be Prevented?

Pneumococcal vaccine prevents pneumococcal pneumonia in high-risk patients, all patients >65 years old, institutionalized elderly, HIV-positive patients, and patients with other severe underlying illness.

How Long Does it Take Patients to Respond to Treatment?

Patients generally improve after 72 hours. X-ray findings can worsen despite clinical improvement, and resolution of x-ray abnormalities lags behind clinical improvement, often taking ≥6 weeks. If a patient is not responding to appropriate therapy, look for a resistant or unexpected organism, an alternate cause of fever, or a complication such as empyema or abscess with cavitation.

Who should be Hospitalized for Treatment?

Admit patients with multiple-lobe involvement, low initial WBC, multiple sites of infection, severe underlying disease, alcoholism, or advanced age. Additionally, admit for signs of early sepsis, including hypotension, orthostasis, tachycardia, tachypnea, or hypoxia.

Case 32-6

A 66-year-old woman with a long history of cigarette use and recent onset of diabetes reports 2 days of worsening cough that started as she was gardening and became productive of purulent, rusty sputum yesterday. She had a severe shaking chill last night. Her vital signs are temperature 38.5° F, HR 80 beats/ min, BP 120/60 mm Hg, and respirations 32.

- A. What are the most likely organisms causing her symptoms?
- B. What other information would you like?
- C. What empiric treatment is appropriate?
- D. After 36 hours, fevers continue to 38.8° C, and WBC remains high. What should you do?
- E. Five days into her stay, her fever reaches 39.4° C. How do you interpret this, and what should you do?

Case 32-7

An 80-year-old woman is brought to your office from her nursing home because she is more confused than usual today. She had been complaining of abdominal pain. Her temperature is 37.0° F, and WBC is 4×10^9/L.

- A. What could this be (list at least seven things)?
- B. Name at least seven tests to help you figure out her diagnosis.
- C. If this is a pneumonia, what organisms do you need to consider?
- D. If this is pneumonia, explain her abdominal pain and lack of fever or leukocytosis.

TUBERCULOSIS

ETIOLOGY

What Causes TB?

TB is an infection caused by a slow-growing aerobic bacillus, *Mycobacterium tuberculosis,* which is not decolorized by acid alcohol and is an acid fast bacillus (AFB).

What are the Risk Factors for TB?

The major risk factors for TB are listed in Box 32-4.

Who is at Risk for Multidrug-Resistant TB?

Most multidrug-resistant TB in the U.S. has occurred in institutions such as prisons and nursing homes and in HIV-infected patients.

Infectious Diseases

BOX 32-4

RISK FACTORS FOR TUBERCULOSIS INFECTION

Major Risk Factors

Close contact with smear-positived patient
HIV infection (or other immunosuppression)
Homelessness

Injection Drug Use

Institutionalization (prison)
Prior residence in endemic area
Africa, Southeast Asia, Central America

Minor Risk Factors

Diabetes mellitus
Gastrectomy
Silicosis

EVALUATION

What is the Purpose of Purified Protein Derivative (PPD) Screening in Healthy-Appearing Patients?

PPD screening identifies patients who have been exposed to TB. A small sample of PPD is placed under the skin and incites an inflammatory reaction if the patient already has immune response against TB, indicating exposure. Because live organisms are effective at evading normal host responses, a positive PPD result also suggests dormant, live bacteria are present as latent infection, waiting for a time of immunosuppression to cause reactivation TB. PPD interpretation depends on the host characteristics and diameter of induration present (Table 32-12). When a patient has a known positive PPD reaction, never retest because subsequent reactions may cause painful inflammation and skin necrosis.

My Patient's Screening PPD is Positive. What should I do Next?

Rule out active infection because treatment of active infection requires multidrug therapy, whereas exposure with latent infection can be treated with isoniazid alone in most cases. Ask about symptoms of TB, including constitutional, pulmonary, GI, and genitourinary symptoms, and about joint pains. Perform a full exam and CXR. Any signs or symptoms that could represent active pulmonary or nonpulmonary TB infection require further work-up.

What are the Typical Symptoms of Active TB Infection?

Classic symptoms are fever, night sweats, weight loss, and cough productive of thick sputum. Hemoptysis and dyspnea are symptoms of

Table 32-12

Interpreting Induration Reaction to Purified Protein Derivative Testing

Reaction	Reading	Patient to Whom PPD Reading Applies
<5 mm	Negative	All patients
≥5 mm	Positive	HIV-infected patients
		Organ transplant patients
		Patients on long-term prednisone
		Recent contacts with TB-infected patients
		X-ray findings suggesting prior TB infection
≥10 mm	Positive	Children <4 years old, children exposed to high-risk adults
		IVDU without HIV infection
		Patients with gastrectomy, malignancy, diabetes, silicosis, renal insufficiency
		Recent immigrants from country with high prevalence of TB
		Staff from AFB lab
		Staff from prisons, nursing homes, hospitals, shelters
≥15 mm	Positive	No known risk factors for TB

PPD, purified protein derivative.

advanced disease. In elderly and HIV-infected patients, symptoms may be more subtle (anorexia, fatigue, confusion, weakness).

When should I Think of TB in the Differential Diagnosis?

Patients who present with typical symptoms and major risk factors should be worked up for TB. Anyone with an upper lobe infiltrate on x-ray also should be considered for work-up. Think of TB (especially reactivation TB) in elderly patients who have infiltrates on x-ray that do not respond to standard antibiotic therapy. Alcoholics are at higher risk for TB because of a higher likelihood of homelessness or incarceration.

What is the Work-Up for TB?

Order a CXR first. If infiltrates are present, especially in the upper lobe, obtain three separate morning sputum samples for AFB smear and culture. Patients admitted to the hospital and undergoing TB work-up should be kept in respiratory isolation until three smears are negative. TB skin testing (PPD) is most helpful when the presentation is atypical. In patients with typical presentations and a suggestive CXR, obtain sputum samples first to avoid a painful large positive PPD. Work-up for nonpulmonary TB infection is rarely needed and is more invasive, requiring sampling affected tissues as indicated: urinalysis for sterile pyuria, urine AFB culture, joint aspiration, liver biopsy, gastric secretion collection, bone marrow biopsy, or bone sampling.

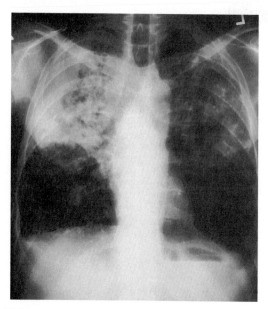

FIGURE 32-2 CXR of TB. Findings of bilateral upper lobe pleural thickening, cavities, and infiltrates (more extensive in the right upper lobe).

What are the Typical X-Ray Findings of TB?

Most TB is reactivation TB with upper lobe infiltrates, cavitation, and pleural thickening (Figure 32-2). Patients with primary infection can develop hilar adenopathy, pleural effusions, or miliary pattern (diffuse small nodules in the lungs, named after millet seeds). HIV-infected patients can have varying x-ray presentations.

TREATMENT

Who should Receive Isoniazid Prophylaxis for Latent Infection?

In general, patients with a newly positive PPD or close contact with smear-positive patients should receive prophylaxis (Box 32-5). Patients with HIV disease should receive prophylaxis if the PPD test shows ≥5 mm of induration.

What Treatment is Warranted for Latent TB Infection?

If evaluation for active TB is negative in a patient with positive PPD, proceed with 9 months of isoniazid prophylaxis, 300 mg/d. LFT (AST, ALT, bilirubin) should be obtained at baseline, and if abnormal at baseline should be repeated monthly while on therapy. All patients taking isoniazid should be monitored monthly for adherence to the medication and asked about symptoms of hepatitis (nausea, vomiting, anorexia, and

BOX 32-5

INDICATIONS FOR ISONIAZID PROPHYLAXIS

PPD positive without prior treatment *and* old positive PPD >15mm
   and age <35
Recent PPD conversion to positive, any age ≥15mm
High risk criteria, (PPD ≥10mm)
   Homeless
   IVDU
   Nursing home or prison resident
   Prior residence in endemic country
   Chronic diseases (silicosis, diabetes, end-stage renal disease)
Very High-risk criteria, any age (PPD ≥5mm)
   CXR consistent with old TB
   Close contact with a smear-positive patient
   HIV-infection
   Prolonged steroid use
   Immunocompromise (organ transplant)

abdominal pain). Isoniazid also can interfere with pyridoxine metabolism, causing peripheral neuropathy; to prevent this complication, many prescribe 25–50 mg/d of vitamin B_6.

What Therapy should a Patient with Active TB Receive?

Multiple drug therapy is the rule because of the risk of drug resistance. Start with four drugs—usually isoniazid, rifampin, pyrazinamide, and ethambutol. Directly observed therapy has a much greater success rate. If the organism turns out to be sensitive to isoniazid and rifampin, ethambutol can be discontinued after 2 months, and the 6-month course can be finished off with isoniazid and rifampin. Thrice-weekly therapy with isoniazide, rifampin, pyrazinamide, and ethambutol under direct observation for 6 months is highly effective. Give vitamin B_6 (see previous question) to avoid neuropathy from isoniazid.

Case 32-8

A 48-year-old man presents with 3 months of 15 lb of weight loss and cough, with occasional hemoptysis. He is a heavy alcohol drinker, has been homeless for the past 2 years, and has spent most of that time in homeless shelters. He was in jail briefly 4 years ago. He has a 40-pack-year smoking history.

A. List possible causes of his symptoms.
B. What features on a CXR would suggest TB?
C. If his work-up reveals TB, what treatment would you choose?

URINARY TRACT INFECTIONS

ETIOLOGY

My Patient has Dysuria. What is the Likely Cause?

Dysuria, urgency, frequency, and occasionally incontinence are symptoms of urethral irritation from UTI. Similar symptoms can occur with vaginitis or urethritis (e.g., *Candida* or HSV infection). Men with prostatitis can present with dysuria.

What Causes UTI?

Twenty percent of women have a UTI during their lifetime. In young women with acute cystitis, the most common bacterial pathogens are *Escherichia coli* and *Staphylococcus saprophyticus*. Sexual intercourse and diaphragm use increase risk. Complicated cystitis is a broad category that includes young women at risk for resistant organisms, elderly or immunocompromised women with acute cystitis, pregnant women, and patients with indwelling catheters. Uncomplicated pyelonephritis is by definition community acquired and has no urologic abnormalities. As with cystitis, *E. coli* is the most common pathogen. Complicated pyelonephritis is an upper tract infection occurring in the setting of urinary catheters, stones, obstruction such as BPH, or recent urinary procedures. Resistant gram-negative rods and *Enterococcus* are important organisms in this condition. Consider *Pseudomonas* with indwelling catheters and recent urologic procedures (TURP, cystoscopy) and *Enterococcus* when broad-spectrum antibiotics such as cephalosporins have been used recently.

EVALUATION

How is Urinalysis Interpreted?

In patients with dysuria, obtain clinic dipstick and lab microscopic analysis of a spun urine sediment. Many dipstick results include LE, which correlates with the presence of pyuria with 95% sensitivity; this does not denote UTI, however. LE and WBC are nonspecific, occurring also in cervicitis, vaginitis, and urethritis. Microscopic hematuria is present in 40%-60% of patients with acute cystitis and is uncommonly found in other causes of acute dysuria, making it a modestly specific indicator of cystitis.

When is Urine Culture Useful?

There is no role for culture in acute cystitis. Send urine for culture and sensitivity in suspected pyelonephritis, in recurrent UTI, or if the urinalysis is equivocal. A positive culture is defined as >100,000 colonies of a single organism. Lower counts, 10^2-10^4, can still be associated with infection; this is termed "acute dysuric syndrome." Screening for asymptomatic bacteriuria is appropriate in pregnant women.

Infectious Diseases

BOX 32-6

FACTORS SUGGESTING OCCULT PYELONEPHRITIS OR COMPLICATED URINARY TRACT INFECTION

Diabetes
Pregnancy
Male patient
Childhood UTI
Elderly patient
Indwelling catheter
Immunosuppression
Urologic anatomic abnormality
Symptoms for >7 days
Recent urinary tract instrumentation or antibiotics

How are Symptoms of Cystitis Different from Pyelonephritis?

Patients with cystitis usually present with dysuria, frequency, urgency, and suprapubic pain, sometimes accompanied by frank hematuria. Fever is not a symptom of isolated cystitis. Patients suspected to have cystitis also should be asked about risks for sexually transmitted disease and about vaginal discharge. If sexually transmitted disease is possible by this history, perform pelvic examination. Pyelonephritis is important to distinguish from cystitis because a longer duration of therapy may be indicated, and treatment failures and complications are more likely. Also termed upper tract infection, pyelonephritis commonly manifests with fever, back or abdominal pain, and costovertebral angle or flank tenderness. Concurrent cystitis symptoms may be present. Other symptoms seen with pyelonephritis are nausea, vomiting, headache, and malaise. Pyelonephritis can be subclinical (without classic symptoms) and should be suspected in patients with risk factors (Box 32-6).

TREATMENT

What is the Best Antibiotic for Cystitis?

For uncomplicated cystitis in young women, short-course therapy with 3 days of trimethoprim-sulfamethoxazole or a quinolone has an excellent cure rate and few side effects. There is increasing resistance to trimethoprim-sulfamethoxazole (15%), so if a patient has persistent symptoms despite treatment with trimethoprim-sulfamethoxazole, check a urine culture. Short-course therapy is not recommended for patients with diabetes or for men; treat these patients for 7 days.

How does Treatment for Complicated Pyelonephritis Differ?

Treat complicated infections with drugs effective against resistant gram-negative rods, including *Pseudomonas*. If urine Gram stain shows gram-positive cocci, cover for *Enterococcus* as well. For empiric therapy, use an aminoglycoside and an antipseudomonal third-generation cephalo-sporin. The best treatment option for enterococcus is ampicillin, but resistance is common. Remove urinary catheters if possible. When cultures are available, narrow antibiotics. For *Pseudomonas,* use two drugs to limit emergence of resistance. Septic shock often accompanies complicated UTIs. Support BP with intravenous fluids, and treat refractory hypotension with vasoactive medications. Relieving any urinary obstruction is a crucial part of therapy.

What Patients with Asymptomatic Bacteriuria should be Treated?

There is no benefit in the screening for or treatment of asymptomatic bacteriuria in almost all patient populations. The only exceptions are pregnant women and patients who are undergoing urologic procedures that would cause mucosal bleeding (especially TURP procedures).

How do I Treat Cystitis or Asymptomatic Bacteriuria in Pregnant Women?

Antibiotics to use in pregnancy include amoxicillin, amoxicillin-clavula-nate, nitrofurantoin, cephalexin, cefixime, fosfomycin, and sulfisoxazole. Quinolones are contraindicated because of adverse effects on fetal cartilage development. Sulfonamides should be avoided in the third trimester. Optimal length of treatment is unclear. Single-dose, 3-day therapy, and 7-day treatment regimens all have been used.

How are Recurrent UTIs Managed?

Recurrence is due either to relapse of the same organism or to reinfection with a new organism. Relapse immediately after short-course therapy warrants 2-week treatment for presumed upper tract disease. For reinfection, self-treatment by patients is reasonable because studies show excellent correlation between patients' symptoms and bacteriologic evidence of UTI. For patients with two to three recurrences per month, prophylactic therapy with daily trimethoprim-sulfamethoxazole has been shown to decrease infections by 95%. Drinking cranberry juice daily can decrease recurrence rates by 50%. Postcoital prophylaxis with trimethoprim-sulfamethoxazole, nitrofurantoin, or a quinolone is another effective option for women who get frequent UTIs associated with sexual activity.

What Treatment is Appropriate for Community-Acquired Pyelonephritis?

The major treatment decision is whether to hospitalize. Admit a patient when vomiting prevents use of oral medications and makes intravenous fluids necessary, and when noncompliance is likely. For uncomplicated pyelonephritis, choose antibiotics with good gram-negative activity, such as aminoglycosides, third-generation cephalosporins, or quinolones. Amoxicillin is a poor choice because 25%-35% of community-acquired

E. coli are resistant. Increasing *E. coli* resistance to trimethoprim-sulfa-methoxazole is occurring, now reported to be about 15%-20%. Trimeth-oprim-sulfamethoxazole is a good treatment option to switch to if results of urine cultures confirm sensitivity. Duration of therapy is contro-versial; most physicians treat acute uncomplicated pyelonephritis for 2 weeks. Initial bacteremia and fevers that persist for several days into therapy are common and should not change treatment.

Case 32-9

A 67-year-old woman presents with dysuria and frequency, but is otherwise healthy. Her past medical history includes breast cancer and hypertension. She is sexually active with her husband. Her vital signs are stable. Urinalysis reveals positive LE, RBC, and WBC.

    A. Is any further evaluation necessary?
    B. What prescription would you write for her?

KEY POINTS – ENCEPHALITIS

◆ Only 1 in 150 individuals infected with West Nile virus has clinical symptoms of CNS disease.

◆ HSV encephalitis may present with personality change, odd behavior, and confusion, along with fever, headache, and vomiting.

◆ Early empiric therapy with intravenous acyclovir is critical for decreasing mortality and diminishing the likelihood and severity of permanent neurologic sequelae.

◆ DNA PCR for HSV on CSF is the preferred diagnostic test for HSV encephalitis.

KEY POINTS – ENDOCARDITIS

◆ Endocarditis in IVDU is usually *S. aureus* infection of the tricuspid valve.

◆ Blood culture is the most important diagnostic procedure in endocarditis.

◆ Echocardigraphy provides useful confirmatory information, but TTE only has a 55%-65% sensitivity.

KEY POINTS – GENITAL INFECTIONS

◆ In any patient with new discharge, perform a genital exam, a microscopic exam in women, chlamydia and gonorrhea tests, and consider RPR and HIV tests.

◆ In asymptomatic high-risk women, perform a pap smear and screen for *Chlamydia* annually.

◆ Urine NAAT is a highly sensitive and specific test for gonorrhea and *Chlamydia.*

◆ Suspect PID in women with pelvic pain, especially if other suggestive features are present.

◆ Genital warts may be easily removed, although the underlying infection persists.

◆ HPV is easily transmitted and is associated with cervical and rectal cancer.

◆ HSV outbreaks can be treated episodically or prevented with daily suppressive therapy, depending on frequency and severity of episodes.

KEY POINTS – HIV INFECTION PRIMARY CARE

◆ Perform skin and oral cavity exam at all visits.

◆ Use HIV viral load to decide when to start antiretrovirals and assess response to treatment.

◆ Use combination therapy, beginning with two NRTI and a PI, or two NRTI and a NNRTI.

◆ Prevent needle-stick injuries—never recap needles, wear gloves, and discard all sharps appropriately.

◆ Typical features of lipodystrophy syndrome are temporal wasting, thin arms and legs, increased central fat deposition, low high-density lipoprotein, high TG, and glucose intolerance.

KEY POINTS – COMPLICATIONS OF HIV INFECTION

◆ Pneumothorax in an AIDS patient should make you think of PCP.

◆ When the $CD4^+$ count is >300, TB presents typically with cough, fever, sputum, and upper lobe infiltrates; when $CD4^+$ count decreases, the presentation is more atypical with hilar adenopathy, lower lobe disease, or miliary TB.

◆ Bacterial pneumonias are common, usually due to *S. pneumoniae* and *H. influenzae;* when the CD4$^+$ count is <100, *P. aeruginosa* becomes a possible pathogen.

◆ Patients with oral candidiasis and dysphagia have a >90% likelihood of candidal esophagitis and should receive empiric fluconazole or ketoconazole.

◆ Consider *C. difficile* as an important cause of diarrhea with HIV infection.

◆ Consider drugs as causes of fever (especially trimethoprim-sulfamethoxazole).

KEY POINTS – MENINGITIS

◆ Obtain CSF to look for meningitis in patients with mental status changes, headache, and fever.

◆ Mental status changes or seizure may be the only symptoms of meningitis in the elderly.

◆ Obtain contrast-enhanced CT before LP if the patient has a seizure, papilledema, focal neurologic exam or in HIV patients with CD4$^+$ <200.

◆ Viral meningitis may increase PMN's in the CSF early in the course of the disease; treat patients with antibiotics until CSF bacterial cultures are negative (24 hours is sufficient).

◆ Treat suspected pneumococcal meningitis with vancomycin plus a third-generation cephalosporin until cultures and sensitivity return.

KEY POINTS – PNEUMONIA

◆ Assess patients with pneumonia for predisposing risk factors, including HIV, alcohol use, and smoking.

◆ Risk factors for poor outcome include low WBC, multiple-lobe involvement, extrapulmonary infection, severe underlying disease (CHF or cancer), and advanced age.

◆ A good sputum Gram stain is more predictive of a true pathogen than sputum culture.

◆ IVDU are at high risk of *S. aureus* pulmonary infection.

(continued)

Infectious Diseases

- Two common causes of pneumonia in healthy young adults are *Mycoplasma* and *Chlamydophila*.
- Pneumococcal strains resistant to penicillin are increasing.

KEY POINTS – TUBERCULOSIS

- Major risk factors for TB include recent exposure to a patient with active TB, injection drug use, HIV infection, homelessness, history of residence in a prison, and emigration from a country where TB is endemic.
- If TB is a possibility in a hospitalized patient, place the patient in an isolation room while you wait for results of three consecutive morning sputum AFB smears.
- Strongly consider TB when a patient has an upper lobe infiltrate on CXR.
- Directly observed therapy has a high success rate and should be used if there are any concerns about adherence to the regimen or problems with follow-up.

KEY POINTS – URINARY TRACT INFECTIONS

- Cystitis does not cause fever.
- In young women with UTI, 3-day trimethoprim-sulfamethoxazole is the preferred treatment.
- Patients with Foley catheters or recent instrumentation of the urinary tract are at high risk for resistant gram-negative rods or enterococcal infection.
- Obtain urine culture for recurrent UTIs and pyelonephritis.

Case Answers

32-1 A.   *Learning objective:* **Delineate a differential diagnosis for new pelvic pain.** Not-to-miss diagnoses include ectopic pregnancy and PID. Other possibilities include vaginitis, cervicitis, appendicitis, cystitis, and endometriosis.>

32-1 B.   *Learning objective:* **Outline work-up for a young woman with pelvic pain.** Perform pelvic bimanual and speculum exams with KOH and saline prep of vaginal fluid. Obtain pregnancy test, urine *Chlamydia* and gonorrhea NAAT, and urinalysis with culture if indicated. Consider CBC, ESR, and pelvic ultrasound or CT if cause not identified and symptoms persist.

32-1 C. *Learning objective:* **Recognize the importance of early empiric therapy for PID.** This woman is young (<25 years old—younger women are more susceptible to PID because of changes in the cervix) and has pelvic pain and cervical motion tenderness on exam. Still obtain urine LCR for gonorrhea and *Chlamydia* and urine culture, but regardless of results, treat with a broad regimen appropriate for PID (third-generation cephalosporin intramuscularly and doxycycline). Repeat exam in 3–5 days to be certain she is improving. Her sexual partner also requires treatment.

32-2 A. *Learning objective:* **Understand when to start antiretroviral therapy and what agents to use.** Current guidelines recommend starting antiretroviral therapy in patients with CD4$^+$ counts <350 or in patients with viral load >55,000. Although this patient has a CD4$^+$ count of 340, his viral load of 75,000 is high warranting treatment with a potent antiretroviral regimen. He has been on zidovudine and didanosine, so he may be resistant to these. It would be appropriate to do resistance testing before starting therapy. Patient adherence is another important thing to evaluate before starting therapy. These regimens are complex and require a high level of patient commitment. Poor compliance can result in only intermittent antiretroviral therapy, which quickly leads to resistance. Noncompliance may be a reason to defer therapy. Combination therapy is the rule with at least three drugs.

32-2 B. *Learning objective:* **Order appropriate routine testing for HIV-infected individuals.** This patient needs a PPD, VDRL, *Toxoplasma* titer, LFT, hepatitis serologies, cholesterol panel, CBC, and platelet count. VDRL is important because of the increased incidence of syphilis (especially in patients with a history of male-male sexual contact or injection drug use). *Toxoplasma* titer assesses risk for developing future infection; patients with positive IgG titers are at greater risk of toxoplasmosis infection. LFT and hepatitis serologies provide a baseline and assist in determining if hepatitis B vaccine is needed. Cholesterol panel provides a baseline for evaluating the effect of PI. CBC provides an important baseline, particularly if zidovudine is restarted (causes anemia and neutropenia). Platelet count is important because of a fairly high incidence of immune-mediated thrombocytopenia in patients with HIV. Vaccines against pneumococcus and hepatitis B (if nonimmune) are warranted. If a patient has hepatitis C, he or she should receive hepatitis A vaccine; otherwise it is optional.

32-3 A. *Learning objective:* **Recognize that the severity of seborrheic dermatitis correlates with immune function and CNS disease.** Seborrheic dermatitis is common in patients with HIV (80% have it at some point). Severity worsens with declining immune function or CNS disease. This holds true even in cases of non–HIV infection, where seborrheic dermatitis is commonly seen in patients with Parkinson's disease.

32-3 B.   *Learning objective:* **Recognize that molluscum suggests declining immunity, and hairy leukoplakia suggests more rapid disease progression.** Molluscum contagiosum is seen usually when $CD4^+$ <100 and is a sign of declining immunity, especially with giant molluscum. Hairy leukoplakia is specific for HIV disease and may be a marker for increased risk of disease progression.

32-3 C.   *Learning objective:* **Discuss the differential diagnosis for headache in an AIDS patient.** This patient presents with headache, encephalopathy, and fever. On physical exam, he has focal findings on the left side. The most likely diagnosis is cerebral toxoplasmosis. This is made even more likely because the patient was not on toxoplasmosis prophylaxis (trimethoprim-sulfamethoxazole is the best prophylactic drug). Other possibilities include CNS lymphoma and progressive multifocal leukoencephalopathy—both cause focal motor findings and can cause encephalopathy but usually not fever.

32-3 D.   *Learning objective:* **Order CNS imaging for AIDS patients with headache and fever.** Because of the focal neurologic exam, CNS imaging is key. Options are contrast CT scan or MRI. MRI is more sensitive (and about 2.5 times as expensive). Progressive multifocal leukoencephalopathy usually does not show up on CT scans, but does on MRI. Serum IgG for *Toxoplasma* is an important part of the work-up. If the MRI scan is negative (which is unlikely), LP would be appropriate.

32-4 A.   *Learning objective:* **Plan appropriate work-up for mental status change in an elderly patient.** This patient needs a glucose level, urinalysis and culture, blood cultures, oxygen saturation, ECG, and CXR. Based on results of these tests, you would next decide if he needs more invasive testing (LP).

32-4 B.   *Learning objective:* **List the most common causes for delirium in the elderly.** This patient has had a sudden change in mental status in the setting of fever and an elevated WBC. Mental status change may be the only symptom of infection in the elderly. The most common causes of acute delirium in the elderly are UTI and pneumonia. Meningitis is a rare cause. Another important cause of delirium is medication side effects. This patient probably has a UTI. If urinalysis and x-ray are normal, LP would be appropriate. Fever makes MI less likely, but always consider this possibility in confused elderly patients.

32-5 A.   *Learning objective:* **Order appropriate tests to evaluate for meningitis.** This patient presents with high fever, seizures, evidence of pneumonia, and alcoholism, important risk factors for pneumococcal disease. Order blood cultures, ABG, and head CT scan. A CT scan should be obtained before LP because the patient is obtunded and can't give a history, and he has seized (increases likelihood of a mass lesion). The risk of herniation is low (6%) even in the setting of increased intracranial pressure, but is a complication worth avoiding. If contrast CT does not show shift, perform LP. Order CSF protein, glucose, WBC count, Gram stain, and culture. A CIE also can be ordered. Give antibiotics before the patient goes to the CT scanner.

32-5 B. *Learning objective:* **Recognize pneumococcal meningitis.** Most pneumococcal meningitis is seeded from a pneumonia, as in this case. *Listeria* and meningococcus are less likely to have concurrent pulmonary infection. This patient could have a brain abscess causing the seizure, seeded from the lung (usually occurs in the setting of a pulmonary shunt or right-to-left cardiac shunt).

32-5 C. *Learning objective:* **Design appropriate empiric therapy for patients with probable pneumococcal meningitis.** This patient should have empiric therapy to cover meningococcus, pneumococcus (because of his pulmonary infiltrate) and *Listeria* (because of his alcohol use). Vancomycin plus ceftriaxone plus ampicillin is appropriate. Vancomycin is given because of increasing penicillin-resistant pneumococcus. Vancomycin controls bacteremia, but does not penetrate the CNS well. Ceftriaxone penetrates the CNS well and is effective against intermediate–penicillin-resistant pneumococcus. Ampicillin is added to cover for *Listeria*. As soon as CSF Gram stain or culture are positive, simplify therapy.

32-6 A. *Learning objective:* **List likely organisms causing pneumonia in an older smoker.** Abrupt onset of cough with rusty sputum and shaking chill suggest community-acquired pneumonia. Pneumococcus is most likely. *Haemophilus, Moraxella,* and, much less likely, *Legionella* also are possible because of her smoking history. Because she does not live in an institution, TB, *Staphylococcus,* and *Pseudomonas* are unlikely. There is no history of alcohol, sedating medications, or neurologic disease to suggest aspiration. Her pulse is unexpectedly low for the degree of fever, a finding called "pulse-temperature dissociation" and sometimes associated with *Legionella,* although this can occur with any pneumonia.

32-6 B. *Learning objective:* **Design appropriate work-up for a patient who likely has pneumonia.** Check vital signs, pulse oximetry, and orthostatic changes in pulse or pressure to determine intravenous fluid requirements and detect early sepsis. Perform lung exam looking for signs of consolidation or effusion (dullness, fremitus, egophony, bronchial breath sounds). Send CBC, electrolytes, creatinine, BUN, blood culture, ABG, sputum Gram stain, and culture. Order a CXR.

32-6 C. *Learning objective:* **Choose appropriate empiric antibiotic coverage based on details of the clinical setting.** A second-generation or third-generation cephalosporin (cefuroxime, cefotetan, ceftriaxone) is adequate to cover potentially beta-lactam–resistant pneumococcus, *Haemophilus,* or *Moraxella.* Although *Legionella* is not as likely, it is potentially life-threatening. Adding high-dose erythromycin to cover *Legionella* is reasonable in light of her smoking (likely lung disease) and pulse-temperature dissociation.

32-6 D.   *Learning objective:* **Recognize the usual course of response to therapy in patients with pneumonia.** Patients may spike fevers 2–4 days into therapy, although in general the peak temperature gradually declines over that time. Leukocytosis may not resolve until 4 days of therapy. Continue current therapy, and monitor for any signs of deterioration. Generally, empiric antibiotics are broad and left unaltered over the first 72 hours of therapy, unless an organism is found, or the patient gets rapidly worse.

32-6 E.   *Learning objective:* **Recognize deviation from the usual course of response to therapy, and design appropriate work-up to detect complications.** Fever should be abating at this point. Look for a resistant organism, an empyema or other complication, drug fever, or a noninfectious cause of fever. Order repeat CXR and blood and sputum cultures. If CXR shows fluid, obtain bilateral decubitus films to see if the fluid is free-flowing (amenable to pleural tap), and perform a pleural tap immediately.

32-7 A.   *Learning objective:* **Recognize altered mental status as a presentation of pneumonia in an elderly patient, and generate a broad differential diagnosis.** Differential diagnosis includes pneumonia, PE, MI, electrolyte disturbance (hyponatremia, hypercalcemia), sepsis (from UTI, ischemic bowel, meningitis, cholecystitis), pancreatitis, and medication.

32-7 B.   *Learning objective:* **Design work-up in an older patient with altered mental status.** Aside from careful history and physical, obtain electrolytes, calcium, amylase, LFT, CXR, oxygen saturation, ABG, ECG, and urinalysis to start with, looking for the entities in answer 3A. Consider LP if fever or elevated WBC is found with no apparent source of infection. Stiff neck or other meningeal signs mandate head CT and LP.

32-7 C.   *Learning objective:* **List most likely organisms causing pneumonia in an elderly patient who resides in a nursing home.** Pneumococcus, *S. aureus, P. aeruginosa,* other gram-negative rods, TB, and anaerobes all are possible causes of infection in this nursing home resident with altered mental status. Alcohol use, poor dentition, and impaired swallowing owing to underlying neurologic disease make aspiration even more likely.

32-7 D.   *Learning objective:* **Describe factors making atypical presentations of pneumonia more likely.** Elderly patients may not have the vigorous immune response necessary to produce sputum,

Infectious Diseases

cough, or fever. Pain localization can be inaccurate, and lower lobe pneumonia can manifest as abdominal pain.

32-8 A. *Learning objective:* **Know the appropriate differential diagnosis for patients with subacute pulmonary symptoms and weight loss.** An appropriate differential diagnosis for this patient would include TB, lung cancer, lung abscess, and HIV-related pulmonary disease. His risk factors for TB include homelessness including spending time in homeless shelters, history of spending time in jail, and to a lesser extent alcoholism. His symptoms are compatible with TB (weight loss, cough, hemoptysis). Lung cancer also is an important diagnostic concern given the combination of hemoptysis, weight loss, and smoking history. His alcoholism puts him at risk for aspiration pneumonia and subsequent development of lung abscess. Typical features of lung abscess include weight loss, cough, and low-grade fevers. This patient should have further questioning about HIV risk factors. HIV disease is more common in individuals who have been in prison. HIV-related pulmonary diseases to consider include PCP and an increased risk for lung cancer.

32-8 B. *Learning objective:* **Know the typical x-ray findings of pulmonary TB.** Upper lobe infiltrates are the hallmark of reactivation TB. Pleural thickening and cavity formation can occur. Elderly patients and patients with advanced HIV disease may have lower lobe infiltrates.

32-8 C. *Learning objective:* **Understand how to treat active TB.** This patient would be best treated with directly observed therapy. Nonadherence to therapy increases the risk of development of drug-resistant TB. It may be most appropriate to admit him to the hospital to start his treatment and set up monitoring. In most cases, patients with TB do not need to be hospitalized to start therapy. His homeless status and alcoholism make hospitalization a good option. An appropriate medication regimen would be four drugs (isoniazid, rifampin, pyrazinamide, and ethambutol) given three times a week with direct observation. Length of therapy would be 6 months, testing at 3 months to ensure the culture is negative. Most patients with TB take daily medications. In patients in whom nonadherence is likely, using thrice-weekly directly observed therapy is preferable because it is easier for the public health system to administer drugs three times a week than daily.

32-9 A. *Learning objective:* **Recognize complicated cystitis and risk factors for other conditions.** This woman is considered to have complicated cystitis based on her age and diabetes. She is likely not taking hormone replacement therapy because of her breast cancer, so she may have atrophic vaginitis causing her symptoms. Although sexually transmitted diseases such as HSV also might present in this way, this is unlikely in this monogamous woman. If she had atypical symptoms or other risk factors, you could consider a gynecologic evaluation. Most important is to ascertain if she has had frequent

UTIs, and if so, whether cultures have been done recently. For this scenario, assume that she has not had recent UTIs.

32-9 B. *Learning objective:* **Outline a treatment regimen for complicated cystitis.** This woman has not been exposed to many antibiotics, so trimethoprim-sulfamethoxazole is a reasonable choice for her. The duration is key—rather than the 3-day course given to uncomplicated cystitis, at least a 7-day course should be given. If her symptoms recur or persist, obtain urine culture and sensitivities, and perform a gynecologic exam if none has been done recently, to evaluate for sexually transmitted diseases and atrophic vaginitis. If the latter is present, you could consult with her oncologist, and consider topical estrogen therapy.

REFERENCES

Endocarditis
Baddour LM, Wilson WR, Bayer AS, et al: Infective endocarditis, diagnosis, antimicrobial therapy, and management of complications. Circulation 2005;111:3167.

Mylonakis E, Calderwood SB: Infective endocarditis in adults. N Engl J Med 2001;345:1318.

Genital Infections
Centers for Disease Control and Prevention: Sexually transmitted diseases treatment guidelines—2002. MMWR Morb Mortal Wkly Rep 2002;51 (no. RR-6).

HIV Infection Primary Care
Yeni PG, Hammer SM, Hirsch MS, et al: Treatment for adult HIV infection: 2004 recommendations of the International AIDS Society—USA Panel. JAMA 2004;292:251.

Meningitis
Sigurdardottir B, Bjornsson OM, Jonsdottir KE, et al: Acute bacterial meningitis in adults: a 20-year overview. Arch Intern Med 1997;157:425.

Tunkel AR, Hartman BJ, Kaplan SL, et al: Practice guidelines for the management of bacterial meningitis. Clin Infect Dis 2004;39(9):1267–1284.

Van de Beek D, De Gans J, Spanjaard L, et al: Clinical features and prognostic factors in adults with bacterial meningitis. N Engl J Med 2004;351(18):1849–1859.

Pneumonia
Mandell LA, Bartlett JG, Dowell SF, et al: Infectious Diseases Society of America: Update of practice guidelines for the management of community-acquired pneumonia in immunocompetent adults. Clin Infect Dis 2003;37:1405.

Marie TJ: Pneumococcal pneumonia: Epidemiology and clinical features. Semin Respir Infect 1999;14:227.

Niederman MS, Mandell LA, Anzueto A, et al: Guidelines for the management of adults with community-acquired pneumonia: Diagnosis, assessment of severity, antimicrobial therapy, and prevention. Am J Respir Crit Care Med 2001;163:1730.

Tuberculosis
Blumberg HM, Burman WJ, Chaisson RE, et al: American Thoracic Society/Centers for Disease Control and Prevention/Infectious Diseases Society of America: Treatment of tuberculosis. Am J Respir Crit Care Med 2003;167:603.

Infectious Diseases

Urinary Tract Infections

Gupta K, Hooton TM, Stamm WE: Increasing antimicrobial resistance and the management of uncomplicated community-acquired urinary tract infections. Ann Intern Med 2001;135:41.

Warren JW, Abrutyn E, Hebel JR, et al: Guidelines for antimicrobial treatment of acute uncomplicated bacterial cystitis and acute pyelonephritis in women. Clin Infect Dis 1999;29:745.

USEFUL WEB SITES

Bioterrorism
CDC web site. http://www.bt.cdc.gov/

Genital Infections
CDC sexually transmitted disease web site. http://www.cdc.gov/std/

HIV Infection Primary Care
2001 USPHS/IDSA guidelines for the prevention of opportunistic infection in persons with human immunodeficiency virus. http://www.aidsinfo.nih.gov

Antiretroviral therapy guidelines: Panel on clinical practices for treatment of HIV infection. Guidelines for the Use of Antiretroviral Agents in HIV-Infected Adults and Adolescents. Washington, DC, U.S Department of Health and Human Services, 2005.
http://www.aidsinfo.nih.gov

Post-exposure prophylaxis information: Updated U.S. Public Health Service guidelines for the management of occupational exposures to HIV and recommendations for post-exposure prophylaxis—September 30, 2005. http://www.aidsinfo.nih.gov

Medical management of HIV infection. http://www.hopkins-aids.edu/

Complications of HIV Infection
Guidelines for the prevention of opportunistic infections among HIV infected persons—2002. Recommendations of the U.S Public Health Service and the Infectious Diseases Society of America. http://aidsinfo.nih.gov/ContentFiles/OIpreventionGL.pdf

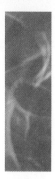

33

Nephrology

DOUGLAS S. PAAUW, LISANNE R. BURKHOLDER,
DAWN E. DEWITT, and MARY B. MIGEON

ACID-BASE DISTURBANCES

ETIOLOGY

What Causes Acid-Base Disturbances?

The body normally maintains arterial blood pH at 7.4. Respiratory or metabolic derangements can alter pH. Hyperventilation removes carbon dioxide (CO_2) and hydrogen ions, creating a respiratory alkalosis. Hypoventilation or airway obstruction raises P_{CO_2} and creates a respiratory acidosis. Metabolic derangements altering pH include ingestion of particular substances, changes in renal bicarbonate processing, and production of endogenous acids such as ketones or lactate (Table 33-1).

What do the Terms Acidemia and Alkalemia Mean?

These terms refer to arterial blood pH. Patients with pH <7.4 are acidemic; patients with pH >7.4 are alkalemic. In contrast, acidosis and alkalosis refer to processes that cause excess accumulation of acid or alkali. Multiple processes can coexist, each affecting pH (Table 33-2).

What are the Causes of Metabolic Acidosis?

Metabolic acidosis is divided into anion gap and non–anion gap acidosis. Anion gap acidosis occurs when an unmeasured anion lowers pH. The mnemonic *MULE PAK* may help you remember the causes of anion gap acidoses: *m*ethanol, *u*remia, *l*actic acidosis, *e*thylene glycol, *p*araldehyde, *a*spirin, *k*etoacidosis. Most common on this list are lactic acidosis (i.e., sepsis) and ketoacidosis, which can be from uncontrolled type 1 DM, starvation, or alcohol ingestion. Non–anion gap acidosis is caused by loss of bicarbonate through the gut or kidney (see Table 33-1).

Table 33-1

Causes of Acid-Base Derangements

Respiratory		Metabolic	
Acidosis (Pco_2 >40)	**Alkalosis** (Pco_2 <40)	**Acidosis** (HCO_3^- <24)	**Alkalosis** (HCO_3^- >24)
Hypoventilation	PE	Anion gap acidosis	Chloride-sensitive
Asthma	Pneumonia	Lactic acid (sepsis)	Vomiting
COPD	Pulmonary edema	Uremia	Volume contraction
	Aspirin	Aspirin	Diuretics
	Hepatic	Ketoacidosis	Chloride-resistant
	insufficiency	Methanol	Cushing's
	Fever	Ethylene glycol	syndrome
	Anxiety	Paraldehyde	Hyperaldosteronism
	Pregnancy		Bartter syndrome
		Non–anion gap	
		acidosis	
		Diarrhea	
		Acetazolamide	
		Topiramate	
		Renal tubular	
		acidosis	

Table 33-2

Interpretation of Key Lab Tests in Patients with Acid-Base Disorders

Value	Normal	Interpretation If High	Interpretation If Low
pH	7.4	Alkalemia	Acidemia
HCO_3^-	24 mEq/L	Metabolic alkalosis	Metabolic acidosis
Pco_2	40 mm Hg	Respiratory acidosis	Respiratory alkalosis

What is Renal Tubular Acidosis?

Renal tubular acidosis occurs when kidneys waste bicarbonate because of malfunctioning tubules. Renal tubular acidosis is proximal (type 2) or distal (types 1 and 4) depending on which tubules are affected. Type 4 is most common and is seen with DM; type 1 is often associated with nephrolithiasis.

What Causes Metabolic Alkalosis?

Metabolic alkalosis is either sodium chloride–responsive or sodium chloride–resistant, depending on whether it corrects with sodium chloride volume infusion. Sodium chloride–responsive alkalosis is common and occurs with vomiting, NG suction, or diuretic-induced volume contraction. In these conditions, urine chloride is low. Sodium chloride–resistant metabolic alkalosis is rare and causes elevated urine

Nephrology

chloride. Examples of this hormonally driven chloride wasting include hyperaldosteronism, Cushing's syndrome, and Bartter syndrome.

What are Primary and Compensatory Acid-Base Processes?

The primary process is the main alteration in pH. The term "acidemia" implies a primary acidosis; "alkalemia" implies a primary alkalosis. Compensatory processes occur when the kidney or respiratory system reacts to correct an altered pH. Respiratory compensation is immediate, whereas renal compensation takes 12–24 hours to kick in.

EVALUATION

Is there a Systematic Way to Approach Acid-Base Problems?

Yes; see Box 33-1. Calculate anion gap routinely in all hospitalized patients. Suspect an acid-base derangement when you see an abnormal respiratory rate, altered bicarbonate (HCO_3^-), elevated anion gap, poor oxygenation, suspected CO_2 retention, or unexplained altered mental status. If any of these are present, draw an ABG for pH and P_{CO_2}. pH, P_{CO_2}, and a chemistry panel (sodium, chloride, and HCO_3^-) allow you to calculate anion gap and identify primary, compensatory, and other concurrent acid-base processes.

My Patient's pH is 7.3, P_{CO_2} is 60 mm Hg, and HCO_3^- is 30 mEq/L. How do I Identify the Primary Process?

Here are a few key principles:

Patients never overcompensate for the primary acid-base derangement.
Respiratory processes alter P_{CO_2} (P_{CO_2} >40 = acidosis, P_{CO_2} <40 = alkalosis).
Metabolic processes alter HCO_3^- (HCO_3^- >24 = alkalosis, HCO_3^- <24 = acidosis).
Change in pH is inversely related to CO_2 and directly related to HCO_3^-.

BOX 33-1

SYSTEMATIC STEPS TO INTERPRETING ACID-BASE PROBLEMS*

- Identify the primary process
- Identify the compensatory process
- Calculate anion gap, correcting for low albumin (even if pH is normal or high)
- If anion gap is elevated, calculate osmolar gap
- If anion gap is elevated, use delta-delta to find simultaneous metabolic derangements
- Use clues in history and physical to determine specific conditions causing alterations

*See text for details.

The pH of 7.3 reveals acidemia, so the primary process is an acidosis. Now you are ready to decide whether the source of the low pH is respiratory (true if P_{CO_2} is high) or metabolic (true if HCO_3^- is low). In this case, the high P_{CO_2} of 60 reveals the primary respiratory acidosis.

So I Found the Primary Process. How Do I Identify a Compensatory Process?

Using the same example, look next at the HCO_3^-. The high HCO_3^- reveals a metabolic alkalosis, which is compensating for the respiratory acidosis. Here's another example: pH = 7.2, P_{CO_2} = 20, and HCO_3^- = 15. The pH reveals acidemia. Low HCO_3^- reveals a primary metabolic acidosis. The low P_{CO_2} reveals compensatory respiratory alkalosis.

How can I Tell if a Patient has Compensated or Uncompensated Respiratory Acidosis?

With sudden-onset respiratory acidosis, pH falls before the kidney has time to compensate. In uncompensated respiratory acidosis, pH decreases 0.08 for each CO_2 increase of 10. In compensated respiratory acidosis, the kidney makes extra HCO_3^-, so the decrease in pH would be less.

How do I Calculate the Anion Gap?

To calculate the anion gap, subtract anions from cations: anion gap = sodium − (chloride + HCO_3^-). The normal anion gap is 8–12. This number represents unmeasured negative charges, mostly on albumin. If albumin is abnormally low, the baseline normal anion gap also is smaller (see later for correction). When unmeasured anions appear (e.g., lactate or ketones), they displace chloride and HCO_3^-, and the anion gap increases. It is significant when anion gap increases by >8 points.

What does a Low Anion Gap Mean, and Why is this Important?

Multiple myeloma, hypoalbuminemia, and lithium provide positively charged, unmeasured cations, which lower the baseline anion gap. This can mask a significant anion gap acidosis. To avoid this, correct the expected anion gap for albumin: If albumin is low, estimate baseline anion gap as three times the albumin level. For example, a calculated anion gap of 14 may look normal; however, when albumin = 2, the baseline anion gap should be expected to be $2 \times 3 = 6$. The change from a baseline expected anion gap of 6 to a measured anion gap of 14 represents a significant anion gap acidosis.

When and How do I Calculate the Osmolal Gap?

When your patient has an anion gap acidosis, calculate the osmolar gap:

Osmolar gap = (measured osmoles) − (calculated osmoles)

where calculated osmoles = 2 (sodium) + $\frac{BUN}{2.8}$ + $\frac{glucose}{18}$.

If the osmolar gap is >10, suspect methanol or ethylene glycol ingestion. Look for oxalate crystals in the urine, seen with ethylene glycol ingestion. Blood levels of these agents can be measured, but wouldn't be available soon enough to be useful.

What is a "Triple Ripple," and How do I Use the "Delta-Delta"?

A triple ripple occurs when multiple acid-base disorders coexist. Use the delta-delta when an anion gap acidosis is present to find a concurrent metabolic alkalosis or non–anion gap acidosis. In an isolated anion gap acidosis, the anion gap should increase from baseline (delta-AG) by the same amount that the HCO_3^- decreases (delta-HCO_3^-). If delta-AG is not the same as delta-HCO_3^-, another metabolic process is present. People put this concept to use in various ways. One way is to add the change in anion gap (= measured gap − normal gap) to the measured HCO_3^- to see if you get a number estimating a normal HCO_3^-. If the result is >24, there is a concurrent metabolic alkalosis. If the result is <24, there is a concurrent non–anion gap acidosis (Table 33-3). Practice this on Case 2 (see later). Be sure to correct the normal anion gap for low albumin levels.

What are Pertinent History and Physical Clues in my Patient with a Low PH?

You must use clues from the history and physical to decide what specific conditions are causing the acid-base disturbances. Alcoholism increases the likelihood of alcoholic ketoacidosis or methanol or ethylene glycol ingestion. Elderly patients are at increased risk for lactic acidosis (e.g., sepsis, bowel necrosis) or inadvertent aspirin overdosage. Patients with a history of suicide attempts are at risk for aspirin, methanol, or ethylene glycol ingestion.

TREATMENT

What should be my Approach to Treatment?

Treat the underlying disorder.

Table 33-3

Finding Concurrent Metabolic Processes Using the Delta-Delta Concept

Change in anion gap should equal change in bicarbonate if there are no other concurrent metabolic processes

When	Then the Patient Has
Change in anion gap* + HCO_3^- = 24	Isolated anion gap acidosis
Change in anion gap + HCO_3^- > 24	Anion gap acidosis plus metabolic alkalosis
Change in anion gap + HCO_3^- < 24	Anion gap acidosis plus non–anion gap acidosis

*Change in anion gap = measured anion gap − normal baseline anion gap.

Case 33-1

A 45-year-old man with a long history of chronic low back pain presents with several days of melena and the following lab results: Na 140, Cl 103, HCO_3^- 15, glucose 108, BUN 20, measured osmoles 295, pH 7.5, Pco_2 20, and Po_2 90. He asks for morphine for his pain.

A. What is his primary acid-base derangement?
B. Is there a compensatory acid-base adjustment, and if so, what is it?
C. Are any other acid-base derangements present?
D. What do you think is going on clinically to cause his acid-base derangements?

Case 33-2

A 21-year-old woman is found unresponsive. Her friends report that she was going to the bathroom all the time and was vomiting profusely earlier in the day. Lab results are as follows: Na 130, Cl 88, HCO_3^- 10, pH 7.1, Pco_2 32, Po_2 88, BUN 28, glucose 720, and osmoles 315.

A. What is her primary acid-base derangement?
B. Is there a compensatory acid-base adjustment, and if so, what is it?
C. Are any other acid-base derangements present?
D. What do you think is going on clinically to cause her acid-base derangements?

ACUTE AND CHRONIC RENAL DISEASE

ETIOLOGY OF ACUTE RENAL FAILURE AND CHRONIC KIDNEY DISEASE

What Causes Acute Renal Failure (ARF)?

ARF is rapid deterioration of renal function resulting in azotemia (elevated BUN and creatinine) and usually oliguria (<400 mL urine output/24 h). Causes are divided into prerenal (40%-80%), intrinsic renal, and postrenal, based on the pathophysiology of injury (Table 33-4).

What Causes Prerenal ARF?

Prerenal azotemia results from inadequate blood supply to glomeruli. This can be due to decreased cardiac output (e.g., CHF), hypovolemia (e.g., bleeding, diarrhea, burns, diuretics), or renovascular problems

Nephrology

Table 33-4

Common Causes of Acute Renal Failure[*]

Location of Injury	Common Causes
Prerenal (40%-80%)	Hypovolemia—bleeding, diarrhea, sepsis, drugs
	Poor perfusion—renal artery stenosis, thrombosis, drugs
	Poor cardiac output—CHF
Postrenal (10%)	Bladder outlet obstruction—BPH, cancer
	Medications—anticholinergics, narcotics
Intrinsic renal (30%-50%)	
Glomeruli	Immune—IgA nephropathy, lupus, Wegener's granulomatosis, Goodpasture's syndrome
	Infectious—HBV, HCV, poststreptococcal infection, HIV, endocarditis
	Toxic—heroin
Interstitial nephritis	Drugs—NSAIDs, penicillins, sulfa drugs
	Infection—pyelonephritis
Acute tubular necrosis	Toxins—radiocontrast, aminoglycosides, myoglobin
	Tubular obstruction—myoglobin, myeloma
	Tubular ischemia—sepsis, hypotension

[*]% of total ARF cases.

(e.g., stenosis, medications). ACEI dilate efferent arterioles; NSAIDs block prostaglandins resulting in afferent arteriolar narrowing.

What is ATN?

Acute tubular necrosis (ATN) is a common cause of ARF that occurs with tubular ischemia from any severe prerenal state, such as septic shock. Nephrotoxins, such as radiocontrast dye and aminoglycosides, are the second major cause. Prehydration, nonionic contrast, and possibly N-acetyl cysteine minimize dye toxicity. Once-daily dosing decreases aminoglycoside toxicity. Other causes of ATN include tubular deposition of myoglobin from rhabdomyolysis (e.g., crush injury, status epilepticus, extreme exertion) or paraproteins from multiple myeloma. Renal function frequently recovers after ATN.

What Causes Glomerulonephritis and Interstitial Nephritis?

Intrinsic renal failure can occur in the glomeruli (glomerulonephritis), the interstitium (interstitial nephritis), or the tubules (ATN). Glomerulonephritis, injury to the glomeruli from any cause, is most commonly immune-mediated (e.g., SLE, poststreptococcal glomerulonephritis, Goodpasture's syndrome, HCV). Interstitial nephritis, inflammation in the interstitial space, can be caused by NSAIDs, antibiotics (e.g., penicillins cephalosporins), and infectious diseases. Patients are often asymptomatic, but may present with fever, rash, and joint pain. Medications or toxins (e.g., contrast agents) should always be considered potential causes of renal injury.

What Toxins Damage the Kidneys?

Toxins can injure the kidney at various sites. NSAIDs cause acute interstitial nephritis and nephrotic syndrome. NSAIDs also decrease renal blood flow by blocking the dilating effect of prostaglandins on the afferent arterioles, a particular problem in patients with low intravascular volumes, such as patients with CHF, cirrhosis, or nephrotic syndrome. Contrast (iodinated dye) nephropathy affects about 40% of patients with pre-existing renal disease or DM. Use of nonionic contrast, prehydration, and N-acetyl cysteine minimize risk. Once-daily dosing decreases aminoglycoside toxicity, which can occur several weeks after use because of binding at the renal cortex.

What is Nephrotic Syndrome?

Nephrotic syndrome is a common final pathway of many intrinsic renal diseases, including DM and HBV. Massive protein loss (>3.5 g/24 h) leads to hypoalbuminemia, edema, hyperlipidemia, and hypercoagulability owing to loss of antithrombin III in the urine.

Why are Patients with DM at Particular Risk for ARF?

Diabetic nephropathy is common in patients with DM (50% of type 1 DM patients; fewer type 2 DM patients) and increases risk for ARF from other causes, especially toxins. High rates of atherosclerosis in patients with DM also increase the likelihood of renal artery stenosis. Diabetic neuropathy may result in atonic bladder, urinary retention, and postrenal azotemia.

What Postrenal Cause of ARF is Most Common?

Postrenal azotemia is caused by obstruction of the urethra or of both ureters. Bladder outlet obstruction is most commonly due to BPH or prostate cancer. Neurogenic bladder dysfunction and obstruction owing to papillary sloughing, stones, or abdominal tumor also can cause ARF. Relief of severe obstruction with a urinary catheter occasionally precipitates postobstructive diuresis (beware of volume and electrolyte depletion).

What are the Most Common Causes of Chronic Kidney Disease, and What Defines this Condition?

Diabetic nephropathy and hypertensive nephropathy are the most common causes of chronic kidney disease, with smoking and age >50 years as important risk factors. Because most patients with chronic kidney disease are asymptomatic, it is important to be alert for patients at risk. Chronic kidney disease is defined as a glomerular filtration rate <60 mL/min/1.73 m^2 for >3 months, or evidence of kidney damage (>30 mg/d of protein, persistent nonurologic hematuria, or abnormal renal biopsy or ultrasound findings). There is debate about the best method of estimating glomerular filtration rate (Cockroft-Gault versus Modification of Diet in Renal Disease). Both methods are imperfect, and 24-hour urine measurement, if complete, is still the most accurate.

EVALUATION

What Signs and Symptoms would Help Me Detect Renal Failure?

Symptoms are nonspecific and are due to accumulation of nitrogenous wastes or volume overload. Patients may have nausea, vomiting, anorexia or cardiopulmonary symptoms, such as chest pain from pericarditis or dyspnea from pulmonary edema. Patients also may report fatigue, confusion, or pruritus. Look for signs of volume overload, such as elevated JVP, cardiac gallop, or pulmonary crackles. Bladder obstruction sometimes can be detected by abdominal mass or suprapubic dullness from a distended bladder. Severe chronic kidney disease may cause pallor from anemia and skin excoriations owing to pruritus.

What are the First Steps in Diagnosing the Cause of ARF?

For acute oliguric renal failure, first rule out obstruction by placing a urinary catheter and obtaining ultrasound to detect hydronephrosis (dilation of ureters or calyces). Next, give normal saline (or diuretics if volume overloaded) to establish urine output. Review medications, and remove nephrotoxins. Collect a fresh urine sample for urine sediment evaluation. Send BUN and creatinine; a ratio >20:1 suggests a prerenal state.

What is an Active Urine Sediment?

"Active urine sediment" refers to the presence of dysmorphic RBC or cellular casts in a fresh, centrifuged urine specimen and indicates intrinsic renal disease. Prerenal sediment usually shows only hyaline or granular casts. ATN is associated with muddy brown casts. Obstruction may lead to infection with WBC. Specific lab tests may be useful when intrinsic renal disease is suspected (Table 33-5), but renal biopsy may be required.

What is a FeNa, and How does it Help Diagnose Prerenal States?

FeNa is the fractional excretion of sodium from serum into the urine. If the FeNa is <1%, the nephron is working hard to retain salt and water, so the patient likely has prerenal azotemia. Conversely, if the FeNa is >2%, the nephron is not able to retain sodium, indicating tubular damage. Diuretics may falsely increase the FeNa. If the FeNa is equivocal, or the patient is on diuretics, a urine sodium <20 mEq/L suggests prerenal disease.

$$FeNa = Cr^S \times Na^U / Cr^U \times Na^S \times 100$$

FeNa <1% = prerenal cause; FeNa >2% = intrinsic renal cause.

What Lab Tests can Help Me Distinguish Chronic from Acute Renal Failure (ARF)?

Patients with chronic renal failure usually have anemia (decreased erythropoietin), low calcium, and small kidneys on ultrasound. With ARF, anemia is less likely, and kidneys are normal size.

Table 33-5

Characteristic Urine Findings and Special Lab Tests for Major Types of Acute Renal Failure

Location of Injury	Urine Dipstick	Urinalysis	Other Lab Tests
Prerenal	Negative*	Hyaline casts	FeNa <1, UNa <20 BUN:Cr ratio >20:1
Postrenal	Negative	Negative	BUN:Cr ratio <20:1 FeNa >2
Intrinsic renal			
Glomerulonephritis	3+ blood 3+ protein	RBC casts Dysmorphic RBC	Consider: antistreptococcal antibody, ANA, ANCA, SPEP, ESR, HIV, uric acid, hepatitis serology, renal biopsy
Interstitial nephritis	1+ blood 1+ protein†	Eosinophils WBC casts	Serum eosinophils
Tubular injury	Negative‡	Muddy brown casts Tubular cells	Urine myoglobin, serum CK

*Persistent prerenal azotemia can cause ATN, so the urinalysis findings are those of ATN.
†Proteinuria <1.5 g/d = interstitial nephritis, >3.5 g/d = nephrotic syndrome.
‡If ATN is due to rhabdomyolysis, the urine dipstick is positive for blood because of cross-reacting myoglobin, but microscopic urinalysis is negative for RBC.
ANCA, antineutrophilic cytoplasmic antibody; Cr, creatinine; FeNa, fractional excretion of sodium; UNa, urinary sodium.

TREATMENT

How is ARF Managed?

Most patients require hospitalization for diagnosis and volume management. Decide whether volume depletion or overload exists. Use daily weights, "ins and outs" including free water losses (approximately 10 mL/kg for adults), and exam to guide volume repletion or diuresis. Watch for infection because risk is increased in patients with ARF. Nutrition is a priority because anorexia is common. Adjust medication doses based on estimated creatinine clearance. With ARF, the creatinine clearance changes rapidly.

$$\text{Creatinine clearance} = (140 - \text{age}) \times \frac{\text{bodyweight(kg)}^*}{72^\dagger} \times \text{serum creatinine.}$$

---

* Multiply by 0.85 for women to correct for lean body mass.
† Substitute 48.816 for 72 if you are using creatinine units of μmol/L.

Nephrology

What Lab Tests should I Follow?

In oliguric ARF, expect daily increases in creatinine of 0.5–1 mg/dL (44–88 μmol/L) and in BUN of 10–20 mg/dL. Acidemia and hyperkalemia are common, so follow electrolytes at least daily. Obtain CBC, uric acid, calcium, magnesium, and phosphate at admission. If renal failure persists, consider rechecking these levels periodically. Check ABG as needed to monitor pH and acidosis.

What should I Know About Managing Patients with Chronic Kidney Disease?

Hypertension and proteinuria are independent risk factors for cardiovascular disease, and aggressive management delays progression of chronic kidney disease. ACEI, angiotensin receptor blockers aldosterone antagonists (spironolactone, eplerenone), and some calcium channel blockers decrease proteinuria beyond that expected from BP control alone (goal <120/80 mm Hg). ACEI and angiotensin receptor blockers are beneficial even when the creatinine is significantly elevated, but hyperkalemia can be a problem. Although protein-restricted diets slow chronic kidney disease progression, benefits are generally outweighed by malnutrition. When glomerular filtration rate is <50, medications should be adjusted, and monitoring for anemia and calcium and phosphate (secondary hyperparathyroidism) should begin. At that point, calcium supplements with meals (phosphate binders), vitamin D supplementation, and erythropoietin may be beneficial. Sleep apnea, RLS, leg cramps, DVT, and anorexia are common complications. Patients should receive pneumococcal and influenza vaccines.

When is Dialysis Required?

When symptomatic renal failure is present, dialysis may be needed, especially in oliguric patients. The indications for referral and emergent dialysis are listed in Box 33-2. Patients can choose hemodialysis or long-term ambulatory peritoneal dialysis, but hemodialysis is used in urgent situations.

Case 33-3

A 59-year-old woman presents with 6 weeks of increasing fatigue, weight loss, and edema. She has a history of mixed connective tissue disease and was hospitalized 4 weeks ago for streptococcal pneumonia. BP is 190/110 mm Hg, and pulse is 104 beats/min. Weight is 104 lb, and BMI is 18. On exam, she has pale conjunctivae; clear lungs; S_1, S_2, and S_4; and 3+ pitting edema to the knees. Stool is Hemoccult negative. Other values are as follows: HCT 28%, K^+ 5.1 mEq/L, albumin 2.5 mg/dL (25 μmol/L), HCO_3^- 19 mg/dL, BUN 46 mg/dL, and Cr 1.9 mg/dL (167 μmol/L). UA shows dysmorphic RBC and oval fat bodies.

A. Identify two major types of renal disease in this patient.

BOX 33-2

INDICATIONS FOR REFERRAL AND DIALYSIS

Indications for Referral to a Nephrologist

Estimated or measured GFR <30 mL/min/1.72 m^2
Rapidly declining renal function (15% decrease in 3 mo)
Proteinuria >1 g/24 h
Glomerular bleeding and elevated creatinine
Uncontrolled hypertension despite treatment
Significant hypocalcemia, hyperphosphatemia, hyperkalemia, or anemia

Indications for Hemodialysis or Peritoneal Dialysis (Nonurgent)

Severe volume overload with CHF
Life-threatening acidosis
Severe electrolyte abnormalities, especially hyperkalemia
Pericarditis
Toxins that can be removed by dialysis

GFR, glomerular filtration rate.

B. What is the differential diagnosis for the cause of her problem, and what further evaluation would you order?
C. Calculate the estimated creatinine clearance for this patient.
D. What management would you recommend for her edema?

Case 33-4

A 66-year-old man who has had type 2 DM for 10 years treated with insulin, metformin, and an ACEI recently started amitriptyline for diabetic neuropathy pain. He reports increasing difficulty starting his urine stream, grogginess, fatigue, and mild nausea over the past week. On exam, he is afebrile, tachycardic, and hypertensive. His abdomen is distended and tender in the suprapubic region, and his prostate is enlarged. Neurologic exam shows decreased sensation to the 10-g monofilament bilaterally in his feet; slightly decreased ankle reflexes; and otherwise normal strength, sensation, and reflexes. BUN is 59 mg/dL, creatinine is 3.8 mg/dL (334 μmol/L) from his baseline of 1.3 mg/dL (114 μmol/L), and CBC is normal. His PSA is 6.3.

A. What are possible diagnoses?
B. What is your first diagnostic step?
C. What further acute and long-term management do you recommend?

Case 33-5

A 42-year-old triathlon competitor returns to a major competition after 1 year off for a hamstring injury. The next day, he presents to the emergency department with diffuse muscle aches, some mild weakness, and dark urine. He reports that he competed well despite being "undertrained" and grueling weather (temperature of 100° F) during the triathlon. He is not hungry or thirsty and feels quite nauseated. He has not urinated since last night. His only medication is ibuprofen; he took 4 tablets (200 mg each) yesterday for his hamstring injury before the race. BP is 130/88 mm Hg lying and 96/82 mm Hg standing; pulse is 76 beats/min increasing to 108 beats/min. Exam shows a well-muscled, healthy-appearing man with tender muscles in the thighs and calves. Neuromuscular exam is otherwise normal. Urine is very dark with a high specific gravity. BUN is 85 mg/dL, and creatinine is 2.9 mg/dL (260 μmol/L).

A. What are the most likely diagnoses?
B. What work-up should he have?
C. What would you expect to find on his sediment exam?
D. How would you manage him?

ELECTROLYTE DISTURBANCES— CALCIUM

ETIOLOGY

What Causes Hypercalcemia and Hypocalcemia?

The causes of hypercalcemia and hypocalcemia are listed in Boxes 33-3 and 33-4. Hyperparathyroidism and malignancy account for 90% of all cases of hypercalcemia; if due to malignancy, the cancer is usually already diagnosed. Apparent hypocalcemia may result from hypoalbuminemia because most serum calcium is bound to albumin. Total calcium decreases by 0.8 mg/dL for every 1 mg/dL decrease in albumin. Lab tests provide corrected or ionized calcium levels that correct for altered albumin levels.

EVALUATION

When should I Suspect Hypercalcemia or Hypocalcemia?

Hypercalcemia causes nonspecific symptoms or may be discovered incidentally. Check calcium in any older patient with confusion, recalcitrant constipation, or polyuria. Other nonspecific signs include lethargy, nausea, vomiting, anorexia, and abdominal pain (from renal stones or pancreatitis). Severe hypercalcemia causes dehydration by diuresis or vomiting or both. Severe or rapidly acquired hypocalcemia causes painful tetany (muscle spasms). Classic findings are Trousseau's sign (carpel spasm with a BP cuff inflated just above systolic pressure) and

---

BOX 33-3

CAUSES OF HYPERCALCEMIA (FROM MOST TO LEAST COMMON)

Primary hyperparathyroidism
Drug induced
    Thiazide diuretics
    Vitamin D excess
Malignancy
    Osteolytic metastasis (breast cancer)
    PTH-like hormone production (lung cancer)
    Direct bone invasion (lymphoma)
Granulomatous disease (TB, sarcoid)
Immobilization

BOX 33-4

CAUSES OF HYPOCALCEMIA

Hypoalbuminemia (apparent hypocalcemia)
Renal failure
Hypoparathyroidism
Low magnesium
Pancreatitis
Multiple blood transfusions (citrate binds calcium)

Chvostek's sign (facial twitching elicited by tapping the facial nerve just anterior to the ear). Lethargy, confusion, and seizures also may occur.

What Evaluation is Warranted in Patients with Calcium Abnormalities?

With hypercalcemia, obtain history and physical for signs of malignancy; evaluate focal findings further. Check CBC, renal function, and intact PTH. Look carefully at the medication list because thiazide diuretics are a common cause of hypercalcemia. For hypocalcemia, ask about neck surgery (inadvertent parathyroid removal) and other autoimmune disorders, which may be associated with hypoparathyroidism. Obtain albumin, magnesium, phosphorus, PTH, vitamin D, and creatinine. PTH is low with primary hypoparathyroidism and hypomagnesemia, but elevated with other causes of hypocalcemia.

What ECG Findings Suggest Calcium Abnormalities?

The QT interval is shortened with hypercalcemia and prolonged with hypocalcemia. Hypocalcemia also worsens ECG findings of digoxin toxicity.

TREATMENT

How do I Treat Hypercalcemia?

For severe hypercalcemia (>13 mg/dL [>3.25 mmol/L]) or symptoms, start with normal saline hydration to replace the volume lost. After volume repletion, add furosemide, then a bisphosphonate or calcitonin if needed. For long-term control, treat the underlying cause.

How do I Replace Calcium in Patients with Hypocalcemia?

Give intravenous calcium gluconate to acutely symptomatic patients. Replace low magnesium. Find and treat underlying causes. Give oral vitamin D and calcium carbonate for hypoparathyroidism.

ELECTROLYTE DISTURBANCES— POTASSIUM

ETIOLOGY

What Causes Elevated Potassium?

Pseudohyperkalemia commonly occurs when RBCs lyse during sample collection, releasing intracellular potassium. Redraw blood with a larger gauge needle, and ensure that the tourniquet is not on too long. Hyperkalemia occurs through one of three ways: too much in, too little excreted, or shift. Patients can rarely take too much potassium in, usually as a result of excessive intravenous replacement. The causes of impaired excretion include some types of renal tubular acidosis, adrenal insufficiency, potassium-sparing diuretics (e.g., spironolactone), ACEI, angiotensin receptor blockers, and trimethoprim-sulfamethoxazole. Trimethoprim-sulfamethoxazole is most likely to cause hyperkalemia when used in elderly patients or at very high doses, such as those used to treat *Pneumocystis carinii*. Causes of hyperkalemia secondary to shift include rhabdomyolysis (muscle cell injury releases intracellular potassium) and extracellular shift of potassium with acidosis.

What Causes Hypokalemia?

Most hypokalemia is due to diuretics; vomiting and diarrhea also are common causes. Magnesium depletion can cause hypokalemia, especially in patients with excessive alcohol use. Medications causing potassium depletion include diuretics, cisplatin, theophylline, aminoglycosides, and amphotericin.

EVALUATION

What Evaluation is Warranted in Patients with Hypokalemia?

Patients on diuretics may not need further tests. Check magnesium when patients use alcohol heavily, or when hypokalemia resists aggressive replacement. With hypertension and hypokalemia, consider adrenal hormone excess.

What Clues on ECG Suggest a Potassium Abnormality?

Hyperkalemia causes peaked T waves, progressing to widened QRS complexes and sine waves as potassium continues to increase. Hypokalemia causes T wave flattening and U waves.

TREATMENT

How should I Treat a Patient with Hyperkalemia?

ECG changes mandate emergent treatment. First, give intravenous calcium gluconate to stabilize cardiac membranes. Next, give intravenous glucose, insulin, and HCO_3^- to drive potassium into the cells. If the patient can make urine, give intravenous furosemide. Kayexalate, a sodium/potassium exchange resin, is given orally or as an enema, but acts slowly. In extremely urgent situations, use dialysis.

How do I Replace Potassium?

Replace orally with potassium chloride or potassium phosphate. If intravenous replacement is required, remember that it commonly causes a burning discomfort, and give no faster than 10 mEq/h.

ELECTROLYTE DISTURBANCES— SODIUM

ETIOLOGY

What Causes Hypernatremia?

Hypernatremia is commonly caused by lack of water. Patients unable to get to water become hypernatremic (e.g., from acute cerebrovascular accident or coma). Occasionally, fluid requirements are too great to maintain adequate intake (e.g., diabetes insipidus).

What Causes Hyponatremia?

Causes are categorized by volume status as hypovolemic, euvolemic, or hypervolemic. In hypovolemic hyponatremia, water and sodium are depleted, and sodium losses exceed volume losses. With hypervolemic hyponatremia, patients have total body excess sodium with even greater excess water in edematous states such as CHF, cirrhosis, or severe hypoalbuminemia from nephrotic syndrome. Euvolemic hyponatremia is most often from SIADH (Table 33-6). Patients with hyponatremia secondary to SIADH usually have low BUN and uric acid levels. Thiazide diuretics are a common cause of euvolemic hyponatremia, with the exact pathogenesis unclear. Pseudohyponatremia occurs with severe hyperlipidemia, hypergammaglobulinemia, or hyperglycemia. For each

Table 33-6

Causes of SIADH

Cause of SIADH	Examples
Severe pulmonary disease	Lung abscess, severe pneumonia, mechanical ventilation with PEEP
Tumor	Small cell lung carcinoma
CNS disorders	Meningitis, encephalitis, tumor
Drugs	Morphine, SSRI, thiazide diuretics, carbamazepine
Endocrine disorders	Hypothyroidism, primary adrenal failure

increase of glucose by 100 mg/dL (6 mmol/L) over a normal glucose level of 100 mg/dL, the serum sodium decreases by 1.6 mEq/L.

EVALUATION

When should I Suspect Sodium Disturbances?

Patients with hypernatremia are often volume depleted and may have altered consciousness preventing them from drinking. Symptoms of hyponatremia include confusion, disorientation, and anorexia. Seizures or coma may occur with severe or rapidly developing hyponatremia. For patients with any sodium derangement, first establish volume status.

What Evaluation is Helpful in Patients with Hyponatremia?

Ask about medications and a recent history of GI losses, pulmonary or CNS disease, or malignancy. Examine vital signs, neck veins, mucous membranes, and skin turgor to help determine volume status (none of these signs are particularly sensitive or specific for hypovolemia). Measure urine sodium. A urine sodium <20 mEq/L suggests poor renal perfusion but a normal kidney, as with CHF or hypovolemia. A urine sodium >40 mEq/L suggests SIADH, renal failure, or other inappropriate wasting of sodium. A concurrent alkalosis may suggest volume contraction from diuretics or emesis. A metabolic acidosis may suggest renal or adrenal failure as the source of hyponatremia. Normal pH would be expected with SIADH and edematous states.

TREATMENT

How do I Treat Hypernatremia?

First, replace volume deficit with normal saline. Next, replace free water deficit with 5% dextrose in water over 36 hours, reducing sodium by 0.5–1 mEq/h. Calculate the free water deficit:

$$\text{Free water deficit} = (\text{serum sodium}/140 - 1) \times 0.6 \times \text{weight in kg}$$

For central diabetes insipidus, replace antidiuretic hormone.

How do I Treat Hyponatremia?

Use water restriction for mild euvolemic hyponatremia. For seizures or coma, correct more rapidly with normal (0.9%) or hypertonic saline (3%) and furosemide. Treat hypovolemic hyponatremia with intravenous normal saline. Treat hypervolemic hyponatremia with salt and water restriction along with diuretics as needed. Increase the serum sodium slowly. Different recommendations exist for exactly how slowly to normalize the low sodium, ranging from 8–12 mEq/24 h maximum to avoid central pontine myelinolysis. No cases of central pontine myelinolysis have been seen with rates of ≤8 mEq/24 h, so this is probably the safest choice of correction rate. If patients have ongoing seizures, some authors recommend more rapid initial correction of the sodium by 1–2 mmol/h for the first few hours and then return to a slower rate. In the acute setting of sodium correction, sodium levels require monitoring every 1–3 hours to avoid too rapid a correction.

How do I Estimate the Change in Serum Sodium that would Occur with Intravenous Fluids I give to Patients with Hyponatremia?

You'll need to know the sodium content of your fluid: 154 mEq is in 1 L of normal saline, and 513 mEq is in 1 L of 3% saline. Use the following formula to calculate the effect of each liter of fluid used:

$$\text{Change in serum sodium} = \text{infusate Na} - \text{serum Na}/ \\ \text{total body water} + 1$$

Total body water, in kilograms, is estimated at 60% of total weight for men, 50% for women and elderly men, and 45% for elderly women. When you calculate the change in serum sodium with each liter, you can see how fast to give the fluid to achieve the rate of change you desire. For example, a man weighing 60 kg has a serum sodium of 110. Each 1 L of 3% normal saline would increase the sodium: $(513 - 113)/([0.6 \times 60] + 1)$, or 10.81 mEq. If you wish to increase the serum sodium by only 8 mEq over 24 hours, you would need to use only about 800 mL out of 1-L bag of 3% saline.

FLUID MANAGEMENT

ETIOLOGY

In Which Situations do Patients need Fluid Administration?

Hospitalized patients unable to drink because of illness or procedures need maintenance fluid, electrolytes, and glucose replacement. Volume-depleted patients need volume resuscitation.

Nephrology

EVALUATION

How do I Evaluate Volume Status?

Look for volume depletion by weight loss, postural hypotension, poor skin turgor, dry mucous membranes, oliguria, and tachycardia. An increased BUN-to-creatinine ratio >20 is also a clue. Look for fluid overload (often a preventable iatrogenic occurrence) by weight gain, jugular venous distention, edema, and rales. Evaluate volume status daily in hospitalized patients.

TREATMENT

How do I Design Maintenance Fluid and Electrolyte Therapy?

Patients unable to eat need approximately 2 L of fluid per day, as ¼ or ½ normal saline with glucose for calories. Standard basal requirements for electrolytes are about 1 mEq/kg/d of Na, K, and Cl with adjustments as needed for excess losses.

How do I Choose Appropriate Resuscitation Fluid for a Patient with Volume Depletion?

Fluid therapy is an exercise in balancing input and output of electrolytes and water. Know the electrolyte content of various solutions (Table 33-7). For volume resuscitation in patients with volume depletion or low BP, choose a fluid with high saline content that would stay in the intravascular space (normal saline or lactated Ringer's solution). Lactated Ringer's solution has potassium, so don't give large volumes to anuric patients. Giving fluid in boluses is preferable to running fluids at a high rate (and forgetting about the continuous infusion); this lowers the risk of iatrogenic volume overload. Frequent exams of fluid

Table 33-7

Electrolyte Concentrations in Various Intravenous Solutions (in mEq/L)

Fluid	Sodium	Potassium	Chloride	Bicarbonate	Lactate
Half-normal saline (0.45%)	77		77		
Normal saline (0.9%)	154		154		
Hypertonic saline (3.0%)	513		513		
Ringer's lactate*	130	4	110		28
Sodium bicarbonate (per amp)	44.5			44.5	
5% dextrose in water[†]					

*Also contains 3 mEq calcium/L.
[†]Has 50 g of dextrose/L water and no other electrolytes.

status are mandatory in patients receiving volume resuscitation to evaluate their response and plan further fluid therapy.

Case 33-6

A 50-year-old man with a history of poorly controlled hypertension and renal failure requiring dialysis three times a week comes to the emergency department because he feels weak and short of breath. He has missed his last three dialysis appointments. Exam shows HR 90, BP 180/100, respiratory rate 22, temperature 98.4° F, oxygen saturation 93%, JVP elevated to 10 cm, bibasilar rales, S_3, and 1+ leg edema. Lab test results are as follows: Na 130, K 8, HCO_3^- 18, Cl 100, BUN 60, and creatinine 8.5. Chest film shows prominent vessels in the upper lung fields.

    A. What is this patient's most life-threatening problem and why?
    B. What would an ECG show?
    C. Name the interventions you could use to manage his hyperkalemia, and state how each works.

Case 33-7

A 60-year-old man is brought to the emergency department with increasing confusion. His history includes multiple myeloma, cigarette use, and hypertension. He takes hydrochlorothiazide, ramipril, and aspirin. On exam, he is not oriented to place or time and is unable to identify that anything is wrong. He appears euvolemic and pale. Temperature is 99° F (37.2° C), respiratory rate is 24, BP is 175/90, and HR is 80. He has decreased breath sounds in the right lower lung field, normal heart sounds, and normal abdominal and neurologic exams.

    A. What two electrolyte disturbances can cause confusion, and why might this patient be at risk for these two particular disturbances?
    B. What else should you consider might be causing this man's confusion?
    C. What diagnostic tests do you wish to order?
    D. After you read the answer to C, how do you want to manage this patient's problem?

HYPERTENSION

ETIOLOGY

How Prevalent is Hypertension?

Hypertension is present in 23% of whites and in 32% of non-Hispanic African Americans. Among patients >65 years old, >50% have systolic or diastolic hypertension or both.

What are the Consequences of Hypertension?

Hypertension is a major risk factor for stroke, intracerebral hemorrhage, CAD, LVH, chronic renal insufficiency, and end-stage renal disease. Other sequelae include erectile dysfunction, decreased visual acuity, and dementia as a consequence of multiple infarcts. Acute markedly elevated BP is life-threatening.

What Proportion of Patients is Adequately Treated for Hypertension?

In the NHANES III study of 16,000 patients, 75% of white patients either were unaware of their hypertension or were inadequately treated. The percentages were higher in African Americans and Mexican Americans. In the latter group, only 15% had controlled hypertension, and half were unaware that they had hypertension.

What BP Reading is Considered Hypertension?

The Joint National Consensus Panel on Hypertension VII (JNC VII) categorizes levels of BP elevation. As BP levels increase, so does the risk of adverse outcomes (Table 33-8).

What are the Risk Factors for Primary Hypertension?

The cause of primary or "essential" hypertension is unknown, although it is correlated with several risk factors, including obesity, family history of hypertension, excessive alcohol use, and African American ethnic descent. Increased salt intake may contribute to, but is not causative of, hypertension.

What are Secondary Causes of Hypertension?

Secondary hypertension accounts for about 5% of hypertension, which, by definition, is caused by an identifiable, treatable structural or endocrine abnormality. Younger patients with hypertension or patients poorly responsive to three or more antihypertensive medications should be considered for screening for secondary causes. The core secondary causes are renal artery stenosis, acute and chronic

Table 33-8

Joint National Committee VII Categorization of Blood Pressure

	Systolic (mm Hg)		Diastolic (mm Hg)
Normal	<120		<80
Prehypertension	120–139	or	80–89
Hypertension			
Stage 1	140–159	or	90–99
Stage 2	>160	or	>100

Table 33-9

Risk Factors and Target Organ Damage in Hypertension

The greater the number of risk factors or the presence of target organ damage increases risk of adverse outcome from hypertension and warrants more aggressive intervention

Risk Factors	Target Organ Damage (TOD)
Smoking	Retinopathy
Hyperlipidemia	Peripheral artery disease
Diabetes	Nephropathy
Age >60	Heart disease (LVH, CAD, CHF)
Men and postmenopausal women	
Family history	

renal insufficiency, pheochromocytoma, sleep apnea, coarctation of the aorta, Cushing's syndrome, and primary hyperaldosteronism. Some medications, such as the antidepressant venlafaxine, can cause hypertension.

What Factors are Important in Risk-Stratifying Patients with Hypertension?

JNC VII recommends risk-stratifying patients to determine how aggressively to begin antihypertensive therapy. Table 33-9 lists the two measures for risk stratification—target organ damage (TOD) and risk factors. Patients with no risk factors are at low immediate risk for adverse cardiovascular events. Patients with one or more risk factors are at intermediate risk of adverse outcome, and patients with proven end-organ disease or DM are at highest risk. This risk stratification determines how rapidly to intervene with medications (Table 33-10).

Table 33-10

Joint National Committee VII Recommendations for When to Initiate Antihypertensive Medication

Blood Pressure Stage	Risk A (None)	Risk B (≥1 risk)	Risk C (DM or TOD)
Prehypertension (120–139 mm Hg or 80–89 mm Hg)	Lifestyle	Lifestyle	Drug
Hypertension stage 1 (140–159 mm Hg or 90–99 mm Hg)	Lifestyle	Lifestyle	Drug
Hypertension stage 2 (>160 mm Hg or >100 mm Hg)	Drug	Drug	Drug

TOD, target organ damage.
DM, diabetes mellitus

Is *Systolic* Hypertension as Important a Risk Factor as Diastolic Hypertension?

Yes. Several large studies have clearly established that, similar to diastolic hypertension, systolic hypertension is a strong risk factor for cardiovascular disease. Clinical trials have shown that treatment of systolic hypertension prevents cardiovascular events.

What is "White Coat" Hypertension?

For roughly 25% of patients with mildly elevated BP in clinic, their outside readings are normal. Long-term studies in these patients have shown mild increases in left ventricular mass, but other than mild physiologic changes, the long-term clinical consequences of white coat hypertension are unknown.

EVALUATION

How do I Measure BP?

The patient should be sitting down for 5 minutes in a calm environment. The patient should not have had caffeine within the past hour or cigarettes within the past half an hour. For accurate measurement, the patient's arm should be at the level of the heart. The height of the cuff should be as wide as the patient's arm. The shirt should be removed so that there is no restrictive clothing, and the patient should not be talking.

How is Hypertension Diagnosed?

A single reading does not constitute hypertension. BP varies from visit to visit, and studies have shown that readings decrease by 10–15 mm Hg between the first and third visits for newly diagnosed patients not yet on medications. The JNC VII recommends measuring BP twice on two separate occasions. In the absence of target organ damage, the patient should not be labeled as hypertensive unless the averaged BP is persistently elevated on at least two visits.

What is the Role of Ambulatory Monitoring?

This device measures a patient's BP repeatedly over a 24-hour period. The automatic cuff inflates every 15 minutes while the patient is awake and every 30–60 minutes while the patient sleeps, obtaining real-world measures of BP. This tool is particularly useful when office and outside BP readings do not match (e.g., white coat hypertension), when patient education with closer monitoring may help adherence, and when patient symptoms suggest the BP is overtreated or there is autonomic dysfunction present (e.g., lightheadedness, presyncope).

What History should I Obtain in Patients with Hypertension?

Ask about symptoms or sequelae of hypertension, including headache, visual changes, and chest pain. Review factors that can exacerbate hypertension, such as alcohol, stimulant (especially cocaine), and salt intake;

hormone or NSAID use; and level of exercise. Screen for causes of secondary hypertension, including daytime somnolence, morning headache, or snoring at night (sleep apnea); young age at diagnosis or claudication (coarctation of the aorta); flushing, anxiety, or episodic hypertension (pheochromocytoma); DM, proximal leg weakness, or depression (Cushing's syndrome); cold and heat intolerance, hair or skin changes, or diarrhea or constipation (thyroid disease); and young age at diagnosis of hypertension, presence of peripheral vascular disease, or rapid onset of severe hypertension in an elderly patient (renal artery stenosis).

What Exams are Important in Patients with Hypertension?

BP: Check the measurement in both arms. If elevated, particularly in a young person, check lower extremity BP, and if pressures are unequal, suspect coarctation of the aorta.

Weight/height: Obesity is a major risk factor for hypertension and for sleep apnea, which can worsen hypertension.

Pulse: Tachycardia may suggest hyperthyroidism, hypoxemia, or CHF.

Skin: Abdominal striae, hirsutism, and purpuric bruises are suggestive of Cushing's syndrome.

HEENT: Perform a funduscopic exam for hypertensive changes of arteriovenous nicking, arterial narrowing, hemorrhages, exudates, or papilledema.

Neck: Check for carotid bruit of atherosclerosis or goiter of hyperthyroidism.

Lungs: Listen for rales of CHF from prolonged hypertension.

Heart: Findings of S_3, S_4, and a heave indicates LVH.

Abdominal: Listen for a bruit indicating renal artery stenosis or mass indicating polycystic kidney disease.

Extremities: Edema from CHF or medication side effect or proximal muscle weakness from Cushing's syndrome may be present.

What Tests are Useful in the Initial Evaluation of Patients with New Hypertension?

The initial evaluation includes ECG, UA, glucose, electrolytes, BUN and creatinine, and lipid panel. ECG screens for signs of prior infarct and for LVH, which is associated with increased mortality, and serves as comparison for future ischemia. UA showing casts, RBC, or protein suggests kidney disease as the cause or result of hypertension. Glucose screens for DM. Decreased potassium suggests hyperaldosteronism or Cushing's syndrome and may worsen BP control. Elevated creatinine suggests renal disease. Lipid panel provides additional information about cardiovascular risk.

TREATMENT

What Benefit would my Patient Receive from BP Treatment?

A meta-analysis of clinical trials with 37,000 patients showed a 42% reduction in stroke and a 14% reduction in CAD. In African American women, the number-needed-to-treat to prevent one cardiovascular event is 21. The findings also are striking in DM, in which tight control of BP (<144/82 mm Hg) versus less tight control (154/87 mm Hg) resulted in a 44% reduction in stroke and a 47% reduction in visual acuity decline in the former group. In renal insufficiency, inadequate BP control relates directly to progression of disease and proteinuria.

What Degree of BP Improvement Occurs with Each Type of Intervention?

The degree of BP improvement is roughly the same for lifestyle modifications and starting medication doses: 5–10 mm Hg.

What Lifestyle Modifications can Make a Difference?

Obesity is a major risk factor for hypertension, and weight loss results in a decrease of 0.3–1 mm Hg for every 1 kg lost. For a patient who loses 10 lb (approximately 5 kg), the BP may decrease by 5 mm Hg. Salt restriction to 2–2.5 g/d may reduce BP an average of 2–5 mm Hg. Aerobic exercise lasting 30–45 minutes most days of the week also has been shown to reduce BP. Alcohol intake of more than two drinks a day increases BP. This seems to be dose dependent; more than five drinks a day has the most impact on BP.

Is it Worth Treating Hypertension in Elderly Patients?

Because elderly patients have a higher baseline risk of cardiovascular events, the benefit of even short-term treatment is higher than in younger patients. In patients >80 years old, the number-needed-to-treat is 21 to prevent a cardiovascular event and 30 to prevent a stroke. While treating hypertension aggressively in these patients, keep a close eye on side effects of multiple medications. It is recommended to keep the diastolic BP >65 mm Hg.

How Soon should I Start Medications in Patients?

Start medication immediately at the time of diagnosis for patients with high normal BP and target organ damage (i.e., retinopathy on funduscopic exam) or DM (see Table 33-10). Also start medications without waiting for a lifestyle modification trial in any patient with a confirmed systolic pressure >160 mm Hg or diastolic pressure >100 mm Hg or both. In all patients, diet and exercise are an important part of therapy.

What is the Goal BP?

For low-risk patients, a target BP <140/90 mm Hg is adequate. For higher risk patients, the target level is lower. In high-risk patients with DM, chronic renal disease, and CAD, the goal is <130/80 mm Hg.

Which Antihypertensive would be Most Effective?

When starting a BP medication, take into consideration the established efficacy, cost, quality of life, and any comorbid conditions. Thiazide diuretics and beta blockers have the longest history of improving morbidity and mortality in hypertension, are inexpensive, and are well tolerated at low doses. These factors make these the starting medications of choice for many patients with hypertension. ACEI are increasingly used for first-line therapy as a result of more recent clinical trials showing reduction in cardiovascular end points and renoprotective effects in DM and chronic renal disease. Antihypertensive action is equivalent to beta blockers and diuretics. NSAIDs can blunt the efficacy of diuretics and ACEI.

What if the Initial Medication Dose is Inadequate to Control the BP?

Antihypertensives are approximately equivalent in their initial efficacy—about 40%-60% of patients respond to the first medication. There are two approaches for what to do next. Either start one medication and increase the dose to maximum, or keep the dose relatively low and combine with other agents for an additive effect and minimization of side effects. For patients in whom the BP needs to decrease either >20 mm Hg systolic or >10 mm Hg diastolic, consider starting two medications. Diuretics enhance the effects of all other classes of antihypertensives.

What Comorbidities Affect Antihypertensive Choice?

For many conditions, data support using specific medications in addition to, or instead of, a diuretic or beta blocker. These include ACEI in CHF, ACEI in DM and renal disease to slow progression of kidney damage, and calcium channel blockers in angina inadequately controlled by beta blockers.

Are Calcium Channel Blockers Safe?

Although studies of short-acting calcium channel blockers suggest an increased risk of MI, these findings have not been replicated with long-acting calcium channel blockers. Long-acting calcium channel blockers are considered safe, but less effective than diuretics, beta blockers, and ACEI. They are most appropriate as fourth-line therapy. One exception is that long-acting calcium channel blockers are equally effective as thiazide diuretics in treating isolated systolic hypertension in elderly patients and in this circumstance can be used as an alternative to diuretics. Never use sublingual nifedipine to control a patient's BP acutely. This is an outdated and potentially dangerous practice because it can reduce the BP too precipitously.

How Often should I Monitor BP Short-Term and Long-Term?

For stage 2 disease (systolic >160 mm Hg, diastolic >100 mm Hg), the patient should be seen again within 1 week to determine whether therapy is effective and control is improving. While adjusting medications and monitoring response and side effects, it is useful to see the patient every 4–6 weeks. Check electrolytes, BUN, and creatinine 1 week after changing an ACEI or diuretic dose. When stable, patients can be seen annually.

What are Possible Reasons that my Patient's BP Is not Improving?

Adherence is frequently challenging for patients with hypertension. To help patients with compliance, attend to their reported side effects, and change medications where possible. Remind them that patients with better BP control often feel better. Simplify medication regimens by limiting the number of medications and the frequency of dosing. Investigate how patients pay for their medications, and work with the pharmacist to devise the most cost-effective and health-effective dose. In a patient with poorly controlled hypertension, the medication may be ineffective; switch to or add another agent. Another major factor in poorly controlled hypertension is volume expansion, in part owing to high levels of salt intake. In patients in whom BP control is not reaching target, reinforce a low-salt diet, refer to a nutritionist, and add a diuretic if not already prescribed. For persistently poor control in an adherent patient on multiple medications, evaluate for secondary causes (of which renal artery stenosis is the most common in this scenario) (Table 33-11).

Are there Specific Side Effects or Unwanted Sequelae of these Medications?

See Table 33-12. Cough accompanying ACEI can be quite severe and affects 10% of whites and 40% of Asians.

When should I Admit Someone for Hypertension?

Admit a patient with elevated BP and acute symptoms or signs of end-organ strain, such as confusion, chest pain, papilledema, hematuria or proteinuria, or pulmonary edema. A BP reading >240/130 mm Hg is associated with significant mortality, so even asymptomatic patients with this level of hypertension should be admitted.

Table 33-11

Reversible Causes of Hypertension and Their Evaluation

Condition	Test
Alcohol use	CAGE questions, serum GGT
Hyperthyroidism	TSH
Sleep apnea	Nocturnal pulse oximetry or sleep study
Cushing's syndrome	24-h urine cortisol
Hyperaldosteronism	Serum renin:aldosterone ratio
Renovascular disease	Spiral CT or magnetic resonance angiography
Pheochromocytoma	24-h urine catecholamines

Table 33-12

Relative Cost and Side Effects of Once-Daily Dosed Antihypertensive Medications

Drug	Cost	Important Side Effects	Also Treats
Diuretic Hydrochlorothiazide Chlorthalidone	$	Frequent urination Decreased potassium Increased lipids at doses >25 mg Increased uric acid	Volume overload Leg edema
Beta Blocker Atenolol Nadolol Propranolol SR	$	Fatigue Decreased exercise tolerance Impotence Asthma Bradycardia	Prevents MI recurrence Migraine (prophylaxis) Angina
ACEI Benazepril Lisinopril	$	Renal insufficiency Teratogen Hyperkalemia Cough (10%-20%) Life-threatening angioedema	CHF Diabetic nephropathy
Alpha Blocker Doxazosin Terazosin	$$	Postural hypotension Headache Weakness	BPH
Calcium Channel Blocker Amlodipine Nifedipine SR Diltiazem CD	$$$	Bradycardia and negative inotropy (only with diltiazem) Constipation Leg edema Reflux	Angina
Angiotensin Receptor Blocker Losartan Valsartan Irbesartan	$$$	Hyperkalemia	CHF with or without nephropathy

Case 33-8

A 42-year-old man presents with a recent ankle sprain. For the pain, he has used ibuprofen. He drinks four beers a night. He has no personal or family history of hypertension. On exam, his BP is 146/92 mm Hg.

 A. What could be elevating his BP?
 B. How soon would you like to see him again?

C. What changes would you like to ask him to make before his next visit?

Case 33-9

A 72-year-old woman comes to see you for the first time. Aside from chronic constipation and occasional gout, she is healthy. Her only real medical problem is high BP, which has been present "for years and years." Her medications are Metamucil, milk of magnesia, and nifedipine 20 mg three times daily. From time to time, she takes a "water pill" for her swollen legs. Her BP is 150/ 84 mm Hg, and her pulse is 59 beats/min.

A. Would you recommend a change in her BP medication, and why or why not?
B. What evaluation would you do?
C. What medication would you choose for her?

Case 33-10

A 57-year-old woman with obesity, DM, and depression sits in your office crying because you have just told her she has hypertension. When she is depressed, she eats potato chips and has gained 30 lb over the past year. She is extremely tired all the time; she fell asleep while driving over to see you. In her family, all her siblings have hypertension and DM. On exam, her BP is 166/ 117 mm Hg. She has stretch marks on her stomach and has lower extremity swelling. Her ECG and UA are normal. Her lab tests show low potassium.

A. Name at least five possible causes of, or contributors to, hypertension in this patient.
B. Would you order any further tests, and if so, why?
C. How would you start to treat her?

KEY POINTS – ACID-BASE DISTURBANCES

◆ With pH <7.4, there is a primary acidosis; with pH>7.4, there is a primary alkalosis.

◆ A low baseline anion gap from low albumin or myeloma may mask significant anion gap acidosis.

◆ If you find a patient breathing deeply and rapidly with no immediately apparent cause, suspect respiratory compensation for sepsis or other metabolic acidosis.

◆ If a significant anion gap is present, check for an osmolal gap.

KEY POINTS – ACUTE AND CHRONIC RENAL FAILURE

◆ With the work-up for ARF, consider prerenal, intrarenal, and postrenal causes.

◆ Acidemia, hyperkalemia, and CHF are common and may necessitate dialysis.

◆ Treatment of ARF involves careful volume and electrolyte management; all medications must be dosed based on creatinine clearance.

◆ Patients with chronic kidney disease should have aggressive management of hypertension and proteinuria.

KEY POINTS – ELECTROLYTE DISTURBANCES— CALCIUM

◆ Patients with hypercalcemia can present nonspecifically; check for it in any confused older patient.

◆ Hypocalcemia potentiates digoxin toxicity.

KEY POINTS – ELECTROLYTE DISTURBANCES— POTASSIUM

◆ Hyperkalemia is due to excess intake, shift from the intracellular compartment (e.g., acidosis, cell injury), or inability to excrete potassium (e.g., renal failure, drugs).

◆ The most important drugs that cause hyperkalemia are ACEI, angiotensin receptor blockers, and potassium-sparing diuretics.

◆ Refractory hypokalemia may be due to coexistent hypomagnesemia.

KEY POINTS – ELECTROLYTE DISTURBANCES— SODIUM

◆ Categorize hyponatremia by volume status.

◆ Treat most mild-to-moderate euvolemic hyponatremia with volume restriction.

◆ Correct sodium imbalances slowly by no more than 1 mEq/h.

Nephrology

KEY POINTS – FLUID MANAGEMENT

◆ Assess fluid status at least once daily in all hospitalized patients.

◆ Use ½ normal saline with glucose and potassium for maintenance fluids.

◆ Use normal saline boluses for fluid resuscitation, and reassess fluid status between boluses.

KEY POINTS – HYPERTENSION

◆ Treatment of hypertension reduces risk of stroke and heart disease.

◆ Goal BP depends on comorbidities: 130/80 mm Hg for DM and other target organ damage and 140/90 mm Hg for patients without other risk factors.

◆ Diet, exercise, and salt reduction all can reduce BP.

◆ Treat other risk factors for cardiovascular disease (smoking cessation, lipid management).

◆ In uncomplicated hypertension, start a diuretic or beta blocker; ACEI's have an increasing role in first-line treatment.

◆ In hypertension complicated by DM or CHF, prescribe an ACEI as first-line treatment.

◆ Hypertension in elderly patients and minorities is less likely to be well controlled.

◆ Treat hypertension in elderly patients, including isolated systolic hypertension, but keep diastolic BP >65 mm Hg.

◆ Admit hypertensive patients with signs or symptoms of end-organ strain or with BP >240/130 mm Hg.

Case Answers

33–1 A. *Learning objective:* **Identify the primary acid-base derangement.** Alkalemia with a pH of 7.5 is a primary respiratory alkalosis because Pco_2 is low.

33–1 B. *Learning objective:* **Recognize that a compensatory metabolic acidosis should be a non–anion gap acidosis.** Low HCO_3^- suggests a metabolic acidosis. One might be tempted to call this compensatory. A compensatory metabolic acidosis should be a non–anion gap acidosis, however, because it is generated by renal HCO_3^- loss. The patient's anion gap acidosis is instead a coexisting primary process.

33–1 C. *Learning objective:* **Identify all coexisting primary acid-base derangements by calculating anion gap, osmolar gap, and delta-delta.** Anion gap is elevated at 22 (= 140 − [103 + 15]), meaning anion gap acidosis is present. Calculated osmoles are 296 (= 2[140] + 28/2.8 + 108/18). Osmolar gap is 1 (= 296 − 295), essentially normal, and rules out osmotically active ingestion. When you add the change in anion gap (22 − 12 = 10) to his HCO_3^- (15), you get 25, close enough to 24 that you can declare there are no other simultaneous metabolic processes.

33–1 D. *Learning objective:* **Interpret acid-base abnormalities in the context of clinical information to develop a reasonable differential diagnosis.** He has been taking large doses of aspirin for back pain. Aspirin causes a primary respiratory alkalosis by stimulating CNS breathing centers to hyperventilate and an anion gap acidosis owing to salicylic acid. His melena is likely from NSAID-induced gastritis. Other less likely explanations of the acid-base derangements would have to invoke two separate processes. Early sepsis could cause an anion gap acidosis with compensatory hyperventilation, although the pH should be <7.4 reflecting the primary acidosis.

33–2 A. *Learning objective:* **Identify the primary acid-base derangement.** The patient has acidemia with a low HCO_3^-, giving her a primary metabolic acidosis.

33–2 B. *Learning objective:* **Identify the compensatory acid base derangement.** Low P_{CO_2} from hyperventilating creates a compensatory respiratory alkalosis.

33–2 C. *Learning objective:* **Identify all coexisting acid-base derangements by calculating anion gap and osmolar gap and comparing the change in anion gap with the change in HCO_3^- (delta-delta).** Anion gap is 32 (= 130 − [88 + 10]). Calculated osmoles are 310 (= 2[130] + 28/2.8 + 720/18). Osmolar gap is 5 (= 315 − 310). Using delta-delta, the increase in anion gap is 20 (= 32 − 12), and when you add this to the HCO_3^-, you get 30 (= 20 + 10). Because this is > 24, a metabolic alkalosis also is present.

33–2 D. *Learning objective:* **Interpret acid-base abnormalities in the context of clinical information.** She has diabetic ketoacidosis (polyuria, polydipsia, high glucose), causing an anion gap acidosis. She has some respiratory compensation, blowing off CO_2 to reduce her acidemia. Additionally, she has a coexisting metabolic alkalosis, probably from vomiting acidic stomach contents.

33–3 A. *Learning objective:* **Recognize a patient with glomerulonephritis and nephrotic syndrome.** This patient has glomerulonephritis as defined by dysmorphic RBC in the urine. RBC casts are definitive, but degenerate quickly and require evaluation of fresh urine. She probably has nephrotic syndrome (edema, hypoalbuminemia, and proteinuria >3.5 g/24 h; you also should note lipiduria [oval fat bodies]), but this should be confirmed.

33–3 B. *Learning objective:* **List the common causes of glomerulonephritis.** The most likely causes of this patient's glomerulonephritis include autoimmune diseases such as Wegener's granulomatosis or SLE, IgA nephropathy, poststreptococcal glomerulonephritis (her pneumonia), or HCV.

33–3 C. *Learning objective:* **Calculate estimated creatinine clearance.** Her creatinine clearance would be estimated at 23.8 mL/min. This is very low and would necessitate evaluation for dialysis in the near future. Medications should be adjusted for decreased renal clearance.

33–3 D. *Learning objective:* **Manage edema in patients with renal disease using loop diuretics and ACEI.** You should begin by prescribing a loop diuretic to decrease volume overload and an ACEI to decrease proteinuria. Although her albumin is low, albumin infusion is not helpful. Monitor potassium and creatinine.

33–4 A. *Learning objective:* **Diagnose urinary retention and ARF related to BPH and precipitated by anticholinergic agents.** This man has some underlying diabetic nephropathy, but the presentation and exam suggest ARF precipitated by amitriptyline. He could have neurogenic bladder, but his exam is consistent mostly with mild diabetic neuropathy.

33–4 B. *Learning objective:* **Order appropriate tests to evaluate urinary outlet obstruction.** The most helpful diagnostic step would be bladder and renal ultrasound. Ultrasound would show obstructions such as nephrolithiasis or tumor, would show whether there is renal calyceal dilation, and would give an estimate of the amount retained.

33–4 C. *Learning objective:* **Appropriately manage acute bladder outlet obstruction.** You should catheterize the patient initially. Although bladder decompression hemorrhage is a medical myth, postobstructive diuresis can result in fluid and electrolyte loss, so careful monitoring is important. Metformin (and ACEI) should be withheld until creatinine is normal and stable. Given his elevated PSA, he should be evaluated for prostate cancer and for TURP. Additionally, it may be better to choose an alternative agent (e.g., carbamazepine rather than amitriptyline) that is not anticholinergic for treatment of his neuropathic pain.

33–5 A. *Learning objective:* **Recognize rhabdomyolysis.** This patient has rhabdomyolysis precipitated by his extreme exertion in combination with his use of ibuprofen and dehydration related to the heat. This is common in athletes and crush injuries, and a similar phenomenon is seen after chemotherapy for high-volume tumors (e.g., acute leukemia). Muscle breakdown results in renal ischemia and tubular obstruction. His case is complicated by probable (prerenal) ATN and NSAID toxicity.

33–5 B. *Learning objective:* **Appropriately evaluate patients with rhab-domyolysis and ARF.** He should have electrolytes, calcium, phosphate, uric acid, and muscle enzymes (CK, myoglobin), UA for myoglobinuria and sediment exam, and an ultrasound.

33–5 C. *Learning objective:* **Recognize urinary sediment findings in ATN and rhabdomyolysis.** He will likely have pigmented casts. He also may have muddy brown casts from ATN.

33–5 D. *Learning objective:* **Appropriately manage ARF and rhabdomyolysis.** He should be catheterized and given bolus normal saline. Muscle breakdown releases potassium, phosphate, and uric acid from cells. Patients develop hypocalcemia secondarily. Forced alkaline-mannitol diuresis is the usual approach, but there is no evidence that this is better than saline hydration, and it may cause calcium-phosphate precipitation, so that approach is clinically acceptable.

33–6 A. *Learning objective:* **Prioritize hyperkalemia as a life-threatening problem.** Hyperkalemia is most life-threatening because of the potential for lethal arrhythmias. Hypertension is likely baseline and can be addressed over days to weeks as long as there is no end-organ damage. Dyspnea, elevated JVP, rales, and edema are signs of moderate fluid overload, which can be addressed with diuretics or hemodialysis over hours to days. Metabolic non–anion gap acidosis is likely chronic secondary to renal failure.

33–6 B. *Learning objective:* **State the ECG findings of hyperkalemia.** Moderate hyperkalemia causes peaked T waves. More severe hyperkalemia widens the QRS, reflecting the increased time for ventricular depolarization. With severe hyperkalemia, ECG looks like a sine wave with peaked T waves and wide QRS indistinguishable from each other in an undulating wave.

33–6 C. *Learning objective:* **Identify interventions for acute hyperkalemia, and state the mechanism of each.** To avoid cardiac arrhythmia, first give intravenous calcium gluconate to stabilize cardiac membranes rapidly. Next, give intravenous glucose (an ampule of 50% dextrose) and insulin (5–10 U) to carry potassium into the intracellular space. Do not give so much insulin as to cause hypoglycemia. Alkalinize with intravenous HCO_3^- for a transient intracellular potassium shift. Kayexalate can be initiated with the acute therapies, but is too slow-acting to reverse severe hyperkalemia. Furosemide helps over hours if the patient is making urine. Use dialysis for severe hyperkalemia, although it takes some time to set up; administer calcium, glucose with insulin, and HCO_3^- while waiting for dialysis to begin.

33–7 A. *Learning objective:* **List hyponatremia and hypercalcemia as the two electrolyte disorders that cause confusion, and recognize clinical situations where these might occur.** Hyponatremia and hypercalcemia are the two electrolyte disturbances that can cause confusion. This patient likely has pneumonia (more common in patients with myeloma), which can lead to SIADH-induced hyponatremia. He is taking a thiazide diuretic, which can cause hyponatremia. Myeloma bone metastases can lead to hypercalcemia as a result of increased bone resorption.

33–7 B. *Learning objective:* **List causes of confusion in older patients.** Aside from hyponatremia and hypercalcemia, other causes of confusion include hypoxia, MI, infection, liver failure, thyrotoxicosis, subdural hematoma, and drugs such as opioids or anticholinergics.

33–7 C. *Learning objective:* **Order appropriate investigations in patients with confusion.** Order oxygen saturation (his was 88%), and if low, consider an ABG. Order ECG (his showed LVH, no ischemia) and CXR (showed right lower lobe consolidation suggestive of pneumonia). Order sodium (his was 115), calcium, liver enzymes, cardiac enzymes, UA, blood cultures, sputum stain and culture, TSH (all normal in him). Review medications. If neurologic exam is focal, consider head CT, although his exam was normal.

33–7 D. *Learning objective:* **Appropriately treat euvolemic hyponatremia by stopping potentially causative medications and with fluid restriction.** Stop the hydrochlorothiazide, and place him on a 1.2-L daily fluid restriction. Monitor for complications of hyponatremia such as seizures, and correct the hyponatremia more aggressively with saline or hypertonic saline infusion if these develop.

33–8 A. *Learning objective:* **Identify factors contributing to hypertension.** NSAID, acute pain, and excessive alcohol use all can contribute to his hypertension.

33–8 B. *Learning objective:* **Design appropriate follow-up for patients in whom mild hypertension is found.** Recheck within the next 2 months or so, before he forgets to return.

33–8 C. *Learning objective:* **Counsel patients appropriately about lifestyle modifications to reduce BP.** With a single measurement under extenuating circumstances, his BP will likely normalize. NSAIDs also are appropriate for short-term management of pain and inflammation. You need to address his alcohol use, however. Regardless of whether it has increased his BP, he is drinking enough to cause significant medical and social sequelae. Intervention in a young man is more likely to succeed than in more chronic alcohol users. Use CAGE questions for further screening.

33–9 A. *Learning objective:* **Recognize side effects of nifedipine, and find alternative treatment for three reasons.** (1) Unacceptable side effects are present (constipation and lower extremity edema are common with calcium channel blockers). (2) Increased mortality occurs with short-acting calcium channel blockers. (3) She has to take a pill three times a day, which may make compliance difficult and may relate to why her BP is still elevated.

33–9 B. *Learning objective:* **Perform appropriate initial evaluation for hypertension in patients with unclear prior evaluation.** With a patient that is new to you, you need to begin at the beginning. If she has not had diet and exercise counseling, review this with her. Examine her for end-organ damage: Perform a careful eye and heart exam, and at minimum obtain a lab panel of electrolytes and renal function. Next, consider whether she could have secondary causes for hypertension. Because her hypertension has been long-standing, further testing is probably not indicated. Her age alone puts her at risk for renal artery stenosis, however, so if more than two medications do not control her BP, consider a renal artery duplex.

33–9 C. *Learning objective:* **Choose appropriate antihypertensive therapy in a patient with gout and bradycardia.** Although her lower extremity edema suggests a low-dose diuretic, the increase in uric acid may cause her gout to flare. A beta blocker also may be a poor choice because her pulse is bradycardic. Many elderly patients have bradycardia or borderline heart block from impaired electrical conduction in the heart (as a consequence of degeneration and aging, not ischemia per se). In patients with a low pulse (<60 beats/min), check an ECG before starting a beta blocker. A calcium channel blocker, such as diltiazem or verapamil, may delay conduction at the atrioventricular node and worsen heart block. An alpha blocker is a cheap alternative, but orthostatic hypotension puts older patients at risk for falls. An ACEI may be the best choice; check renal function after 1 week of therapy. If her lower extremity edema is from CHF secondary to long-standing hypertension with hypertrophic cardiomyopathy, an ACEI is the first choice for afterload reduction.

33–10 A. *Learning objective:* **Identify features on history and physical that suggest reasons for hypertension.** Potential factors include family history, obesity, Cushing's syndrome (depression, obesity, DM, stretch marks, and low potassium), hyperaldosteronism, and sleep apnea (fatigue, falling asleep while driving, central obesity).

33–10 B. *Learning objective:* **Order appropriate tests for suspected secondary causes of hypertension in an obese patient with hypokalemia.** Perform serial work-up beginning with a 24-hour cortisol because she has several stigmata of Cushing's syndrome. Other tests to do in serial fashion include renal artery study (DM puts her at risk for vascular disease), an aldosterone-to-renin ratio (low potassium also occurs with hyperaldosteronism), and a sleep study looking for sleep apnea (prevalent in 40% of obese women).

33–10 C. *Learning objective:* **Begin treatment for hypertension with lifestyle modification.** Lifestyle modification is imperative in this patient. Weight loss and exercise would help not only her hypertension, but also her DM. A 10-lb weight loss can make a big change in medication requirements. This patient has stage 2 hypertension, so medications are indicated while she works on her lifestyle changes. Control other risk factors for coronary heart disease by checking cholesterol, treating DM, and starting estrogen replacement (unless contraindicated).

REFERENCES

Hypertension
Chobanian AV, Bakris GL, Black HR, et al: The Seventh Report of the Joint National Committee on Prevention, Detection, Evaluation, and Treatment of High Blood Pressure: The JNC 7 Report. JAMA 2003;289:2560.

Acute and Chronic Renal Failure
Aust Fam Physician 2005;34 (11), (entire issue).

Fluid Management
Adrogue HJ, Madias NE: Hyponatremia. N Engl J Med 2000;342:1581.
Kapoor M, Chan GZ: Fluid and electrolyte abnormalities. Crit Care Clin 2001;17:503.

USEFUL WEB SITE

Acute and Chronic Disturbances
The National Kidney Foundation web site. www.kidney.org

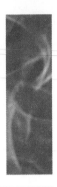

34

Neurology

GENEVIEVE L. PAGALILAUAN and ERIC E. KRAUS

 NEUROLOGIC EXAM

What should I Cover in the Screening Neurologic Exam?

Perform a screening neurologic exam (Box 34-1) on all patients requiring a "full physical" in the hospital and the clinic. This includes assessment of mental status, cranial nerves, strength (scale 0–5), sensation, reflexes (scale 0–4) (Box 34-2), and coordination. If the patient can ambulate, assess gait. This exam should take no more than 3–5 minutes to perform on an alert, cooperative patient. Tell your patient why you are doing each step, for example, "I'm going to test your coordination. Touch my finger, now touch your nose, now go back and forth." Box 34-1 summarizes a normal screening exam.

When do I Need to Perform a More Detailed Neurologic Exam?

If the screening neurologic exam is abnormal, or if the patient presents with a neurologic problem, a more detailed exam is warranted and can be tailored to fit the circumstances (Table 34-1).

 ALTERED MENTAL STATUS

ETIOLOGY

What Causes Altered Mental Status?

Altered mental status is a spectrum ranging from normal to coma. Avoid imprecise terms such as "lethargic," "stuporous," or "obtunded." Instead, describe the level of stimulus required to arouse the patient (e.g., wakens to voice, unarousable to noxious stimuli) and the degree of drowsiness (e.g., falls asleep after several minutes of conversation). Coma means that there is no purposeful response to the environment and requires significant lesions in both cerebral hemispheres or in the

Neurology

BOX 34-1

SAMPLE NORMAL SCREENING NEUROLOGIC EXAM

Mental status—alert and oriented to person, place, and time
Cranial nerves—pupils equal, round, reactive to light and accommodation (PERRLA), extraocular movements intact (EOMI), facial sensation and movement normal, palate elevation symmetric, tongue midline and strong (or cranial nerves II-XII intact)
Sensation—intact to vibration in the toes and light touch in all four extremities
Motor—5 out of 5 strength in all four extremity muscle groups
Coordination—intact to finger-nose-finger; gait normal
Reflexes—symmetric and 2/4 at biceps, triceps, knees, and ankles; 1/4 at brachioradialis; toes down-going

---

BOX 34-2

GRADING MOTOR STRENGTH AND REFLEXES

Motor Strength

0 = no movement
1 = trace movement
2 = movement when the force of gravity removed
3 = able to move against gravity, but not resistance
4 = able to move against resistance, but weaker than expected for age and size
5 = full strength against resistance

Reflexes

0 = no movement
1 = diminished
2 = normal
3 = increased
4 = clonus

---

reticular activation system (RAS) in the brainstem. Lesser degrees of altered mental status can arise from metabolic or toxic derangements or structural problems (Table 34-2).

EVALUATION

What Historical Clues are Helpful In Determining the Cause of Confusion?

Ask family, friends, and emergency medical staff for clues. Abrupt onset suggests a discrete event, such as stroke or seizure, whereas more gradual onset suggests a diffuse metabolic process. Onset with a worst-ever headache

Table 34-1

Additional Neurologic Exams for Specific Conditions

Condition	Neurologic Exam	Observe and Record
Stupor or coma	Responsiveness	Level of stimulus required to rouse patient—voice, shaking, noxious stimuli
	Motor response	Appropriate withdrawal or posturing to noxious stimuli
	Pupil size and response	Size in mm; direct and consensual response to light
	Eye movements	Centered, disconjugate, or conjugate gaze deviation; doll's eyes; or cold water calorics. Clear cervical spine first before doing doll's eyes maneuvers
	Corneal reflexes	Blink elicited when cornea touched with Q-tip
	Breathing	Cheyne-Stokes respirations, neurogenic hyperventilation, apneustic or ataxic respirations
Stroke	Simultaneous double stimuli	Left side neglect is found in patients with right parietal lesions
	Language	Normal, dysarthric, or aphasic
	Carotid auscultation	Listen for carotid bruits
	Romberg	Stand up straight with eyes closed
	Pronator drift	Keep arms extended out at shoulder height with palms up; abnormal if one palm or arm turns downward
	Gait	Symmetry, stride, arm swing, stance (wide or narrow)
Memory loss	Mini-mental status exam	30-point mini-mental status exam
Decreased sensation	Pain and temperature	Sharp toothpick; cold metal
	Proprioception	Toe up or down
	Light touch	Identify pattern—dermatomal, stocking-glove
	Monofilament testing	

suggests subarachnoid hemorrhage (SAH). Progression from an initial focal deficit is a clue to the location of a structural problem. Ask about potential precipitating factors, such as trauma, alcohol withdrawal, or prescription or illicit drug overdose. Obtain pill bottles from the patient's home if possible. A past medical history of DM, seizures, stroke, liver, and kidney disease also provides a clue to possible causes of altered mental status. For elderly patients, confusion is often the final common presenting pathway for numerous conditions, including MI, urosepsis, and pneumonia. Even if

Table 34-2

Causes of Altered Mental Status

	Common Causes	**Less Common Causes**
Metabolic or Toxic	Anoxia (hypoperfusion, hypoxia)	Adrenal insufficiency
	Drugs (prescription, over-the-counter, illicit)	Hypertensive encephalopathy
	Electrolytes (Ca^{++}, Na^{+}, glucose)	Hypothyroidism
	Epilepsy	Vitamin B_{12} deficiency
	Infection (UTI, pneumonia)	
	Liver failure	
	MI	
Structural	CNS trauma	CNS tumor
	Infection (meningitis, encephalitis)	CNS abscess
	Stroke, hemorrhagic or ischemic	

the history is atypical for these common ailments, maintain a high suspicion, and rule them out routinely.

How do I Recognize the Difference between Delirium, Psychosis, and Dementia?

Delirium is transient and characterized by fluctuating confusion and loss of attentiveness over the course of hours to days. It may present with either hyperactive (physical agitation, hallucinations) or hypoactive (lethargy, daytime sleeping) symptoms. Have a high suspicion for delirium in patients with risk factors such as advanced age, hospitalization or institutionalization, history of dementia or cognitive impairment, multiple systemic illnesses, multiple medications, acute infection, and recent surgery. Delirium causes mortality risk to double, but usually resolves with treatment of the underlying cause; in the elderly, infection is a particularly common cause. **Psychosis** may look like delirium, but has no underlying metabolic derangement. In contrast, **dementia** is a confused state in which patients remain attentive. Dementia is chronic, persistent, and slowly progressive with memory loss as a prominent feature (Table 34-3).

Table 34-3

Features Distinguishing Delirium from Dementia

	Delirium	**Dementia**
Level of consciousness	Impaired	Normal*
Clinical course	Acute, fluctuates over hours	Slowly progresses over years
Autonomic hyperactivity	Present	Absent
Prognosis	Usually reversible	Usually irreversible

*Patients usually retain normal level of consciousness until very late in the course of dementia.

Table 34-4

Evaluation and Management of Comatose Patients

Immediate Issues for Stabilization	Urgent Issues after Stabilization	Later Issues
Stabilize airway, breathing and circulation	History	Correct electrolytes
Vital signs including pulse oximetry	Thorough neurologic exam	Correct acid-base imbalances
Cervical spine films to clear neck	ABG, CBC, renal and liver function, electrolytes, UA, toxicology screen	CXR
Naloxone 0.4–1.2 mg IV	Head CT with or without contrast	Other lab tests if indicated
Thiamine 100 mg IV*	LP if indicated	EEG if indicated
Glucose 25 gm IV*	ECG and rule out MI with cardiac enzymes, especially in elderly patients	
Rapid exam for trauma, neurologic deficits	Antibiotics if meningitis suspected	

*Always give thiamine *before* glucose.

What Studies should I Order in a Confused Patient?

Order ECG, oxygen saturation, CBC, electrolytes, renal and liver function, glucose, and UA to detect a metabolic cause for altered mental status (Table 34-4). If no abnormality is found, order the following only as indicated by the specific case: alcohol or drug levels, toxicology screening, ABG, carboxyhemoglobin levels, and head CT. Most mass lesions or bleeds in the cerebral hemispheres are easy to detect on CT; however 5% of SAH can be missed on an early CT scan. A negative CT scan in a patient thought to have SAH requires LP to look for bloody CSF. Also perform LP in any patient with fever and altered mental status, unless a good explanation for both is quickly found.

How do I Evaluate a Comatose Patient?

Prioritize your approach (see Table 34-4) to address urgent issues first. Focus the neurologic exam on level of consciousness; breathing pattern; and motor response to central (finger in the styloid foramen) and peripheral (pressing on nailbeds) stimuli, noxious stimuli, pupillary responses, and eye movement with doll's eyes maneuver and cold water caloric testing (see Table 34-1). Bilateral hemispheric injury can cause Cheyne-Stokes respiration, a rhythmic waxing and waning of respiratory rate and volume. Focal brainstem injuries can cause central neurogenic hyperventilation, apneustic breathing (prominent pauses), or ataxic breathing (randomly, irregular, deep and shallow breathing). Eyes may deviate conjugately toward an ipsilateral hemispheric structural lesion. The doll's eyes maneuver is performed on comatose patients with intact cervical spine by watching eye movements when the head is rotated rapidly to one side. A positive test (normal) occurs when the eyes move in their sockets to remain fixed on a point on the ceiling even though the head is turned. It indicates an intact brainstem in a comatose patient, but conscious patients can suppress it. A negative test (abnormal) means the eyes stay fixed in the socket despite head turning and indicates damage to the pontine gaze center of the brainstem, or the patient is awake and suppressing the reflex.

What Information Helps Determine Likely Outcome in a Comatose Patient?

Use prognostic information to counsel families. Good prognosis is associated with drug intoxication (90% survival), intact pupillary and oculo-motor reflexes, and rapid initial clinical improvement. Poor prognosis is associated with loss of pupillary, corneal, and oculovestibular reflexes for >6 hours after onset of insult (95% mortality); unwitnessed cardiac arrest; prolonged resuscitation; nontraumatic coma with failure to improve after 4 days; and traumatic coma in the elderly. Mortality in a comatose patient is 75% with SAH; 50% with head injury; and 40%-50% with cardiac arrest, tumor, infection, or metabolic insult. Permanent, severe impairment occurs in 15%-25% of coma survivors. Brain death can be determined by clinical exam showing coma, no response to central stimulus, and absence of brainstem activity and is supported further by lack of reversible causes and a positive apnea test (the patient's P_{CO_2} is allowed to increase >20 mm Hg of baseline and there is no respiration).

TREATMENT

How do I Treat a Patient with Altered Mental Status?

For patients with severe mental status alterations, often you must make therapeutic interventions urgently even before diagnostic work-up is complete (see Table 34-4). The first priorities are airway, breathing, and cardiac function (ABCs); intubate if necessary to protect the airway. For severe alterations in mental status, begin rapid empiric treatment with naloxone to reverse potential respiratory depression from opiates, then sequentially give thiamine and glucose to reverse Wernicke's encephalopathy and hypo-glycemia. Don't give glucose before thiamine in a chronic alcohol user; this can precipitate Wernicke's encephalopathy. After these urgent interventions, treat the underlying cause. If meningitis is suspected, give immediate intravenous antibiotics even before LP is completed, to optimize outcome.

STROKE

ETIOLOGY

How Important is Stroke as a Disease?

The age-dependent incidence of stroke is 1–2 per 1000 population per year. Among mortality rates, stroke ranks third after heart disease and cancer. Among disability rates, stroke ranks first.

Neurology

What Causes Ischemic Stroke?

Stroke can be either ischemic or hemorrhagic. **Ischemic stroke** is a disruption of blood flow, food (glucose), or oxygen to the brain resulting in cerebral dysfunction. TIA is a variant of stroke in which the neurologic deficit lasts <24 hours, and on imaging there is no infarct. Ischemic strokes can be due to emboli, thrombosis, hypoperfusion, or myriad other, rarer causes (e.g., vasculitis, hypoxia). Emboli can originate from arteries or veins, often in the setting of a hypercoagulable state. Thrombosis can occur in vessels of different sizes. Closure of larger vessels usually is due to rupture of atherosclerotic plaque, although trauma, radiation, arterial dissection, fibromuscular dysplasia, inflammation, and other etiologies can play a role. **Lacunes** are deep, small vessel strokes that likely result from closure of deep penetrating arteries. Lacunes are caused by emboli, carotid disease, and 25% of the time other etiologies. Risk factors include hypertension, DM, and smoking. Hypoperfusion leads to damage primarily in vascular border zones, such as between the anterior and middle or posterior and middle cerebral artery circulations. These are regions where two different blood vessels cross or anastomose and in which the perfusion pressure is the lowest. Stroke can occur more slowly in this situation. Carotid atherosclerosis can lead to stroke by any of the three mechanisms described earlier (thrombosis, emboli, or hypoperfusion), and effective prevention of recurrence is possible by carotid endarterectomy.

What Causes Hemorrhagic Stroke?

Hemorrhagic stroke is caused by a disruption of blood vessel integrity, although hematologic derangements may contribute. It is classified as subarachnoid or intracranial depending on the location of bleeding. Hemorrhagic stroke should be distinguished from hemorrhagic conversion, which refers to bleeding into an area of ischemic stroke. In approximately 30% of patients with stroke, no etiology is found.

What Other Diseases can Look Like Stroke?

Stroke must be distinguished from other diseases, such as subdural or epidural hematoma, migraine, seizure, tumor, toxic/metabolic encephalopathy, infections, spinal stenosis, and peripheral neuromuscular disease.

What are the Risk Factors for Stroke?

The most important risk factor is age; the most modifiable risk factor is hypertension. Other common and important risk factors are atrial fibrillation, hypercholesterolemia, smoking, DM, CHF, and heavy alcohol use.

EVALUATION

What is the Primary Goal of Stroke Evaluation?

The goal is to minimize damage of the current stroke and prevent future strokes by risk factor modification and medication. The latter requires an understanding of the stroke cause, so if possible determine the underlying mechanism as embolic, thrombotic, hypoperfusion, hemorrhagic, or other.

How is Timing of Onset Helpful?

Timing of onset lends important clues. Most strokes present with acute, maximal symptoms at onset. "Stroke in evolution" and "stuttering stroke" are less common and involve deficits worsening or fluctuating over hours to days. Such presentations suggest a propagating arterial or venous thrombus, recurrent emboli, vasculitis, development of edema, enlarging hematoma, or hypoperfusion. Deficits lasting less than 24 hours are TIA and are considered warning signs of potential future stroke.

How does the Pattern of Deficits give Clues about the Location of a Stroke?

Patterns of deficits are helpful in predicting the type, size, and location of stroke (Table 34-5). Strokes deep in the brain or brainstem are usually lacunar or hemorrhagic, and although they involve small areas of brain, they cause significant deficits because local nerve tracks are compact. A pure motor stroke involving the left face, arm, and leg is usually due to a small vessel stroke in the right internal capsule or right basis pontis.

Strokes that occur in a cortical location are usually embolic or thrombotic and involve larger vessels, involve larger areas of brain, and cause broader symptoms. If they affect only a branch of a cerebral artery, they may cause more focal deficits depending on which hemisphere is involved. Whether a patient is left or right brain dominant can be determined by handedness. Most people are right-handed and left brain dominant, and left brain controls language, and right brain controls visuospatial processing. In a right-handed patient, a left MCA branch stroke can affect language as an expressive or receptive aphasia. A right brain MCA branch stroke may affect visual or spatial functions, causing neglect of a limb or difficulty recognizing objects by feel. Dysarthria, in contrast to aphasias, is a motor deficit in speech, which can occur with deep motor tract or cortical motor area stroke on either side of the brain.

How does Headache Play a Role in Patients with Stroke?

"The worst headache of my life" is often a presenting symptom of subarachnoid bleeding from a ruptured berry aneurysm (usually in the circle of Willis). SAH can be accompanied by vomiting, meningismus (stiff neck, Kernig's and Brudzinski's signs), focal neurologic deficits, or rapid loss of consciousness. Headache also may be prominent in hemorrhage deeper within the brain. In cerebral venous thrombosis, headache is a major feature. In contrast, in ischemic stroke, headache is present only in 20%, is typically mild, and is not the primary symptom.

Table 34-5

Classic Patterns of Stroke Deficits

Deficit	Brain Distribution Involved
Strength	
Face, arm, and leg weakness	Deep lacunes in internal capsule or basis pontis
Focal hand and arm weakness	Cortical stroke, contralateral MCA branch
Speech	
Expressive aphasia	Cortical stroke, dominant brain Broca's area
Receptive aphasia	Cortical stroke, dominant brain Wernicke's area
Dysarthria	Deep motor tract or cortical motor area stroke
Vision	
Visual field deficit	Parietal optic tract (MCA) or occipital lobe (posterior cerebral artery)
Combined	
Weakness or sensory loss on arm and face, with visual field cut	Proximal contralateral MCA stroke
Other	
Altered consciousness	Large hemispheric strokes, brainstem strokes
Vomiting, vertigo, ataxia, CN palsies	Posterior circulation stroke (vertebrobasilar artery)
Stroke Mimickers	
Worst headache ever with meningismus	Subarachnoid bleed from ruptured aneurysm
Unilateral vision loss (amaurosis fugax)	Not brain, but retina from retinal artery embolism from carotid stenosis
Variable	Migraines

Neurology

What Work-Up Should be Done in the Emergency Department?

Complete a focused history and physical within 10 minutes of the patient arriving in the emergency department. Include time of onset, symptoms, course, risk factors, medications, past medical problems, mental status, language, visual fields, cranial nerves, strength, sensory function, reflexes, cerebellar function, gait, and cardiac function. Listen for carotid bruits and cardiac abnormalities. Assess vital signs; most patients are hypertensive to some degree even if that is not a baseline issue. Order ECG, head CT, and lab tests (Table 34-6). Rapidly review head CT results, and consult a neurologist regarding the clinical criteria for thrombolysis because tPA may be beneficial in some stroke patients if used within 3 hours of symptom onset. Additional history and physical can be performed after this decision is made. Controversy exists concerning which patients to admit to expedite further work-up. Strongly consider admitting any patient with stroke, including TIA, if

Table 34-6

Common Studies in Acute Stroke

Study	Potential Findings
ECG	Atrial fibrillation, myocardial ischemia or MI
Noncontrast head CT	Ischemia or hemorrhage, deep versus cortical distribution May be normal in first 6–24 h
Diffusion-weighted MRI	Distinguishes new or old ischemic stroke; sensitive even in first few hours of presentation
Lab Tests	
Electrolytes, glucose, magnesium	Metabolic cause
CBC, platelets	Infection Hyperviscosity Bleeding problem (PT and PTT if tPA or heparin is being considered)

Neurology

the onset was within the last 48 hours. If stroke onset was >48 hours ago, admission depends on the emergency department work-up, suspected or known cause, deficits, and social support. TIA should be worked up aggressively. Time is of the essence because the stroke risk is highest in the first few days to weeks after a TIA.

What Secondary Work-Up should be Considered?

After an initial evaluation in the emergency department, try to categorize the stroke, and limit the secondary work-up appropriately, usually with the assistance of a neurologist. One of the most useful studies is diffusion-weighted MRI because it can distinguish new from old stroke and help predict a cause. Carotid duplex is important because carotid disease can be involved in many stroke categories, and treatment is available for high-grade stenosis. In patients <40 years old without structural lesions, consider a check for hypercoagulability disorders, including antiphospholipid antibodies, heparin-induced thrombocytopenia (HIT), lupus anticoagulant, sickle cell, hyperhomocysteinemia, and protein C and S deficiencies. Other tests used are echocardiography, transcranial Doppler, Holter monitor, angiography, rheumatologic lab tests (ESR, ANA, antineutrophilic cytoplasmic antibody), syphilis serologies, and LP (especially to rule out SAH).

TREATMENT

How do I Treat Ischemic Stroke in the Acute Setting?

The most immediate decision concerns thrombolytic therapy. The major drawback of using tPA is the 10-fold greater risk of intracerebral hemorrhage (6.4% with tPA compared with 0.6% in patients treated more traditionally). Many patients do not meet the within-3-hours-of-onset

BOX 34-3

GENERAL PRINCIPLES IN THE TREATMENT OF ACUTE ISCHEMIC STROKE

Avoid hypotension
Treat hypertension with labetalol only if BP >210/120 mm Hg
Keep oxygen saturation >92%
Maintain glucose control <150 mg/dL with insulin drip
Treat fever with acetaminophen
Correct volume depletion with normal saline
Keep Mg^{++} >2 mg/dL
Prevent DVT
Prevent aspiration if at risk (NPO)

criteria. Other acute stroke management principles are listed in Box 34-3. Higher BP is required to perfuse brain tissues near areas of injury in the days after a stroke. Gently reduce systolic pressures >210 mm Hg with labetalol; do not use diuretics because these lower intravascular volume. Use isotonic maintenance fluids such as normal saline to avoid dehydration. Keep glucose <150 mg/dL (using an insulin drip, if necessary), magnesium >2 mg/dL, and temperature normal (with acetaminophen) for the first 48 hours because abnormalities in any of these areas worsen outcome. Monitor for and treat complications such as pneumonia, UTI, and DVT. Heparin is indicated only in specific situations (consult a neurologist); its use is debated because it carries a higher risk of hemorrhagic conversion, especially in strokes involving large distributions. Heparin should not be bolused in neurology patients; the PTT goal is 50–80, lower than for other medical problems. Finally, start aspirin early if not beginning thrombolysis or anticoagulation. For all stroke patients, perform frequent vital signs and neurologic exams in the first hours to days to monitor for extension or complications of the initial stroke.

How do I Treat Hemorrhagic Stroke in the Acute Setting?

Acute stabilization of ABCs is the same as with ischemic stroke; reversal of the underlying bleeding diathesis is key. If the patient is taking warfarin, use vitamin K or fresh frozen plasma to normalize the PT INR. If on antiplatelet agents or thrombocytopenic, administer platelets. Keep systolic pressure 140–160 mm Hg with nitroprusside or labetalol. Some patients require decreased intracranial pressure with surgical decompression with or without hematoma evacuation, mannitol, or mechanical hyperventilation to prevent uncal and brainstem herniation.

How can I Prevent Stroke?

Primary prevention (preventing the patient's first stroke) is addressed through treatment of risk factors, such as hypertension, DM, and hyperlipidemia (with a statin), and behavioral change, such as smoking

Table 34-7

Secondary Prevention of Stroke

Etiology	Treatment
Embolic Stroke	
Atrial fibrillation	Anticoagulation
CHF	Anticoagulation
Septic embolus	Antibiotics
Antiphospholipid antibody syndrome	Anticoagulation (INR 3–4)
Carotid Stenosis	
<70% stenosis	Antiplatelet and statin
>70% stenosis and symptomatic	Endarterectomy, antiplatelet, and statin
Thrombotic Stroke	
Large vessel stroke	Antiplatelet or anticoagulation
Small vessel lacunar stroke	Antiplatelet
Hemorrhagic Stroke	
Amyloid angiopathy	BP control, avoid aspirin or warfarin
Hypertensive	BP control long-term

cessation. Where indicated (e.g., known hypercoagulable state), begin antiplatelet therapy or anticoagulation. When a patient has had a stroke, begin secondary prevention; stroke risk in these patients is at least 5% per year. If possible, identify the cause of the stroke, and treat appropriately (Table 34-7). In patients for whom a cause is not identified, it is reasonable to start a daily aspirin. Aspirin is generally the antiplatelet therapy of first choice because of ease of administration, low cost, low risk, and universal access. Doses of 75–325 mg are equally effective. When stroke occurs on aspirin (an "aspirin failure"), alternative antiplatelet therapy includes clopidogrel (Plavix) alone (adding aspirin increases bleeding risk without increasing effectiveness), or combination aspirin plus dipyridamole (Aggrenox). Long-term excellent blood pressure control is extremely important in patients who have had a stroke. Ticlopidine (Ticlid) is a third choice because of cost and side effects. Warfarin (Coumadin) is indicated for stroke despite antiplatelet therapy and for atrial fibrillation, where stroke risk is reduced by 64% over placebo in certain groups. Keep in mind the bleeding risks, however. Finally, rehabilitation is a crucial component in the treatment of stroke.

When is Surgery Indicated?

Refer patients with vascular malformations to a surgeon, particularly patients with carotid stenosis of ≥70% *in combination with* symptoms referable to that artery's vascular distribution. In 2-year follow-up, such patients managed medically have a 26% risk of stroke, whereas patients managed surgically have a 9% risk of stroke. Hospitals and surgeons have varying complication rates; this may significantly alter the risk-to-benefit profile. In asymptomatic patients and symptomatic patients with milder carotid stenosis, benefit is less clear. Stenting, angioplasty, and bypass for large vessel stenosis all are being explored.

SEIZURE

ETIOLOGY

What Causes Seizure?

Seizures are paroxysmal, transient electrical discharges of groups of neurons within the brain. Approximately 10% of the population experience one or a few provoked seizures within their lifetime, often related to one of many structural or metabolic derangements, such as CNS infection, childhood fever, hypoglycemia, electrolyte disturbance, CNS hypoperfusion, alcohol or benzodiazepine withdrawal, illicit drug use, medication overdose or side effect, and closed head injury. **Epilepsy** is defined as recurrent seizures without an easily reversible cause and affects approximately 1% of the population. Causes of epilepsy include genetics, stroke, tumor, trauma, degenerative diseases, and idiopathic. Epilepsy can manifest at any age.

What Types of Seizures are There?

Seizures are broadly classified as primarily generalized or partial as determined by a history and EEG. **Primarily generalized seizures** result from a synchronized discharge of the whole brain at the same time. Onset is almost invariably before the age of 18, and current wisdom is that the seizures often have a genetic basis. Generalized seizure subtypes include tonic-clonic, absence, myotonic, and atonic. The classic tonic-clonic seizure begins with a stiff phase of tonic muscle contraction lasting several seconds, followed by generalized rhythmic jerking movements (clonus) during which the individual loses consciousness. Incontinence of bowel or bladder or tongue trauma may occur, although these are nonspecific features of loss of consciousness from any cause. With absence seizures, patients stare blankly without loss of posture or shaking. With atonic seizures, also known as drop attacks, patients abruptly lose postural tone. A prolonged postictal period of extreme sleepiness and confusion is typical for tonic-clonic seizures. In contrast, there is no postictal state after absence or atonic seizures, and patients are able to return to normal function immediately. **Partial seizures** result from a focal cortical discharge. The spread of this focal discharge and the area of brain involved predict the symptoms and signs associated with the seizure. If full consciousness is maintained, the seizure is referred to as simple partial. An abnormal smell is a classic example of a simple partial seizure when the temporal smell centers are involved. If consciousness is reduced, this indicates a larger area of brain involvement, and seizure is referred to as complex partial. When partial seizures secondarily generalize, the result is a tonic-clonic seizure, which can be indistinguishable from a primarily generalized tonic-clonic seizure. Partial complex seizures often manifest as staring episodes, which can be confused with absence seizures. Distinguishing primarily generalized from partial seizures is important because many treatments are specific for one but not the other.

What Else can Look Like a Seizure?

The differential diagnosis for seizure includes migraine, sleep disorders, syncope, stroke, movement disorders, and psychological causes.

EVALUATION

What Work-up is Warranted in Patients Presenting with Their First Seizure?

Individualize the work-up, with a focus on looking for a treatable cause. As usual, the history and physical are most important to rule in a seizure and to rule out disorders that mimic epilepsy. Determine the exact sequence of events, especially whether the first movements were generalized or focal. Seizure and syncope can be associated with loss of consciousness, but seizure and not syncope would have a postictal period longer than a few minutes. Ask about possible precipitants, such as alcohol or benzodiazepine withdrawal, drug overdose, or cocaine use. Look for signs of trauma, tongue laceration, or incontinence. Note vital signs. Order lab tests and other diagnostic testing only to investigate your clinical suspicions (Table 34-8). Hospitalize the patient for an underlying illness, recurrent seizures, slow recovery, poor social situation, or nobody to watch the patient.

When a Patient with Known Epilepsy has a Seizure, What Work-up is Warranted?

Obtain drug levels, and compare with the patient's known therapeutic level. Correct low levels. Most new anticonvulsants do not have helpful drug levels; doses are increased until the desired effect is obtained, or side effects are intolerable. The history dictates if other work-up is needed, but this is generally not the case.

TREATMENT

What is a Rational Approach to Treating Seizures?

Designing rational seizure therapy requires you to address three questions: (1) Are the seizures provoked and reversible? (2) If this is the first seizure, what are the chances more will occur? (3) If more seizures are likely, is there a rational therapy? A single tonic-clonic seizure provoked by an identifiable reversible cause should be managed with correction of the underlying problem and does not warrant an anticonvulsant medication. Seizures likely to recur (i.e., owing to slow resolution of the underlying derangement) warrant phenytoin, which can be given initially as an intravenous loading dose of 18 mg/kg. Side effects include

Neurology

Table 34-8

First Seizure Evaluation

Test	Looking for
Lab Tests	
CBC	Infection
Glucose	Hypoglycemia
Electrolytes, calcium, magnesium	Abnormal levels
Toxicology screen	Intoxication
Imaging	
Urgent—CT with and without contrast	Bleeding, trauma, tumor, stroke, signs of infection
Nonurgent—MRI	Better for all of the above, plus vascular malformations
LP*	Cancer
	Infection
	Rare—Behçet's syndrome, CNS sarcoidosis
	Limitation—postictal CSF pleocytosis <80 may occur for days
EEG*	Seizure confirmation and classification
	Information to guide drug therapy and prognosis
	Limitations—sensitivity of 50%-70%, 2% have a false-positive (sensitivity increased by sleep EEG or repeating EEG × 2–3; 24 h closed circuit television EEG monitoring may be helpful)

*Not always required.

hypotension with rapid loading, rash, and rare but potentially life-threatening leukopenia or hepatitis. Phenytoin is a notorious cause of drug fevers. Continuous seizing (status epilepticus) requires a more rapid-acting drug, such as diazepam in 5-mg intravenous boluses.

Predicting a second seizure must take multiple factors into account. If no cause is found, and the EEG is normal, the risk of a second seizure in the next 2 years is about 25%. If there is an identifiable cause or the EEG is positive, the risk is 50%-80%. When the decision is made to use medication, issues to consider include type of seizure, ease of use, side effects, drug monitoring, drug interactions, and cost. Multiple medications are available for the different classes of seizures (Table 34-9). Except for ethosuximide, most of the drugs in the three lists are interchangeable. Although valproic acid is the best drug for many generalized seizure disorders, it does have efficacy in partial seizures. Likewise, phenytoin is an excellent drug for partial seizures and can be used for generalized onset tonic-clonic seizures, although not for myoclonic or absence seizures. Surgical options are occasionally warranted, but beyond the scope of this chapter.

Table 34-9

Treatment of Seizures

	First-line Therapy	Second-line Therapy
Partial Seizures		
Simple complex	Phenytoin, carbamazepine	Lamotrigine
Tonic-clonic, secondary	Phenytoin, carbamazepine	Lamotrigine
Primarily Generalized Seizures		
Tonic-clonic, primary	Valproic acid, carbemazepine	Phenytoin, topiramate
Myoclonic	Valproic acid	Lamotrigine, benzodiazepines
Atonic	Valproic acid	
Absence	Ethosuximide	Valproic acid

MOTOR WEAKNESS

What about Presentation and Diagnosis of Diseases Causing Motor Weakness?

Table 34-10 summarizes the presentation and diagnosis of some diseases causing motor weakness.

Table 34-10

Motor Deficit Syndromes

Syndrome	Presentation	Diagnosis
Amyotrophic lateral sclerosis	Mixed upper and lower motor neuron deficits cause progressive weakness, twitching, wasting, muscle cramps; may involve tongue, palate, gag reflex; spares extraocular muscles; death after 3–5 y	Clinical picture, electrodiagnostic testing
Botulism	Fulminating weakness 12–72 h after ingestion of contaminated food (usually home-canned food); begins with diplopia, ptosis, facial weakness, dysphagia; progresses to respiratory difficulty; no sensory deficits	Test food and stool for *Clostridium botulinum*; repetitive nerve stimulation increases motor response

(continued)

Neurology

Table 34-10

Motor Deficit Syndromes (Continued)

Syndrome	Presentation	Diagnosis
Multiple sclerosis	Focal episodes of weakness, numbness, unsteadiness, visual change, hyperreflexia; episodes relapse and remit over days to months or may be progressive with persistent deficits	MRI shows focal scattered demyelinating plaques in the brain, spinal cord, optic nerves CSF for oligoclonal bands Prolonged evoked potential latencies
Guillain-Barré syndrome	Symmetric ascending weakness beginning in legs and progressing upward at varying rates; usually accompanied by sensory complaints, autonomic disturbances, respiratory muscle involvement	CSF shows increased protein, normal cell count; electrodiagnostic testing shows conduction slowing of sensory and motor nerves
Myasthenia gravis	Weakness that occurs with activity and abates with rest; diplopia and ptosis are almost invariable; sensory is normal	Repetitive nerve stimulation decreases motor response, Acetylcholine receptor antibodies
Poliomyelitis	Prodromal flulike illness followed by focal, asymmetric, rapid-onset weakness; aseptic meningitis; myalgias	RNA virus can be isolated from nasal cultures, stool, CSF

Case 34-1

A 39-year-old man with history of Parkinson's disease is brought to the emergency department with 2 days of worsening mental status. He is oriented to person and year and attempts to get off of the gurney during the interview. His wife says he was complaining of difficulty emptying his bladder since starting a cold medication 5 days ago. On exam, temperature is 100° F (37.7° C), BP is 100/60 mm Hg, and HR is 110 beats/min. He is orthostatic with standing with notable rhinorrhea, but clear lungs. He grimaces with palpation inferior to the umbilicus. His neurologic exam is notable for intact cranial nerves, cogwheeling, a resting tremor, and rigidity right side greater than left.

A. Is this delirium or dementia?
B. What additional history would you obtain from his wife?
C. What studies would you order?
D. Preliminary results show WBC 10, BUN 45, Creatinine 1.8, UA 3+ leukocytes, and bacteria. What treatment would you institute?

Case 34-2

A 39-year-old man 1 hour ago reported nausea and headache to his wife. He began vomiting and developed progressive weakness of his face, right arm, and right leg over the next 30 minutes. His speech began to slur, and now she has to shake him to get him to respond. On exam, BP is 200/120 mm Hg, there is a right facial droop, left pupil is 2 mm larger than right pupil, and there is right upper extremity and right lower extremity hemiparesis. The patient is increasingly difficult to arouse.

A. What do you do first?

B. What is your differential diagnosis?

C. Noncontrast CT scan shows a bright 3-cm lesion next to the left putamen consistent with an intracranial hemorrhage. What additional information do you need from his wife?

D. What additional studies would you obtain, and what interventions would you start immediately?

KEY POINTS – NEUROLOGIC EXAM

◆ Master a 5-minute screening neurologic exam for inpatient admissions and outpatient physicals.

◆ Focus the neurologic exam depending on the clinical situation.

KEY POINTS – ALTERED MENTAL STATUS

◆ Patients with coma need rapid, prioritized evaluation and management.

◆ Altered mental status with fever suggests meningitis, unless pneumonia or UTI is obvious.

◆ Delirium is an acute alteration in mental status that may fluctuate and is usually caused by a medication, infection, or other reversible metabolic or toxic abnormality.

KEY POINTS – STROKE

◆ Hypertension is the most modifiable risk factor for stroke.

◆ Categorizing stroke can help limit the work-up and lead to appropriate treatment.

◆ Aspirin therapy is often the correct choice for secondary stroke prevention.

◆ Do not aggressively reduce BP in patients presenting with ischemic stroke.

KEY POINTS – SEIZURE

◆ Obtain a history and EEG to classify a seizure as partial or primarily generalized.

◆ First-time seizures require evaluation for cause.

◆ Rational therapy is possible; get to know phenytoin well.

Case Answers

34-1 A. *Learning objective:* **Recognize delirium.** The acute onset over 2 days suggests delirium. His underlying Parkinson's disease can be associated with cognitive impairment and may make him more susceptible to delirium from other causes.

34-1 B. *Learning objective:* **Obtain pertinent history in a delirious patient.** Find out about his baseline mental status and function and current and recently added medications. In this case, anticholinergic medications common in over-the-counter cold medications can worsen or cause urinary obstruction and worsen mental status. Parkinson's medications can contribute to delirium, especially if any are new or recently increased. Ask about problems with urination or UTI. Question him about alcohol and substance use or withdrawal and trauma.

34-1 C. *Learning objective:* **Describe the initial work-up for a delirious patient.** In this case, reasonable testing would include CBC, C-reactive protein, UA, glucose, electrolytes, creatinine, urine and blood cultures, PVR bladder scan, and CXR. Consider ECG.

34-1 D. *Learning objective:* **Outline a treatment plan for a delirious patient with potential urosepsis, and recognize anticholinergic medications as a common culprit in the elderly.** Stop all unnecessary medications, and consult a neurologist about his Parkinson's medications. Place a Foley catheter to drain the bladder. Start empiric antibiotics to cover a presumed urosepsis. Begin intravenous and oral volume resuscitation. Start frequent reorientation; avoid restraints, but start fall precautions.

34-2 A. *Learning objective:* **Recognize the presentation of SAH, and appropriately prioritize airway protection and head CT.** Check a gag reflex, and ensure that he is protecting his airway. Monitor vital signs frequently. Intubate and ventilate the patient if necessary, then bring him for immediate noncontrast head CT.

34-2 B. *Learning objective:* **Recognize probable intracranial bleeding in a young patient with sudden neurologic demise.** Differential diagnoses include intracerebral hemorrhage, SAH, ischemic stroke, and epidural hematoma.

Neurology

34-2 C. *Learning objective:* **Identify key history in a patient with stroke.** Find out about prior medical problems, such as hypertension, atrial fibrillation, history of cancers, alcohol use, or stimulant use (e.g., cocaine). Ask about his usual medications. Because hypertensive intracerebral hemorrhage carries an almost 50% mortality, you may want to discuss his resuscitation/code status with his family.

34-2 D. *Learning objective:* **Describe initial work-up and management of stroke.** Obtain CBC with platelets, INR and PTT, ECG, and ABG if ventilated or considering intubating. Consult a neurologist immediately. Start BP lowering with labetalol for a goal systolic pressure of 140–160 mm Hg in patients with documented intracranial bleeding. If INR is elevated >1.5, start reversal with fresh frozen plasma or prothrombin complex concentrates and vitamin K (vitamin K takes 24 hours to be effective). The risk of embolic stroke in atrial fibrillation is about 4% per year without warfarin. If the reason for anticoagulation was a mitral position mechanical valve, the risk for embolic stroke off warfarin is 8% per year. If platelets are <50,000, transfuse platelets.

REFERENCE

Seizure
Brown TR, Holmes GL: Primary care: Epilepsy. N Engl J Med 2001;344:1145.

USEFUL WEB SITE

Dementia
http://www.aan.com.offcampus.lib.washington.edu/professionals/practice/pdfs/
  dementia_guideline.pdf

35

Palliative Care

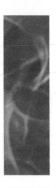

MELISSA M. HAGMAN

What is Palliative Care?

Palliative care is a subspecialty of medicine that uses a multidisciplinary approach to provide comfortable end-of-life care to patients and support for their families and friends.

How do I Know if Palliative Care Might be Appropriate for a Patient?

Consider talking with a patient about palliative care if you would not be surprised if he or she died within a year. Any care (including antibiotics, chemotherapy, and other aggressive interventions) aimed at maximizing a patient's comfort can be included in a palliative care plan. To begin a discussion, first ask permission to talk with the patient about his or her perspective on his or her illness. Ask questions to help define the patient's goals and aid the patient in selecting a care plan that best fits those goals. Frame the discussion so that the patient knows that he or she is the expert on his or her goals, and that the health care providers are the experts in matching therapy to those goals. Consider asking: How do you understand your situation? What are you hoping for? What are your fears or concerns? What gives you strength? Who are the people that support you? What are your past experiences with severe illness? Is there anything else about you or your beliefs that you would like to share?

How can I Manage Pain at End of Life?

For mild pain, begin with nonopioid pain medications, such as acetaminophen or NSAIDs. For more severe or uncontrolled pain, add an opioid. Use adjuvant therapy to augment the benefit of opioids and reduce the necessary opioid dose. Examples of adjuvant treatments include heat and cold therapy, massage, repositioning, antidepressants, anticonvulsants (gabapentin), antispasmotics (oxybutynin), radiation therapy, nerve blocks, support groups, and pastoral counseling. Steroids are particularly helpful for bone pain from metastases or for headaches resulting from increased intracranial pressure. Use noninvasive routes of medication administration whenever possible. Patients on opioids

483

> ### BOX 35-1
>
> **CAUSES OF DYSPNEA AT END OF LIFE (MNEMONIC BREATH AIR) AND POTENTIAL TREATMENTS**
>
> Oxygen supplementation may be useful for many of these causes.
>
> **Causes of Dyspnea and Treatment Options**
>
> Bronchospasm—treat with bronchodilators, steroids
> Rales—treat with diuretics, antibiotics
> Effusion—treat with diuretics, therapeutic thoracentesis
> Airway obstruction—treat with suction, stent placement
> Thick secretions—treat with guaifenesin, fluids
> Hemoglobin low—treat with transfusion
> Anxiety—treat with benzodiazepines, opioids, support groups
> Interpersonal issues—treat with counseling
> Religious concerns—treat with pastoral care

should be proactively treated to prevent constipation. Nausea and itching from opioids usually subside in several days if patients are able to continue on the drug while tolerance develops. Other side effects, such as myoclonus, can develop after longer use of an opioid; treat by switching patients to a different opioid.

How can I Manage Dyspnea at End of Life?

Oxygen and opioids are useful for most causes of dyspnea. In addition, the American Academy of Hospice and Palliative Medicine (www.AAHPM.org) suggests "BREATH AIR" as a mnemonic for causes of dyspnea in patients at the end of life and possibly helpful interventions (Box 35-1). Atropine or scopolamine can be used to reduce secretions.

What is the Principle of Double Effect?

In palliative care, an action having both a good and a bad effect is allowable if the following conditions are met: The act itself is good or at least morally neutral; only the good effect is intended; the good effect is not the result of the bad effect; there is no alternative method of achieving the good effect; there is an appropriately grave reason for taking the action. For example, in a patient with severe shortness of breath not relieved by other measures, opioids may be necessary to treat air hunger and provide comfort. The intended good effect is to relieve the dyspnea. The unintended bad effect is that the opioid also may blunt the patient's respiratory drive.

What if a Patient can no Longer Eat or Drink?

Patients usually lose their appetite as death nears. Family and friends may worry that their loved one is starving, but decrease in appetite is normal as the body prepares itself for death. Parenteral or enteral feeding in patients at the end of life may contribute to pulmonary edema and increase the risk of nausea or aspiration. In most cases, keeping the mouth and lips moist in patients who are no longer eating is all that is necessary to ensure their comfort.

Case 35-1

A 68-year-old man with metastatic renal cell carcinoma and chronic renal failure refused his hemodialysis run today.

    A. Would it be appropriate to talk with this patient about palliative care?
    B. How would you talk with him about palliative care?

Case 35-2

A 71-year-old woman with end-stage liver disease is receiving comfort care. Her hepatic encephalopathy has worsened to the point where she is no longer able to eat or drink. The family is concerned that she is going to "starve to death." What will you tell them?

KEY POINTS

◆ Palliative care is a multidisciplinary specialty that focuses on supporting patients and their loved ones as the patients live the end of their lives.

◆ Palliative care does not mean "no care."

◆ Adjuvant treatments can reduce the amount of opioid needed for pain control and decrease unwanted opioid side effects.

Case Answers

35-1 A. *Learning objective:* **Identify when it is appropriate to talk with patients about end-of-life care.** It would not be surprising if this patient were to die within the next year, and his refusal of dialysis merits investigation. Some patients self-discontinue treatments that they find to be too burdensome. This patient would likely benefit from a palliative care discussion.

35-1 B. *Learning objective:* **Outline how to talk with patients about end-of-life care.** Begin by asking permission to talk with the patient about his understanding of his situation. Elicit information about his hopes, fears, sources of strength, and past experiences with severe illness. Work to match the patient's medical care to his stated goals. In some cases, this might mean a transition to comfort care.

35-2.   *Learning objective:* **Talk with patient and family regarding feeding at the end of life.** Begin by acknowledging that feeding someone is one of the most basic ways in which people show love for one another. As patients near death, however, most lose their appetite and stop eating. At this point, they are not uncomfortable because they are not hungry. Using a wet cloth to keep patients' lips and tongue moist helps prevent the discomfort of dry mouth.

REFERENCES

Manning HL: Dyspnea treatment. Respir Care 2000;45:1342.
Perron V, Schonwetter RS: Assessment and management of pain in palliative care patients. Cancer Control 2001;8:15.

USEFUL WEB SITE

American Academy of Hospice and Palliative Care. www.AAHPM.org

Palliative Care

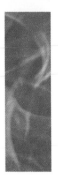

36

Psychiatry

MARY B. MIGEON

 DEPRESSION

ETIOLOGY

How Common is Depression?

Of all causes of death and disability worldwide, depression ranks fourth. Lifetime risk for major depression is 7%-12% in men and 20%-25% in women. Primary care providers recognize only one third to one half of patients with major depression. In one study, 30% of patients presenting with a physical symptom had either depression or anxiety.

Do Medications or Other Substances Cause Depression?

Many medications have been associated with depression, but a clear causal relationship is rare. Medications that are causal in depression should be stopped (Box 36-1). Alcoholism is no more frequent in depressed patients as the general population; however, patients with alcoholism have much higher rates of depression—30% at time of presentation. This suggests that alcoholism is not the result of a patient's attempt to medicate depression with alcohol, but instead the ongoing alcohol abuse results in depression. Some studies support the opposite view—that patients medicate their ongoing psychiatric illness with alcohol.

What is the Interaction of Grief and Depression?

Acute grief, such as over the death of a spouse, has similar symptoms to depression—sorrow, tearfulness, depressed mood, lack of interest, and trouble sleeping. Individuals with normal grief usually maintain self-esteem, and their grief reaction resolves within several months, whereas individuals with grief-related depression may have feelings of worthlessness, and their symptoms can persist for prolonged periods if untreated. In the year after a loss, 15%-35% of grievers develop depression, with resolution in 94%. When grief-related depression is treated with an SSRI, the symptoms of depression resolve, but the intensity of the grief

487

BOX 36-1

MEDICATIONS ASSOCIATED WITH DEPRESSION

Causal

Centrally acting antihypertensives—reserpine, methyldopa, clonidine
CNS depressants—alcohol, sedatives, opiates, psychedelics
Corticosteroids

Possibly Causal

Propranolol
Oral contraceptives, progesterone
Levodopa

---

does not. This may reassure patients who do not wish to "medicate" their loss.

What are Some Subtypes of Depression?

Major depressive disorder is a serious illness with presence of multiple severe symptoms (see later). A subtype, depression with atypical features, includes symptoms of hypersomnia, overeating, lethargy, and rejection sensitivity. One example of this subtype is seasonal affective disorder, which occurs during the short days of winter in far Northern and Southern Hemisphere climates. Another subtype is postpartum depression, occurring 2 weeks to 6 months after delivery. Adjustment disorder with depressed mood occurs in reaction to some identifiable stressor or loss and is usually accompanied by anger and guilt. Dysthymia is a chronic, persistent depressed mood lasting ≥ 2 years, with fewer and milder symptoms than major depression.

What Medical Conditions are Associated with Depression?

Hypothyroidism, Cushing's syndrome, and vitamin B_{12} deficiency are clearly associated with depression. Treatment of these conditions results in improvement or resolution of depression. Many chronic medical conditions are associated with increased rate of depression, although no causative role has been established (Box 36-2). Cancer has the highest incidence (hazard ratio 3.6), followed by chronic lung disease and heart disease (hazard ratio 2.2 for chronic lung disease and 1.5 for heart disease). In most cases, rates of depression are highest shortly after diagnosis and gradually decrease.

EVALUATION

What are the Criteria for Diagnosis of Depression?

Depression is common, but frequently missed. To make the diagnosis of depression, either depressed mood or loss of interest must be present.

BOX 36-2

MEDICAL CONDITIONS AND THEIR ASSOCIATED RISK OF DEPRESSION

Stroke	50%
Diabetes with end-organ damage	70%
MI	40%-65%
Cancer (varies with type and severity)	
Pancreatic	50%
Acute leukemia awaiting transplant	<2%

Include one of these as a question in your review of symptoms. In addition, five of the criteria listed in Box 36-3 should be present for ≥2 weeks. In elderly individuals, irritability, agitation, diminished cognitive function, and sleep disruption are more likely than frank depressed mood. In adolescents, irritability may be the predominant mood state. Ask about suicidality and symptoms suggesting a history of mania or psychosis. Further questions include substance or alcohol abuse history, family or personal history of depression, and recent stressors.

How Can I ask my Patients About Depression Without Making Them Defensive?

It is helpful to question patients about the more physiologic symptoms of depression, such as sleep, food intake, and energy. For example, "How are you sleeping?" investigates the classic pattern of early

BOX 36-3

CRITERIA FOR MAJOR DEPRESSION

Five of the following nine criteria are required to be present for >2 weeks, in the setting of depressed mood or loss of interest or both, for a diagnosis of major depression.

Depressed mood
Anhedonia (loss of interest in most, if not all, activities)
Weight loss or gain (5% of body weight in 1 month)
Appetite loss or gain
Insomnia or hypersomnia
Psychomotor agitation or retardation
Fatigue or loss of energy nearly every day
Feelings of worthlessness or inappropriate guilt
Trouble concentrating, indecision
Recurrent thoughts of death or suicide

morning awakening. You can define depression as a physiologic state that causes the physical symptoms the patient is experiencing before entering into a discussion of mood. This may help patients understand depression as a physiologic condition, rather than something that is "all in their head."

When Should I be Concerned About Bipolar Disorder?

Screen any patient with depressive symptoms for bipolar disorder by asking about any prior or current episodes of symptoms suggesting mania, including hyperactivity, irritability, flight of ideas, hypersexual behavior, impulsivity, spending large amounts of money, sleeplessness, or grandiosity. It is important to rule out bipolar disorder before treating patients for depression because antidepressants may trigger an acute manic episode. Refer patients with a personal history suggesting manic episodes to a psychiatrist to confirm a diagnosis and start treatment.

Should I get any Lab Tests on Patients with Depression?

Because of the potentially causative role, it is reasonable to check TSH and to consider a metabolic panel, including glucose. For patients with elevated glucose, elevated bicarbonate, and low potassium or with cushingoid body habitus (or both), consider 24-hour urine cortisol testing to look for Cushing's syndrome.

If I ask About Suicidal Thoughts, Would This Make My Patient More Likely to Try Suicide?

There is no evidence that asking patients about suicidality makes them more likely to commit suicide. Although these thoughts are common in depression, ask about specific plans and access to means (i.e., guns). Assess risk further by asking about ongoing alcohol or substance abuse, prior personal or family history of suicide attempts, and psychotic symptoms. If a patient is suicidal with a clear plan, contact a social worker or psychiatrist right away so that he or she can assist in admitting the patient for acute inpatient care. Contract with patients for "no self-harm" by having them sign a piece of paper stating that they will not harm themselves.

TREATMENT

Why is Depression Important to Treat?

In addition to the death and disability from depression itself, evidence is mounting that depression has a significant impact on other medical conditions. In one study of patients with MI, concurrent depression was an independent risk factor for mortality equivalent to left ventricular dysfunction. Whether this is due to decreased compliance with medications or other factors is unknown. Although depression may spontaneously remit, untreated depression also may wax and wane, resulting in dysthymia and depression that is more resistant to therapy.

Psychiatry

What are Treatment Options Other Than Traditional Allopathic Medications?

Evidence exists that **psychotherapy** and medications achieve approximately equivalent response rates of 50%-70%. Also, there seems to be a synergistic effect with psychotherapy and medications. Some data suggest that relapse rates are decreased when a patient receives cognitive therapy. Half an hour of **aerobic exercise** three to five times a week has been effective in several studies, although increased social activity may have confounded the results. **St. John's wort** may be effective for mild depression, but is not effective for major depression based on a randomized controlled trial. For seasonal affective disorder, an effective treatment is **light therapy** with a high-intensity, 10,000-lux light box for 15–30 minutes daily during the darker winter months.

Can I Prescribe Medications for Depression Without a Psychiatrist's Help?

Primary care physicians can and should treat uncomplicated cases of depression. In more severe cases with suicidality, poor response to medicine, and complicating psychiatric conditions such as personality disorder, mania, or delusions, refer the patient to a psychiatrist.

What Medication should I Use?

The most common medications currently used to treat depression are SSRIs. A study of SSRIs (sertraline, fluoxetine, and paroxetine) in nearly 600 depressed patients in the general medicine outpatient setting showed two thirds of patients recovered by 9 months. If the patient did not respond to the first SSRI tried, there was a high likelihood of success with switching to a second agent. All three medications had similar rates of side effects, generally related to mild GI distress, agitation, or headache. The serotonin and norepinephrine uptake inhibitors venlafaxine and duloxetine have similar efficacy, but are more expensive currently. Venlafaxine can increase BP. TCA medications are equally effective for depression. Side effects include sedation, dry mouth, constipation, orthostatic hypotension, and potential for cardiac arrhythmia. The last effect makes TCA dangerous in overdose; SSRIs are relatively safe in overdose. Another effect from SSRIs may be sexual side effects, which can range from mild to severe difficulty achieving orgasm. Bupropion, a heterocyclic antidepressant, preserves sexual function in most cases.

How Shall I Counsel My Patient About Starting Medications?

Counsel patients at the outset that side effects often precede symptom improvement. Ask patients to commit to a 4-week medication trial. Compliance is improved if you have the patient return for a visit in 1–2 weeks. Counsel patients that if the first medication is not effective by 2–4 weeks, or isn't tolerated, there are many options for treatment.

How Long are Medications Required?

First-episode depression should be treated for 6–9 months or until symptoms have completely resolved, whichever is longer. When stopping an antidepressant, taper the dose to the lowest possible dosage before cessation. Tapering the medication is important for paroxetine in particular; abrupt cessation may result in a self-limited but unpleasant withdrawal syndrome of dysequilibrium. If depression recurs shortly after cessation, longer term therapy is necessary. With a third recurrence of depression, lifelong medication is recommended.

When Should I Combine Medications?

For marked sleep disturbance, add a low dose of a sedating antidepressant at bedtime, such as 10–25 mg of doxepin or 50 mg of trazodone. Use caution with benzodiazepines for insomnia, even briefly, because of their addictive potential. Do not try to combine high-dose antidepressants; monoamine oxidase inhibitors with SSRIs can be lethal (see serotonin syndrome later). Refer to a psychiatrist for refractory depression. Low-dose bupropion or lithium and T3 (thyroid hormone) are increasingly used as an adjuncts to SSRI treatment, particularly for refractory depression.

When Should I Start an Antidepressant Other Than an SSRI?

In patients with chronic pain, particularly neuropathic pain, medication options are TCA, duloxetine, venlafaxine, and bupropion. Although SSRIs treat the depression that often accompanies chronic pain, they are less effective than the previously listed medications for the pain itself. If there is a history of significant sexual dysfunction, consider selecting another class of drug rather than SSRIs, such as bupropion. Depression itself often manifests with decreased libido. For smokers interested in cessation, data support bupropion as an aid. Mirtazapine is sedating and can cause weight gain. It is helpful in depressed patients who have lost weight and need to regain the weight. It also is an option in patients who have severe insomnia as part of their depression.

When Should I Prescribe Benzodiazepines for Anxious Patients?

Generalized anxiety disorder is a relatively uncommon condition. By contrast, depression manifesting as anxiety is common. A patient who seems anxious or overly concerned about his or her medical condition needs an evaluation for anxiety and depression. Benzodiazepines can be used to treat a patient's insomnia and agitation short-term until the antidepressant begins to take effect. Because of the addiction risk with benzodiazepines, this should be done cautiously, with explicit intention to convert completely to an antidepressant.

What is a Depressed Patient's Prognosis?

Most depression resolves at 1 year without any intervention. Antidepressants or psychotherapy or both shorten this interval to 1–2 months. Of

Psychiatry

patients, 50% are cured with first-time therapy, and depression never recurs. In 50% of patients, depression does return when medications are stopped. Of patients who experience recurrence, another 50% never have another episode. Ten percent of patients with depression have chronic symptoms.

What Would Happen if My Patient Stopped His or Her Medication Abruptly?

With some antidepressants, there is a withdrawal syndrome. This is most profound with shorter acting SSRIs, such as paroxetine, from which withdrawal can precipitate sudden episodes of dysequilibrium and imbalance. This resolves in about 1 week after discontinuation of the medication.

What is Serotonin Syndrome?

Serotonin syndrome causes agitation, mental status changes, diarrhea, and autonomic changes such as hypertension and fever and occurs when serotonin-producing or serotonin-sparing medications are combined. Although there have been case reports of numerous medications, the most common culprits are SSRIs with either monoamine oxidase inhibitors or high-dose TCA. SSRIs combined with cocaine and reserpines also may result in this syndrome.

KEY POINTS

◆ Depression is common and responds to medications, counseling, and exercise.

◆ Most patients can be managed in the primary care setting.

◆ Suicidality, symptoms of mania, and poor response to therapy require referral to psychiatry.

Case 36-1

A 78-year-old woman with DM and hypertension is brought to the clinic by her son, who is concerned about her memory and her lack of interest in her life. She is agitated with him and vehemently denies she is depressed and states that she is just "tired." Her mini-mental score is 27/30, and her neurologic exam is grossly normal

    A. What is your differential diagnosis?
    B. What further questions do you want to ask?
    C. What further testing would you order?
    D. If her lab tests and exam are normal, what medication might you recommend?

Case 36-2

A 24-year-old man comes to the clinic after breaking up with his girlfriend. He reports several weeks of sleeplessness, agitation, poor appetite, and trouble concentrating on his graduate studies. He feels he is depressed and states that his father has been depressed. When pressed, he acknowledges feeling suicidal once a few weeks ago. He adamantly refuses any medication.

- A. Does he meet criteria for depression?
- B. What further questions do you want to ask to assess his suicide risk?
- C. What questions can you ask him about his concern about medications?
- D. What options can you provide him for treatment for his depression?

Case Answers

36-1 A.   *Learning objective:* **Outline a differential diagnosis for an elderly woman with mild memory deficits.** Early Alzheimer's disease, multi-infarct dementia, electrolyte abnormalities, polypharmacy, vitamin B_{12} deficiency, alcohol abuse, pulmonary or genitourinary infections, thyroid disease, subdural hemorrhage, and depression all might be contributing factors in this woman. Recognize that absence of depressed mood does not exclude the diagnosis of depression.

36-1 B.   *Learning objective:* **Devise questions for the history in a woman in whom you suspect depression may be a possibility.** Ask about sleep pattern, anhedonia, depressed mood, suicidality, change in appetite, weight loss or gain, concentration, and excessive guilt. To investigate nonpsychiatric causes further, inquire about recent blood glucose recordings (has she had hypoglycemic episodes); balance or gait difficulties suggesting stroke or vitamin B_{12} deficiency; falls contributing to subdural hemorrhage; or heat or cold intolerance, constipation, or other findings of thyroid disease. Because a family history of depression makes this condition more likely, ask patients about family history of depression or bipolar disorder. Also ask about family history of dementia or stroke.

36-1 C.   *Learning objective:* **Order appropriate lab tests when considering depression in an elderly patient.** Order TSH, electrolytes, and calcium; consider a CXR or UA if chest or genitourinary symptoms are present, respectively. If there are abnormalities on the neurologic exam or a recent fall, consider a contrast head CT scan.

36-1 D.   *Learning objective:* **Identify a trial of SSRI as a reasonable course in an elderly patient with cognitive deficits, otherwise normal lab tests and exam, and findings consistent with depression.** In this patient, start an SSRI with cautions about side effects and expected response within 4 weeks. If she does not improve, consider switching to a second agent. Retest memory when and if depressive symptoms improve.

36-2 A. *Learning objective:* **List criteria for depression.** This patient has at least five criteria: depressed mood, sleep disruption, agitation, trouble concentrating, decreased appetite, and suicidality.

36-2 B. *Learning objective:* **Clarify risk of suicide in a depressed patient.** Ask him about suicidal ideation and any specific plans. Find out whether he has access to guns or prescription medications.

36-2 C. *Learning objective:* **When patients are reluctant to take medications, explore the source of their resistance.** Ask this young man about his father's response to medications because older treatments were often not well tolerated and at times ineffective. Inquire further about manic-depressive symptoms in him and his father. Ask if he has been on medications previously, and how he responded. Inquire as to his attitude about depression and medical therapy; many patients consider depression a character flaw.

36-2 D. *Learning objective:* **Identify alternative methods of treating depression.** This young man needs intensive treatment for his depression, but it is his right to refuse medication. Offer him counseling as an option, particularly given his acute grief over his ended relationship. Provide him with several names and phone numbers of reliable therapists. Recommend that he abstain from all alcohol and substance abuse. He should exercise to a good sweat three to five times a week.

REFERENCES

Kroenke K, West SL, Swindle R, et al: Similar effectiveness of paroxetine, fluoxetine, and sertraline in primary care: A randomized trial. JAMA 2001;286:2947.

Schulberg HC, Katon W, Simon GE, et al: Treating major depression in primary care practice: An update of the Agency for Health Care Policy and Research Practice Guidelines. Arch Gen Psychiatry 1998;55:1121.

Snow V, Lascher S, Mottur-Pilson C: Pharmacologic treatment of acute depression and dysthymia. Ann Intern Med 2000;132:738.

Williams JW Jr, Barrett J, Oxman T, et al: Treatment of dysthymia and minor depression in primary care: A randomized controlled trial in older adults. JAMA 2000;284:1519.

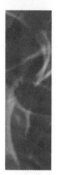

37

Pulmonary Diseases

KARNA GENDO, ROBERT R. KEMPAINEN, and
LINDSEY S. KLAFF

 ASTHMA

ETIOLOGY

What is Asthma?

Asthma is a chronic inflammatory disorder of the airways. Inflammation increases airway responsiveness and changes airway architecture by airway epithelium denudation, collagen deposition beneath the basement membrane, airway edema, inflammatory cell infiltration (especially mast cells, eosinophils, and T lymphocytes), hypertrophy of bronchial smooth muscle and mucous glands, and plugging of small airways with thick mucus. Symptoms include wheezing, dyspnea, chest tightness, and cough, particularly at night or in the early morning (or both) and are associated with variable airflow obstruction that is at least partly reversible spontaneously or with treatment. Currently, approximately 5% of the population has asthma. The highest asthma mortality rates are among African Americans 15 to 24 years old. Each year, approximately 470,000 hospital admissions and 5000 deaths in the U.S. are attributed to asthma.

What can Precipitate Symptoms?

Patients with allergic asthma have worsening of symptoms after exposure to allergens, such as pollens, animal proteins, dust mites, and molds. Nonspecific precipitants of asthma include tobacco smoke, exercise, upper respiratory tract infections, rhinitis, sinusitis, postnasal drip, aspiration, gastroesophageal reflux, cold air, and stress. Agents in the workplace can trigger occupational asthma, and symptoms may occur weeks to years after initial exposure and sensitization. Certain individuals may experience asthma symptoms after exposure to aspirin or NSAIDs. Aspirin-induced asthma often occurs as a triad of nasal polyps, aspirin sensitivity, and wheezing (Samter's triad).

496

What Causes Wheezing?

Wheezing is caused by oscillation of opposing walls of an airway that is narrowed almost to the point of closure. In patients referred to a pulmonary outpatient clinic, postnasal drip syndrome was the most common cause of wheeze. It is important to be aware that "All that wheezes is not asthma, all that is asthma does not always wheeze, and all that wheezes is obstruction." Many conditions are associated with wheezing and bronchial hyperresponsiveness (Box 37-1).

Why is Asthma Classified by Severity?

To guide therapy, the National Asthma Education Project Program suggests categorizing asthma severity as mild-intermittent, mild-persistent, moderate-persistent, or severe-persistent (Table 37-1). Although these categories describe the chronic condition, even patients with mild-intermittent disease can have exacerbations severe enough to warrant hospitalization.

EVALUATION

How Can I Use the History in the Diagnosis of Asthma?

Symptoms of asthma include cough, wheeze, dyspnea, chest discomfort, phlegm production, and hyperventilation syndrome. These symptoms

BOX 37-1

CONDITIONS ASSOCIATED WITH WHEEZING AND BRONCHIAL HYPERRESPONSIVENESS

Common Causes

- Allergic rhinitis
- Apparently normal patients
- COPD
- First-degree relatives of asthma patients
- GERD
- Irritant exposure
- Left ventricular failure
- Postviral reactive airway disease
- Smoking

Less Common Causes

- Chronic eosinophilic pneumonia
- Churg-Strauss syndrome
- Cystic fibrosis
- Extrathoracic obstruction, including vocal cord dysfunction
- Mechanical obstruction—tracheal stenosis, tracheomalacia, neoplasm or inflammatory mass, foreign body
- Quadriplegia or high paraplegia
- Pulmonary embolism
- Sarcoidosis

Table 37-1

NAEPP* Classification of Asthma and Suggested Pharmacotherapy

Asthma Severity	Symptoms	Nighttime Symptoms	Lung Function	Pharmacotherapy
Mild intermittent step 1	≤2×/wk Asymptomatic between exacerbations	≤2×/mo	FEV_1 ≥80%	Short-acting beta$_2$ agonists as needed
Mild persistent step 2	≥2×/wk, but <1×/d May have exertional asthma	≥2×/mo	FEV_1 ≥80%	Low-dose ICS, leukotriene modifiers, theophylline, cromolyn, or nedocromil
Moderate persistent step 3	Daily symptoms Exacerbations ≥2 days a week or lasting days	≥1×/mo	FEV_1 ≥60% but <80%	Low-dose/medium-dose ICS LABA Medium-dose ICS Low-dose/medium-dose ICS plus either leukotriene modifier or theophylline
Severe persistent step 4	Continual symptoms Reduced physical activity Frequent exacerbations	Frequent	FEV_1 ≤60%	High-dose ICS and LABA plus systemic corticosteroids if needed Consider monoclonal anti-IgE

Note: Top severity within any category determines classification. All four classifications may have severe and life-threatening exacerbations.

FEV_1, forced expiratory volume in 1 second; ICS, inhaled corticosteroid; LABA, long-acting beta$_2$ agonist.

*National Asthma Education and Prevention Project.

tend to be episodic and respond favorably to specific asthma treatment. Several studies have evaluated the diagnostic characteristics of the "classic triad" of symptoms and found that 35% of patients with persistent wheezing, 24% of patients with chronic cough, and 29% of patients with chronic dyspnea were eventually diagnosed with asthma. In patients presenting with chronic dyspnea, a history of wheezing had a PPV of 42% and a NPV of 83%. Wheezing on physical exam is a poor predictor of the severity of airflow obstruction in asthma. It alerts one to the likely presence of some degree of airway narrowing and the need to measure lung function.

How do I Document Reversible Airway Obstruction?

Office spirometry suggests airway obstruction when forced expiratory volume in 1 second (FEV_1) or FEV_1/forced vital capacity (FVC) ratio or both are reduced to <80% predicted. Significant reversibility of airflow obstruction is defined by an increase of $\geq$12% and 200 mL in FEV_1 or $\geq$15% and 200 mL in FVC after inhaling a short-acting bronchodilator. The absence of improvement in airflow after use of albuterol is not proof of irreversible airflow obstruction, however, and asthmatics with a normal FEV_1 can have increases in FEV_1 after bronchodilator use.

What if a Patient has a History Suggestive of Asthma but Normal Spirometry?

The diagnosis of asthma can be supported with the use of methacholine challenge testing, or peak flow monitoring. A low PC20 (the concentration of inhaled methacholine needed to cause a 20% decrease in FEV_1) on methacholine challenge testing supports a diagnosis of asthma. The use of methacholine challenge testing is limited by its labor-intensity, cost, small risk of inducing severe bronchospasm, and 25% positive test result in patients with allergic rhinitis without asthma. A reliable series of peak flow measurements over 2 weeks that documents >20% variability (especially when reductions are associated with asthmatic symptoms) supports the diagnosis of asthma. The use of peak flow monitoring is limited by its significant dependence on patient effort.

What Key Questions Should I Ask a Patient with Asthma?

- Description of symptoms—when they occur (e.g., day or night, season of the year, during final exams), how long they last, what triggers them, what makes them better, and where they occur (e.g., at work, at home, on the softball field); symptoms at nighttime, with exercise intolerance, with cough, or suggestive of GERD
- Past asthma history—prior emergency department visits, hospitalizations, intubations, childhood symptoms
- Other allergy history—allergic rhinitis, eczema, urticaria, previous skin testing, or allergies to aspirin or NSAIDs

- Family medical history—asthma or other allergy-like syndromes in parents and siblings
- Home environment—carpets, dust collectors (e.g., books, stuffed animals), plants, pets
- Work environment—chemical exposures, animal exposures, workday symptoms improve off work and on vacation
- Medication use—current and past prescriptions, over-the-counter and alternative therapies. Beta blocker and NSAID use is especially important
- Use of tobacco or inhaled street drugs—often make asthma more difficult to treat

What are the Key Features of an Outpatient Evaluation for Asthma?

Obtain history by asking key questions to gauge severity of symptoms. Physical exam usually shows normal vital signs and breath sounds that range from normal to diffuse end-expiratory wheezing. The expiratory phase time may be prolonged. There may be signs of other allergic disease, such as conjunctival erythema or dermatitis. Also use the exam to rule out cardiac disease or other significant lung disease. Office spirometry is essential; many patients with seemingly mild symptoms can have alarmingly compromised lung function. CXR can exclude other diagnoses, but is not recommended as a routine initial test. Eosinophilia is neither sensitive nor specific. Allergy skin testing (or in vitro specific IgE tests, i.e., ImmunoCAP) may help identify specific allergens to avoid or may guide immunotherapy. Ask the patient to keep an asthma diary, including peak flow monitoring, to assist with diagnosis and guide treatment. Periodic assessment of psychosocial status, adherence and compliance, medication side effects and review of written asthma action plan also are helpful.

TREATMENT

What are the Goals of Asthma Therapy?

The goals of asthma therapy are to prevent chronic and troublesome symptoms, maintain normal or near-normal pulmonary function and activity levels, prevent recurrent exacerbations and permanent pulmonary impairment, and provide optimal pharmacotherapy with minimal or no adverse effects. Well-controlled asthma is defined as symptoms twice a week or less; rescue bronchodilator use twice a week or less; normal or personal best peak flow or FEV_1; no nighttime or early morning awakening; and no limitations on exercise, work, or school.

What is the Best Therapy for Chronic Asthma?

Asthma requires a three-pronged approach: (1) control inflammation, (2) relieve acute bronchoconstriction, and (3) control precipitants (Table 37-2). For all but the mildest intermittent asthma, you must address all three components. Patient education and a patient action plan are essential to successful long-term therapy. The amount of

Table 37-2		
Three Fundamental Components of Asthma Therapy		
	Examples	**When to Use**
Control Inflammation	Corticosteroid: inhaled, oral, or intravenous Leukotriene antagonist Mast cell stabilizer Anti-IgE/omalizumab (q2–4wk)	Daily
Relieve Bronchoconstriction	Beta$_2$ agonist inhaler Anticholinergic inhaler Theophylline tablet	As needed for symptoms
Control Precipitants	Environmental modifications such as carpet removal, cockroach extermination, pet removal, allergen-impermeable mattress/pillow/box spring covers, bedding washing in hot water, HEPA filter vacuuming, dilute chlorine bleach cleaning of bathroom and kitchen, HEPA air filters GERD therapy Allergy referral for testing and immunotherapy Influenza, pneumococcal vaccines Intranasal steroids for rhinitis Smoking cessation Allergic rhinitis/sinusitis treatment Remove occupational triggers	In all cases, as dictated by exposures, allergies, and comorbidities

HEPA, high-efficiency particulate air

anti-inflammatory medication and frequency of dosing are dictated by asthma severity and control. Inhaled corticosteroids are the preferred anti-inflammatory medications because they significantly improve lung function, symptoms, and mortality and have a low side-effect profile. Leukotriene antagonists modestly improve symptoms and lung function by decreasing airway inflammation and bronchoconstriction, especially in exercise-induced and aspirin-induced asthma (Table 37-3). To relieve acute bronchoconstriction, use beta$_2$ agonists, such as albuterol and metaproterenol, which relax airway smooth muscle. Salmeterol is a long-acting beta$_2$ agonist with a slow onset of action; it is useful in preventing nocturnal wheezing, but is not helpful in relieving acute bronchoconstriction. Theophylline is a less potent bronchodilating adenosine antagonist with a narrow therapeutic index. Cromolyn and nedocromil are less potent mast cell stabilizers, which prevent

Table 37-3

Medications Used in Asthma

ICS*

Beclomethasone (Vanceril, Beclovent)	2–4 puffs bid-qid (40 μg, 80 μg) max 320 μg
Triamcinolone (Azmacort)	2 puffs tid-qid or 4 puffs bid (100 μg)
Flunisolide HFA (Aerobid)	2 puffs bid (160 μg)
Budesonide (Pulmicort)	1–2 puffs bid (200 μg)
Fluticasone (Flovent)	2–4 puffs bid (110 μg, 220 μg)
Mometasone (Asmanex)	1–2 inhalations qPM-bid (220 μg)

Leukotriene Antagonists†

Montelukast (Singulair)	10 mg PO qd
Zafirlukast (Accolate)	20 mg PO bid 1 h before or 2 h after meals
Zileuton (Zyflo)	600 mg PO qid (check LFT for the first 3 mo)

Mast Cell Stabilizers

Cromolyn (Intal)	2–4 puffs tid-qid
Nedocromil (Tilade)	2–4 puffs bid-qid

Monoclonal Antibody

Omalizumab (Xolair)	150–375 mg subcutaneously q2–4wk

Short-Acting Beta$_2$ Agonists

Albuterol (Proventil, Ventolin)	2–4 puffs q4–6h prn for symptoms or before exercise
Levalbuterol (Xopenex HFA)	2 puffs q4–6h prn for asthma symptoms
Pirbuterol (Maxair)	1–2 puffs q4–6h prn for asthma symptoms
Metaproterenol (Alupent)	2–3 puffs q3–4h prn for asthma symptoms

Anticholinergic Agents

Ipratropium (Atrovent)	1–2 puffs q4–6h prn for asthma symptoms

LABA

Salmeterol (Serevent Diskus)	1 inhalation bid
Formoterol (Foradil)	1 inhalation bid

Methylxanthines

Theophylline (Theo-Dur and others)	100–400 mg PO bid; follow serum levels

Combined ICS/LABA

Fluticasone/salmeterol (Advair)	1 inhalation bid (100, 250, 500/50)

ICS, inhaled corticosteroid; LABA, long-acting beta$_2$ agonist.
*Listed from minimum to maximum potency.
†Rare cases of eosinophilic vasculitis (Churg-Strauss syndrome) have occurred among patients withdrawn from oral steroids after beginning a leukotriene antagonist.

bronchospasm and airway inflammation from allergens and exercise when taken before exposure. For patients intolerant of beta$_2$ agonists, inhaled anticholinergics, such as ipratropium, can provide short-term relief. Combined use of beta$_2$ agonists and anticholinergics used in

Table 37-4
Suggested Hospital Admission Criteria for Asthma

Failure of outpatient or emergency department treatment
Persistent and worsening dyspnea or wheeze
FEV_1 or PEFR <50%-70% predicted
Comorbid diseases
Hypoxia or hypercarbia on ABG
Altered mental status
Complications of pneumothorax, pneumomediastinum, pneumonia, or fatigue
Factors that should favor admission
    Prior intubation
    Recent emergency department visit
    Multiple emergency department visits or hospitalizations
    Symptoms for >1 wk
    Current use of systemic steroids
    Inadequate follow-up mechanisms
    Psychiatric illness
    Inability to speak in full sentences
    Use of accessory muscles for breathing

FEV_1, forced expiratory volume in 1 second; PEFR, peak expiratory flow rate.

treating acute asthma in the emergency department can reduce the hospital admission rate (Table 37-4).

How do you Treat Acute Asthma Exacerbations?

Each patient should have a written action plan that guides initial self-management based on peak flow measurements. Mild exacerbations are treated with increases in inhaled beta$_2$ agonist frequency, increased inhaled steroids, and control or avoidance of precipitants; antibiotics if indicated, oral steroid therapy, and a plan for when to go to the emergency department are additional treatment considerations. For severe acute asthma exacerbation, emergency department management is warranted for immediate systemic corticosteroids, given as oral prednisone 40–60 mg (or 1 mg/kg) or intravenous methylprednisolone 60–125 mg. This takes effect in 4–6 hours. Give repeated nebulized albuterol (combined with ipratropium, if necessary) and supplemental oxygen if the patient is hypoxic. Epinephrine can be considered in severe exacerbations if inhaled bronchodilators are ineffective. Intravenous magnesium can be considered for severe, acute exacerbations. The use of intravenous aminophylline is limited by its toxicity and lack of additional bronchodilation compared with standard care with beta$_2$ agonists. Observe for signs of improvement, and measure the peak flow before discharging. If clinically improved and stable, discharge on oral steroids at 40–60 mg daily with a rapid taper over the ensuing week, and increase the intensity of anti-inflammatory treatment to prevent a recurrence of symptoms.

What Medications Should I Avoid or Use Cautiously in Patients with Asthma?

Aspirin, NSAIDs, beta blockers (including glaucoma eye drops), medications possessing anticholinesterase properties (i.e., myasthenia gravis treatment agents), and parasympathomimetic agents (e.g., pilocarpine) can worsen bronchospasm to varying degrees in patients with asthma. More recent studies have suggested, however, that cardioselective beta blockers are safe for patients with asthma.

What can be Done for a Severe Asthmatic Who Does Not Respond to Usual Therapy?

Observe the patient's metered-dose inhaler technique, and review medication adherence. Review the known asthma precipitants, and try to identify others. Send for allergy testing. Try a trial of therapy for GERD, even if asymptomatic, with H_2 blockers or PPIs. Reconsider the diagnosis; other less common diseases, such as cardiac ischemia, vocal cord dysfunction, allergic bronchopulmonary aspergillosis, cystic fibrosis, alpha-1-antitrypsin deficiency, or endobronchial lesions, may be present. Refer to a pulmonary specialist for further treatment recommendations and evaluation. There are rare asthmatics who are dependent on or resistant to corticosteroids. These patients can be treated with other agents, such as omalizumab or methotrexate, after other diagnoses have been ruled out.

What are the Side Effects of Steroids?

Oral steroids in the short-term can cause psychosis, hypertension, hypokalemia, and glucose intolerance. Long-term use of oral steroids or of high dose inhaled steroids (usually >1000 µg/d) can cause osteoporosis, immunosuppression, elevated intraocular pressure, avascular necrosis, and cataracts. Using spacers and mouth rinsing can minimize systemic absorption of inhaled steroids. Ciclesonide is a new-generation inhaled steroid with unique pharmacologic characteristics resulting in reduced local adverse effects, lack of cortisol suppression, greatly reduced systemic effects, and the option for once-daily dosing.

When Should an Asthmatic with an Acute Exacerbation be Hospitalized?

Admission can be considered for patients with failure of outpatient treatment, persistent and worsening dyspnea, FEV_1 or peak expiratory flow rate <50% predicted, comorbid diseases, hypoxia or hypercarbia on ABG, and altered mental status (see Table 37-4). When deciding whether to hospitalize, always err on the side of patient safety.

Case 37-1

A 30-year-old woman complains of increasing difficulty controlling her asthma since moving to a new house. She has had asthma since childhood and has managed well with occasional use of her albuterol inhaler until recently, when she has used it almost daily. She reports frequent coughing and occasional chest tightness, with nighttime awakenings because of asthma symptoms.

A. What further history would be helpful?
B. What are your next steps in therapy?
C. What information do you share regarding the risks and benefits of treatment?

Case 37-2

A 52-year-old woman with asthma calls you stating that for the last 3 days she has been feeling wheezy and short of breath. About 1 week ago, she had URI symptoms after visiting her grandchild. You try to ask her some questions on the phone, but she is able to answer you only in short two- to three-word answers.

A. What do you do?
B. How should she be evaluated?
C. Should this patient be hospitalized?

Answers appear on pages 516–517.

CHRONIC OBSTRUCTIVE PULMONARY DISEASE

ETIOLOGY

What is COPD?

COPD is a chronic, typically progressive disorder characterized by persistent respiratory symptoms in the presence of partially irreversible airflow obstruction. The cough and dyspnea experienced by patients with COPD result from chronic bronchitis and emphysema, the primary disease processes of COPD. **Chronic bronchitis** is diagnosed clinically and is defined as the presence of a productive cough on most days for a minimum of 3 months per year for at least 2 consecutive years in the absence of another discernible cause. **Emphysema** is characterized by permanent enlargement and destruction of the alveolar airspaces and respiratory bronchioles with loss of the surrounding pulmonary capillaries. Most patients with COPD have varying degrees of chronic bronchitis and emphysema. Although an "asthmatic" or reversible component is often present, some degree of irreversible airflow obstruction persists. Episodic, completely reversible airflow limitation suggests asthma rather than COPD. Irreversible airflow obstruction develops in a few asthmatics, blurring the lines between asthma and COPD. Sputum production can occur with asthma and COPD and is not a helpful discriminator.

What are Risk Factors for COPD?

Of the risks for developing COPD, 80%-90% comes from cigarette smoking. Pipe and cigar smokers have a risk intermediate between cigarette smokers and nonsmokers. Only 10%-15% of smokers develop clinically significant COPD, however, indicating the importance of genetic factors in the pathogenesis of COPD. Other risk factors for COPD include alpha-1-antitrypsin deficiency, air pollution, exposure to occupational dusts and chemicals, intravenous methylphenidate (Ritalin) use, and possibly childhood respiratory infections.

What Causes COPD Exacerbations?

COPD exacerbations are characterized by increases in cough, sputum production, sputum purulence, and dyspnea. Respiratory tract infections are a known trigger, but the relative importance of viral and bacterial pathogens is controversial. Noncompliance with medications and environmental factors such as exposure to dusts, fumes, pollens, and tobacco smoke and weather changes also play a role. In about one third of patients, the cause is unknown.

EVALUATION

How do Patients with COPD Present?

The presence of chronic cough, sputum production, and dyspnea in the setting of chronic tobacco use is highly suggestive of COPD. Cough is the most common symptom and may precede airflow limitation by many years. Patients tend to present to the physician with exertional dyspnea, however, at which point extensive, irreversible airway destruction may be present. To diagnose COPD earlier in the course of disease, obtain spirometry in all patients with chronic cough and exposure to risk factors, regardless of whether dyspnea is present. Differential diagnosis for the presentation of cough and dyspnea includes asthma, CHF, bronchiectasis, pneumonia, malignancy, and pulmonary embolism.

What Exam Findings Suggest COPD?

Exam findings of COPD include decreased breath sounds, wheezes, rhonchi, and prolonged expiration. Look for tobacco staining of the fingertips or teeth. In advanced disease, look for barrel-shaped chest, pursed lip breathing, emaciation, and accessory muscle use. Cor pulmonale is defined as right ventricular enlargement caused by lung disease. This often accompanies late COPD, in which destruction of the pulmonary vascular bed, along with vasoconstriction from chronic hypoxemia and hypercapnia, increases pulmonary arterial pressures and right ventricular afterload. The resulting right ventricular hypertrophy and pulmonary hypertension manifest as a loud S_2 and right-sided gallop or murmur or both. Sustained cor pulmonale results in right heart failure with elevated neck veins, hepatic congestion manifesting as an enlarged tender liver, and lower extremity edema.

What Tests are Appropriate for the Evaluation of COPD?

Postbronchodilator spirometry reveals an FEV_1/FVC ratio <0.70, indicating airflow obstruction, which, in the proper clinical setting, confirms the diagnosis of COPD. The American Thoracic Society has suggested using the postbronchodilator percentage of predicted FEV_1 to judge severity of COPD: FEV_1 >80%, mild; 50%-80%, moderate; 30%-50% severe; <30%, very severe. In patients with advanced disease, obtain an ABG to assess hypoxemia and to establish baseline degree of carbon dioxide retention. CXR may reveal flattened diaphragms and bullae, but these findings are nondiagnostic, and radiographs are primarily useful for excluding other diagnoses.

What are Common Complications of COPD?

Anorexia and weight loss are common in advanced disease. Poor nutrition, steroid use, and smoking all increase the risk of osteoporosis. Depression and anxiety frequently accompany COPD, but often go unrecognized despite a significant effect on quality of life. Polycythemia may develop in response to chronic hypoxemia. Advanced COPD is almost invariably accompanied by cor pulmonale. Structural changes of the right heart, along with hypoxemia and high doses of beta agonist bronchodilators, trigger a variety of arrhythmias (e.g., multifocal atrial tachycardia, atrial fibrillation, VT, and premature beats). Pneumothorax is more common in COPD; even small pneumothoraces can cause life-threatening respiratory failure in patients with limited ventilatory reserve. Leaks are often slow to heal and may require surgical management.

TREATMENT

What Nonpharmacologic Interventions are Available for Stable COPD?

Smoking cessation is the most effective means of slowing the progression of disease and should be pursued aggressively in all smokers. Reduction or elimination of occupational exposures is important in patients with work-related disease. Yearly influenza vaccination reduces COPD morbidity and mortality. Less compelling evidence is available for pneumococcal vaccine, but the Advisory Committee on Immunization Practices (ACIP) recommends it for patients with COPD. Long-term continuous oxygen therapy improves survival in patients with severe hypoxemia (Pao_2 ≤55 mm Hg or oxygen saturation <88%) and in patients with Pao_2 ≤59 mm Hg plus cor pulmonale or polycythemia. Intermittent oxygen is appropriate for patients who experience desaturation exclusively during exercise or sleep. Pulmonary rehabilitation, a comprehensive program to address deconditioning, weight loss, medication compliance, and psychosocial well-being, improves exercise tolerance and decreases symptoms at all stages of disease. Carefully selected patients with severe, debilitating disease may benefit from lung volume reduction surgery or lung transplantation.

What Pharmacologic Options are Available for Stable COPD?

Pharmacotherapy improves symptoms and reduces the frequency of exacerbations, but does not alter the progressive decline in lung function. Inhaled bronchodilators are first-line therapy for all symptomatic patients. Availability and patient response dictate whether a short-acting beta$_2$ agonist, such as albuterol, or an anticholinergic, such as ipratropium bromide, is used initially. Combining drugs from each class has an additive effect. Long-acting beta$_2$ agonists or a long-acting anticholinergic, tiotropium, or both are appropriate for patients requiring frequent use of short-acting bronchodilators or experiencing frequent exacerbations. Because of toxicity risk, methylxanthines, such as theophylline, generally are used as second-line bronchodilators. The use of inhaled corticosteroids in stable COPD is controversial. Symptomatic patients with either a combination of severe disease and frequent exacerbations or an objective response to a 6-week trial of therapy (FEV$_1$ improvement of 15% and at least 200 mL) are most likely to benefit. It is important to review proper inhaler technique periodically and encourage the use of spacer devices.

What Therapies are Appropriate for Exacerbations of COPD?

The initial management of a COPD exacerbation consists of a rapid assessment for an alternative diagnosis, while providing treatments that decrease the need for intubation (Table 37-5). Hypoxemia typically corrects easily with low levels of supplemental oxygen; oxygen saturation around 90% is adequate. Steroids reduce the need for hospitalization and shorten hospital stays. Antibiotics are frequently used for the triad of increased dyspnea, sputum production, and sputum purulence, although data supporting this are limited.

What is the Role of Noninvasive Ventilation?

Noninvasive positive pressure ventilation (NIPPV) plays an increasingly important role in the management of COPD exacerbations. Early initiation of NIPPV in patients with moderate-to-severe respiratory distress improves gas exchange and reduces mortality and the need for mechanical ventilation. NIPPV is labor-intensive and requires close monitoring by experienced personnel. The decision to proceed to intubation is complex and multifactorial. In general, patients with progressive respiratory failure and distress despite maximal medical therapy and a 1- to 2-hour trial of NIPPV should be intubated unless their preference is to forego mechanical ventilation.

Case 37-3

A 48-year-old woman presents to the clinic for the first time with a 4-year history of asthma. Exercise is consistently limited by dyspnea to walking three or four blocks. She is a former smoker with a 30-pack-year history. Her symptoms persist despite long-term prednisone 10 mg/d and albuterol metered-dose inhaler 14 puffs/d. On exam, she is lean and alert, with normal vital signs and oxygen saturation. Breath sounds are clear but decreased, and the ratio of expiratory to inspiratory time is increased to 3:1. Heart sounds are distant, JVP is 7 cm H$_2$O, and

Table 37-5

Management of Acute COPD Exacerbations

Initial
Assess severity
  VS, RR, ABG, WOB, LOC
NIPPV for moderate-to-severe exacerbation
  Contraindications—severely decreased LOC, increased secretions, respiratory arrest,
    facial deformity/surgery, cardiovascular instability, upper GI bleed
Consider intubation if not suitable for NIPPV
  Review patient preferences
Consider alternative diagnoses
  Exam, CXR, ECG, laboratories
  Differential diagnoses—CHF, pneumonia, pneumothorax, MI, arrhythmias,
    pulmonary embolism, aspiration
Supplemental oxygen to keep oxygen saturation >90%
Consider repeat ABG to evaluate increased CO_2
High-dose beta$_2$ agonist
  Albuterol 4–6 puffs via spacer or nebulizer q20min

Subsequent
Add intravenous or oral steroids
  Methylprednisolone or prednisone
  Dose variable (e.g., 60–125 mg bid-qid with a rapid taper over 2 wk)
Add anticholinergic
  Ipratropium bromide 2 puffs q2–4h via spacer or 500 μg nebulizer q2–4h *or*
  Tiotropium
Consider antibiotics*
Consider intravenous methylxanthine
  Aminophylline—watch for toxicity

*If increased volume or purulence or both of sputum.
VS, vital signs; RR, respiratory rate; ABG, arterial blood gas; WOB, work of breathing;
LOC, level of consciousness.

extremities are without edema or clubbing. CXR shows a flattened diaphragm and
hyperlucency in the lower lung fields consistent with bullous disease. Spirometry
reveals moderate obstruction with FEV_1/FVC ratio of 60% and FEV_1 of 1.2 L (55%
of predicted). There is no improvement after bronchodilator.

    A. Is the patient more likely to have COPD or asthma?
    B. What risk factors for COPD besides tobacco use should be considered in
       this patient?
    C. What changes in her medications, if any, would you recommend?

Case 37-4

A 68-year-old man with a history of COPD and 50-pack-years of tobacco use
has an FEV_1 that is 25% of predicted. On exam, he is barrel-chested, using

accessory muscles at rest, and has markedly prolonged expiration with diffusely decreased breath sounds. Heart sounds are distant, and JVP is about 12 cm H_2O. He has hepatomegaly and bilateral lower extremity edema. ABG are pH 7.37, Pa_{CO_2} 55 mm Hg, Pa_{O_2} 56 mm Hg, with serum bicarbonate of 35 mEq/L. He is on inhaled bronchodilators and has infrequent exacerbations.

A. What would you expect the remainder of his pulmonary functions tests to show: FEV_1/FVC, TLC, and DLCO?
B. Is long-term oxygen therapy indicated in this patient?
C. What intervention would slow progression of his COPD most effectively?

PULMONARY EMBOLISM

ETIOLOGY

What Causes Pulmonary Embolism?

Pulmonary embolism is an underrecognized and potentially fatal condition; most PEs are not diagnosed before death. The major origin of PE, accounting for 90% of cases, is DVT of the lower extremities. Untreated, 50% of proximal lower extremity DVT embolize to the lungs. Risk factors for DVT and PE include Virchow's triad of hypercoagulability, immobility, and endothelial injury (Box 37-2).

BOX 37-2

RISK FACTORS FOR PULMONARY EMBOLUS

Venous Stasis

◆ Prolonged immobilization
◆ Recent surgery
◆ Obesity
◆ CHF, MI

Hypercoagulability

◆ Malignancy
◆ Inherited abnormality of clotting factors
◆ OCPs, pregnancy
◆ Nephrotic syndrome

Blood Vessel Intimal Damage

◆ Lower extremity surgery, trauma
◆ Age >60

EVALUATION

How do Patients with Pulmonary Embolism Present?

Some patients with pulmonary embolism are completely asymptomatic. In others, the symptoms are nonspecific. Patients may present with chest pain (typically pleuritic), dyspnea, cough, hemoptysis, or syncope. Common findings on exam include tachypnea, tachycardia, low-grade fever, cyanosis, diaphoresis, accentuated S_2, right ventricular heave, and crackles. Rarely one may hear an S_3 gallop or pulmonary friction rub if a PE causes infarcted lung tissue at the pleural surface. A massive PE also may cause cardiopulmonary collapse. Unilateral lower extremity edema can be a clue to the original DVT, although most patients with PE have no leg symptoms.

What Initial Tests should I Order When I Suspect a PE?

Initial work-up includes standard tests for dyspnea: CBC, chemistry panel, ABG, CXR, pulse oximetry, ECG, and possibly brain natriuretic peptide (BNP) if you also are considering CHF. ABG may be normal with a PE, but usually shows an alveolar-arterial difference (A-a gradient) >20 mm Hg (Box 37-3) and a respiratory alkalosis (hypoxia causes patients to hyperventilate, decreases carbon dioxide, and raises pH). CXR may be normal or may show atelectasis, pleural effusion, infiltrates, or elevation of a hemidiaphragm. It also may identify another diagnosis, such as pneumonia, pneumothorax, or CHF. Rarely on CXR with PE, you might see the "classic signs," such as Hampton's hump, a triangular infarct from occlusion of a pulmonary artery, or Westermark's sign, a prominent central pulmonary artery with decreased peripheral vascularity. The ECG in patients with PE most commonly shows sinus tachycardia or nonspecific ST/T wave

---

BOX 37-3

Alveolar Oxygen Concentration (P_{AO_2})

P_{AO_2} $= F_{IO_2}(PB - 47) - P_{CO_2}/0.8$

         $=$ approximately 100 at sea level when normal

Where: PB $=$ atmospheric pressure $= 760$ mm Hg at sea level

F_{IO_2} $=$ fraction of inspired oxygen $= 0.21$ at sea level

P_{aO_2} $=$ arterial oxygen concentration $=$ blood gas P_{O_2}

P_{CO_2} $=$ arterial carbon dioxide concentration

Alveolar-Arterial Oxygen Gradient (A-a gradient)

         A-a gradient $= P_{AO_2} - P_{aO_2}$

changes. Pulmonary embolism also may cause atrial arrhythmias, right heart strain, right axis deviation, right bundle branch block, or "S1, Q3, and T3" pattern (S wave in lead I and Q wave and flipped T wave in lead III).

When should I Pursue Further Testing for Pulmonary Embolism, and What Tests should I Order?

The level of clinical suspicion based on risk factors, history, physical, and initial tests is key in guiding further work-up. Criteria were created to determine the likelihood of a patient having a DVT (Box 37-4). If a patient has a low probability of a PE, the D-dimer, a fibrin degradation product, is a useful blood test to exclude a PE when the D-dimer is negative. A positive test does not diagnose a PE. The most appropriate initial

---

BOX 37-4

WELLS CRITERIA: CLINICAL MODEL FOR PREDICTING THE PRETEST PROBABILITY OF A DEEP VENOUS THROMBOSIS

Clinical Characteristic	Score
Active cancer	1
Paralysis, paresis, or recent plaster immobilization of lower extremities	1
Recently bedridden for ≥3 d, or major surgery within 12 wk	1
Localized tenderness along distribution of deep venous system	1
Entire leg swollen	1
Calf swelling at least 3 cm larger than that on asymptomatic side (measured 10 cm below tibial tuberosity)	1
Pitting edema confined to symptomatic leg	1
Collateral superficial veins	1
Previously documented DVT	1
Alternative diagnosis at least as likely as DVT	−2

Score ≥2—DVT likely
Score <2—DVT unlikely

From Wells PS, Anderson PR, Rodger M, et al: Evaluation of D-dimer in the diagnosis of suspected deep-vein thrombosis. N Engl J Med 2003;349: 1227.

imaging modality for pulmonary embolism is controversial because of rapidly advancing technologies. There are four imaging options: Doppler ultrasound of the leg, ventilation-perfusion scan of the chest, CT angiogram of the pulmonary arteries, and pulmonary angiogram. Doppler ultrasound of the lower extremities detects 95% of proximal leg clots and obviates the need for further tests if positive. A negative ultrasound does not rule out a PE, however. CT angiogram, previously called spiral or helical CT scan, is a minimally invasive option for diagnosing PE. The negative predictive value of a normal CT angiogram is 98%. This technology is now the most common initial imaging test for pulmonary embolus. Further, the CT scan provides useful information of alternative diagnoses. V/Q scan, ventilation-perfusion scan, is a nuclear medicine test that is read as normal or nondiagnostic or high probability. Most V/Q scans are read as indeterminate due to underlying pulmonary changes, and therefore do not contribute to diagnosis. However, these scans still have a role when renal insufficiency rules out the use of intravenous contrast material in CT angiogram or pulmonary angiogram. Pulmonary angiogram is currently the "gold standard" for diagnosing PE. This is an invasive test and is used only when other studies are nondiagnostic.

TREATMENT

How do I Treat Pulmonary Embolism?

Stabilize the airway, breathing, and circulation, and administer oxygen. Start intravenous unfractionated heparin or subcutaneous LMWH if there are no contraindications (Box 37-5). If clinical suspicion for PE is high, treatment should be started even before a definitive diagnosis is made. Start warfarin after PE is confirmed, and continue heparin or LMWH until the INR is 2–3 (usually 5 days). Treatment usually lasts 6 months, although warfarin may be continued indefinitely if risk is not modifiable (e.g., cancer, inherited hypercoagulable state). If there is a concern for an inherited hypercoagulable state (family history or recurrent thrombotic event), consider pursuing this work-up.

What Other Treatment Options Exist?

For patients with a massive PE who may be hypotensive or severely hypoxemic, thrombolytic therapy is recommended to lyse the clot and improve hemodynamics. These patients have an extremely high mortality rate. Inferior vena caval filters can be placed when patients have absolute contraindications to anticoagulation (see Box 37-5) or recurrent PE on appropriate anticoagulation. The filter is a wire barrier that is placed under angiographic guidance into the inferior vena cava. It allows blood flow, but stops larger clots from proceeding to the lungs.

BOX 37-5

CONTRAINDICATIONS TO THE USE OF HEPARIN

Absolute Contraindications

◆ Active internal bleeding
◆ Intracranial bleeding
◆ Intracranial lesions likely to bleed
◆ Severe heparin-induced thrombocytopenia (HIT)
◆ Malignant hypertension

Relative Contraindications

◆ Hemorrhagic diathesis
◆ Recent stroke
◆ Recent major surgery
◆ Severe hypertension
◆ Bacterial endocarditis
◆ Thrombocytopenia
◆ Peptic ulcer disease (PUD)

Case 37-5

A 40-year-old woman presents with dyspnea over the last 24 hours. She has a cough and a low-grade fever, but no chest pain or abdominal pain. She recently returned from a trip to Vietnam. Past medical history includes asthma. She uses an albuterol inhaler occasionally and OCP. She quit smoking 5 years ago, but she admits that she has started smoking again over the last 2 months because she has been "feeling stressed." On physical exam, she is an obese woman who appears mildly dyspneic, speaking in full sentences. Temperature is 38° C, pulse is 105 beats/min, BP is 150/70 mm Hg, respiratory rate is 22, and oxygen saturation is 93% on room air. Chest exam reveals occasional crackles at the right base. Cardiac exam is regular without murmurs. Extremity exam is difficult given body habitus, but you measure her calves, and one is 5 cm larger than the other. WBC is 10.5, hematocrit is 38%, and creatinine is 0.8.

A. What is your differential diagnosis for this patient's shortness of breath?
B. What are her risk factors for pulmonary embolism?
C. What further evaluation do you perform?
D. You diagnose a PE. How do you treat her?

Case 37-6

A 75-year-old man with stage III colon cancer falls and develops a small subdural hematoma. He is observed in the hospital, and his subdural hematoma is stable. He has no other medical history and has never smoked or consumed alcohol. On the third hospital day, he becomes confused and pulls out his intravenous catheter. He is unable to describe any symptoms. On exam, he appears agitated and cannot follow commands. Temperature is 38.1° C, pulse is 110 beats/min, BP is 110/60 mm Hg, respiratory rate is 26, and oxygen saturation is 86% on room air. His lungs are clear, and HR is tachycardic but regular and without murmurs. JVP is difficult to assess. He has 1+ edema in his legs bilaterally. His WBC count is 12,000, hematocrit is 29, and creatinine is 2.1. A brain natriuretic peptide is 75. Cardiac enzymes are normal. CXR shows low lung volumes, but no infiltrate. ECG shows sinus tachycardia, but no ST changes.

    A. What is your differential diagnosis?
    B. What are this patient's risk factors for a PE?
    C. Your suspicion for a PE is high; what do you do at this time?
    D. You diagnose a PE; what are your treatment options?

KEY POINTS – ASTHMA

◆ Asthma is a disease of chronic airway inflammation triggered by a wide array of precipitants.

◆ Treatment for asthma should always include an inhaled corticosteroid whenever possible, bronchodilators for symptom relief, and modification of the precipitants.

◆ Treat asthma exacerbations with systemic steroids and increased bronchodilators.

KEY POINTS – COPD

◆ COPD is a chronic, progressive disease characterized by largely fixed airflow obstruction.

◆ Smoking cessation is the most important intervention in slowing progression of COPD.

◆ A variety of medications can ameliorate symptoms, but none alters the decline in lung function.

◆ Supplemental oxygen reduces mortality in patients with COPD and severe hypoxemia.

◆ NIPPV reduces the need for intubation and improves mortality in selected patients.

KEY POINTS – PULMONARY EMBOLISM

◆ Pulmonary embolism is a potentially life-threatening disease; the signs and symptoms are nonspecific, so you must have a high index of suspicion, especially in patients with risk factors.

◆ CT pulmonary angiogram, ventilation-perfusion scan, lower extremity duplex ultrasound, and pulmonary angiogram all are imaging methods that can be used to confirm the diagnosis of PE.

◆ Anticoagulate with intravenous unfractionated heparin or subcutaneous LMWH when clinical suspicion is high, and there are no contraindications as you pursue the PE work-up.

Case Answers

37-1 A. *Learning objective:* **In new or worsening asthma, ask about pre-cipitants.** In this patient's new house, are there carpets, wood stoves, pets (either previously or currently)? Is she newly exposed to cigarette smoke? Has she changed jobs, now with an occupa-tional exposure? Do her symptoms resolve when she travels back to her prior residence, suggesting allergies or exposures? Has she been sick recently with upper respiratory symptoms?

37-1 B. *Learning objective:* **Identify the indications, risks, and benefits of regular use of inhaled corticosteroids.** In light of her increase in symptom frequency, exacerbations, and nighttime symptoms, she is classified as having at least mild persistent asthma. An anti-inflammatory therapy is necessary, specifically an inhaled corti-costeroid. Inhaled corticosteroids provide the most potent and con-sistently effective long-term control of asthma by inhibiting production of cytokines and other inflammatory mediators, reversing airway inflammation and decreasing airway hyperresponsiveness.

37-1 C. *Learning objective:* **Outline the risks and benefits of inhaled cor-ticosteroid therapy.** Inhaled steroids would decrease her symp-toms and would prevent the remodeling that leads to irreversible pulmonary damage. Although the negative impact of low-dose inhaled steroids is unclear, long-term use of high-dose inhaled ster-oids (usually >1000 μg/d) can cause osteoporosis, immunosuppres-sion, elevated intraocular pressure, altered bone homeostasis, and cataract formation. Minimize systemic absorption by mouth-rinsing after each administration and by use of spacer devices. For all patients, recommend preventive measures for osteoporosis and consider DXA screening (see Chapter 40).

37-2 A. *Learning objective:* **Recognize signs of severe asthma exacerba-tion and outline an action plan.** This patient has a severe asthma exacerbation. Her ability to speak only in short sentences is an early sign of impending respiratory failure. Instruct her to take 60 mg of prednisone if she has some at home and to go to an emergency department immediately. She should not drive herself, and an emergency medical team should be called if necessary.

37-2 B. *Learning objective:* **Describe the evaluation and treatment for acute asthma exacerbation.** Check vital signs, give intravenous corticosteroids, and begin continuous albuterol via nebulizer. Follow serial vital signs, including pulsus paradoxus (significant decrease in systolic pressure with inspiration). Look for use of accessory muscles of respiration and paradoxical abdominal motion. Observe the expiratory-to-inspiratory ratio, often increased with airway obstruction. Listen to the lungs for air movement and wheezing. Obtain ABG. Although URI is the most likely precipitant, consider a CXR to look for signs of pneumonia and an ECG to evaluate for cardiac ischemia. Sputum can be thick and greenish even in the absence of infection, but a sputum culture might be helpful. Watch for trends in vital signs and exam. With any sign of worsening, hospitalize immediately, preferably in an ICU.

37-2 C. *Learning objective:* **Recognize respiratory failure in severe asthma exacerbations.** Common signs of impending respiratory failure include the presence of a worsening pulsus paradoxus; decrease in respiratory rate or use of accessory muscles, which suggests fatigue; and prolongation of the expiratory phase leading to an increased expiratory-to-inspiratory ratio. Wheezing is often a difficult sign to interpret because a patient who has severely compromised air movement may have *no* wheezing or air movement. As she improves, diffuse wheezing may appear. Obtain an ABG, and hospitalize for significant hypoxemia or hypercarbia. It is important to recognize early respiratory failure and intubate with mechanical ventilation in a controlled setting, not after the patient exhibits hemodynamic compromise.

37-3 A. *Learning objective:* **Distinguish COPD from asthma.** This patient almost certainly has COPD rather than asthma. Her consistent (rather than episodic) dyspnea on exertion, tobacco history, age of symptom onset, suggestion of bullous disease on CXR, and fixed obstructive defect on spirometry all favor the diagnosis of COPD.

37-3 B. *Learning objective:* **List the risk factors for COPD.** Although her COPD may be entirely the result of smoking, the basilar predominance of bullous changes on CXR and diagnosis before age 45 raise the possibility of alpha-1-antitrypsin deficiency, a rare genetic disorder. Low serum enzyme levels make the diagnosis. Intravenous injection of crushed methylphenidate (Ritalin) tablets is an even more rare cause of early-onset, basilar-predominant emphysema.

37-3 C. *Learning objective:* **Devise a medication regimen appropriate for a patient with stable COPD.** The highest priority in this patient is weaning her off prednisone. Long-term oral steroids are not indicated for the treatment of COPD and have serious chronic side effects. The patient is using a large amount of albuterol; the addition of a long-acting beta$_2$ agonist or a scheduled anticholinergic inhaler or both is appropriate. Theophylline is an option if there is an inadequate response to first-line bronchodilators. If she's symptomatic despite these interventions, a trial of inhaled corticosteroid is reasonable. If her FEV$_1$ fails to improve, however, inhaled steroid should be discontinued because there is an increased risk of osteoporosis associated with long-term use. The patient may benefit from enzyme augmentation therapy if she has alpha-1-antitrypsin deficiency.

37-4 A.   *Learning objective:* **Patients with COPD have airflow obstruction, and his FEV$_1$/FVC should be <70%.** His FEV$_1$ at 25% of predicted is consistent with severe disease, and his lung volumes likely would include an increased TLC indicating hyperinflation and an elevated residual volume as a result of air trapping. DLCO is usually severely decreased in patients with severe emphysema, reflecting destruction of the lung parenchyma. A relatively preserved DLCO should prompt consideration of a large reversible component to airflow obstruction as seen in patients with asthma. The chronic, compensated carbon dioxide retention and hypoxemia seen on his ABG are consistent with his advanced disease.

37-4 B.   *Learning objective:* **State the indications for supplemental oxygen in COPD patients.** Long-term oxygen therapy for >15 h/d reduces mortality in chronically hypoxemic patients with COPD and is indicated in this patient. Long-term oxygen therapy is indicated for all patients with Pao$_2$ ≤55 mm Hg or with Pao$_2$ 55–60 mm Hg in the presence of pulmonary hypertension, right heart failure, or polycythemia (HCT >55%). The patient's exam is consistent with cor pulmonale and right heart failure. Intermittent supplemental oxygen may improve quality of life in patients who experience desaturate during exercise or sleep, but has not been shown to improve mortality.

37-4 C.   *Learning objective:* **Identify smoking cessation as the most effective way to slow progression of COPD.** Smoking cessation is the most effective way to slow disease progression. This patient's prognosis is poor. The FEV$_1$ is the best predictor of mortality in patients with COPD. This patient has an estimated 5-year survival of only about 30%, however. Although the course of disease varies among individuals with comparable degrees of airflow obstruction, this patient's hypoxemia and cor pulmonale place him at greater risk of mortality.

37-5 A.   *Learning objective:* **List a differential diagnosis for dyspnea.** The differential diagnosis for dyspnea in an obese woman with hypertension, tobacco use, asthma, and recent travel is broad. Possible pulmonary causes include pulmonary embolism especially given her risks of obesity, tobacco use, prolonged immobilization, and OCP use. An asthma exacerbation would be possible given her history. She also may have COPD given her tobacco history. Cardiac causes include coronary artery disease (an "anginal equivalent") versus heart failure. Infectious causes include community-acquired pneumonia, influenza or other viruses, or possibly an endemic infection from Vietnam, such as tuberculosis. Other causes include anxiety and deconditioning.

37-5 B.   *Learning objective:* **Identify risk factors for a PE.** Risk factors for a PE include obesity, tobacco use, recent immobility during plane travel, and OCP use.

37-5 C.   *Learning objective:* **Order appropriate work-up in patients with dyspnea.** Order ECG to look for evidence of ischemia and a CXR to assess for pneumonia or pulmonary edema. Check a D-dimer—if negative, a PE is less likely; if positive, more testing is necessary to diagnose or rule out a PE, such as CT pulmonary angiogram, ultrasound of the leg, or ventilation-perfusion scan. In addition, consider ordering brain natriuretic peptide (BNP) to assess for heart failure and an ABG to calculate the A-a gradient. This patient has multiple risk factors, so it is appropriate to skip the D-dimer and proceed to a more definitive imaging study for PE.

37-5 D.   *Learning objective:* **Design treatment for a PE in a hemodynamically stable patient.** Because the patient's renal function is normal, treatment options include LMWH or intravenous heparin accompanied by warfarin. She probably should be admitted to the hospital, although there is increasing evidence that some patients with a PE may be treated at home. Treatment with LMWH or unfractionated heparin should continue until her INR is 2–3. Treatment should continue for approximately 6 months. Consider stopping her OCP given her clot and tobacco use. If she had a prior history of DVT, consider pursuing a hypercoagulability work-up and indefinite anticoagulation to decrease the risk of another recurrence.

37-6 A.   *Learning objective:* **List the differential diagnosis for a hospitalized patient with hypoxia and delirium.** The differential diagnosis for an elderly hospitalized patient who becomes delirious and hypoxemic includes infectious causes such as a nosocomial pneumonia or a community-acquired pneumonia that was not initially recognized. Other infections also could cause delirium (UTI, intravenous line infection, skin breakdown), and one could see hypoxia with sepsis-related lung injury. Noninfectious causes include pulmonary embolism, myocardial infarction with resultant heart failure (elderly patients may not complain of chest pain), and excessive sedation owing to narcotics.

37-6 B.   *Learning objective:* **Identify risk factors for pulmonary embolism.** Risk factors include immobility and malignancy.

37-6 C. *Learning objective:* **Order appropriate work-up for a PE.** A D-dimer would not be appropriate in this patient because he is an inpatient and at high risk. A CT pulmonary angiogram and pulmonary angiogram also are not good options because he has an elevated creatinine. An ultrasound of his lower extremities or a ventilation-perfusion scan or both would be appropriate.

37-6 D. *Learning objective:* **Choose appropriate treatment for a PE in a patient with a contraindication for anticoagulation.** Because this patient has a new subdural hematoma, anticoagulation is contraindicated. An inferior vena cava filter can be placed by interventional radiology to prevent further emboli.

REFERENCES

Asthma
Attaining optimal asthma control: A practice parameter. J Allergy Clin Immunol 2005;116:S3.
Dahl R: Systemic side effects of inhaled corticosteroids in patients with asthma. Respir Med 2006;100:1392.
Salpeter SR, Ormiston TM, Salpeter EE: Cardioselective beta-blockers in patients with reactive airway disease: A meta-analysis. Ann Intern Med 2002;137:715.

Chronic Obstructive Pulmonary Disease
ATS/ERS Task Force: Standards for the diagnosis and treatment of patients with COPD: A summary position of the ATS/ERS position paper. Eur Respir J 2004;23:932.
Pauwels RA, Buist AS, Calverley PM, et al: Global strategy for the diagnosis, management, and prevention of chronic obstructive pulmonary disease. Am J Respir Crit Care Med 2001;163:1256.

USEFUL WEB SITES

Asthma
New Guidelines for the Diagnosis and Management of Asthma from the National Asthma Education and Prevention Program updating the 1991 Expert Panel Report of the National Heart, Lung, and Blood Institute. July 1997. NIH Pub. No. 97–4051. http://www.nhlbi.nih.gov/guidelines/asthma/asthgdln.pdf
http://www.nlm.nih.gov/medlineplus/asthma.html

Chronic Obstructive Pulmonary Disease
American Thoracic Society, COPD section. http://www-test.thoracic.org/COPD

Pulmonary Embolism
American Thoracic Society consensus statement. www.ats.org
Management of Deep Vein Thrombosis and Pulmonary Embolism. www.americanheart.org/presenter.jhtml?identifier=1200000

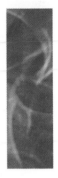

38

Rheumatology

DOUGLAS S. PAAUW, GREGORY C. GARDNER, and LISANNE R. BURKHOLDER

GOUT

ETIOLOGY

What Causes Gout?

Gout is an inflammatory arthritis caused by the deposition of monosodium urate crystals in a joint. Crystals form because of either underexcretion (90%) or overproduction of uric acid. Risk factors for gout include medications, alcohol use, obesity, hereditary predisposition (extremely common in individuals from Samoa and the Philippines) and hyperuricemia, although not all of these patients develop gout. Less common precipitants of gout include lead poisoning and tumor lysis syndrome (seen during chemotherapy for various cancers).

What Medications Cause Increases in Uric Acid?

Diuretics are the most commonly used medications that trigger gout. Low-dose aspirin, cyclosporine, and niacin also are important precipitants of gout.

What are Common Triggers for a Gouty Attack in Patients with a History of Gout?

Rapid changes in urate level can trigger gout. Decreased uric acid secretion and fluid shifts are contributing factors associated with physiologic stresses, such as surgery, trauma, medical illness, and new medications that decrease uric acid secretion. Hospitalization can trigger acute gout attacks in patients with a prior history of gout. Physical activities such as running and long walks may precede gouty attacks in the first MTP joint. Occasionally, starting therapy with allopurinol precipitates or worsens a gouty attack. For this reason, allopurinol is not started during an acute attack.

521

EVALUATION

What is the Typical Presentation of Gout?

Men much more commonly have gout than women. The most common first site of involvement is the MTP joint of the great toe (>50% of initial gout attacks). In >80% of cases, the first episode of gout is monarticular. The pain is great and is exacerbated by minimal pressure even of bed sheets on the joint. Erythema and warmth of the affected joint are typical. The onset of pain is usually sudden and often involves only one joint. In older patients, it is common for gout to occur in joints with known osteoarthritis. Less typically, an ankle, foot, or knee also can be the site of acute gout; hips and shoulders are hardly ever affected.

What Symptoms and Signs would I See with a Severe Attack of Gout?

Common findings are fever, multiple joint involvement, tachycardia, and an increased WBC. These patients are frequently misdiagnosed as having an infection.

How do I Diagnose Gout?

WBC and ESR are usually elevated during acute attacks, but are nonspecific. The diagnosis is made by aspirating the involved joint and examining the fluid under polarized microscopy. Urate crystals are needle-shaped or rod-shaped and are intracellular, in neutrophils, and extracellular. They are strongly negatively birefringent when examined under compensated polarized microscopy. Most patients with gout have a high uric acid level (>7 mg/dL). Occasionally, uric acid levels are depressed during an acute attack; repeat the uric acid level in patients after the attack subsides. In patients with an established diagnosis of gout and recurrent episodes, there is no need to tap the joint again unless clinical features suggest the possibility of a septic joint (fever, chills, lack of response to gout therapy).

What Happens to Patients with Long-Standing Gout?

Patients may have acute attacks separated by long symptom-free periods. Gouty arthritis also can become chronic, with urate deposition in joints and periarticular tissues that can lead to chronic, destructive, deforming arthritis. With chronic joint destruction, x-rays may show classic "rat-bite" erosions, which look like punched-out areas of bone loss with an associated overhanging rim of cortical bone. Gout crystals can precipitate in the subcutaneous tissues causing deforming tophi. The digits and ears are the most common sites for tophi.

TREATMENT

How Should I Treat an Acute Attack of Gout?

The mainstay for treatment is NSAIDs (e.g., indomethacin 50 mg three times a day). Be extremely careful to avoid using NSAIDs in patients with contraindications, such as CHF, renal insufficiency, history of gastric or duodenal ulcer, or allergy to aspirin or NSAIDs. The alternatives for treatment of acute gout are prednisone (a 5- to 7-day course) or joint injection with corticosteroids. Treatment-dose colchicine should not be used in patients with renal insufficiency. Colchicine causes severe diarrhea at treatment doses and is the least attractive option for treating gout.

Who Should Receive Long-Term Medication to Prevent Gouty Attack?

Patients who have had more than two attacks of gout within 1 year are reasonable candidates. After a first attack, 75% of patients have a second attack within 2 years; patients with more than two attacks are likely to have more recurrences.

What Therapy Should be Used for Preventing Attacks?

Allopurinol and probenecid are effective in preventing recurrent acute attacks and in resorbing chronic tophaceous deposits. Allopurinol decreases production of uric acid, whereas probenecid decreases renal reabsorption of filtered urate. Probenecid works only with intact renal function. Do not start either drug during an acute attack because they can prolong or worsen the attack. Allopurinol is the preferred drug in patients who overproduce urate, have urate stones, or have renal insufficiency. Allopurinol can infrequently cause rash, vasculitis, and hepatitis. Low-dose colchicine (0.6 mg/d) is an effective therapy to bridge the gap between acute treatment and starting a prophylactic drug.

Case 38-1

A 39-year-old man with type 1 DM presents with severe pain in the left foot. On exam, he has erythema over the first MTP joint of the left foot. Lab results are as follows: BUN 39, creatinine 3.3, glucose 350, HCT 35, and WBC 4.6. Joint fluid shows crystals consistent with urate. Uric acid is 8.8, and hemoglobin A1C is 10.

    A. What therapy would you use?

Case 38-2

A 61-year-old man is evaluated for an acute episode of gout involving the right knee. Three months ago and 1 year ago, he had gouty attacks involving his left great toe. Medical problems include hypertension and renal insufficiency (creatinine 2.4).

    A. What therapy would you recommend?
    B. What would be an appropriate plan to help prevent future attacks of gout?

RHEUMATOID ARTHRITIS

ETIOLOGY

What is RA?

RA is a chronic autoimmune disease of unclear etiology that causes synovial inflammation with erosion of articular cartilage and bone. Worldwide prevalence is 1%, with women developing RA three times as frequently as men. It occurs in all age groups, although it generally increases with age. The course of RA varies, but it usually causes significant morbidity and decreased longevity.

EVALUATION

What are the Most Common Symptoms of RA?

RA is usually a symmetric polyarthritis involving characteristic peripheral joints, especially the MCP and MTP joints (Figure 38-1). Lumbosacral and distal interphalangeal joints are rarely involved. The inflamed joints produce a deep, aching discomfort. Stiffness is most severe in the morning or after periods of inactivity and characteristically lasts ≥1 hour. Constitutional symptoms may precede overt arthritis and

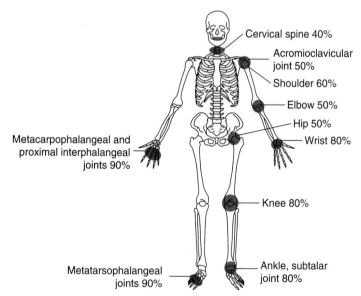

FIGURE 38-1 Joints commonly involved in RA (pattern of involvement is usually symmetrical and involves the MCP, MTP, and proximal interphalangeal joints).

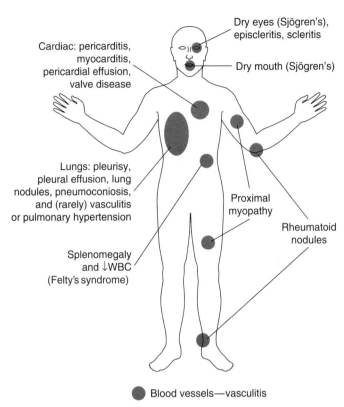

Dry eyes (Sjögren's), episcleritis, scleritis

Cardiac: pericarditis, myocarditis, pericardial effusion, valve disease

Dry mouth (Sjögren's)

Lungs: pleurisy, pleural effusion, lung nodules, pneumoconiosis, and (rarely) vasculitis or pulmonary hypertension

Proximal myopathy

Rheumatoid nodules

Splenomegaly and ↓WBC (Felty's syndrome)

● Blood vessels—vasculitis

FIGURE 38-2 Extra-articular manifestations of RA.

include weight loss, low-grade fever, and fatigue. Twenty percent of patients develop extra-articular manifestations (Figure 38-2).

What Should I Look for on the Musculoskeletal Examination?

Palpate each joint for effusions, synovial swelling, and tenderness. Presence of synovial proliferation gives the joint a boggy consistency and diffuse tenderness. In comparison, tendinitis and bursitis cause focal pain without boggy synovial swelling. Also check active and passive ROM; in tendinitis, only active ROM is painful, whereas with joint involvement, passive *and* active ROM are painful. Detailed measurements of ROM are rarely necessary. Describe ROM as normal; slightly, moderately, or markedly limited; or fused. Rheumatoid nodules may be found at sites of pressure, such as the posterior elbow and over the Achilles tendon. Watch for common deformities, including ulnar deviation of fingers, subluxation of MCP joints, swan neck and boutonnière deformities of the fingers and cock-up deformities of the toes (Figure 38-3). Asymptomatic flexion contractures (easily noticed in superficial joints such as the elbow) suggest active synovitis.

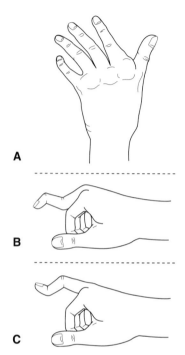

FIGURE 38-3 Characteristic joint deformities seen in RA. **A,** Ulnar deviation. **B,** Swan neck deformity. **C,** Boutonnière deformity.

What Might I see on Neurologic Exam of a Patient with RA?

Check for paresthesias of the hands and feet because compressive neuropathies are common secondary to active synovitis (e.g., carpal tunnel syndrome). The cervical spine can become unstable owing to erosive synovitis, particularly at the atlantoaxial junction (C1–2). If localized pain and x-ray findings suggest this is the case, perform a careful neurologic exam at every visit. Patients with significant C1–2 subluxation can have chronic, progressive pyramidal tract (upper motor neuron) compression leading to weakness, spasticity, and pathologic reflexes. Sudden, acute cervical cord compression also can occur after only minor trauma or as a complication of intubation for surgery.

How do I Diagnose RA?

RA is a clinical diagnosis requiring presence of at least four of seven criteria, listed in Box 38-1.

What Lab Tests Should I Order if I Suspect RA?

Order rheumatoid factor, an IgM antibody specifically active against IgG. Although RF is present in 80% of adults with RA, it is nonspecific

BOX 38-1

REVISED CRITERIA (1987) FOR DIAGNOSIS OF RHEUMATOID ARTHRITIS

♦ Four criteria are required for diagnosis
♦ Criteria 1–4 must be present for ≥6 wk
  1. Morning stiffness lasting at least 1 h
  2. Arthritis in at least three joints
  3. Arthritis of the hand joints
  4. Symmetrical arthritis
  5. Rheumatoid nodules
  6. Positive serum rheumatoid factors
  7. X-ray changes typical of RA

(found in many other inflammatory conditions) and suggests RA only if other clinical criteria are present (see Box 38-1). High titers are associated with worse joint disease and extra-articular manifestations (see Figure 38-2). When rheumatoid factor is positive, you never need to check it again because it does not correlate with disease activity or response to treatment. ESR and C-reactive protein are typically elevated and roughly correlate with disease activity (although normal values do not rule out RA). Other helpful lab tests to monitor include HCT because anemia of chronic disease is common in active RA. Anti–cyclic citrullinated peptide (anti-CCP) antibody is positive in many patients with RA. It is frequently positive early in the disease before rheumatoid factor is positive and has greater specificity than rheumatoid factor for RA (90%-96% specificity).

What will I See on a Joint Aspiration with RA?

Joint aspirations in patients with RA show inflammation (WBC 3000–35,000 with predominantly PMN). Tap a joint if you are uncertain of the diagnosis of RA (and are looking for evidence of another disease process, such as gout), or if you think the joint might be infected. Have a low threshold for tapping a joint that is persistently or excessively inflamed compared with the patient's other joints because patients with RA are at risk for joint infections.

Are X-Rays Helpful in Diagnosis of RA?

X-rays early in the disease usually are normal or show juxta-articular osteopenia and are not helpful for diagnosis. It may take months to years for erosive changes, including joint space narrowing and joint margin erosions, to develop on x-ray. X-rays have an important role in monitoring disease progression, however.

What are Potential Extra-Articular Manifestations of RA?

Extra-articular manifestations include interstitial lung disease, rheumatoid nodules (lung, cardiac, subcutaneous tissue), pleuropericarditis, myocarditis, neuropathy from compression (cervical spine instability, carpel tunnel syndrome) or vasculitis (skin ulcers, mononeuritis multiplex), vasculitis skin or vessel changes, scleritis, episcleritis, splenomegaly, Sjögren's syndrome, osteoporosis, myositis, neutropenia, thrombocytopenia, anemia, and cricoarytenoid abnormalities leading to hoarseness and upper airway obstruction.

What Evaluation is Warranted on Routine Follow-Up of Patients with Known RA?

Assess disease activity by looking for signs of active inflammation (e.g., synovial swelling, joint erythema or warmth, and morning stiffness of 1 hour duration). Assess disease severity by asking about the number of joints involved, the severity of pain and fatigue, and the presence of extra-articular manifestations. Compare level of function between visits by identifying an activity that the patient can perform only marginally well (e.g., combing hair, slicing bread, walking more than two blocks), and have the patient describe the level of function with this activity at each visit. Also ask about onset of any new extra-articular manifestations. Elevations in C-reactive protein and ESR levels and decreases in albumin and hemoglobin levels all correlate with disease activity. A high rheumatoid factor portends worse prognosis overall, but does not fluctuate with disease activity. Mild disease is indicated by at least three joints involved without extra-articular manifestations. Moderate disease is indicated 6–20 joints with signs of early inflammation on x-rays (periarticular osteopenia and swelling). Severe disease involves any one or more of the following: >20 joints, anemia, hypoalbuminemia, erosions on x-rays, or extra-articular disease.

TREATMENT

Are Any Nonpharmacologic Therapies Recommended for Patients with RA?

Patient education and counseling are key to ensure a good therapeutic alliance because treatments often require adjustment and can cause toxicities. Advise periods of rest for symptoms of severe fatigue or to decrease joint wear and tear during periods of joint inflammation. Regular exercise and ROM improves function, maintains joint mobility, and prevents muscle and bone loss. Physical therapy maneuvers with ultrasound, heat or cold applications, ROM exercises, and splinting painful joints can reduce pain and increase function. Weight loss is advised for obese patients to decrease joint stress. Bone loss is common from the effects of RA directly and from steroids used to decrease inflammation and treat complications. Calcium 1000–1500 mg/d and vitamin D 800 IU/d are essential. Bisphosphonates also may be used to protect against further bone loss.

What Medicines are Used to Treat RA?

There is no cure for RA, but early medical therapy—in addition to alleviating pain—delays or possibly prevents joint deformities. There are two main categories of medications: NSAIDs and disease modifying anti-rheumatic drugs (DMARDs). NSAIDs relieve symptoms, but do not delay joint destruction. In the past, patients were treated initially with NSAIDs, and DMARDs were started late in the disease. The focus now is on early treatment with DMARDs, to halt the underlying inflammation and delay or prevent joint destruction. No DMARD is universally effective in all patients, and they frequently have to be discontinued because of side effects. Specific DMARDs are tried in a stepwise manner, often in combinations, until inflammation is suppressed as indicated by ESR and C-reactive protein or symptoms. Hydroxychloroquine is usually the first DMARD given and in patients with mild disease may be effective alone. In patients with aggressive RA, methotrexate is the most often used DMARD and is usually given in combination with hydroxychloroquine. The treatment of RA has improved dramatically with the advent of the biologic agents—tumor necrosis factor (TNF)–alpha inhibitors and IL-RA. TNF-alpha inhibitors are etanercept, infliximab, and odalimumab. Because these agents inhibit inflammatory cytokines that are used in normal inflammatory responses to infection, patients should be advised to seek medical attention if they develop serious fever and chills. It has been shown that patients on TNF-alpha inhibitors are at greater risk for tuberculosis. Other more toxic agents added or substituted when first-line agents fail include gold salts, penicillamine, sulfasalazine, prednisone, cyclophosphamide, cyclosporine, chlorambucil, and azathioprine.

What Surgical Therapies are Used for Patients with RA?

Advances in orthopedic surgery have had a profound effect on the quality of life of patients with RA. Surgical synovectomy of a joint may temporarily improve symptoms, decrease joint destruction seen early in disease, remove debris interfering with normal function, and prevent tendon rupture. Total joint replacement of larger joints (hips, knees, and shoulders) can markedly increase function and decrease pain. Other surgical options include repair of ruptured tendons, correction of valgus or varus deformities of the knee to realign weight-bearing bones, joint fusion to stabilize joints not easily replaced (e.g., ankle, wrist, thumb, or cervical spine), correction of severe contractures, and metatarsal head excision to alleviate severe forefoot pain and improve gait.

Case 38-3

A 35-year-old woman reports gradual onset over the past 2 months of fatigue, pain involving the MCP, proximal interphalangeal, and wrist joints and morning stiffness lasting 1 hour. On exam, MCP, proximal interphalangeal, and wrist joints are swollen bilaterally. The joints are tender and slightly warm.

A. What is your differential diagnosis?
B. What lab tests would you order?
C. What do you recommend for treatment?

Case 38-4

A 45-year-old woman is taking 7.5 mg of prednisone a day for seropositive RA with multiple joint deformities. She reports that she cannot raise her left foot. On exam, she is slightly cushingoid. There is 2+ swelling of the MCP, proximal interphalangeal, wrist, and ankle joints, and ulnar deviation, boutonnière, and swan neck deformities. Flexion and extension of the wrist are markedly reduced. Her toes are cocked up. She cannot dorsiflex her left foot.

A. What is the differential diagnosis of the left footdrop?
B. What tests would you obtain?
C. What do you recommend for treatment?

SYSTEMIC LUPUS ERYTHEMATOSUS

ETIOLOGY

What is SLE?

SLE is a chronic immune disorder that involves many organ systems and causes a wide variety of symptoms. The severity ranges from nearly asymptomatic to life-threatening. Many patients have mild disease with a variety of skin lesions, alopecia, or arthritis, but some patients have serious complications, including renal failure, organic psychosis, and vasculitis. Survival rate in SLE is approximately 90% over the first 10 years. Involvement of the kidneys or CNS is an unfavorable prognostic sign. Major causes of death are renal failure, infection (often due to the use of immunosuppressive drugs), and CAD.

Who gets SLE?

SLE is most common among women of childbearing age, with a 9:1 female-to-male ratio. African American women are affected three times more commonly than whites, although blacks in Africa hardly ever get SLE. It usually develops between ages 13 and 40, but can occur at any age. Genetic factors are important because SLE is more common in relatives of affected patients.

What Causes SLE?

SLE is an autoimmune disease. For unidentified reasons, autoantibodies (Table 38-1) cause tissue injury when they are directed at a specific cell type (e.g., RBC), or if they form antigen-antibody (immune) complexes. Circulating immune complexes are deposited in blood vessels initiating a cascade of complement-mediated injury. Certain drugs can cause a reversible drug-induced SLE; common drugs include hydralazine, procainamide, and isoniazid.

Table 38-1	

Important Antibodies in Lupus and Their Frequency	
Antibody	**Frequency (%)**
Anti–double-stranded DNA	70
If positive, it is likely patient has lupus (high specificity)	
Often increases with flares (doubling or increase of 30 in	
<10 wk suggests disease flare)	
Anti-Smith antibody	30
Nearly pathognomonic for SLE when it is present	
Anti-RNP antibody	40
Can be present in other rheumatologic conditions	
Anti-Ro antibody (SS-A)	30
Children of mothers with anti-Ro are at risk of neonatal lupus	
and congenital heart block	
Anti-La antibody (SS-B)	10
Can be present in other rheumatologic conditions	
Antihistone antibody	70
Positive in 95% of patients with drug-induced SLE and 20% of	
patients with idiopathic SLE	
Anticardiolipin antibody	40
Strongly associated with stroke and venous and arterial	
clotting in lupus patients; many have the skin finding of	
livedo reticularis	

Does Pregnancy Exacerbate SLE?

Active disease at conception is likely to worsen during pregnancy, but patients already in remission usually complete pregnancy without a clinical exacerbation. Nearly half of all SLE patients deliver prematurely, often by emergency cesarean section. Patients with a positive anti-Ro antibody are at risk of delivering a child with neonatal SLE or congenital heart block. Phospholipid antibody syndrome may occur in association with SLE and can cause fetal loss.

EVALUATION

What are the Most Common Manifestations of SLE?

The most common presenting symptom is symmetric arthritis, seen in about 65% of patients at presentation. Morning stiffness and distribution of joints involved are similar to RA. Other common manifestations are fatigue, skin rashes (some photosensitive), renal insufficiency, fevers, and hematologic cytopenias. Think of the possibility of SLE in a young woman presenting with thrombocytopenia. An ANA should always be checked in the work-up of patients with severe thrombocytopenia. Although fatigue is common in patients with SLE, fatigue also may be due to other concurrent medical or psychiatric conditions and should not be ignored. Less common manifestations of disease include

Table 38-2

Diagnosing Lupus (1982 American Rheumatism Association Criteria)*

	Symptom, Sign, or Lab Abnormality	Frequency (%)
S	Serositis—pleuritis, pericarditis	56
O	Oral or nasopharyngeal ulcers—painless	27
A	Arthritis—nonerosive, two or more peripheral joints	86
P	Photosensitivity—erythematous skin rash, raised or flat	43
B	Blood dyscrasias	
	Hemolytic anemia (with reticulocytosis)	30
	Leukopenia (WBC <4000) on two or more occasions	40
	Lymphopenia (<1500) on two or more occasions	
	Thrombocytopenia (<100,000) in the absence of offending drugs	30
R	Renal—proteinuria, casts	50
A	Antinuclear antibody—in absence of drugs known to cause lupus	>95
I	Immunologic disorders	
	Anti–double-stranded DNA	70
	Anti-Smith—antibody to Smith nuclear antigen	30
	False-positive VDRL × 6 mo, negative FTA-ABS	
N	Neurologic disorder—seizures, psychosis	50
M	Malar rash—flat or raised erythema, spares nasolabial folds	
D	Discoid rash—raised erythematous, scaling, follicular plugging, atrophic scarring	

*Classic lupus is considered present when many criteria are met; definite lupus, when four criteria are met; probable lupus, when three criteria are met; and possible lupus, when only two criteria are met.

pericarditis, pleuritis, oral ulcers, and psychiatric disturbances (Table 38-2). The disease characteristically has episodic flares and remissions. Symptoms during flares can occur on a spectrum from catastrophic to low grade.

What Questions Should I Ask if I Think a Patient May Have SLE?

Ask a thorough review of symptoms, including specifically about the many possible manifestations of SLE in various organs. If the patient has three or more possible manifestations of SLE, further testing with an ANA is warranted.

What are Features of Drug-Induced SLE?

Arthralgias, pleuritis, and pericarditis are common in drug-induced SLE (e.g., with hydralazine or procainamide), but renal and CNS manifestations are rare. Discontinuation of the drug typically resolves the syndrome. Nearly all patients with drug-induced SLE have a positive antihistone antibody (95%), but anti–double-stranded DNA, found in 70% of patients with idiopathic SLE, is almost always absent.

Table 38-3

Drugs Commonly Used in Lupus Treatment

Drug	Use
NSAIDs	Mild arthritis or serositis
Steroids	
High dose	Potentially life-threatening severe neuropsychiatric conditions, pulmonary hemorrhage, rapidly progressing renal failure
Low dose	Hemolytic anemia, thrombocytopenia, NSAID-resistant arthritis, mild glomerulonephritis
Hydroxychloroquine	Mild disease, dermatitis, arthritis; steroid-sparing
Cyclophosphamide*	Severe organ involvement, glomerulonephritis, CNS disease
Azathioprine†	Potentially life-threatening disease, severe vasculitis, nephritis

*Cyclophosphamide can cause GI and bone marrow toxicity. Intravenous treatment can cause nausea and vomiting. Reversible alopecia occurs in 50% of patients. Infertility also can result.

†Azathioprine is less effective, but safer than cyclophosphamide and takes 3 months for the full effect. It can cause bone marrow toxicity. Long-term use may result in a slightly higher rate of certain malignancies.

How do I Diagnose SLE?

No one clinical abnormality or lab test establishes the diagnosis of SLE. In 1982, the American College of Rheumatism developed a classification system of 11 criteria (Table 38-3). SLE is diagnosed when patients meet at least 4 of these 11 criteria, either serially or at the same time. ANA is positive in nearly all patients with SLE and is the best screening test, although it also can be positive with many other chronic inflammatory conditions.

What Complications can Occur?

Infection can be difficult to distinguish from a lupus flare. ESR, double-stranded DNA, and complement may be more abnormal with a flare than with infection. Osteonecrosis of the hips and knees, osteoporosis, and premature CAD all occur owing to long-term steroid use. Congenital heart block and neonatal SLE can occur when maternal anti-Ro antibodies are present. Stroke is a devastating complication, usually occurring in patients who have anticardiolipin antibody.

TREATMENT

What Medications can be Used for Patients with SLE?

There is no cure for SLE. The goal of treatment is to relieve symptoms, suppress inflammation, and prevent future pathology (see Table 38-3). The risk-to-benefit ratio of potentially toxic drugs must be tailored to each individual. General measures involve rest and avoidance of stressful emotional experiences, sunlight, and drugs such as OCPs that can trigger SLE flares. Patients with SLE should always wear sunscreen when they are exposed to sunlight.

What Features Suggest a Better or Worse Prognosis for Patients with SLE?

The following are associated with worse prognosis: renal disease, hypertension, male gender, young age or older age of onset, black race (perhaps as a function of socioeconomic status), poor socioeconomic status, antiphospholipid antibodies, and highly active disease.

Case 38-5

A 30-year-old African American woman reports 6 months of fatigue and painful swollen wrists, fingers, knees, and ankles worst for the first 30 minutes after she gets out of bed. Her past medical history includes intermittent episodes of rash after sun exposure, sharp chest pain, painless sores on the roof of her mouth, and a spontaneous abortion. Exam reveals normal vital signs and an erythematous rash over her cheeks and nose that spares the nasolabial folds. Joint exam reveals tender but mild spongy swelling of the wrist, MCP, and ankle joints bilaterally.

  A. What is the most likely diagnosis, and what are some other possible diagnoses?

  B. Which of the 11 criteria of SLE does this patient meet?

  C. Which labs should you send next, and how will they affect your management of this patient?

  D. What initial therapy would you recommend for this patient?

VASCULITIS

ETIOLOGY

What Causes Vasculitis?

Vasculitis results from inflammation of blood vessels, usually secondary to immune complex deposition. This inflammation affects the organ involved (e.g., renal failure in the kidney, purpuric rash in the skin, aortitis in large vessel disease, footdrop in vasculitic neuropathy). Vasculitis can occur as a primary process or in association with various systemic diseases, such as RA or SLE. Where immune complexes play a role, size and charge may be important in determining which vessels and organ systems are involved. A good example of immune complex–mediated vasculitis is chronic hepatitis B and C infections causing renal failure and rash. Purpuric rash of cutaneous vasculitis can result from bacteremia with *Neisseria gonorrhoeae, Neisseria meningitidis,* or

Table 38-4

Examples of Vasculitis Categorized by Size of Vessel Typically Affected

Large Vessel	Medium Vessel	Small Vessel
Giant cell/temporal arteritis	Polyarteritis nodosa (PAN)	Hypersensitivity—drugs, hepatitis C, Henoch-Schönlein purpura (HSP), subacute bacterial endocarditis (SBE)
Takayasu arteritis	Churg-Strauss syndrome	Wegener's granulomatosis
Systemic disease—RA, ankylosing spondylitis, syphilis	Connective tissue disease–associated—RA, lupus	Microscopic polyarteritis nodosa (MPAN)

Rickettsia. The cell type (lymphocytes, neutrophils, or eosinophils) also helps determine the pattern of vascular inflammation.

How are the Various Forms of Vasculitis Classified?

Classification is currently based on size of the vessels involved (large, medium, and small) with three major syndromes in each category (Table 38-4).

What Illnesses can Mimic Vasculitis?

Atrial myxoma and endocarditis can present with fever, weight loss, strokelike symptoms, purpuric rash, Raynaud's phenomenon, and an elevated ESR. Meningococcemia, HIV infection, and hepatitis B infection also can cause vasculitic rashes and systemic symptoms. Cholesterol emboli may cause livedo reticularis (a diffuse, lacy, violaceous skin discoloration) and nonpalpable purpura along with an elevated ESR, renal insufficiency, active urinary sediment, pancreatitis, and eosinophilia. Cocaine use also may cause a vasculitis or cause digital ischemia owing to vasospasm that mimics vasculitic lesions.

EVALUATION

When Should I Consider Vasculitis in the Differential Diagnosis?

Abnormalities of several organ systems at the same time, such as the kidneys (renal failure), skin (palpable purpura), and nerves (footdrop), are a classic feature of many forms of vasculitis. Systemic symptoms, such as fever, anorexia, and weight loss, are common. Diagnosis usually hinges on a biopsy specimen showing vessel inflammation. Footdrop and wristdrop are specific potential signs of vasculitis.

How does Large Vessel Vasculitis Manifest?

Giant cell arteritis (temporal arteritis) is seen in individuals >55 years old, especially individuals of Northern European extraction. Symptoms include headache, jaw claudication (pain in the chewing muscles with chewing), transient or permanent loss of vision, tenderness over the temporal scalp, fever, and weight loss. Many patients with giant cell arteritis have anemia. Polymyalgia rheumatica accompanies temporal arteritis in 50% of patients and is characterized by proximal muscle pain without weakness (which distinguishes it from polymyositis). ESR is usually >100 mm/h. Diagnosis of giant cell arteritis is suggested by the clinical picture and confirmed by temporal artery biopsy. Takayasu arteritis is most often reported in young women (especially Asian) and is one of the major causes of renovascular hypertension in Asian young adults. Inflammation and stenosis occur in the aorta and vessels arising from the aortic arch. Renal and CNS arteries also can be affected. ESR is elevated. Diagnosis is by arteriogram. Large artery involvement, especially of the proximal aorta, can be seen in miscellaneous systemic diseases, such as ankylosing spondylitis, reactive arthritis, syphilis, relapsing polychondritis, and rarely RA.

How does Medium Vessel Vasculitis Present?

Polyarteritis nodosa (PAN) affects small and medium-sized muscular arteries. Target organs include the CNS, peripheral nerves, intestines, and kidneys. An isolated cutaneous form also exists. PAN may be associated with chronic HBV, hairy cell leukemia, HIV infection, or amphetamine abuse. ESR is often elevated, and an active urinary sediment is frequently present. Diagnosis is based on arteriogram showing vasculitis, with or without aneurysms especially in renal arteries. Biopsy of nerve, muscle, or testicular tissue is often useful. Churg-Strauss vasculitis affects similar vessels as PAN with less renal and much more pulmonary involvement. Distinctive features include a history of asthma in almost all patients, formation of granulomas, and eosinophilic infiltrates in the lungs and vessels. Diagnosis is similar to PAN. Connective tissue diseases, such as RA or SLE, may have an associated PAN-like vasculitis.

How does Small Vessel Vasculitis Present?

Wegener's granulomatosis classically involves a triad of upper respiratory tract, lung, and kidneys, but may present in a more limited fashion. Skin, eyes, and joints also may be involved. Antineutrophil cytoplasmic antibody is usually positive, with a cytoplasmic pattern of staining, called "c-ANCA." This serology has not replaced the need for open lung biopsy to confirm diagnosis. Wegener's granulomatosis can be a culprit causing chronic sinusitis or a saddle nose deformity. Microscopic PAN is a small vessel version of PAN with similar organ involvement. c-ANCA and p-ANCA (perinuclear antineutrophil cytoplasmic antibody) patterns are seen in these patients. Hypersensitivity vasculitis comprises a group of different diseases that typically cause a leukocytoclastic vasculitis of the skin, characterized by neutrophilic infiltrate with neutrophil fragmentation in and around the small capillaries and venules. Skin is most often involved, showing petechiae or purpura, especially on the lower extremities. Kidneys and bowel also can be involved depending on the cause. Etiologies include drugs (penicillin, sulfa) and other causes of serum sickness, SBE, HSP, mixed essential cryoglobulinemia (now known to be caused primarily by HCV), and other connective tissue diseases (Table 38-5).

Table 38-5

Common Clinical Manifestations of Vasculitic Syndromes

Syndrome	CNS	Lung	Kidney	Skin	Nerve
Large Vessel					
Temporal arteritis	Headache, blindness, rare stroke			Rare scalp infarct	
Takayasu's arteritis	Eye disease, strokes		Renovascular hypertension	Rare	
Medium Vessel					
PAN	Strokes	Infiltrates, hemoptysis	Hematuria to renal failure	Ulcers, ischemic digits, livedo reticularis	Mononeuritis multiplex, peripheral neuropathy
Churg-Strauss syndrome	Strokes	Infiltrates very common, history of asthma	Rare	Similar to PAN	Similar to PAN
Small Vessel					
Hypersensitivity vasculitis	Rare	Rare infiltrates	Glomerulonephritis seen with several syndromes	Leukocytoclastic vasculitis typical	Peripheral neuropathy
Wegener's	Eye involvement, rare strokes	Infiltrates, nodules, cavitating lesions	Glomerulonephritis very common	Purpura, petechiae common	Peripheral neuropathy
MPAN	Rare stroke	Infiltrates	Glomerulonephritis common	Purpura, petechiae common	Peripheral neuropathy

What Other Vasculitis Syndromes Should I be Aware of?

Primary CNS vasculitis is a small and medium vessel vasculitis limited to the CNS that can cause stroke in young adults. It is seen in patients who abuse amphetamines, in patients after recent herpes infection involving the eye, or in patients with Hodgkin's lymphoma. Thromboangiitis obliterans (Buerger's disease) occurs most often in men who smoke and may represent a hypersensitivity to nicotine. It is characterized by panarteritis or panphlebitis with thrombosis and typically involves medium and small vessels of the lower extremities. Symptoms may include claudication (painful leg muscles with walking), Raynaud's-like phenomena, and superficial thrombophlebitis.

TREATMENT

Treat giant cell arteritis with high-dose steroids to prevent blindness, which can occur suddenly. Steroids and methotrexate are used for Takayasu arteritis, with surgery if necessary to bypass stenotic vessels. Treat PAN, microscopic PAN, and primary CNS vasculitis with steroids and cyclophosphamide. Cyclophosphamide is the drug of choice for Wegener's granulomatosis; methotrexate also may be useful. Some patients with mild, limited disease also may respond to TMP-SMX. For Buerger's disease, counsel patients to stop smoking; surgery and immunosuppressive therapy may be beneficial in some patients.

Case 38-6

A 63-year-old white woman with a history of hypothyroidism and hypertension reports feeling unwell for 1 month. She has lost 5 lb and has had frequent low-grade fevers and stiffness in the shoulders and low back when she awakes in the morning. She has a past history of migraine headaches, but over the last month she has had a more persistent right-sided headache. She attributes her weight loss to the fact that her jaw gets tired as she eats. She takes estrogen, progesterone, thyroxine, and acetaminophen with codeine. Exam reveals BP 140/85 mm Hg in both arms, weight 154 lb, temperature 38° C, mild tenderness of the right temporal scalp, and mildly reduced ROM in both shoulders.

- A. What is the most likely diagnosis?
- B. What are the appropriate diagnostic tests?
- C. What would you recommend for treatment?

Case 38-7

A 45-year-old white woman with a history of joint pain and positive rheumatoid factor presents with "red bumps all over her legs." She reports using intravenous drugs as a teenager for 6 months. Current medication is ibuprofen 400 mg three times daily. On exam, there is no evidence of active swelling of joints of the hands, wrists, or feet. There are numerous palpable petechiae on the lower extremities below the knees.

    A. What is the likely diagnosis?
    B. What are the appropriate diagnostic tests?
    C. What would you recommend for treatment?

KEY POINTS – GOUT

◆ Common medications that trigger gout are diuretics and niacin.

◆ Do not start allopurinol during an acute attack.

◆ Treat acute gout with NSAIDs except in patients with renal insufficiency or PUD.

KEY POINTS – RHEUMATOID ARTHRITIS

◆ RA causes symmetric arthritis of peripheral joints, especially MCP and MTP joints.

◆ With RA, prolonged stiffness is most severe in the morning or after periods of inactivity.

◆ Extra-articular manifestations occur in 20% of patients with RA (usually in patients with increased rheumatoid factor).

◆ Early treatment with a DMARD, alone or in combination with other DMARDs, is essential to prevent destructive changes in patients with RA.

◆ Surgical therapy (e.g., joint replacement) is effective for severely damaged joints.

KEY POINTS – SYSTEMIC LUPUS ERYTHEMATOSUS

◆ SLE is diagnosed clinically by satisfying at least 4 of 11 diagnostic criteria.

◆ ANA is nearly always positive with SLE (>95% sensitivity), but some patients with a positive ANA do not have SLE (not very specific).

(continued)

Rheumatology

- Anti–double-stranded DNA has low sensitivity and high specificity; only 70% of patients with SLE have anti–double-stranded DNA, but when it is present, the patient usually has SLE.
- Double-stranded DNA levels predict flares when they are elevated, but ANA levels do not.
- Photosensitivity is a very common problem in SLE.

KEY POINTS – VASCULITIS

- Headache or fever of unknown origin in an elderly patient could be due to giant cell arteritis.
- Aortic insufficiency in a young man could be from ankylosing spondylitis or a reactive arthritis.
- Acute onset of footdrop or wristdrop could be PAN.
- PMR is an important cause of shoulder and neck pain and stiffness in elderly patients; about 10%-20% of these patients develop giant cell arteritis.
- Petechiae and purpura associated with vasculitis are raised and palpable; in contrast, noninflammatory disorders, such as platelet abnormalities, cause nonpalpable purpura.
- Think about primary CNS vasculitis in a young patient with a stroke.
- PAN is often associated with chronic HBV.
- HCV is an important cause of small vessel vasculitis by formation of cryoglobulins.

Case Answers

38-1 A. *Learning objective:* **Choose appropriate therapy for acute gout with attention to risk factors.** This patient has an acute attack of gout. Decisions about treatment are complicated by his other medical problems. He should not receive NSAIDs because of his renal insufficiency. Colchicine also is more toxic in patients with renal insufficiency. Steroid treatment would likely markedly increase blood glucose levels, which seem to be under poor control (hemoglobin A_{1c} 10 plus random glucose of 350). Injecting his joint with steroids is the best option.

38-2 A. *Learning objective:* **Choose appropriate therapy for acute gout with attention to risk factors.** This patient comes in with a gouty attack involving a major joint (knee). He has chronic renal insufficiency and hypertension complicating his treatment options. An NSAID is usually the first choice, but should not be used in this patient because of renal insufficiency. NSAIDs also could make his antihypertensive regimen less effective. Colchicine in full treatment doses is more toxic in patients with renal insufficiency and should be avoided. The best option would be a knee injection with corticosteroid (10–20 mg of triamcinolone would work well). Another option would be a 5- to 7-day course of oral prednisone.

38-2 B. *Learning objective:* **Decide when to institute prophylactic medication to prevent gout attacks, and decide on the best treatment options.** This patient has had three attacks in the past year. He would benefit from preventive treatment because he is extremely likely to have recurrences. The timing of starting therapy with urate-lowering medication is important. Therapy should not be started during an acute attack because it may prolong the acute attack. Low-dose colchicine (0.6 mg/d) can be used to bridge the gap between the acute attack and beginning urate-lowering therapy. Allopurinol is the best option because probenecid is effective only in patients with normal renal function.

38-3 A. *Learning objective:* **Recognize early manifestations of RA, and be aware of other disorders that might mimic RA.** RA is the most likely diagnosis, but patients with SLE may have a similar presentation. The presence of objective joint swelling rules out fibromyalgia alone as the cause of her symptoms. Duration of symptoms rules out viral disorders associated with arthritis, such as parvovirus B19.

38-3 B. *Learning objective:* **Order appropriate lab tests in a patient newly diagnosed with RA.** CBC is indicated because some patients may have anemia as part of RA. ESR and C-reactive protein may be elevated; normal studies do not exclude RA. Rheumatoid factor is indicated. This test is more for prognostic value than diagnosis because many other disorders can have rheumatoid factor. High titers of rheumatoid factor are associated with a worse prognosis, in particular, worse joint disease and risk of extra-articular features. A high titer of ANA with a negative or slightly positive rheumatoid factor would point more to the diagnosis of SLE. X-rays of the hands in early RA are usually normal except for juxta-articular osteopenia. In more aggressive disease, marginal joint erosions may be present.

38-3 C. *Learning objective:* **Recognize the importance of early treatment of RA.** In a patient with active synovitis and positive rheumatoid factor, early treatment is important. Patients are usually initially placed on hydroxychloroquine 400 mg/d followed immediately by methotrexate given once per week starting with a dose of 7.5 mg. An NSAID may give symptomatic relief.

38-4 A. *Learning objective:* **Recognize extra-articular manifestations of RA.** Patients with RA may develop extra-articular manifestations, such as rheumatoid vasculitis, peripheral neuropathy often secondary to vasculitis, compression neuropathies such as carpal tunnel syndrome, rheumatoid nodules including pulmonary nodules, or

Felty's syndrome characterized by leukopenia and splenomegaly. This patient has a neuropathy secondary to rheumatoid vasculitis. Extra-articular manifestations including vasculitis are usually associated with high titers of rheumatoid factor. In the differential diagnosis, footdrop is a peroneal nerve compression caused by prolonged crossing of the legs or radiculopathy.

38-4 B. *Learning objective:* **Order appropriate tests for a new, significant neuropathy.** Nerve conduction test distinguishes a vasculitic neuropathy from a compression syndrome neuropathy. ESR is usually elevated in these patients, and rheumatoid factor is generally strongly positive.

38-4 C. *Learning objective:* **Choose appropriate treatment for this disorder.** Treat patients with neuropathy secondary to rheumatoid vasculitis with prednisone 60 mg/d and cyclophosphamide 1–2 mg/kg/d. Prednisone is gradually reduced. After 3 months of cyclophosphamide treatment, azathioprine can be substituted.

38-5 A. *Learning objective:* **List the common causes of polyarticular symmetric inflammatory arthritis, and recognize other features suggestive of SLE.** Possible causes of polyarticular symmetric joint inflammation include postviral arthritis, SLE, RA, psoriatic arthritis, or reactive arthritis. Other features of the patient's presentation (oral ulcers, photosensitivity, pleuritis, spontaneous abortion) suggest SLE and are not characteristic of the other conditions on this list.

38-5 B. *Learning objective:* **Know and use diagnostic criteria for SLE.** This patient meets five criteria for SLE—oral ulcers, arthritis, photosensitivity, malar rash, and probable serositis (episodes of chest pain). If ANA is positive, SLE is a nearly certain diagnosis.

38-5 C. *Learning objective:* **Order appropriate lab tests to evaluate a patient with probable SLE.** Order ANA with autoantibody reflexive panel, CBC with differential, PTT, ESR, complement levels (C3, C4, and CH50), RPR or VDRL, BUN, creatinine, and urinalysis. A positive ANA and anti–double-stranded DNA, in combination with her symptoms, make SLE highly likely. Low complement levels and an elevated ESR suggest disease activity. Elevated BUN and creatinine or active urine sediment indicates renal involvement. Prolonged PTT or falsely positive VDRL or RPR suggests antiphospholipid antibody syndrome (APAS). CBC is important to detect thrombocytopenia, anemia, and leukopenia (treatable complications of SLE). She has a positive ANA and anti–double-stranded DNA, ESR of 50, and low complement level.

38-5 D. *Learning objective:* **Design appropriate therapy for mild SLE.** In choosing therapy, you must balance the risks and benefits of each medication. Because this patient has relatively mild disease (i.e., no serious or life-threatening organ involvement, such as rapidly progressing renal disease or psychosis), start with an NSAID and hydroxychloroquine (the least toxic medications). If she does not improve, consider adding low-dose steroids.

38-6 A. *Learning objective:* **Recognize the presentation of giant cell arteritis.** The most likely diagnosis is giant cell arteritis, given the patient's age, morning shoulder stiffness and pain, headache (likely temporal), and jaw claudication.

38-6 B. *Learning objective:* **Order appropriate diagnostic tests for temporal arteritis.** The patient needs an ESR to confirm the inflammatory nature of her symptoms and a temporal artery biopsy.

38-6 C. *Learning objective:* **Appropriately treat giant cell arteritis.** Prednisone in a dose of 40–60 mg/d is the usual therapy given to prevent blindness. Patients with jaw claudication are at increased risk of visual changes, which can be permanent; some physicians add low-dose aspirin to the regimen at least initially.

38-7 A. *Learning objective:* **Recognize the presentation of small vessel vasculitis.** A patient with "RA" who does not really have RA but has polyarticular joint symptoms along with palpable petechiae should make one consider HCV. The patient's history of use of intravenous drugs earlier in life is important. Other causes of joint pain and petechiae could include SLE, HBV, or endocarditis.

38-7 B. *Learning objective:* **Order appropriate diagnostic tests to look for hepatitis and endocarditis in patients with palpable purpura.** LFTs are inadequate in most cases. Serologies for hepatitis B and C with PCR to confirm viral presence if HCV is positive and a blood culture and a good listen to the heart would be helpful for endocarditis. Rheumatoid factor is commonly positive in hepatitis C patients, as are cryoglobulins

38-7 C. *Learning objective:* **Treat hepatitis C–associated vasculitis.** Treatment of hepatitis C is beyond the scope of this chapter, but for the associated small vessel vasculitis such as the one presented, NSAIDs may be sufficient. If not, colchicine, low-dose prednisone (<15 mg), hydroxychloroquine (200–400 mg/d), or dapsone may be effective.

Rheumatology

REFERENCES

Gout

Agudelo CA, Wise CM: Gout: Diagnosis, pathogenesis, and clinical manifestations. Curr Opin Rheumatol 2001;13:234.

Simpkin PA: Gout and hyperuricemia. Curr Opin Rheumatol 1997;9:268.

Rheumatoid Arthritis

Lee DM, Weinblatt ME: Rheumatoid arthritis. Lancet 2001;358:903.

Pisetsky DS, St. Clair EW: Progress in the treatment of rheumatoid arthritis. JAMA 2001;286:2787.

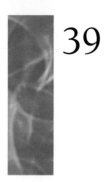

39

Substance Abuse

DOUGLAS S. PAAUW and AMY BAERNSTEIN

 ALCOHOL

ETIOLOGY

How Common are Alcohol-Related Problems?

Up to half of all men have temporary alcohol-related problems, and 10%-20% of men and 5%-10% of women have persistent alcohol-related problems, defined as alcohol use causing legal, marital, physical, or interpersonal problems.

Why do Patients Who use Alcohol have Electrolyte Problems?

Chronic use of alcohol causes renal magnesium wasting from tubular cells. Magnesium is important in maintaining a normal potassium level; low magnesium levels lead to potassium loss and hypokalemia. Adequate magnesium levels also are important in normal PTH production and release. With hypomagnesemia, inadequate PTH levels lead to low 1,25-dihydroxyvitamin D, calcium, and phosphate levels. Poor nutrition decreases phosphate intake, and phosphate loss in the urine occurs in hypomagnesemia.

Why do Patients with Alcoholism Develop Alcoholic Ketoacidosis?

Alcoholic ketoacidosis occurs in a patient who habitually drinks heavily, but has stopped drinking 1–2 days before presentation. The patient often has not had anything to eat or drink over the preceding 12–24 hours owing to nausea and abdominal pain. ABG shows a moderate acidosis, chemistry shows a low HCO_3^-, and serum ketones are elevated with predominance of beta-hydroxybutyrate. During the starvation state, counter-regulatory hormones produce a marked increase in serum free fatty acids. Alcohol suppresses ketogenesis initially, but as the alcohol level falls, there is rapid conversion of fatty acids to ketones.

EVALUATION

How can I Recognize and Diagnose Alcohol-Related Problems?

Suspect alcohol abuse in patients with trauma, motor vehicle accidents, or unexplained abdominal pain. Also, consider alcohol use in patients with hypertension or osteoporosis because alcohol is an important secondary cause of hypertension and osteoporosis, especially in men. Ask all patients if they consume alcohol. If the answer is no, ask if they have had problems with alcohol in the past. Patients who are currently using alcohol can be screened with CAGE questions (Box 39-1). CAGE questions have a sensitivity of 80% and a specificity of 85% if a cutoff of two or more positive responses is used; they are less sensitive in women and ethnic minorities. Men who drink >14 drinks a week and women who drink >7 drinks a week are at risk for problem drinking.

What Cardiovascular Abnormalities are Seen with Alcohol Abuse?

There is a firm link between chronic alcohol consumption and hypertension. This is seen in patients who drink three or more drinks a day and is a common cause of secondary hypertension. "Holiday heart" is a syndrome of paroxysmal arrhythmias, the most common of which is atrial fibrillation, described in alcohol binge drinkers. Other arrhythmias include atrial flutter, paroxysmal atrial tachycardia, and VT. Alcohol is an important cause in 50% of congestive cardiomyopathies. There is some reversibility with cessation of alcohol use.

What are the Acute and Chronic Effects of Alcohol on the Liver?

The manifestation of alcoholic hepatitis from an acute alcohol binge ranges from asymptomatic LFT abnormalities to florid, acute, life-threatening liver failure. Usually, the presentation is insidious with anorexia, nausea, vomiting, abdominal pain, and low-grade fever. Physical exam usually reveals an enlarged, tender liver. Evidence of portal hypertension (severe hemorrhoids, ascites, GI bleeding from esophageal varices) and hepatic encephalopathy may be present in severe cases. Liver enzymes are mildly or moderately elevated, AST more so than ALT (Table 39-1). Cirrhosis develops in 10%-20% of chronic alcoholics.

Substance Abuse

BOX 39-1

CAGE QUESTIONS USED TO SCREEN FOR ALCOHOL ABUSE

Have you ever felt you should Cut down on your drinking?
Have people Annoyed you by criticizing your drinking?
Have you ever felt Guilty about your drinking?
Have you ever started the day by having a drink to get going or to calm your nerves? (Eye opener)

Table 39-1

Laboratory Abnormalities Seen with Heavy Regular Alcohol Use

Abnormal Lab Test	Cause
Hematology	
Anemia	
Microcytic	Iron deficiency due to GI blood loss
Macrocytic (mildly increased MCV)	Liver disease/direct effect on stem cells
(markedly increased MCV)	Folate deficiency
Thrombocytopenia	Decreased platelet survival or hypersplenism or both due to cirrhosis
Leukopenia	Decreased marrow production of WBC
Abdominal	
Increased AST > increased ALT (AST rarely ever >300)	Alcoholic hepatitis
Increased GGT	"Alcohol use test," very sensitive to alcohol use
Decreased albumin	Alcoholic hepatitis or cirrhosis
Increased PT	
Increased amylase	Pancreatitis
Minerals/Electrolytes	
Decreased magnesium	Renal tubular magnesium wasting
Decreased potassium	Renal potassium loss worsened by magnesium deficiency
Decreased calcium	Hypomagnesemia decreases PTH release, causing poor GI calcium absorption
Decreased phosphate	Poor nutrition, increased urinary loss

It develops at a lower daily alcohol intake in women because of 50% less alcohol dehydrogenase in their stomachs and resulting decreased immediate metabolism of alcohol. In many patients, cirrhosis is unrecognized until a life-threatening complication, such as esophageal variceal bleeding, occurs. Check liver synthetic function with PT and albumin.

What are the Different CNS Complications Seen with Alcohol Use?

Acute intoxication can cause ataxia, incoordination, and drowsiness. Large amounts of alcohol, especially in individuals without chronic use, can cause coma. Wernicke-Korsakoff syndrome is a nutritional neurologic disorder caused by thiamine deficiency. It commonly goes unrecognized. The clinical manifestations of Wernicke's encephalopathy are acute onset of oculomotor abnormalities (bilateral abducens palsy, nystagmus, total ophthalmoplegia), ataxia, and global confusional state. Other symptoms that can occur include hypothermia, hypotension, and coma. All of these symptoms may reverse with administration of thiamine. Eighty percent of patients with Wernicke's encephalopathy who survive develop Korsakoff's psychosis, which is characterized by retrograde and anterograde amnesia. Confabulation, the fabrication of stories, may be present. A significant proportion of patients with Korsakoff's psychosis do not recover and require long-term institutionalization. Chronic alcohol use can cause peripheral neuropathy, which involves the feet first, then the hands in a "stocking and glove" distribution.

What are the Symptoms of Alcohol Withdrawal?

Most patients with chronic alcohol use have mild withdrawal symptoms of tremor, sleep disturbance, and increased anxiety. In addition, tachycardia and increased temperature can occur. A few (<5%) can have severe withdrawal with marked confusion and hallucinations (delirium tremors). Alcohol withdrawal seizures occur in a few patients, usually in the first 2 days after cessation of alcohol. A prior history of withdrawal seizures increases the risk of recurrence with subsequent episodes of withdrawal.

TREATMENT

How is Alcohol Withdrawal Treated?

For mild withdrawal symptoms of tachycardia and jitteriness, a beta blocker can be helpful. Benzodiazepines are the mainstay of treatment of alcohol withdrawal. Longer acting benzodiazepines such as diazepam are effective, but are more likely to cause prolonged sedation secondary to drug accumulation. Lorazepam has an intermediate half-life and better elimination in elderly patients and in patients with renal insufficiency. Symptom-triggered therapy, where patients receive medication when their symptom score is above a certain threshold is effective and requires less medication than a fixed-dose schedule for treatment of alcohol withdrawal.

What Other Treatments Should be Given to Hospitalized Alcoholics?

Most patients have magnesium deficiency and should receive intravenous magnesium. All patients should receive intravenous thiamine 100 mg daily for three doses and a daily multiple vitamin with folate.

When Should I Hospitalize a Patient with Complications of Alcohol Use?

Hospitalize patients with the following:

- Alcohol withdrawal with mental status changes or unstable vital signs
- Metabolic disturbances that are severe (hypokalemia, alcoholic ketoacidosis)
- Severe alcoholic hepatitis with recurrent emesis or signs of portal hypertension or encephalopathy
- A desire for inpatient alcohol treatment to facilitate transfer to an alcohol treatment program

Case 39-1

A 39-year-old man with a history of alcohol abuse presents with nausea, vomiting, and abdominal pain. He has had low-grade fevers as well and has been drinking 18–24 beers a day.

  A. What is your differential diagnosis for his abdominal pain?
  B. What lab tests would you order?
  C. His potassium is 2.9. What other electrolytes would you expect to be abnormal?

Case 39-2

A 49-year-old man with a 20-year history of alcohol abuse is admitted with confusion and weakness. His last drink was 24 hours ago. He usually drinks three to four bottles of wine daily. On exam he is tremulous with a pulse of 128 and BP of 160/100. He is oriented only to person. Lab results are as follows: Na 136, K 3, HCO_3^- 13, BUN 20, creatinine 1, glucose 60, chloride 98, serum osmolality 280.

  A. What is the most likely cause for his metabolic acidosis? How would you treat it?
  B. What is appropriate therapy for his alcohol withdrawal?

Answers appear on pages 553–555.

 COCAINE

ETIOLOGY
How and Why do People Use Cocaine?

Cocaine is derived from the leaves of the coca plant and has been chewed as a stimulant for thousands of years. The user gains a euphoric sense of boundless energy and self-confidence. Users can be hypersexual, angry, or violent. The drug is metabolized quickly, and the high is followed by a "crash," during which the user feels depressed and irritable. Drug craving sets in during this period. Powdered cocaine can be used intranasally (snorted), which gives a less intense high and is most expensive. Dissolved in water, cocaine can be injected intravenously, which gives an immediate and intense high. When no vein is available, cocaine can be injected subcutaneously ("skin-popping") or intramuscularly ("muscling"). "Crack" is a cheap smokable form of cocaine that gives a brief but intense high and is highly addictive. Its introduction in the 1980s was associated with a surge in drug-related crime, violence, and social problems across the U.S.

EVALUATION

How do I Know Cocaine is Causing a Patient's Problem?

Ask every patient about drug and alcohol use. Patients who do not offer information about their drug use at first will sometimes admit it if you tell them how important it is to treat their immediate problem. Urine drug screens detect cocaine for at least 48 hours after use.

What are the Medical Complications of Cocaine?

Cocaine causes centrally mediated sympathetic overdrive, with tachycardia, hypertension, and vasospasm of coronary and cerebral arteries. Seizures, hypertensive encephalopathy, and ischemic and hemorrhagic strokes are common neurologic sequelae. Chest pain and dysrhythmias, such as SVT, VT, and ventricular fibrillation, are the most common cardiac complications. Rhabdomyolysis, acidosis, fever, and coma are additional sequelae that can be rapidly fatal. Less serious are nonhealing scabs and shallow skin ulcers that result from uncontrollable picking and the sensation of bugs on the skin (formication) that occurs even in noninjection users and epistaxis and septal necrosis in intranasal users.

If Cocaine is a Stimulant, Why do Users Present with Decreased Consciousness?

At very high doses, cocaine's local anesthetic effect predominates over its stimulant effect and causes life-threatening coma. Also, individuals who have been on a cocaine binge become profoundly lethargic for hours or days after they stop, a condition called "postcocaine depression" or "cocaine washed-out syndrome."

TREATMENT

How do I Treat Cocaine-Related Medical Problems?

Intravenous diazepam is the primary treatment for most types of cocaine toxicity. By decreasing centrally mediated sympathetic overdrive, diazepam reduces agitation, seizures, hypertension, tachycardia, and vasospasm-mediated chest pain. Even VT and ventricular fibrillation, if cocaine-induced, should be treated with diazepam in addition to the usual defibrillation. If diazepam alone does not control BP, labetalol and nitroprusside are good choices. Pure beta blocker drugs, such as esmolol and metoprolol, cause unopposed alpha adrenergic stimulation and worsen the situation. A patient with chest pain that resolves with diazepam and shows no ischemic ECG changes can be safely discharged, but ischemic changes on ECG and elevated cardiac enzymes require admission and standard therapy for acute MI. Rhabdomyolysis, confirmed by a high serum CPK and positive urine myoglobin, can be fatal and requires intravenous diazepam, intravenous bicarbonate, and aggressive hydration.

HEROIN

ETIOLOGY

How and Why are Opioid Drugs Abused?

Opioids are naturally derived or synthetic drugs that mimic the effects of opium, producing pain relief, relaxation, sleep, and a powerful sense of well-being. These are also called narcotics. Oral narcotics, extensively used for medical pain relief, can be abused. A much more potent "high" comes from intravenous use. Heroin is the most commonly injected narcotic, but morphine, meperidine, and fentanyl also are available. Heroin also may be smoked or snorted. A "speedball" refers to injecting heroin and cocaine together.

EVALUATION

What are the Toxic Effects of Heroin?

A heroin overdose occurs when the user takes enough heroin to suppress the respiratory drive. The individual is found unconscious and apneic with pinpoint pupils. Prolonged apnea leads to hypoxic brain injury and may be complicated by aspiration, hypothermia, or rhabdomyolysis from prolonged immobility. With frequent use, tolerance develops to the respiratory depressant effect of opioids. A common situation for heroin overdose is a user who has been abstinent for a period of time and then uses the same amount to which he or she was previously accustomed. Noncardiogenic pulmonary edema can occur after intravenous narcotic use in new and experienced users. Its etiology is unknown.

How can I Identify Heroin Overdose?

Most overdose patients are treated by prehospital personnel with naloxone, an opioid antagonist, and are alert when they reach the hospital. Naloxone can be used safely on any unconscious patient as a diagnostic maneuver; a response proves opioid intoxication.

How can I Identify Heroin Withdrawal?

Narcotic withdrawal begins as soon as a chronic user misses an expected dose. The longest acting opioids, such as methadone, produce the longest lasting withdrawal syndrome. Along with dysphoria and drug craving, physical symptoms include some or all of the following: nausea, vomiting, diarrhea, abdominal cramping and pain, lacrimation, rhinorrhea, yawning, chills, diaphoresis, myalgias, piloerection (goose flesh—thus "quitting cold turkey"), and involuntary muscle jerks ("kicking the habit"). Fever is not part of narcotic withdrawal, and any heroin user with a fever needs an aggressive search for an infection.

Substance Abuse

TREATMENT

When Should I Treat Heroin Overdose?

A patient who has hypoxia as a result of slow or ineffective respirations needs naloxone (intravenous or intramuscular). If the patient does not immediately recover normal mental status, consider intubation to protect the airway and provide adequate air exchange. It is essential to consider other causes of depressed mental status in this case. Patients successfully treated with naloxone may become sleepy as the drug wears off, but if they are successfully oxygenating 1 hour after naloxone was given, are fully arousable, and have no infectious complications of their injection drug use, they may be safely discharged. Overdose of long-acting narcotics, usually methadone, requires frequent redosing of naloxone, and the patient should be admitted.

How can I Treat Heroin Withdrawal in a Hospitalized Patient?

The symptoms of withdrawal are alleviated by substituting a longer acting narcotic, such as methadone for heroin. Withdrawal from methadone also occurs, but a hospitalization can be a transition to a structured detoxification program or a long-term methadone maintenance program. Although heroin withdrawal is intensely uncomfortable, in contrast to alcohol or benzodiazepine withdrawal the syndrome is not physically dangerous. Clonidine is an alternative to methadone because it lessens narcotic withdrawal symptoms.

INFECTIOUS COMPLICATIONS OF PARENTERAL DRUG ABUSE

ETIOLOGY

What Types of Infections Affect Intravenous Drug Users?

Shared needles transmit viral infections from user to user, including HBV, HCV (present in about 80% of IDU), and HIV. Nonsterile injection also causes local bacterial infections, including open ulcers from "skin popping," deeper skin abscesses and cellulitis from intravenous use, and large, deep intramuscular abscesses from "muscling." Injected cocaine causes local vasoconstriction and tissue necrosis, so cocaine-related abscesses are generally larger and more difficult to heal. Bacterial cultures reveal *Staphylococcus, Streptococcus, Pseudomonas,* and oral flora including anaerobes (in users who lick their needles). Tetanus may be present. Every injection causes a transient bacteremia, with the potential for developing endocarditis, meningitis, septic PE, and lumbar osteomyelitis or epidural abscess. A depressed gag reflex during heroin use makes aspiration pneumonia common. Socioeconomic factors and poor immune function increase the risk of TB.

Substance Abuse

EVALUATION

How do Bacterial Infections Differ in Drug Users?

Because of impaired immunity, elevated WBC and fever are often absent in drug users with a serious infection. Cellulitis, abscesses, and osteomyelitis are best diagnosed by exam. CXR is essential in diagnosing pneumonia, although individuals with AIDS may have pneumonia with a normal film. If fever is present in an IDU, it strongly suggests infection.

What Primary Care Might Specifically Benefit Patients Who Use Intravenous Drugs?

Primary care for the IDU is an emerging concept currently lacking supporting data; these patients' high risk of acquiring and transmitting a variety of infections makes the following steps sound reasonable. Screen for HIV; hepatitis A, B, and C; and TB (by purified protein derivative). For patients who have not been exposed to hepatitis A or B, vaccinate. Hepatitis A vaccine is especially important in patients who have hepatitis C. Make sure patients have received tetanus boosters, as IDU is a higher risk group for developing tetanus. Pneumococcal vaccine also may be warranted. Because 50% of female IDU participate in prostitution, regular screening for gonorrhea, *Chlamydia,* and cervical cancer also is wise.

TREATMENT

Who Needs Hospitalization for a Drug-Associated Bacterial Infection?

Any IDU with a fever >38.5° C should be hospitalized and treated presumptively for endocarditis with nafcillin and gentamicin. If another infection is present that could account for the fever, such as pneumonia or cellulitis, it is appropriate to tailor antibiotics to that illness while ruling out endocarditis with blood cultures. Cellulitis alone or an abscess that can be drained in the clinic can be treated on an outpatient basis with oral antibiotics, such as cephalexin or dicloxacillin. If methicillin-resistant *Staphylococcus aureus* is common in your location, a non–penicillin-derived antibiotic with gram-positive coverage, such as TMP-SMX, should be chosen instead. Abscesses should be repacked once or twice a day.

Case 39-3

A 19-year-old college student comes to you because of arm pain. Her left antecubital fossa has a 6 cm × 10 cm area of erythema, induration, warmth, and tenderness. You can easily see multiple tiny needle punctures along the vein. You suspect this is a complication of injection drug abuse.

A. How would you approach asking her about drug use?
B. What structures may be affected by this infection?
C. What therapies are appropriate? How does her drug use change your management?

Substance Abuse

Case 39-4

A 43-year-old man sees you in the office for chronic abdominal pain and
constipation. He has seen multiple physicians for this problem, but no diagnosis
has been found. He is angry because his last physician suggested that his main
problem is addiction to pain pills. He has been taking large quantities of oral
narcotics for many years, prescribed for multiple musculoskeletal pains.

  A. If this assessment is correct, what do you think would happen if he
     stopped taking all opiates?
  B. How would you counsel this patient?

KEY POINTS – ALCOHOL

◆ Multiple mineral and electrolyte disorders occur with chronic alcohol
  use; hypomagnesemia is probably the most important and leads to
  hypokalemia and hypocalcemia.

◆ Alcoholic hepatitis can mimic acute cholecystitis with fever,
  leukocytosis, and RUQ pain.

◆ Transaminases are usually only modestly elevated with AST > ALT in
  alcoholic hepatitis.

◆ Alcohol use is an extremely common cause of secondary hypertension in
  the U.S.

KEY POINTS – INFECTIOUS COMPLICATIONS OF PARENTERAL DRUG ABUSE

◆ Cocaine has many potentially fatal toxic effects, most mediated by
  sympathetic overdrive.

◆ Heroin overdose causes respiratory depression and is reversible with
  naloxone.

◆ Heroin, cocaine, and methamphetamine do not have physically dangerous
  withdrawal syndromes, in contrast to alcohol or benzodiazepines

Case Answers

39-1 A. *Learning objective:* **State the common causes of abdominal pain
associated with alcohol use.** Nausea, vomiting, low-grade fevers,
and abdominal pain are likely due to alcoholic hepatitis. Pancreatitis
also is possible. Gastritis from alcohol use is less likely.

39-1 B. *Learning objective:* **Order appropriate tests for evaluating abdominal pain in a patient with history of alcohol abuse.** Order transaminases, bilirubin, amylase, alkaline phosphatase, and CBC. If he has alcoholic hepatitis, you would expect AST to be two to three times greater than ALT. Pancreatic amylase would be elevated if he has acute pancreatitis. A CBC looks for a low HCT (GI tract bleeding) and an elevated WBC (seen with alcoholic hepatitis and pancreatitis). Consider a CXR to look for aspiration pneumonia.

39-1 C. *Learning objective:* **Understand common electrolyte disorders associated with heavy alcohol use.** Low magnesium, calcium, potassium, and phosphate levels are likely in the setting of chronic alcohol use.

39-2 A. *Learning objective:* **Recognize alcoholic ketoacidosis.** This patient has an anion gap acidosis in the setting of heavy alcohol use. Consider an ingestion of methanol or ethylene glycol in addition to alcoholic ketoacidosis in your differential diagnosis. The lack of an osmolal gap makes those ingestions unlikely. Treat alcoholic ketoacidosis with fluid resuscitation containing glucose. Check a magnesium level, replace electrolytes, and give thiamine and a multivitamin with folate.

39-2 B. *Learning objective:* **Treat alcohol withdrawal appropriately.** He should receive benzodiazepines in adequate doses, which may require dosing every 2–4 hours initially. He probably also would benefit from a beta blocker because he is tachycardic and hypertensive.

39-3 A. *Learning objective:* **Outline an appropriate drug history.** Questions about drug use should be integrated into the rest of the history. Ensure that your patient feels safe with you and sees you as nonjudgmental and respectful of her confidentiality. If she does not initially report injection drug use, ask her again, emphasizing that the information is essential in properly diagnosing and treating her arm infection.

39-3 B. *Learning objective:* **Describe the infectious complications of intravenous drug use.** This infection is probably cellulitis, an infection of the skin. Examine carefully, however, for signs of abscess (an area of fluctuance), septic arthritis (joint effusion and extreme pain on passive ROM), osteomyelitis (changes on x-ray or bone scan), and endocarditis (high fever and sometimes a heart murmur).

39-3 C. *Learning objective:* **Treat intravenous drug use–associated infections.** If this patient has cellulitis alone, has a fever <38.5° C, and is able to tolerate food and medicine, prescribe oral dicloxacillin or cephalexin, and arrange for a follow-up exam within a few days. Small abscesses may be drained in the office and treated the same way. Patients with large abscesses, septic arthritis, osteomyelitis, or endocarditis should be admitted for intravenous antibiotics and further evaluation. Patients with vomiting and dehydration likewise should be admitted. In either case, a drug-related infection is a time when your patient may be most motivated to start drug treatment. Consider counseling, screening, and vaccination or screening for hepatitis A, B, and C, and HIV. Anticipate heroin withdrawal in daily users of this drug who are hospitalized.

39-4 A. *Learning objective:* **Describe opiate withdrawal.** You can expect that over a period of days this patient will develop some or all of the following: dilated pupils, rhinorrhea, muscle cramps, bone and joint aches, abdominal cramps, nausea, vomiting, diarrhea, and piloerection. You would not expect him to have fever, tachycardia, or hypertension as a result of opiate withdrawal; these findings would require further evaluation.

39-4 B. *Learning objective:* **Devise an approach to a patient with chronic drug use.** You may be able to help this patient most by providing information and resources in a nonaccusatory, nonjudgmental way. Establishing trust over several visits and keeping appropriate boundaries with him also would help. Tapering the opiate dose slowly would minimize the withdrawal symptoms. Addressing the underlying addiction is essential.

REFERENCES

Alcohol

Chang PH, Steinberg MB: Alcohol withdrawal. Med Clin North Am 2001; 85:1191.

Kosten TR, O'Connor PG: Management of drug and alcohol withdrawal. N Engl J Med 2003;348:1786.

Infectious Complications of Parenteral Drug Abuse

Emerg Med Clin North Am 1990;8.

USEFUL WEB SITE

Infectious Complications of Parenteral Drug Abuse

National Institute on Drug Abuse (NIDA). http://165.112.78.61/NIDAHome.html

Substance Abuse

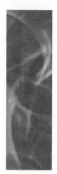

40

Women's Health

HEIDI S. POWELL, ANNE EACKER, MARY B. LAYA, ELIZA L. SUTTON, and MARY B. MIGEON

ABNORMAL PAP SMEARS

ETIOLOGY

What Causes Abnormal Pap Smears?

The Papanicolaou test (Pap smear), which can be done with a conventional smear or with a liquid-based technique, is the most widely available screening test for cervical cancer. Risk factors for abnormal Pap smears, also known as cervical dysplasia, include multiple sexual partners, early age of sexual intercourse (<17 years old), history of sexually transmitted diseases, HIV infection, promiscuity of male partner, tobacco use, and OCP use. Certain subtypes of HPV play a key role in most cases of cervical dysplasia. Other reasons for abnormal Pap smears include hormonal changes, inflammation related to vaginal infections, and artifacts related to Pap smear collection. Such changes may be identified by the cytopathologist.

EVALUATION

When should Cervical Cancer Screening Start, and How Often should Pap Smears be Obtained?

Cervical cancer screening should begin 3 years after a woman becomes sexually active or at age 21. Annual screening should be done until there have been three consecutive normal Pap smears. Subsequently, the screening interval can be increased to every 2–3 years in most women. Screening should be discontinued when a woman is 65 years old, has had three consecutive normal Pap smears within the previous 10 years, and is not at high risk for cervical cancer. Any woman who has not had regular screening, even if she is >65 years old, should be screened if she is otherwise healthy. Women who have had a hysterectomy for benign reasons do not need Pap smears.

How is the Pap Smear Result Interpreted?

Most cytopathologists use the Bethesda System for reporting Pap smear findings. This system reports "squamous intraepithelial cell" lesions (cervical dysplastic changes) separately from "specimen adequacy" and "benign cellular changes." Cervical dysplasia is a precancerous condition, requiring follow-up surveillance to detect progression to cancer. Cervical dysplasia is usually reported as ASCUS, LGSIL, or HGSIL. Each finding should be triaged for appropriate follow-up as outlined in Figure 40-1 with HPV testing, surveillance Pap smears, or colposcopy. Colposcopy allows the clinician to view the cervix under low-power magnification and to obtain a biopsy specimen of cervical tissue to confirm cytologic findings of the Pap smear.

What Role does HPV Subtyping Play in Managing Cervical Dysplasia?

HPV strains have been differentiated into high-risk, intermediate-risk, and low-risk subtypes for causing cervical cancer. High-risk subtypes, especially HPV 16 and HPV 18, are strongly correlated with carcinoma in situ or invasive carcinoma. HPV subtyping is useful for triaging patients with ASCUS for colposcopy and for follow-up surveillance in a woman who has had a previously abnormal Pap smear. Routine screening for HPV is not indicated for all women at this time because it is often transient in young women, and positive results would result in unnecessary follow-up testing. The U.S. Food and Drug Administration has approved HPV testing in combination with cervical cytology as a screening tool for cervical cancer in women >30 years old. If both of these tests are negative, the woman can wait 3 years to be screened again, even if she has multiple new sexual partners. A vaccine is available for HPV and is recommended for girls and women ages 13–26 but can be administered as early as 9 years old.

TREATMENT

How is Cervical Dysplasia Treated?

Treatment options depend on the extent of disease and invasive potential. Ablative therapy includes cryotherapy and laser vaporization. Excisional therapy includes cold knife conization, laser conization, and LEEP. Excisional therapy is indicated when patients have more severe dysplastic changes, when the transformation zone is not well visualized, or when further histologic evaluation is needed.

Case 40-1

A 33-year-old woman had a normal pelvic exam 3 weeks ago. Her Pap smear returns as ASCUS. She has no history of abnormal Pap smears.

A. How would you follow up on this test result?
B. Is routine screening for HPV recommended for all women?

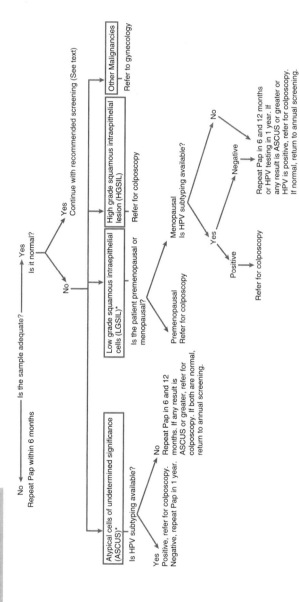

FIGURE 40-1 Algorithm for management of abnormal Pap smears. *Alternative options for the following populations: **Adolescents (13–21 years old) with ASCUS or LGSIL:** Forego initial HPV testing because HPV is often transient in this age group, and positive results lead to unnecessary colposcopies. Instead, repeat Pap at 6 and 12 months or HPV testing in 1 year. If any results are ASCUS or greater or HPV is positive, refer for colposcopy. If normal, repeat Pap in 1 year. **Postmenopausal women with ASCUS or LGSIL:** If HPV is negative, and there are signs of atrophy, treat with estrogen vaginal cream for 3 weeks with follow-up Pap 1 week later. If abnormal, repeat Pap in 4–6 months. If normal, return to annual screening. If either Pap is ASCUS or greater, refer for colposcopy.

Case 40-2

A 72-year-old woman establishes care with you. She is healthy and in a monogamous relationship. The last time she had a Pap smear was when she was in her 50s.

    A. Does she need a Pap smear?

    B. At what age can cervical cancer screening be discontinued?

ABNORMAL UTERINE BLEEDING

ETIOLOGY

How is Abnormal Bleeding Defined?

Normal menarche usually occurs before age 16 with a cycle repeating every 24–35 days and menstrual flow lasting 4–6 days. Abnormal bleeding includes any change in menstrual cycle frequency, duration, or amount of flow and intermenstrual bleeding. Abnormalities in bleeding are characterized using specific terminology (Table 40-1).

What are Common Causes of Abnormal Uterine Bleeding?

The differential diagnosis depends on age and bleeding pattern. Always consider pregnancy and its complications with any abnormal bleeding pattern in a woman of any age. Aside from pregnancy, causes may be structural, hormonal, infectious, pharmacologic, or systemic (Table 40-2). In adolescents, the most common cause is anovulation, manifested as irregular menses, but other causes include coagulopathy with heavy menstrual

Table 40-1

Terminology Used to Describe Abnormal Patterns of Menstrual Bleeding

Terminology	Pattern
Amenorrhea	Lack of menses for ≥90 d
Menorrhagia (hypermenorrhea)	Heavy bleeding at regular intervals with menstrual cycle (bleeding lasts >7 d and amount is >80 mL/d or 6 pads/d)
Metrorrhagia	Irregular bleeding (can be too frequent or too infrequent)
Oligomenorrhea	Infrequent bleeding
Intermenstrual bleeding	Bleeding between regular menstrual cycles
Polymenorrhea	Regular bleeding at intervals <21 d
Dysfunctional uterine bleeding (DUB)	Excessive uterine bleeding in the absence of identifiable organic pathology, not during a usual cyclic bleed

Women's Health

Women's Health

Table 40-2
Common Causes of Abnormal Vaginal Bleeding Based on Bleeding Pattern

	Menorrhagia	Metrorrhagia	Postcoital	Postmenopausal
		Type of Bleeding		
Structural Causes	Fibroid Polyp Coagulation disorder Copper IUD	Polyp, especially endocervical	Polyp, especially endocervical	Atrophy

Hormonal Causes		DUB
		Anovulation
		  Polycystic ovary syndrome (PCOS)
		  Anorexia
		  Thyroid disorders		

Neoplastic Causes	Cervical or endometrial cancer	Cervical or endometrial cancer	Cervical cancer	Endometrial cancer
Infectious Causes		Endometritis	Cervicitis	
Pharmacologic Causes	Anticoagulants Chemotherapy	Progestin-only contraceptives Combined hormonal contraceptives Psychotropic drugs		Systemic estrogen therapy Systemic estrogen- progestin therapy

bleeding and infection with intermenstrual spotting or postcoital bleeding. Hyperthyroidism and hypothyroidism can cause menstrual irregularities, including menorrhagia and less frequent menses. In premenopausal women, causes are more varied, including those already mentioned, but pregnancy and malignancy are the "do-not-miss" diagnoses. Anatomic problems, such as endometrial polyps and uterine fibroids, can cause heavy bleeding, usually during menses without changing menstrual cycle timing. Postcoital bleeding is usually due to a cervical abnormality, such as polyp, cervicitis, or cervical cancer. Irregular and infrequent bleeding that has persisted since onset of menarche is likely due to PCOS. In postmenopausal women, bleeding is often due to atrophic changes, but 10% have endometrial cancer.

What Causes Anovulation, and How does This Affect the Menstrual Cycle?

Anovulation is common in adolescent girls and in women approaching menopause. Cycles that vary by >10 days from one to the next are likely anovulatory. Anovulation can occur suddenly or transiently with excessive weight changes, stress, illness, or endocrine disorders that disrupt function of the hypothalamic-pituitary axis. It also can be chronic, as in PCOS. Patients with chronic anovulation have unpredictable, often infrequent and heavy bleeding owing to unopposed estrogen exposure (without ovulation, there is no progesterone produced). The unopposed estrogen causes buildup and unpredictable periodic sloughing of the endometrial lining and possible increased risk of endometrial cancer.

Why do Some Patients have Abnormal Bleeding with Hormonal Contraception?

The low doses of estrogen in today's combined hormonal methods (pill, ring, patch) result in a fragile and atrophic endometrial lining. This leads to breakthrough bleeding or spotting between periods, which is especially common in the first few months of use. Progestin-only regimens, including Depo-Provera, the "mini pill," and the Mirena IUD, also cause unpredictable bleeding, especially in the first 6 months of use. Overall menstrual blood loss is less with all of these hormonal methods than with no hormonal method.

EVALUATION

How do I Evaluate Patients with Abnormal Uterine Bleeding?

Ask about precipitating factors (intercourse, trauma), duration of the problem, pattern and amount of bleeding, use of birth control, and associated symptoms such as pain or fever. Quantifying vaginal bleeding can be a challenge. It may help to ask how many pads or tampons the patient has required over a 24-hour period. Medication history also is key (see Table 40-2). Perform a pelvic exam to look for anatomic or infectious causes, such as endocervical polyp or cervicitis. Verify normal secondary sexual characteristics, and look for virilization or hirsutism.

Include orthostatic BP and pulse if bleeding is brisk. Patients presenting with changes over one or two cycles with an otherwise unremarkable history and physical can keep a menstrual log because the pattern of bleeding helps guide diagnostic work-up.

What Should my Approach be for Evaluating Postmenopausal Bleeding?

Bleeding occurring after menopause is concerning for malignancy. Perform a pelvic exam looking for any cervical abnormalities needing biopsy, obtain a Pap smear, and schedule for a transvaginal ultrasound. Endometrial biopsy may be required if bleeding persists or recurs even if other tests are negative. Postmenopausal bleeding is a common problem in women on estrogen-progestin therapy, especially within the first 6 months of continuous therapy. Adjustment of the hormonal regimen within the first 6 months of therapy without further evaluation is reasonable, but evaluate as described if bleeding persists or recurs.

What Investigations should I Order?

Order tests selectively based on history, physical, and menopausal status. A urine pregnancy test should always be ordered in women at risk. TSH can almost always be justified as well. If ectopic pregnancy is suspected, send a serum β-HCG level and order urgent pelvic ultrasound. Consider screening for *Chlamydia trachomatis* in any woman who is sexually active, especially if she has postcoital bleeding or new breakthrough bleeding on contraception. Check HCT if excessive bleeding is reported; consider platelets and coagulation studies if an underlying medical condition or the clinical picture suggests a clotting problem. In addition, prolactin, LH, and FSH can be helpful if an underlying endocrine problem is suspected. Hyperprolactinemia can cause either amenorrhea or anovulatory bleeding. Hypothalamic hypopituitarism may be suggested on the basis of amenorrhea with low body weight. Consider PCOS in patients with hirsutism, obesity, glucose intolerance, and long-standing menstrual irregularity. Cervical cultures for *Chlamydia* and gonorrhea may be taken during the pelvic exam if PID or endometritis is suspected; alternatively, obtain first-void urine to test for gonorrhea and *Chlamydia*. Transvaginal ultrasound or endometrial biopsy or both are required to evaluate for endometrial hyperplasia or malignancy in postmenopausal patients and may be indicated in younger women as well.

TREATMENT

What is the Treatment for Abnormal Uterine Bleeding?

Management of abnormal uterine bleeding should be directed at resolving the underlying problem. Urgent cessation of bleeding with surgical intervention is rarely needed. Urgent medical treatment to stop prolonged bleeding may be desirable on the basis of severe anemia or patient convenience. Short-term cessation of bleeding often can be achieved with a course of progesterone (medroxyprogesterone 10 mg daily × 10 days). OCP (or the ring or patch) can be used to regulate bleeding cycles in chronic anovulatory states such as PCOS and hypothalamic dysfunction. *Trichomonas* or other sexually transmitted disease diagnoses should be treated with appropriate antibiotics and should prompt consideration of testing for other sexually transmitted diseases, including syphilis and HIV. Cervical polyps easily visualized can be removed by simple twisting with ringed forceps. Endometrial polyps require more invasive techniques for removal. Fibroids may be followed, although they should be removed if they are growing rapidly or causing significant anemia. Endometrial cancer usually requires hysterectomy. Patients with heavy, prolonged DUB should receive hormonal therapy with estrogen or progesterone to stop the bleeding, then remain on OCP if there are no contraindications.

When Should I Hospitalize or Refer?

Indications for urgent referral and hospitalization include excessive vaginal bleeding causing hemodynamic changes, a significant drop in blood count, or suspicion of ectopic pregnancy.

Case 40-3

A nulliparous 22-year-old woman presents for routine annual exam. She reached menarche at age 11 and has always had irregular periods, which generally come two to four times a year. She is not interested in birth control and she assumes that because she has irregular periods, she cannot get pregnant. She uses topical tretinoin for acne. On exam, height is 64 inches, weight is 180 lb, and she has mild hirsutism of her face and acanthosis nigricans on her posterior neck. Normal secondary sex characteristics are present, and there is no evidence of virilization.

   A. How would you evaluate this patient for her irregular menses?
   B. What other conditions would you wish to exclude?
   C. How would you counsel her regarding treatment?

BREAST HEALTH

ETIOLOGY

What Benign and Malignant Findings can Occur in Breast Tissue?

Benign causes of lumps include simple cysts and fibroadenomas. Atypical hyperplasia, although benign, is a risk factor for subsequent development of cancer. Carcinoma in situ and invasive carcinoma of the ducts or lobules or both are malignant lesions.

Women's Health

What is Mastalgia?

Mastalgia (breast pain) occurs in 80% of women during their reproductive years; 20% of women experience moderate-to-severe breast pain. Bilateral cyclic tenderness is most common in the premenstrual period and does not require further evaluation. Although only 6% of cancers manifest with pain, persistent, focal pain requires biopsy.

What are Risk Factors for Breast Cancer?

Breast cancer kills >40,000 annually in the U.S., but women may live many years with breast cancer. Age is an important risk factor; approximately 75% of breast cancer patients >50 years old have no risk factors aside from age. Other risk factors include early menarche, late menopause, nulliparity, and atypical cells on prior breast biopsy. A family history of premenopausal breast cancer in two or more first-degree relatives may suggest the presence of a genetic predisposition to breast cancer.

EVALUATION

What Screening is Recommended for Breast Cancer?

Screening patients >50 years old with annual examination and mammogram decreases mortality from breast cancer by 30%. Mammography for women 40–50 years old is reasonable, but benefits are smaller, and the risk of false-positive findings is greater. Screen earlier in women with very high risk (*BRCA1* or *BRCA2* gene mutation, first-degree relative, or atypia on breast biopsy specimen).

How do I Perform a Good Breast Examination?

Inspect and palpate both breasts, axillae, and subareolar areas. Using the pads of two fingers and a circular motion, swirl through the layers of the breast tissue to the chest wall. Examine the entire breast systematically using a vertical stripe pattern. Document exact location, size, and quality of any breast exam findings. Comparing one side with the other reduces uncertainty about what is normal versus abnormal.

What Clinical Presentations are Worrisome for Underlying Cancer?

Any palpable breast lump, asymmetric thickening, or focal pain should be regarded with suspicion. Breast cancer risk factors do not substantially alter pretest probabilities of cancer and should not play a role in the decision to evaluate. Work-up is indicated for any focal finding or symptom. It is impossible to distinguish benign from malignant conditions on physical exam, but the presence of any of the following raises concern for malignancy (most breast cancers show none of these):

- A mass fixed to the chest wall
- Dimpling of the skin overlying the breast
- Recent-onset unilateral nipple inversion
- Spontaneous nipple discharge, especially if clear or bloody

- Scaly lesions of the nipple
- Failure of breast inflammation to respond promptly to antibiotics
- Persistent, focal breast pain

What are the First Steps in the Work-Up of a Breast Lump, Thickening, or Focal Pain?

Order a diagnostic mammogram in all patients ≥25 years old. This differs from a screening mammogram in that it requires more time, additional views, and direct supervision by a mammographer. Breast ultrasound, an important adjunct to the evaluation of breast masses, reliably identifies benign simple cysts, helps characterize solid lesions and direct biopsy, and is used diagnostically in women <25 years old because more dense tissue makes mammogram less accurate. When mammogram or ultrasound shows a clearly benign finding (simple cyst or calcified fibroadenoma), no further evaluation is needed.

When should a Biopsy be Done?

Refer patients with lumps fixed to the chest or associated with dimpling for surgical biopsy. Patients with lesions suspicious for cancer on imaging also should undergo core needle biopsy under ultrasound or stereotactic guidance. Other palpable masses or focal thickenings warrant close follow-up by repeat exam or FNA, even if mammography findings are normal. FNA is not a true biopsy, but it is a useful procedure for sampling cells when clinical and radiographic suspicion for malignancy is low. An abnormal FNA mandates biopsy. A mass with negative "triple test" findings (negative FNA, negative mammogram, and low-suspicion clinical breast exam) has <3% chance of being a missed cancer and can be followed without biopsy.

What is the Appropriate Follow-Up for Focal Breast Problems with Normal Imaging?

Because 10% of breast cancers are not detectable on mammography, plan close clinical follow-up. Have a low threshold for consultation with a breast specialist.

How does Staging Determine Prognosis in Breast Cancer Patients?

Many prognostic factors help determine therapy. Your patient's prognosis is better if her tumor is small, if it has estrogen receptors, and if it has few S (synthesis) phase cells (the pathologist determines this). The most important prognostic factor is the absolute number of positive axillary lymph nodes.

TREATMENT

How are Simple Cysts and Fibroadenomas Managed?

For simple cysts shown on ultrasound, no further follow-up is necessary. If the cyst is bothersome or interferes with examination, it can be reduced through aspiration of fluid. Biopsy may be needed for complex cysts. Fibroadenomas should be biopsied or followed for stability for 24 months. Refer patients for resection when they have fibroadenomas that are >2 cm in size, or if they have grown rapidly or are painful.

What Alleviates Breast Pain?

A well-fitting bra, low-fat diet, and reduction in caffeine intake may be effective, but data are limited. Treat infection with antibiotics and abscess with drainage.

What is the Best Treatment for a Breast Cancer Lump?

Surgical resection is required for all breast cancers. Lumpectomy with radiation is as effective as modified radical mastectomy in most patients. Adjuvant therapy refers to the use of hormone therapy chemotherapy or immunotherapy after definitive surgical treatment. Adjuvant hormone therapy with tamoxifen or an aromatase inhibitor or both is used for estrogen receptor–positive tumors. Adjuvant systemic chemotherapy is recommended for tumors >1 cm, node-positive cancers, and node-negative cancers with high-risk immunohistochemistry.

How is Metastatic Breast Cancer Treated?

Metastatic breast cancer is unlikely to be cured, but local and systemic therapies can improve survival and quality of life. Hormonal manipulation is helpful in estrogen receptor–positive patients—oophorectomy for premenopausal women and tamoxifen or aromatase inhibitors or both for postmenopausal women. Immunotherapy with trastuzumab, a monoclonal antibody against the *HER2/neu* gene, is indicated for patients with *HER-2/neu*-positive tumors. Chemotherapy is used for highly aggressive, unresponsive, or widely metastatic disease.

How Effective is Therapy?

The breast cancer death rate has declined since 1990 as a result of treatment advances and early detection. The overall 10-year disease-free survival is 80%. Survival decreases with larger tumor size, poor immunohistologic grade, and number of positive lymph nodes. Many patients now live with breast cancer, a disease that can be effectively managed if not cured.

Case 40-4

A 48-year-old woman reports a month-long history of a sensation of fullness in the upper outer quadrant of her left breast. You detect a 2-cm lump with indistinct margins that is mobile and without overlying skin dimpling.

A. What is the first step in the evaluation?
B. If the diagnostic evaluation is negative, what follow-up should be planned?
C. What should prompt a referral to a breast surgeon?

Women's Health

Case 40-5

A 28-year-old woman presents with a 2.5-cm, mobile, slightly tender mass in the inferior left breast. Mammogram is negative, although breast tissue is very dense.

A. What other tests are indicated?
B. What is appropriate follow-up if studies suggest a fibroadenoma?
C. What is appropriate follow-up if studies suggest a simple cyst?

MENOPAUSE

ETIOLOGY

What is Menopause?

Natural menopause is the permanent cessation of menses and marks a woman's entry into the postreproductive phase of life. The final menstrual period is defined retrospectively after 12 consecutive months of amenorrhea. The menopause transition includes the years before the final menstrual period when variability of the menstrual cycles increases. This transition period and the 12 months after the final menstrual period are defined as the perimenopause. The perimenopause is a period of physiologic disruption owing to fluctuating levels of hormones and symptoms. After menopause, CAD and osteoporosis increase significantly.

What is a Hot Flash?

A hot flash is a symptom complex caused by the sudden downward resetting of the central core temperature set-point. This results in a sensation of heat and the initiation of heat-dissipating mechanisms, such as vasodilation, sweating, and a reflex tachycardia. Hot flashes are more frequent and can be quite severe in the perimenopause and decline in subsequent years. They are a common reason women seek care at perimenopause.

Can Menopause Cause Depression?

Major depression and anxiety disorders are not associated with menopause and are less prevalent than earlier in life. Mood swings may be associated with sleep problems leading to daytime irritability, forgetfulness, and fatigue. Perimenopause also is a time of profound social and psychological change for women—children leave home, elderly parents need assistance, work roles may change, and relationships with spouses may change. The stresses and health effects of these life events may be falsely attributed to coincidental biologic changes associated with menopause. Major depression, if present, requires treatment and would not respond to hormone therapy alone.

Why is Osteoporosis Particularly Prevalent In Postmenopausal Women?

Although men and women show age-related decline in bone mineral density after age 40, most women have an accelerated phase of bone loss associated with the cessation of ovarian estrogen production in the 5 years after menopause. Men are protected against osteoporosis because they achieve higher peak bone mass, and they do not have an abrupt decline in sex hormones.

EVALUATION

How does One Determine if a Woman is Perimenopausal?

Perimenopause can be identified clinically by a combination of age and characteristic symptoms. The median age of onset of the menopausal transition occurs at 47.5 and the final menstrual period at 51 years. The characteristic symptoms of hot flashes, sleep disturbance, and mood swings peak in perimenopause and diminish in the years following. Vaginal dryness and urinary frequency manifest later in the transition and in the postmenopausal years. Classic symptoms do not occur in every woman, may precede the transition by years, and may be caused by other conditions.

Are Blood Tests Helpful in Defining Perimenopause?

Blood tests such as FSH have no place in defining this phase of life in nonhysterectomized women. FSH levels fluctuate markedly during this time and do not reliably correlate with stage of perimenopause or predict transition events. By contrast, women who have undergone hysterectomy do not manifest menstrual changes, so an elevated FSH is helpful in deciding when to begin hormone replacement. Unusual patterns, such as cycle irregularity at an early age, warrant further testing for unexpected pregnancy, thyroid disease, and hyperprolactinemia with β-HCG, TSH, and prolactin levels.

What are the Expected Bleeding Patterns in the Transition Phase?

Most commonly, menstrual cycles become further apart and the volume of menstrual blood flow is reduced reflecting the waning production of estrogen by the ovaries and the increasing frequency of anovulatory cycles. In 10% of women, menses cease abruptly.

What Bleeding Patterns Should Prompt Further Evaluation?

Heavy menstrual bleeding, prolonged menses (>7 days), and more than two cycles in 1 month should prompt investigation for endocrine (hypothyroidism) or structural abnormalities. Endovaginal ultrasound detects uterine fibroids and uterine polyps, which may cause heavy bleeding. In addition, ultrasound is useful for ruling out endometrial carcinoma. An endometrial stripe of <5 mm makes endometrial cancer extremely unlikely. Endometrial sampling using a pipelle catheter also can detect endometrial hyperplasia or carcinoma.

TREATMENT

What are the Options for Treatment of Perimenopausal Symptoms?

Hot flashes, mood swings, and sleep disturbances are most effectively treated with hormone replacement therapy (HRT). The relatively new SERMs, such as raloxifene, do not prevent hot flashes. Other treatment modalities are less effective, but may be useful in women who cannot or do not wish to take HRT. These include clonidine, soy products, vitamin E, and environmental control such as maintenance of cool ambient temperature and cotton clothing. Many alternative medicines are available, but to date none has shown effectiveness. Data suggest that estrogen may increase risk of second MI in patients with prior MI and may increase breast cancer risk slightly after ≥5 years of use. Women should be counseled on these potential harms before initiating HRT.

What are the Currently Available Replacement Hormones?

For women with an intact uterus, HRT should consist of an estrogen and a progestin, the latter to protect against endometrial proliferation and uterine cancer. The most commonly used estrogens in the U.S. are conjugated equine estrogen (oral), micronized estradiol (oral), 17-beta estradiol (transdermal patches and vaginal creams), and piperazine estrone sulfate (oral). The available progestins are medroxyprogesterone acetate and micronized progesterone (Table 40-3).

Table 40-3

Estrogen and Progestin Preparations Commonly Used in Perimenopause

	Method	Usual Dose Range and Frequency	Cost (Relative)
Estrogens			
Estradiol	Oral	0.5 mg or 1 mg daily	$
17-beta estradiol	Transdermal	0.05 mg/d or 0.1 mg/d patch, changed 1–2 ×/wk	$$
Conjugated equine estrogen	Oral	0.3 mg, 0.45 mg, or 0.625 mg daily	$$$
Progestins			
Medroxyprogesterone acetate	Oral	2.5 mg or 5 mg daily or 5 mg daily on 14 consecutive days/mo	$
Micronized oral progesterone	Oral	100 mg daily or 200 mg daily on 14 consecutive days/mo	$$$

What Replacement Therapy Regimens are Currently Used?

One of the aforementioned estrogens is usually taken daily. Progestins may be given cyclically (e.g., medroxyprogesterone acetate 5 mg days 1–14) or continuously (e.g., 2.5 mg daily). The cyclic regimens should result in regular bleeding starting day 9 or later and are particularly useful in an early perimenopausal patient to regulate cycles. The daily continuous regimen should lead to amenorrhea after the first 6–12 months of therapy. Out of phase bleeding should result in adjustment of the regimen or evaluation of the endometrium by ultrasound or endometrial biopsy to rule out hyperplasia or cancer. Adjustment in the estrogen-progesterone regimen is an appropriate approach if bleeding occurs within the first 6 months of replacement therapy. If bleeding continues beyond 6 months, work-up with endovaginal ultrasound or endometrial biopsy is appropriate. For isolated vaginal symptoms, the estrogen ring is an appropriate alternative, is placed vaginally by the patient, and releases hormone locally. The ring is changed by the patient every 3 months.

What are the Benefits and Risks of HRT?

Based on prior large observational studies and basic science research, HRT has been thought to be protective against cardiovascular disease through a variety of mechanisms. More recent randomized trials call this belief into question, however. It is unclear whether these benefits are limited to certain women, and whether they outweigh the risks of estrogen administration when relative contraindications to HRT exist, such as family history of breast cancer. Large-scale randomized clinical trials are ongoing to examine these issues. Data from a prior study, the Women's Health Initiative, are presented in Table 40-4.

Table 40-4

Change in Absolute Risk (per 10,000 Woman-Years) from Menopausal Hormone Therapy

	CEE* + MPA[†]	CEE* Alone
Coronary heart disease	+ 7	NS
Stroke	+ 8	+ 12
DVT or pulmonary embolism	+ 8	NS
Breast cancer (invasive)	+ 8	NS
Hip fracture	− 6	− 6
Colon cancer	− 6	NS
Global index (any significant event)	+ 19	NS

*CEE = conjugated equine estrogen 0.625 mg/d.
[†]MPA = medroxyprogesterone acetate 2.5 mg/d.
NS, no significant difference from placebo group.
Data from Rossouw J, Anderson G, Prentice R, et al: Risks and benefits of estrogen plus progestin in healthy postmenopausal women: Principal results from the Women's Health Initiative randomized controlled trial. JAMA 2002;288:321–333.

Case 40-6

A 48-year-old woman seeks care for a 6-month history of bothersome hot flashes and infrequent menses. She is otherwise in good health and has a normal physical exam.

- A. What tests are required to assure she is in the menopause transition?
- B. What type of HRT would you prescribe?
- C. Three months later, she reports prolonged menses lasting 14 days. What should you do next?
- D. What other regimen might you prescribe?

 OSTEOPOROSIS

ETIOLOGY

What is Osteoporosis?

Osteoporosis is a state of low bone mass and skeletal fragility owing to microarchitectural deterioration of bone tissue. Osteopenia is a precursor to osteoporosis.

Why is Osteoporosis a Problem?

Long-term sequelae of osteoporosis include fractures of the hip, spine, and other bones; chronic fracture pain; and kyphosis with compression of internal organs from repeated vertebral compression fractures. The most severe result of osteoporosis is hip fractures, occurring in 15% of elderly women. Only one third of patients with hip fracture return to prefracture independence. As the population ages, the number of hip fractures is expected to triple by 2040.

Who gets Osteoporosis?

Osteoporosis affects an estimated 30% of postmenopausal white and Asian women in the U.S. Rates are lower, although not inconsequential, among other groups. Approximately 10% of African American women and 13%-16% of Hispanic women ≥50 years old have osteoporosis. Women are four times as likely to get osteoporosis as men, although men have more disability after hip fracture. In men, as with postmenopausal women, hypogonadism accelerates bone loss. Alcoholism also is a major risk factor in men.

What are Other Secondary Causes of Osteoporosis?

Early menopause (e.g., with oophorectomy), corticosteroid therapy, vitamin D deficiency, celiac disease, hyperthyroidism, and hyperparathyroidism can cause bone loss.

What are Risk Factors for Osteoporosis?

Key, easily identifiable risk factors include the following:

- Age
- Family history of fracture in first-degree relative (particularly before age 80)
- Personal history of fracture after age 40
- Current cigarette smoking
- Low body weight (<127 lb)

Additional risk factors include white or Asian ethnic descent. Lifestyle issues also play an important role, including inadequate vitamin D and calcium intake, tobacco and alcohol use, and sedentary habits. Osteoporosis also is associated with hyperthyroidism, hyperparathyroidism, and chronic inflammatory conditions, such as collagen vascular diseases. Medications such as corticosteroids, heparin, anticonvulsants, and methotrexate also predispose to the development of osteoporosis.

EVALUATION

Who Should be Screened for Osteoporosis?

Recommendations vary, but screening for premenopausal women is not indicated. The National Osteoporosis Foundation recommends screening all women >65 years old and postmenopausal women >50 years old with one or more risk factors. A more conservative, evidence-based organization, the U.S. Preventive Services Task Force, revised their screening recommendations as follows: Women ≥65 years old should receive screening routinely. In women with risk factors as outlined previously, they recommend screening begin at age 60. Earlier screening is not endorsed.

How is Osteoporosis Diagnosed?

Diagnosis is made by T-score on DXA scan of <−2.5 *or* by fragility fracture regardless of T-score (Box 40-1). A fragility fracture is a fracture that occurs with minimal or no trauma (e.g., a vertebral compression fracture). Ultrasound also has been used to measure bone density at the heel or elbow. Although the method correlates with fracture risk, it has limited precision, and peripheral site bone loss may lag. Also, results have not been standardized to treatment recommendations. Patients require confirmatory DXA scan.

BOX 40-1

INTERPRETATION OF DXA SCAN RESULTS

T-score >−1 = normal
T-score −1 to −2.5 = osteopenia
T-score <−2.5 = osteoporosis

Women's Health

What are T-scores and Z-scores?

The T-score represents the patient's bone density in standard deviations compared with an average 25-year-old woman. The Z-score is the age-matched result. The T-score has been chosen as the marker for osteoporosis.

What Site is Best to View with DXA Scan, and How Often Should the DXA Scan be Repeated?

Site of DXA measurement (hip, spine, or wrist) best predicts fracture at that site. Hip bone mineral density is the best predictor of future hip fracture. Hip DXA measurement also is the best *overall* fracture risk predictor. Recommendations for frequency of monitoring vary. A conservative approach that avoids artifactual variation in readings is as follows: repeat DXA scan every 2–5 years unless you expect rapid loss, such as with steroid use.

TREATMENT

When Should Treatment be Started?

Although common sense would dictate that treatment should start before full osteoporosis develops, a large-scale national study found benefit only in patients with T-score <−2.5 (i.e., in patients with full-scale osteoporosis). Nonetheless, the current National Osteoporosis Foundation (NOF) recommendations are listed in Box 40-2. These guidelines may be revised, so visit the NOF web site for the most recent information.

What are Options for Treatment?

Calcium, vitamin D, and weight-bearing exercise are baseline treatments in any patient with osteoporosis and for prevention in all women (Box 40-3). First-line pharmacologic treatments are bisphosphonates. The bisphosphonates alendronate and risedronate show fracture reduction rates of 50%, and both are available on a once-weekly dosing regimen. Optimal duration of therapy is unknown. Whether bone loss resumes when therapy is stopped is controversial. Bisphosphonates may cause erosive esophagitis, so patients must take precautions to remain upright for 30 minutes after intake. Intravenous formulations are under

---

BOX 40-2

WHEN TO START OSTEOPOROSIS TREATMENT

T-score <−2
Or
T-score <−1.5 plus one or more risk factors
Or
Fragility fracture regardless of T-score result

BOX 40-3

RECOMMENDED TOTAL DAILY INTAKE FOR CALCIUM AND VITAMIN D

Calcium

- 800 mg for children 4–8 years old
- 1300 mg for children and young adults 9–18 years old
- 1000 mg for adults 19–50 years old
- 1200 mg for adults >50 years old

Vitamin D*

- 200 IU daily for children and adults <50 years old
- 400 IU daily for adults 50–70 years old
- 600 IU daily for adults >70 years old
- 800 IU daily for adults who are homebound or institutionalized

*Less vitamin D may be required if sunlight is abundant and no sunscreen is used.

study for osteoporosis use (e.g., zoledronate can be dosed as an intravenous infusion one to four times per year). This drug is not yet approved by the Food and Drug Administration for osteoporosis. Osteonecrosis of the jaw rarely has been associated with bisphosphonates, particularly with the intravenous forms. The selective estrogen receptor modulator raloxifene decreases vertebral fracture risk and lowers low-density lipoprotein. Similar to bisphosphonates, raloxifene is a good choice for osteoporosis prevention. For frank osteoporosis, bisphosphonates have stronger data. A similar agent to raloxifene, tamoxifen, is used in breast cancer and has weaker, although perhaps adequate bone density loss prevention. Before the results of the Women's Health Initiative, estrogen replacement was considered first-line therapy in the prevention and treatment of osteoporosis. The added benefits of controlling hot flashes and reducing vulvar atrophy made it a welcome option for many women. Data from the Women's Health Initiative revealed, however, that estrogen-progestin therapy increases the risk of breast cancer, stroke, and venous thromboembolic events. Nonetheless, these events accrue over time, and for women with strong postmenopausal symptoms, shorter term estrogen therapy is the best choice. Uterine cancer is increased with postmenopausal estrogen use, but can be offset by simultaneous progesterone use. Bone density loss resumes when the hormone therapy is stopped. For men with hypogonadism, testosterone is first-line therapy. Regarding monitoring response to therapy, DXA every 2 years is reasonable. Benefit to bone may be separate from actual changes in bone density figures. Precision error in DXA measurement is 2% in the spine and 4%-6% in the hip. Biochemical markers of bone turnovers vary, although the scale of change after starting antiresorptive therapy may be large enough to overcome this. Nonetheless, these tests are of questionable use.

Can Osteoporosis be Prevented?

Prevention of osteoporosis is more effective in reducing morbidity and mortality than treatment of established disease. It is crucial to identify in adolescence and early adulthood the conditions that may predispose toward inadequate bone mass development; peak bone mass is reached in the late 20s for women and mid-30s for men. Conditions include eating disorders, hypothalamic conditions leading to amenorrhea, tobacco and alcohol use, sedentary lifestyle, intolerance of dairy products, and vitamin D deficiency. Smoking cessation is vital. For elderly patients, fall prevention is crucial. Providers should be aware that gait instability, poor vision, unsafe home environment, and medications that alter consciousness are potentially avoidable precursors in this population. Hip protectors for individuals at increased risk of falls have been shown to prevent fracture. Prevention should start in the teenage years or earlier with vitamin D and calcium (see Box 40-3). Further benefit is gained from weight-bearing exercise on sites susceptible to fracture (i.e., walking for hip and spine density, weights for wrists).

Case 40-7

A 62-year-old Asian woman with eczema, reflux, and tobacco use is in the office for her annual health maintenance exam. She is lactose intolerant and does not exercise. On exam, she weighs 120 lb, has normal vital signs, and stooped posture, which she reports is similar to her mother's posture.

A. What are her risk factors for osteoporosis?
B. Should she be screened?
C. What test would you use for screening?
D. Before her test results, what treatment would you recommend?

Case 40-8

A 57-year-old woman has a screening DXA scan because she has a family history of osteoporosis. Her T-score is −2.3. She is not having menopausal symptoms currently. She has a history of spontaneous DVT.

A. Does she have osteoporosis or osteopenia?
B. Does she require treatment?
C. What treatment would you recommend?

KEY POINTS – ABNORMAL PAP SMEAR

◆ Risk factors associated with cervical dysplasia include HPV infection, early first intercourse, multiple sexual partners, promiscuity of male partners, OCP use, and tobacco use.

◆ Refer for colposcopy when HGSIL is identified or when ASCUS is found on follow-up surveillance Pap smears.

◆ Use high-risk HPV type testing in triaging ASCUS.

◆ Women who have had a hysterectomy for benign causes do not need Pap smears.

◆ Screening can be discontinued in women at age 65 if they have had three consecutive normal Pap smears within the previous 10 years and are not at high risk for cervical cancer.

KEY POINTS – ABNORMAL UTERINE BLEEDING

◆ Use targeted, stepwise lab testing to rule out common diagnoses first.

◆ Refer for hospitalization or urgent gynecologic evaluation if hemodynamically significant bleeding or possible ectopic pregnancy is present.

◆ Suspect endometrial cancer if postmenopausal bleeding is present.

KEY POINTS – BREAST HEALTH

◆ Most breast cancer occurs in the absence of risk factors aside from age.

◆ Physical exam cannot reliably distinguish benign from malignant breast conditions.

◆ Begin with diagnostic mammography for evaluation of most breast complaints in women >25 years old.

◆ Palpable masses must be followed up with repeat exams or FNA even if mammogram findings are normal.

KEY POINTS – MENOPAUSE

◆ The symptoms of perimenopause are hot flashes, sleep disturbances, mood swings, and irregular menses; not all women require or desire treatment.

Women's Health

◆ Evaluate heavy or frequent bleeding out of phase in the perimenopause for uterine pathology by endovaginal ultrasound or endometrial biopsy.

KEY POINTS – OSTEOPOROSIS

◆ Main risk factors for osteoporosis are age, female sex, low weight (<127 lb), family or personal history of fracture, and cigarette smoking.

◆ Screen for osteoporosis with DXA scan in women >65 years old and women >50 years old with risk factors.

◆ Diagnosis of osteoporosis is made by DXA scan T-score <−2.5 or by fragility fracture regardless of T-score.

◆ Prevent osteoporosis with adequate vitamin D and calcium intake and reasonable weight-bearing exercise starting in the teenage years.

◆ Bisphosphonates are the main pharmacologic therapy for osteoporosis.

Case Answers

40-1 A. *Learning objective:* **Know how to manage ASCUS results on a Pap smear.** This patient should have HPV (high-risk) testing done if it is available. If her Pap smear was collected using the ThinPrep technique, HPV testing can be performed on that sample without having the patient return to the clinic for another test. A negative HPV test has a very high negative predictive value (98%) in women who have ASCUS on Pap smear. If her test is negative, she can wait 1 year for a follow-up Pap smear. If her test is positive, she should be referred for colposcopy. If HPV testing is unavailable, she should return for follow-up Pap smears at 6 and 12 months. If both are normal, she can return to annual testing. If there is an abnormal result, she should be referred for colposcopy.

40-1 B. *Learning objective:* **Understand when to use HPV testing.** Routine screening for HPV is not recommended for all women at this time. HPV often is transient in young women, and a positive result may result in unnecessary testing. HPV testing is recommended when Pap smear results are nondiagnostic (ASCUS). It is not indicated for LSIL or HSIL because >80% of these lesions are associated with a positive HPV result, and it wouldn't alter the patient's management (except in postmenopausal women with LGSIL). HPV testing combined with cervical cytology can be used as a screening tool for cervical cancer in women >30 years old. If both of these tests are negative, the patient can wait 3 years to be screened again, even if she has multiple new sexual partners.

40-2 A. *Learning objective:* **Identify women at risk for cervical cancer.** Yes, she needs a Pap smear. More than 60% of cervical cancer cases in the U.S. are in women who have not received routine screening. One quarter of all cervical cancers occur in women >65 years old owing to lack of screening.

40-2 B. *Learning objective:* **Know when to discontinue cervical cancer screening.** The U.S. Preventive Services Task Force recommends discontinuation of screening in women at age 65 who have had three consecutive normal Pap smears within the last 10 years and who are not at high risk for cervical cancer. Screening should be continued annually in elderly women who are in reasonably good health but who have immunosuppression, HIV, history of in utero exposure to diethylstilbestrol, multiple sexual partners, or history of cervical cancer.

40-3 A. *Learning objective:* **Identify a clinical scenario suggestive of PCOS.** This patient's primary oligomenorrhea, hirsutism, obesity, and acanthosis nigricans are strongly suggestive of PCOS. This is a poorly understood condition with heterogeneous presentation. Despite the suggestive name, the anatomic finding of polycystic ovaries is variably present. Significant controversy surrounds the basic pathophysiologic mechanism of disease. Most experts agree that there is inappropriate feedback involving the ovarian-pituitary axis, leading to relative hyperandrogenism. An LH-to-FSH ratio of >2:1 can be confirmatory; however, its absence would not rule PCOS out. It is unnecessary to perform a pelvic ultrasound. A TSH and prolactin level should be done to rule out thyroid and pituitary disease.

40-3 B. *Learning objective:* **Recognize the association of insulin resistance and endometrial cancer in patients with PCOS.** PCOS has been associated with insulin resistance and endometrial cancer. Exclude these by fasting glucose and endometrial monitoring by ultrasound or biopsy (guidelines for frequency or mode of screening don't currently exist).

40-3 C. *Learning objective:* **Prescribe OCPs to prevent unwanted pregnancy, regulate cycles, and prevent atypical endometrial changes.** Amenorrhea or oligomenorrhea can lead to endometrial hyperplasia and atypia. Patients with PCOS should receive OCPs to help regulate endometrial shedding; this also protects against pregnancy because infertility cannot be assumed. Patients who do not desire contraception may choose instead to use cyclic medroxyprogesterone to induce menstruation every 3 months.

40-4 A. *Learning objective:* **Design appropriate work-up for a breast lump.** Order diagnostic mammogram. Unless a clearly benign finding is noted, perform ultrasound and FNA.

40-4 B. *Learning objective:* **Plan follow-up when work-up for a breast lump is negative.** A negative "triple test"—physical exam without suspicious features, negative mammogram, and benign FNA—reduces, but does not eliminate, the possibility of cancer. Perform follow-up exams every 3–6 months for at least 1 year to ensure stability.

40-4 C. *Learning objective:* **Recognize indications for referral of patients with abnormal breast findings.** Suspicious mammogram, ultrasound, or FNA should prompt early referral. Referral also is indicated if the mass enlarges over time.

40-5 A. *Learning objective:* **Identify the role of ultrasound in work-up of abnormal breast lesions.** Ultrasound is useful, especially when mammogram is difficult to interpret because of high breast density. Alternatively, FNA results may reveal a cyst or cytology consistent with a fibroadenoma.

40-5 B. *Learning objective:* **Appropriately manage a fibroadenoma.** Fibroadenomas are benign, disorganized breast tissue. Indications for removal are size >2 cm, rapid growth, and discomfort.

40-5 C. *Learning objective:* **Appropriately manage a simple breast cyst.** If ultrasound of the mass clearly shows a simple cyst, no further follow-up is necessary. If the mass is bothersome to the patient or interferes with mammography or physical exam, aspirate under ultrasound guidance.

40-6 A. *Learning objective:* **Recognize that menopause is a clinical diagnosis.** No further testing is required.

40-6 B. *Learning objective:* **Design HRT for a perimenopausal woman.** A cyclic regimen might be preferred in women in the transition whose ovaries continue to produce some sex hormones at irregular intervals. It may be possible to regulate cycles with this regimen. Review risks and benefits with the patient before initiating HRT.

40-6 C. *Learning objective:* **Understand importance and method of evaluating out-of-phase or prolonged bleeding in a woman on HRT >6–12 months.** Consider an endometrial biopsy or pelvic ultrasound to evaluate the endometrial lining and rule out hyperplasia, malignancy, or structural abnormality such as a polyp or fibroid.

40-6 D. *Learning objective:* **Use progestin to stabilize endometrium.** If the endometrial biopsy and uterine ultrasound are normal, the next step is to increase progestin to foster transformation of the proliferating endometrium. Alternatively, very-low-dose OCP can be used to capture cycles completely and provide regular bleeding.

40-7 A. *Learning objective:* **List osteoporosis risk factors.** This patient has several clear risk factors: weight <127 lb, current smoking, and probably family history given her mother's posture (dowager's hump, or kyphosis, from chronic vertebral compression fractures). In addition, she does not exercise and most likely has low vitamin D intake owing to her lactose intolerance.

40-7 B. *Learning objective:* **Be familiar with current NOF osteoporosis screening recommendations.** The NOF recommendations applied to this case are as follows: This patient is not >65 years old, when the NOF (and USPSTF) recommends all women should be screened for osteoporosis. She has several risk factors for osteoporosis, however, and so should have been screened after age 50—12 years ago.

40-7 C.   *Learning objective:* **State the best screening test for osteoporosis.** DXA scan is the standardized test for osteoporosis. Other tests, such as urine metabolic markers of bone turnover or heel or wrist ultrasound obtained at malls, may indicate the possibility of osteoporosis, but are not reliable enough to direct treatment. Rather, their results may prompt the DXA scan, which is the standardized measure of osteoporosis. Another option in this patient is to obtain a lateral CXR to screen for compression fractures. If present, and no secondary cause is suspected (i.e., pathologic fracture of multiple myeloma), the fragility fracture would make the diagnosis of osteoporosis without a DXA scan required.

40-7 D.   *Learning objective:* **Identify nonpharmacologic measures for osteoporosis prevention.** The patient should stop smoking, which would decrease her risk for osteoporosis and potentially improve her reflux symptoms. She should begin weight-bearing exercise and start taking vitamin D and calcium daily.

40-8 A.   *Learning objective:* **Interpret T-score result.** The T-score of −2.3 indicates 2.3 standard deviations below the average bone density of a 25-year-old white woman. This is consistent with osteopenia, which is defined as T-score between −1 and −2.5.

40-8 B.   *Learning objective:* **Outline when to begin pharmacologic treatment in osteopenia.** Although this patient does not have osteoporosis, treatment should be started based on current NOF guidelines because her T-score is <−2. Because of her risk factor of family history, therapy would be started for a T-score of −1.5. These guidelines are under review and may become slightly more stringent in the next year or so. See the NOF web site at the end of the chapter for current recommendations.

40-8 C.   *Learning objective:* **Design pharmacologic treatment for osteoporosis in this patient with a history of DVT.** Because of this patient's history of DVT, hormone therapy is inappropriate. In her case, a bisphosphonate would be an excellent choice. Alendronate 70 mg a week would be reasonable. As with all osteoporosis prevention and treatment, ascertain that the patient is getting adequate vitamin D, calcium, and weight-bearing exercise.

REFERENCES

Abnormal Pap Smear

Cox JT: The clinician's view: Role of human papillomavirus testing in the American Society for Colposcopy and Cervical Pathology Guidelines for the

Women's Health

Management of Abnormal Cervical Cytology and Cervical Cancer Precursors. Arch Pathol Lab Med 2003;127:950.

Solomon D, Davey D, Kurman R, et al: The 2001 Bethesda System: Terminology for reporting results of cervical cytology. JAMA 2002;287:2114.

Abnormal Uterine Bleeding

Hardiman P, Pillay OS, Atiomo W: Polycystic ovary syndrome and endometrial carcinoma. Lancet 2003;361:1810–1812.

Osteoporosis

Kado DM, Browner WS, Palermo L, et al: Vertebral fractures and mortality in older women: A prospective study. Study of Osteoporotic Fractures Research Group. Arch Intern Med 1999;159:1215.

USEFUL WEB SITES

Osteoporosis
www.osteoed.org
www.nof.org

Practice Examination

Answers appear on page 602.

1. A 57-year-old man has been recently diagnosed with hypertension. Other than his BP of 160/100 mm Hg, he has no concerning findings on physical exam. An ECG, UA, basic chemistry panel, and lipid panel are normal. Past medical history is significant for a prior episode of gout and asthma. Despite a 6-month course of nonpharmacologic management, his BP remains elevated. What is the most appropriate treatment?

   A. Thiazide diuretics

   B. Alpha blockers

   C. Beta blocker

   D. ACEI

   E. Nitrates

2. A 70-year-old woman with hypertension reports shortness of breath, orthopnea, and PND. She denies chest pain or syncope, but has a cough producing frothy sputum. On exam, HR is 104 beats/min, BP is 100/76 mm Hg, respirations are 26, and oxygen saturation is 92% on room air. Her JVP is 14 cm, and she has bibasilar crackles, an S_3, and pitting edema to her knees bilaterally. Which study would you order next?

   A. ETT

   B. Cardiac catheterization

   C. Echocardiogram

   D. Coxsackievirus titers

   E. Dipyridamole-thallium scan

3. A 50-year-old alcoholic is found lying in an alley. He is brought to the emergency department where an alcohol level is 100. Additional lab tests show a BUN of 71 and creatinine of 5.2, up from his baseline of 1.1. A urine dipstick shows 3+ blood, but is otherwise negative. Urine microscopy shows no RBC or WBC, but occasional renal tubular cells and muddy brown casts. The cause of his renal failure is most likely:

   A. Hepatitis B

   B. Multiple myeloma

   C. Interstitial nephritis

   D. Rhabdomyolysis

   E. Urinary obstruction

4. A 33-year-old man is referred for a renal artery duplex as a part of a hypertension evaluation. The test comes back positive. The

renal artery duplex is highly sensitive (92%) and specific (94%) for renal artery stenosis as a cause of hypertension. The incidence of renal artery stenosis in the population is 2%. Which statement is accurate in interpreting the results of the test for the patient?

A. The test rules in the diagnosis of renal artery stenosis because of its high sensitivity.

B. The test rules out the diagnosis of renal artery stenosis because of its high specificity.

C. The high sensitivity and specificity reliably predict the accuracy of the diagnosis.

D. The low disease incidence results in a low PPV for the test.

E. The low disease incidence results in a low NPV for the test.

5. A 28-year-old woman comes to clinic reporting that she has had three disabling headaches this month. She describes a pattern of unilateral throbbing with associated nausea and vomiting. The headache was so disabling that she had to lie down. She is worried that she may have a brain tumor or stroke. What is the most likely cause of this headache?

A. SAH

B. Cluster headache

C. Tension type headache

D. Migraine headache

E. Brain tumor

6. A sexually active, athletic 23-year-old man comes to the clinic with an exquisitely painful right knee. The patient reports that the knee has become progressively painful over the last day, and he notes swelling and warmth to the touch. Small amounts of knee flexion and extension cause extreme pain. What is the most appropriate initial diagnostic study?

A. Knee films

B. Arthrocentesis

C. Uric acid

D. CBC

E. MRI

7. A 20-year-old college student presents to the student health service with sore throat, low-grade fever, and fatigue. Physical reveals bilateral lymphadenopathy of the neck, axilla, and groin. She has previously been in excellent health and denies weight loss or night sweats. CBC and differential show many atypical lymphocytes. What is the most likely cause of this student's illness?

A. Gonorrhea

B. HIV

C. Mononucleosis

D. Hodgkin's disease

E. HSV

8. A 34-year-old man with a long history of alcohol abuse presents to the clinic with nausea and abdominal pain. He has been drinking heavily (beer and vodka) for the past 3 weeks, but stopped yesterday because of severe pain and nausea. What abnormalities would you expect to see?

   A. Low phosphate, high magnesium, low bicarbonate, high amylase, high calcium

   B. Low phosphate, low magnesium, low bicarbonate, high amylase, low calcium

   C. High phosphate, high magnesium, high bicarbonate, high amylase, low calcium

   D. Low phosphate, low magnesium, high bicarbonate, normal amylase, low calcium

   E. High phosphate, low magnesium, low bicarbonate, high amylase, high calcium

9. A 72-year-old World War II veteran is hospitalized with CHF. He develops pain involving the great toe shortly after admission. The toe is red, warm, and extremely painful to the touch. His medications are furosemide, lisinopril, and carvedilol. He informs you that this is probably a recurrence of his gout. Which medication would you choose in initially treating this patient?

   A. Indomethacin

   B. Prednisone

   C. Allopurinol

   D. Probenecid

   E. Do not treat without arthrocentesis

10. A 45-year-old man comes to the clinic for a general physical. You note that he was diagnosed with ulcerative colitis at age 25. He reports that he hasn't had many problems with the colitis over the years. He denies melena, hematochezia, or change in stool pattern. The most appropriate recommendation for colorectal cancer screening in this patient is:

    A. Annual digital rectal exam

    B. Annual stool occult blood testing

    C. Flexible sigmoidoscopy

    D. Colonoscopy

    E. Delay screening until age 50

11. A 40-year-old woman has a WBC of 40,000 and a high serum leukocyte alkaline phosphatase score. What is the most appropriate next step in her work-up?

A. Referral for possible bone marrow transplant
B. Infection work-up
C. Begin hydroxyurea
D. Chromosome analysis
E. Bone marrow biopsy

12. A 65-year-old man presents with hemoptysis, dyspnea, and cough. He recently quit smoking. CXR shows a mediastinal mass. CT scan confirms the mass, and an additional lesion is found in the liver. A biopsy specimen of the mediastinal mass is obtained confirming a diagnosis of NSCLC. What is the most appropriate intervention at this point?

A. Begin chemotherapy
B. Referral for surgical resection
C. Biopsy of the liver lesion
D. Further staging including head CT and bone scan
E. Referral for hospice services

13. An unstable patient is airlifted to your medical center. The referring physician notes that the patient had a metabolic acidosis. The osmolar gap was 15, and oxalate crystals were seen in the urine. The most likely cause of this patient's acidosis is:

A. Uremia
B. Aspirin ingestion
C. Ketoacidosis
D. Sepsis
E. Ethylene glycol ingestion

14. A 43-year-old woman with a 23-year history of type 1 DM is seen in the clinic with fatigue and postprandial nausea. Her lab test results are Na 136, Cl 112, K 5.5, HCO_3^- 14, BUN 16, creatinine 1.3, glucose 146, and hemoglobin A_{1C} 6.8. What is the most likely cause for the patient's low HCO_3^-?

A. DKA
B. Renal tubular acidosis
C. Lactic acidosis
D. Recurrent vomiting
E. Aspirin ingestion

15. A 23-year-old, previously healthy man has onset of nausea, vomiting, fever, and headache. He appears lethargic and has difficulty answering questions. He is oriented only to name. His neurologic exam is nonfocal. A head CT with contrast administration is unremarkable. LP shows RBC's and 40 WBC with 95% lymphocytes. What is the most appropriate immediate intervention at this point?

A. Intravenous acyclovir
B. MRI

C. Intravenous amphotericin B

D. Intravenous vancomycin

E. Intravenous ciprofloxacin

16. A 49-year-old man has worsening hypertension over the past 6 months. Home BP readings have been 180–200/100–110. Three years ago, he had a normal BP. His physical is unremarkable. His lab test results are Na 138, K 2.9, BUN 10, creatinine 1.2, and glucose 90. A renal duplex scan is negative. What would be the next best step?

   A. No testing; treat essential hypertension

   B. Aldosterone-to-renin ratio

   C. 24-hour urine catecholamines

   D. TSH

   E. Abdominal CT scan

17. A 29-year-old alcoholic presents with fever, headache, and mental status changes. His physical exam is significant for nuchal rigidity, Kernig's sign, and disorientation on mental status exam. His lab test results are HCT 36, MCV 104, and WBC 23,000. What organism is the most likely cause of his symptoms?

   A. *Streptococcus pneumoniae*

   B. *Neisseria meningitidis*

   C. *Haemophilus influenzae*

   D. *Listeria monocytogenes*

   E. Coxsackievirus

18. A 70-year-old woman with a history of advanced osteoarthritis of the knees and hips presents with chest pressure, which occurs with emotional distress and exertion. The chest pressure does not radiate, and she has no associated dyspnea. ECG shows left bundle branch block. What diagnostic test would be most helpful?

   A. ETT

   B. ETT with thallium

   C. Echocardiogram

   D. Dipyridamole-thallium scan

   E. Exercise echocardiogram

19. A 44-year-old alcoholic reports the sudden onset of severe abdominal pain that doubled him over. He states it felt like "someone shot me in the belly." He had recently had some more generalized abdominal pain and had been taking aspirin and alcohol to kill that pain. On exam, BP is 80/50 mm Hg, and pulse is 130. Abdomen is rigid. Which of the following abdominal x-ray findings would be most worrisome and likely in this scenario.

   A. Subdiaphragmatic "free" air

   B. Multiple pancreatic calcifications

C. Dilated small bowel with air-fluid levels

D. Markedly dilated colon

E. Pneumatosis intestinalis (air in the bowel wall)

20. A 50-year-old woman with a history of heavy alcohol use presents to her primary care physician with new-onset abdominal swelling. She denies any pain or fever. On physical exam, her BP is 96/70, HR is 110, and she has evidence of shifting dullness in the abdomen. The most appropriate way to evaluate the cause of her ascites is:

A. Abdominal CT scan

B. Abdominal ultrasound

C. Pelvic ultrasound

D. Paracentesis

E. Colonoscopy

21. A 45-year-old man with long-standing cirrhosis secondary to HBV comes to the clinic to establish care. He denies any weight loss, abdominal swelling, or pain. Which tumor marker would be the best screen for hepatocellular carcinoma?

A. β-HCG

B. CEA

C. AFP

D. CA-125

E. BRCA1

22. A 69-year-old man with a history of COPD is hospitalized in an ICU with respiratory failure. He is on a ventilator for 5 days. On the sixth day, he becomes febrile, and a blood culture reveals *Pseudomonas aeruginosa*. Sputum cultures grow *Escherichia coli* and *P. aeruginosa*. What is the most appropriate antibiotic for this patient?

A. TMP-SMX

B. Ceftriaxone

C. Ampicillin-sulbactam

D. Ceftazidime

E. Vancomycin

23. An 80-year-old man with hypercholesterolemia and atrial fibrillation presents with diffuse abdominal pain. The pain has been increasing throughout the day and is now accompanied by maroon stools. Exam shows a temperature of 38.6° C and a soft abdomen with mild diffuse abdominal tenderness. There is no guarding or rebound, and the stool is guaiac-positive. Lab tests show a mild leukocytosis and a metabolic acidosis. What is the most appropriate next test for this patient?

A. Mesenteric duplex
B. Abdominal CT scan
C. Abdominal ultrasound
D. HIDA scan
E. Exploratory laparotomy

24. A 72-year-old man presents for evaluation of fatigue. He states that he drinks one fifth of whiskey each day and has a poor diet. Lab tests show HCT of 28 with MCV of 109. Which of the following would you expect to see on his peripheral blood smear?

A. Schistocytes
B. Teardrops
C. Döhle's bodies
D. Hypersegmented neutrophils
E. Spherocytes

25. A 40-year-old woman reports a cough for the last 8 months. She does not smoke or take any medications, and she denies fever or hemoptysis. Over the last year she has gained 20 lb because her new job does not allow time for exercise. Her cough tends to be worse after dinner and when she is trying to go to sleep at night. She recently stopped drinking alcohol and thinks that the cough improved some after stopping. What is the most appropriate initial therapy based on her history?

A. Azithromycin
B. Diphenhydramine
C. Nasal steroid spray
D. Albuterol metered-dose inhaler
E. Omeprazole

26. A 33-year-old woman reports intermittent loose stools for the past year. Her symptoms are associated with crampy abdominal pain and a bloating sensation. Defecation seems to relieve the discomfort. She has not noticed any blood in her stool. When her symptoms are flaring, she sometimes has three to five bowel movements a day to control the discomfort. She is not waking up at night with pain or having bowel movements at night. Between episodes, however, she is often constipated. The most likely cause of this patient's diarrhea is:

A. Inflammatory bowel disease
B. Irritable bowel syndrome
C. *Giardia lamblia* infection
D. Lactose intolerance
E. Celiac sprue

27. A 72-year-old woman reports 2 weeks of episodic dizziness. She describes the room "spinning in circles" when she gets in and out

of bed or if she looks up toward the ceiling. The episodes typically last <2 minutes. She denies any hearing problems or tinnitus. On exam, a Hallpike-Dix maneuver produces rotary nystagmus. The most likely cause of this patient's symptoms is:

A. Benign positional vertigo

B. Acute labyrinthitis

C. Meniere's syndrome

D. Brainstem ischemia

E. Acoustic neuroma

28. A 30-year-old man presents with chest pain. He describes the pain as crushing substernal chest pressure radiating to his left arm. It started 1 hour after eating lunch and is associated with nausea and sweatiness. On exam, he is pale and diaphoretic, but has normal vital signs and a normal heart and lung exam. An ECG during the exam is normal, but his pain improves 10 minutes after taking a sublingual nitroglycerin tablet. The most likely etiology of this patient's chest pain is:

A. MI

B. PE

C. Esophageal spasm

D. Aortic dissection

E. Pericarditis

29. A 59-year-old Peruvian woman reports nausea and achy epigastric pain for the last 2 months. She does not drink alcohol or take any medications and has not had any vomiting or diarrhea. A serum *H. pylori* serology is positive. Which of the following causes of dyspepsia would respond to *H. pylori* eradication?

A. GERD

B. Irritable bowel syndrome

C. Chronic pancreatitis

D. Diabetic gastroparesis

E. Peptic ulcer disease

30. A 31-year-old construction worker reports that she feels tired all the time. She has trouble getting through the workday and worries that she may have a serious illness. Her fatigue has worsened since she was recently promoted to foreman, a job that involves longer work hours and a higher stress level. Which of the following symptoms are concerning for a physical rather than a psychological cause of her fatigue?

A. Symptoms relieved by sleep

B. Symptoms increased during periods of stress

C. Symptoms better later in the day

D. Symptoms for the last 10 months

E. Symptoms that began at the time her father died

31. A 50-year-old woman with long-standing alcohol abuse and cirrhosis presents with hematemesis. Her BP is 120/80; her HR is 95; and she has spider telangiectasias, palmar erythema, and splenomegaly. HCT is 28. EGD shows bleeding esophageal varices that are successfully banded. She improves over the next several days in the hospital and is able to be discharged home. In addition to abstinence from alcohol, what is the best prophylaxis against a repeat variceal bleed?

   A. Omeprazole

   B. Lisinopril

   C. Perphenazine

   D. Nadolol

   E. Metoclopramide

32. A 31-year-old woman presents with pain and swelling in her wrists and hands. She also has pain in the ball of her foot. She has a history of pneumococcal pneumonia with sepsis 1 year ago and two prior spontaneous abortions in the past 4 years. On exam, she has spongy, tender swelling in the wrist, MCP, and MTP joints. Her lab test results are HCT 33, platelets 114,000, BUN 20, creatinine 1.2, and UA 2+ protein with 10–30 RBC/high-power field. Which lab test is the most likely to confirm a diagnosis?

   A. ANA

   B. Rheumatoid factor

   C. ESR

   D. cANCA

   E. Total complement (CH50)

33. A 40-year-old man comes in to establish care. He has no chronic diseases and has had no preventive health screening. Review of systems reveals no concerning symptoms, and his physical exam is normal. Which screening test would be most appropriate to do in this patient?

   A. PSA

   B. *Helicobacter pylori* serologies

   C. Total cholesterol

   D. Fecal occult blood test

   E. Flexible sigmoidoscopy

34. A 50-year-old man reports pain in his lower back since lifting a heavy crate. He rested and took ibuprofen without relief. He has restricted his activity and is worried that he may not be able to ski this winter because of his pain. What would be most concerning for a dangerous cause of this patient's low back pain?

A. New onset of marked constipation
B. No improvement after 2 weeks of ibuprofen
C. No relief with weekly chiropractic intervention
D. Pain in the lower back with straight leg raise
E. Worsened symptoms after 7 days of bed rest

35. A 20-year-old man with C3 HIV disease (CD$_4$ count 29/viral load 23,000) returns to the clinic for discussion of therapy options. He is interested in treatment and has not missed previous clinic visits. What therapy do you recommend?

    A. No antiretroviral therapy
    B. Zidovudine
    C. Tenofovir + lamivudine
    D. Zidovudine + lamivudine
    E. Efavirenz + zidovudine + lamivudine

36. A 32-year-old HIV-positive patient reports difficulty swallowing for 3 days. Swallowing also is very painful. Her CD4$^+$ count was 100 last month, but she has done well other than occasional oral thrush. She takes TMP-SMX, tenofovir, lamivudine, ritonavir, and atazanavir. Her exam is remarkable for a temperature of 38.5° F and oral thrush. The most likely cause of this patient's symptoms is:

    A. Hairy leukoplakia
    B. CMV esophagitis
    C. HSV esophagitis
    D. Candidal esophagitis
    E. GERD

37. A 25-year-old woman presents with 4 days of dysuria and frequency. She has had no fevers or flank pain. She has one sexual partner with no new partners in the past 12 months. A chlamydia test was negative 9 months ago. Physical exam is unremarkable. What test or tests should be ordered?

    A. UA
    B. UA and urine culture
    C. UA, urine culture, and *Chlamydia* culture
    D. UA, urine culture, and gonorrhea and *Chlamydia* culture
    E. Urine culture

38. A 37-year-old man with C3 HIV disease and a history of injection drug use presents with fever, weight loss, and nonproductive cough. He has adenopathy in the axilla and neck. His CD4$^+$ count is 80 with a viral load of 75,000. His CXR shows bilateral hilar and paratracheal adenopathy. No infiltrates are present. What is the most likely cause?

    A. *Pneumocystis carinii*
    B. Sarcoidosis

C. *Mycobacterium tuberculosis*
D. Endocarditis
E. Persistent generalized lymphadenopathy

39. A 41-year-old man presents with a long history of recurrent sinusitis reports a new episode of nasal discharge, cough, and fatigue. On physical exam, he has crusted blood in the nares and a tender right maxillary sinus with opacification on transillumination. CXR reveals bilateral nodules. His lab test results are HCT 33, WBC 10,000, BUN 33, and creatinine 2.6. UA shows 2+ protein, 0–3 WBC, and 30–50 RBC. What test is the most likely to explain his sinus disease and lab findings?

   A. ANA
   B. Anticardiolipin antibody
   C. ESR
   D. cANCA
   E. CEA

40. A 27-year-old elementary school teacher is seen for evaluation of fever and cough. She has had a nonproductive cough for the past 5 days, myalgias, sore throat, and fevers (T_{max}101.8). On exam, she has rhonchi and wheezes in the right lower lobe. Lab tests show WBC 10.8 and HCT 37. CXR shows a subsegmental right lower lobe infiltrate. What is the most likely organism?

   A. *Haemophilus influenzae*
   B. Influenza A
   C. Mixed anaerobes
   D. *Mycoplasma pneumoniae*
   E. *Streptococcus pneumoniae*

41. A 79-year-old woman presents with fever, nausea, vomiting, jaundice, and RUQ pain. Lab tests show bilirubin 2.5, alkaline phosphatase 360, and WBC 23,000. Ultrasound shows gallstones and dilated common bile duct. What is the most appropriate course of action?

   A. Consult surgery for urgent cholecystectomy
   B. Treat with intravenous azithromycin
   C. Treat with intravenous cefazolin
   D. Treat with intravenous ampicillin
   E. Consult a gastroenterologist for emergent ERCP

42. A 33-year-old IDU presents with a 3-day history of cough, fever, and pleuritic chest pain. Cardiac exam reveals a grade II/VI systolic murmur, normal skin exam, and bilateral rhonchi on chest auscultation. CXR shows bilateral, patchy peripheral infiltrates. What test is most important for making a diagnosis?

A. Two sets of blood cultures
B. Chest CT scan
C. Sputum Gram stain
D. Echocardiogram
E. Sputum culture

43. A 33-year-old woman presents with fatigue and weight gain. She reports a family history of hypothyroidism. Which set of clinical features would be most consistent with hypothyroidism?

    A. Macroglossia, tachypnea, increased CPK, amenorrhea
    B. Amenorrhea, bradycardia, increased cholesterol, cool skin
    C. Macroglossia, tachycardia, increased cholesterol, menorrhagia
    D. Menorrhagia, increased CPK, increased cholesterol, carpal tunnel syndrome
    E. Amenorrhea, decreased cholesterol, bradycardia, macroglossia

44. A 47-year-old obese man presents for his annual physical. He reports a family history of type 2 DM. A screening fasting blood glucose is 200. He begins a diet and loses 10 lb over 3 months, and a repeat fasting blood glucose is 160 with a hemoglobin A1C of 7.8. Cholesterol is 220 with TG of 400 and high-density lipoprotein of 30. What is the best initial therapy for this patient?

    A. Insulin
    B. Metformin
    C. Metformin + sulfonylurea
    D. Rosiglitazone
    E. Sulfonylurea + rosiglitazone

45. A 45-year-old woman with type 1 DM for 18 years presents as a new patient for evaluation. Her physical is remarkable for nonproliferative diabetic retinopathy and a BP of 146/92. Lab results show hemoglobin A_{1C} 7, BUN 12, and creatinine 0.8. UA shows trace protein. What would you recommend for this patient?

    A. Follow BP; no treatment at this time
    B. Begin hydrochlorothiazide
    C. Begin ACEI
    D. Begin calcium channel blocker
    E. Begin β-blocker

46. A 34-year-old pregnant woman from Cambodia in her second trimester presents with increasing dyspnea on exertion. She also has coughed up occasional bloody sputum. On exam, she has a low-pitched diastolic murmur heard best at the apex. What is the most likely diagnosis?

    A. Bacterial pneumonia
    B. Primary pulmonary hypertension

C. Aortic regurgitation

D. Aortic stenosis

E. Mitral stenosis

47. A 25-year-old man with HIV infection and a CD4$^+$ count of 100 presents with fever, headache, confusion, and mild photophobia. Funduscopic exam reveals normal optic discs, and the patient has a nonfocal neurologic examination. Diagnostic evaluation should begin with which of the following?

A. LP

B. Contrast head CT scan

C. Monitor clinical symptoms

D. Begin intravenous acyclovir

E. Begin intravenous amphotericin

48. A 54-year-old man presents to the hospital with a 6-month history of fever, night sweats, and weight loss. CT reveals evidence of multiple tumors confined above the diaphragm. Biopsy reveals low-grade lymphoma. What is the correct stage of this patient's NHL?

A. I

B. IB

C. II

D. IIB

E. IIIB

49. A 55-year-old man with type 2 DM reports progressive lower extremity pain over the last 3 months. The pain is bilateral and varies from burning to an uncomfortable tingling sensation. It started in his feet and has progressed to involve both ankles. The pain is most bothersome at night. On exam, an ABI is 1.1, and he has decreased vibration and proprioception in his feet. What is the most likely cause of this patient's leg pain?

A. Peripheral vascular disease

B. Venous obstruction

C. Nocturnal cramps

D. Multiple myeloma

E. Diabetic peripheral neuropathy

50. A 30-year-old woman smoker reports 3 days of left lower extremity swelling. She denies any trauma to the leg and states that in the last day it has started aching as well. She also has developed a low-grade temperature, but denies chills, sweats, or rash. Which of the following would increase her risk of DVT the most?

A. Corticosteroid therapy

B. History of asthma

C. History of MI

D. History of nephrotic syndrome

E. Laparoscopic cholecystectomy

51. A 59-year-old executive presents with shortness of breath, cough, and sharp right chest pain 2 days after returning from Europe where he spent a working holiday. He has a history of hypertension and hypercholesterolemia. Exam shows pulse 99 and BP 138/88. JVP is 8 cm. Cardiac exam shows S_1, S_2, and a 2/6 systolic murmur heard best at the right and left midsternal border without radiation. Lung exam is unremarkable. He has trace edema at the ankles. Which finding on this patients' CXR would be most helpful in confirming the diagnosis?

   A. Silhouette sign

   B. Enlarged left atrium

   C. Left pleural effusion

   D. Kerley B lines

   E. Normal chest

52. A head CT before performing LP is needed in each of the following scenarios except:

   A. A 43-year-old woman with a history of breast cancer who presents with headache, vomiting, and fever

   B. A 32-year-old HIV-positive man with a $CD4^+$ count of 20 who presents with fever and new-onset headache

   C. A 45-year-old man with fever, headache, and a normal neurologic exam

   D. A 23-year-old woman who had a seizure and now is febrile

   E. A 19-year-old man who presents with fever and confusion and is unable to give a history because of his depressed mental status

53. Informed consent before performing the necessary procedure is needed in each of the following situations except:

   A. A 45-year-old man presents with hypotension and a ruptured abdominal aortic aneurysm on imaging studies. The surgeons want to take him to the operating room for an emergent operation.

   B. A 51-year-old man with cirrhosis presents with ascites and is encephalopathic. He is admitted to the hospital for mental status changes. You would like to do a paracentesis to rule out SBP.

   C. A 23-year-old man presents with fever, lethargy, and headache. He is disoriented. You want to perform LP for evaluation of possible meningitis.

   D. A 17-year-old girl from Cambodia presents with chest discomfort and cough. A CXR shows a large free-flowing right-sided effusion. You would like to perform a thoracentesis for evaluation.

54. A 50-year-old man complains of a lump in his neck. He has noted a lump for several weeks on his right neck. He otherwise feels well. He has a history of hypertension and hyperlipidemia. He has smoked one pack per day for the last 33 years. On exam, a 2.5-cm mobile mass in his right neck is palpated. It is firm, not fluctuant, and not warm. The remainder of his exam is unremarkable. His CXR is clear. What is the next step in his care?

A. CBC with differential

B. *Toxoplasma* titers

C. Monospot

D. Re-evaluate in 3 months

E. Surgery evaluation for biopsy

55. An 83-year-old man, generally in good health, presents to the hospital with a fractured left humerus sustained in a fall at home. He reports that he was feeling well until he was cooking breakfast when he suddenly found himself on the floor. He denies associated chest pain, dyspnea, or dizziness. He currently has no symptoms except left arm pain. His BP is 148/88 mm Hg, and heart rate is 68 beats/min. His rhythm strip is shown in Figure 1. The appropriate treatment for this patient is:

A. Pain control and operative repair of humeral fracture

B. Aspirin and a beta blocker for presumed acute coronary syndrome

C. Hospital admission with telemetry monitoring, temporary pacer, and plans for permanent pacemaker placement

D. Amiodarone loading

E. Immediate cardioversion

56. A 45-year-old man comes to see you about dyspnea. He is having trouble coaching his son's soccer team, something he has done for several years without difficulty. He has type 2 DM and arthritis of his knees, but is otherwise well. Exam reveals a healthy-appearing tan man in no distress. BP is 122/80, and pulse is 100. JVP is 9 cm with S_1, S_2, and S_4 and no murmurs heard on cardiac auscultation. Lungs show crackles at the bases bilaterally, and his liver edge is felt 2 cm below the costal margin. He is tan under his underclothes and has small, firm testicles. Glucose is 194 mg/dL, and his transaminases are three times normal. The test most likely to be helpful in establishing the diagnosis is:

A. TSH

B. Serum testosterone

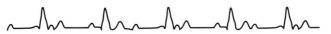

FIGURE 1 Figure 1, question 55.

C. Coxsackievirus serology

D. 24-hour urine protein

E. Iron saturation

57. The most likely inheritance pattern for this man's condition (see Question 56) is:

A. Autosomal dominant

B. Autosomal recessive

C. X-linked

D. Sporadic mutation

E. Partial penetrance

58. A 54-year-old man with CAD complains of chest pain at rest over the past 2 days. He was diagnosed with CAD 2 years ago and has been medically managed since then with aspirin, a beta blocker, and sublingual nitroglycerin. Up until the past 2 days he had experienced angina only with intense exertion. In the past 2 days, however, he has had five or six episodes of angina, two of which occurred when he was sitting quietly. His most recent chest pain occurred earlier in the day and resolved after he took 3 nitroglycerin tablets. He is now pain-free. On exam, he appears well. BP is 150/95 mm Hg, and HR is 85 beats/min. Physical exam is otherwise normal. His ECG shows nonspecific T wave inversions in the inferior leads (II, III, AVF). You decide to:

A. Increase his beta blocker dose and discharge him from clinic

B. Check a troponin level and if normal plan to discharge him from clinic on an increased dose of his beta blocker

C. Add clopidogrel to his medical regimen

D. Admit him to the hospital

E. Order an ETT, and refer him to cardiology.

59. A 56-year-old man is being discharged from the hospital after an inferior wall MI. His discharge medications include aspirin, nitroglycerin, atorvastatin, omeprazole, and sertraline. Which medication would provide a mortality benefit to this patient?

A. Amlodipine

B. Clopidogrel

C. Warfarin

D. Metoprolol

E. Digoxin

60. A 56-year-old man develops severe hypertension during anesthesia induction for routine laparoscopic cholecystectomy. The surgery is cancelled. He has a history of labile hypertension for several years with occasions of palpitations and sweating. Review of the chart shows mild glucose intolerance and postural hypotension on some

occasions. His physical exam is otherwise unremarkable. Which lab test is likely to be abnormal?

A. Serum aldosterone-to-renin ratio

B. TSH

C. Urine metanephrines

D. ACTH

E. Serum potassium

61. A 32-year-old woman has been treated repeatedly with high-dose prednisone for severe steroid-dependent bronchoconstrictive disease. As her breathing improves, and the steroids are tapered, she frequently develops weakness, fatigue, abdominal pain, and hypotension. Which lab test would you do?

A. TSH

B. Cosyntropin stimulation test

C. Colonoscopy

D. Serum calcium

E. 24-hour urine free cortisol

62. A 28-year-old woman with pernicious anemia and hypothyroidism presents with weakness and increased skin pigmentation. She has lost weight in the last year. Her medicines are levothyroxine 0.112 mg orally daily and vitamin B_{12} 1 mg intramuscularly monthly. Her BP is 100/60, and a previous breast biopsy scar is darkly pigmented. CBC is normal, and TSH is 1.2 mU/L. Electrolytes are significant for sodium 134 mEq/L, potassium 5.3 mEq/L, CO_2 19 mEq/L, and glucose 64 mg/dL. Which lab test do you anticipate would be abnormal?

A. Aldosterone-to-renin ratio

B. Iron and TIBC

C. C-peptide

D. ACTH

E. 25-Hydroxyvitamin D

63. A 43-year-old accountant who has had type 1 DM since age 7 comes to the clinic for care of recent severe hypoglycemia. He has been previously well, with a hemoglobin A_{1C} of 7%. He has been using NPH insulin twice daily before breakfast and dinner and has been taking rapid insulin aspart with each meal. He exercises regularly and has mild "hypos" (glucose 40-50 mg/dL). He has had two recent blackouts. The first occurred when there was a delay in receiving his lunch meal in a restaurant; the second occurred at midnight when he was at home with his fiancée who was visiting for the weekend. In both instances, he needed the help of another person. He is very concerned because he is planning to get married soon, and the second episode frightened his fiancée. The most likely cause of his hypoglycemic events is:

A. Noncompliance with insulin
B. Munchausen syndrome
C. Poor injection technique
D. His insulin is peaking when he is not eating
E. Obsessive-compulsive disorder with overly tight glucose control

64. The best initial treatment change at this time is:

A. Switch his NPH to insulin glargine
B. Switch his insulin aspart to regular insulin
C. Decrease his NPH insulin
D. Decrease his insulin aspart
E. Switch him to an insulin pump

65. A 54-year-old man with hypertension on a beta blocker has a BP of 145/82, TC 290, TG 400, low-density lipoprotein estimated at 175, and high-density lipoprotein 34. He is 15 lb overweight. His risk of developing CHD over 10 years is 21%. You advise him that his cholesterol is too high and suggest:

A. A 12-week trial of lifestyle modification with diet and exercise
B. A fibrate to treat his elevated TG and reassess low-density lipoprotein in 3 months
C. He has two cardiovascular risk factors, so low-density lipoprotein goal is <130
D. Diet and exercise and start a statin at the same visit.
E. Repeat his cholesterol level in 1 year after he loses 15 lb

66. A 49-year-old woman returns to the clinic for follow-up. She was recently diagnosed with type 2 DM. She is currently on Prempro for hot flashes and lisinopril for hypertension. Over the past 3 months she has lost 12 lb through diet and exercise. Her blood glucose is now under good control. Her BP is 122/75. Fasting lipid panel shows TC 207, TG 220 (high), low-density lipoprotein 125, and high-density lipoprotein 38. Previous low-density lipoprotein was 140. Which of the following treatments would you recommend?

A. Start niacin 2-3 g/d in divided doses.
B. Start atorvastatin 10 mg nightly.
C. Congratulate her on her good work. No further therapy is warranted because her low-density lipoprotein is less than her target of 130.
D. Start gemfibrozil 600 mg twice daily.
E. Increase her dose of Prempro with the hopes that it will decrease her low-density lipoprotein and increase her high-density lipoprotein.

67. A 42-year-old woman with type 1 DM since age 9 has no known complications from her DM. Her hemoglobin A_{1C} is 7.5. Recently, she

presented with arthralgias and a rash and was found to have mildly elevated liver enzymes. Evaluation revealed HCV. BP is 144/92, and temperature is 37.8° C; pulse and exam are normal except for some warmth over both knees and elbows and a mildly tender liver edge. Creatinine is found to be elevated for the first time at 2.3 mg/dL. LFT show ALT 320 mg/dL and AST 290 mg/dL. The most likely abnormal finding on this patient's urine sediment exam is:

A. Uric acid crystals

B. Oxalate crystals

C. WBC casts

D. RBC casts

E. Pigmented casts

68. A 65-year-old woman presents to the emergency department with 60 minutes of difficulty speaking. She has a history of hypertension, hyperlipidemia, and tobacco use. On exam, BP is 180/100, HR is 98, and temperature is 36.6° C. She has bilateral carotid bruits and a regular rhythm without murmur. On neurologic exam, she follows directions, but has difficulty naming objects, and there are multiple pauses in her attempts to speak. She has a right facial droop, but her other cranial nerves are intact. Head CT shows no bleed. She qualifies for tPA and has substantial improvement of her aphasia with speech therapy. What is the most appropriate secondary work-up and intervention?

A. Echocardiogram and warfarin

B. MRI and asprin-dipyridamole

C. Carotid duplex and possible carotid endarterectomy

D. Hypercoagulability work-up and aspirin

E. Transcranial Doppler and clopidogrel

69. A 42-year-old man without significant medical problems complained of cramping in his leg with activity and several falls when hiking over the last 2 months. On review of systems, he has also noticed a couple of choking episodes with solid food over the last 3 weeks. On exam, his cranial nerves are intact, as is his cognition; strength is 3/5 with left ankle dorsiflexion; his left toe is up-going; and he has notable fasciculations over his left anterior tibialis. What is the most likely cause of his neurologic problem?

A. Multiple sclerosis

B. Amyotrophic lateral sclerosis

C. Stroke

D. Guillain-Barré syndrome

E. Lumbar radiculopathy

70. A 32-year-old woman reports acute shortness of breath that occurred at rest and right-sided pleuritic chest pain. She has a

history of SLE, three spontaneous abortions, and a DVT in her early 20s at which time she was given anticoagulation for 6 months. She is currently taking hydroxychloroquine and smokes 1 pack per day, but does not drink alcohol. Temperature is 37.9° C, BP is 130/80, pulse is 100, respiratory rate is 22, and oxygen saturation is 95% on room air. She is a healthy-appearing woman with a malar rash. Cardiac exam shows tachycardia and no JVD or lower extremity edema. Lung exam is clear. A CBC, electrolytes, and UA measured in clinic last week are normal. What would be the most appropriate next step?

A. Initiate heparin therapy, and order a CT pulmonary angiogram
B. Order thrombolytic therapy
C. Consult interventional radiology for an inferior vena caval filter placement
D. Initiate heparin therapy, and order a pulmonary angiogram
E. Order a D-dimer.

71. A 52-year-old man with multiple myeloma without any cardiac history becomes acutely dyspneic in the waiting room. You are particularly concerned about a PE. You obtain an ECG. What would you most likely see on the ECG?

A. Left bundle branch block
B. S in 1, Q in 3, and a flipped T in 3
C. Sinus tachycardia
D. Sinus bradycardia
E. Right bundle branch block

Answers and Explanations

1. **D: ACEI (Hypertension).** The patient has hypertension with appropriate attempt at nonpharmacologic management. An ACEI would be the best choice in this case. He should not receive a thiazide because it may precipitate more gout attacks. A beta blocker would be contraindicated because of his asthma history. Alpha blockers and nitrates are not appropriate first-line antihypertensive drugs.

2. **C: Echocardiogram (CHF).** The patient has clinical signs and symptoms of CHF; an echocardiogram would help clarify the degree and cause of the heart failure. ETT, cardiac catheterization, and persantine-thallium scan all are diagnostic tests for CAD. Coxsackievirus can cause a myopericarditis, but would be an inappropriate initial test.

3. **D: Rhabdomyolysis (Renal failure).** This patient has ARF. His rapid rise in creatinine would be consistent with rhabdomyolysis, pressure necrosis of muscles. This diagnosis is suggested by the fact that he was found down (was immobile causing persistent pressure

necrosis of muscle) and that his dipstick was positive for blood but no RBC were seen on microscopic evaluation. The 3+ blood without RBC is due to myoglobin released from crushed muscle.

4. **D: Low PPV (Sensitivity and specificity).** PPV refers to the percentage of patients with a positive test who actually have the disease in question (true positives/all positive tests). When the prevalence of disease is low, it makes it much more likely that a positive test is due to error rather than being a true positive, resulting in a low PPV. Highly sensitive tests can help rule out diagnoses ("SnOut"), whereas highly specific tests can help rule in diagnosis ("SpIn"). Even highly sensitive and specific tests are unreliable, however, in the setting of very high or very low pretest probabilities. NPV refers to the percentage of patients with a negative test who are disease-free; a low disease prevalence results in a high NPV.

5. **D: Migraine (Headache).** This patient has symptoms typical of migraine headache. The intermittent nature, unilateral location, throbbing quality, and disabling severity all suggest migraine headache. The associated GI symptoms also are common with migraine. Tension headache is usually not unilateral and is not disabling. Cluster headache usually occurs in men and is marked by short, severe, recurrent headaches usually around the eye. The headache of SAH usually is not recurrent and is often catastrophic.

6. **B: Arthrocentesis (Joint pain).** The patient is a young man with acute knee pain and swelling. With no trauma history, the most likely causes would be either gonococcal arthritis or reactive arthritis (Reiter's syndrome). The best diagnostic test would be an arthrocentesis with culture and cell count of the joint fluid.

7. **C: Mononucleosis (Lymphadenopathy).** This young woman has mononucleosis. It is extremely common in this age group; clinical symptoms after infection with EBV occur in 50%-70% of patients 15-24 years old compared with only 10% of children. The clinical features this patient has of fever, sore throat, adenopathy, and fatigue are typical of mononucleosis. The presence of atypical lymphocytes also strongly suggests mononucleosis. Hodgkin's disease could cause fever and adenopathy, but would be an unlikely cause of sore throat; it is also far rarer. Acute HIV infection mimics mononucleosis in that it can cause fever, sore throat, and lymphadenopathy. No significant risk factors for HIV were given in this case.

8. **B: Low phosphate, low magnesium, low bicarbonate, high amylase, low calcium (Alcohol).** With chronic alcohol abuse, the renal tubules waste magnesium leading to total body magnesium depletion. With low magnesium, phosphate is lost in the urine (and is already low owing to poor dietary intake). Low magnesium also results in low potassium and decreased PTH release with consequent decreases in calcium. High amylase occurs with alcohol-induced pancreatitis. Low bicarbonate occurs with alcoholic ketoacidosis, essentially a starvation state.

9. **B: Prednisone (Gout).** This patient has typical features of gout. He is on a diuretic for his CHF, which is likely triggering his gout by raising the serum uric acid level. He should not be treated with indomethacin because it would likely exacerbate his CHF through fluid retention, and he would be at higher risk for nephrotoxicity. Probenecid and allopurinol are inappropriate treatments for acute gouty attack. They should be used for prevention and not started during an acute attack. The correct treatment would be prednisone.

10. **D: Colonoscopy (Colon cancer).** Patients with ulcerative colitis are at an increased risk for colorectal cancer. Most guidelines recommend screening colonoscopies every 1-3 years starting 8 years after onset of disease (or starting at 15 years for isolated left-sided colitis). For a patient with average risk, a colonoscopy every 10 years (*or* annual fecal occult blood testing or flexible sigmoidoscopy or both every 3-5 years) is recommended for colorectal cancer screening starting at age 50.

11. **B: Infection work-up (Leukemia).** A high leukocyte alkaline phosphatase score indicates a leukemoid reaction—an acute WBC response to infection such as TB. In leukemia, the leukocyte alkaline phosphatase would not be elevated.

12. **D: Head CT and bone scan (Lung cancer).** The management of NSCLC depends heavily on the extent of disease (stage). Early-stage disease can be treated successfully with surgical resection alone, whereas the treatment for advanced disease is chemotherapy or radiation therapy or both. A complete staging work-up including head CT and bone scan is necessary before deciding on a treatment course. This patient may eventually need a biopsy of the liver lesion to determine if it represents a metastasis, but it would be prudent to perform noninvasive testing first to evaluate for other possible metastases. If there is evidence of lesions elsewhere, a liver biopsy would not be necessary.

13. **E: Ethylene glycol (Acid-base disturbances).** All of the answer choices are causes of metabolic acidosis with elevated anion gap. Patients with elevated anion gaps should have an osmolar gap calculated. This patient's osmolar gap was elevated (>15); major causes are methanol or ethylene glycol ingestion. The oxalate crystals suggest ethylene glycol ingestion. This is a life-threatening poisoning; management includes inhibition of alcohol dehydrogenase (with intravenous fomepizole or ethanol) to reduce production of toxic metabolites, hemodialysis, and aggressive supportive care.

14. **B: Renal tubular acidosis (Acid-base disturbances).** This patient has a long-standing history of type 1 DM and has a non–anion gap acidosis. She also has an elevated potassium, suggesting that her non–anion gap acidosis is due to a type 4 renal tubular acidosis (hyporenin hypoaldosterone renal tubular acidosis). Type 4 renal tubular acidosis is quite common in patients who have long-standing DM.

DKA, lactic acidosis, and aspirin ingestion all would cause an anion gap acidosis. Recurrent vomiting would cause a metabolic alkalosis.

15. **A: IV acyclovir (Encephalitis).** This patient has symptoms suggestive of a CNS infection, possibly encephalitis. The blood and lymphocytosis on LP suggest possible HSV type 1 infection. Immediate acyclovir is appropriate when this diagnosis is suspected. It is unlikely that he has bacterial meningitis, and the antibiotic options of ciprofloxacin and vancomycin would be inappropriate if he did.

16. **B: Aldosterone-to-renin ratio (Hypertension).** Secondary causes of hypertension should be suspected in patients with young age of onset or severe or refractory hypertension. This patient's BP are markedly elevated. His low serum potassium is suggestive of primary hyperaldosteronism, a common cause of secondary hypertension, and checking an aldosterone-to-renin ratio would be an appropriate first step. Pheochromocytoma (24-hour urine catecholamines) and hyperthyroidism or hypothyroidism (TSH) are less common causes of secondary hypertension. An abdominal CT scan looking for adrenal masses would be an inappropriate screening test in the absence of biochemical markers of hyperaldosteronism, pheochromocytoma, or hypercortisolism.

17. **A: *Streptococcus pneumoniae* (Meningitis).** This patient likely has meningitis. *Streptococcus pneumoniae* is the most common cause of bacterial meningitis; alcohol is a risk factor. The elevated MCV (along with the patient's history) is consistent with chronic alcohol use. All of the other pathogens are less common causes of meningitis. *Neisseria meningitidis* affects mainly younger adults; terminal complement deficiency is another risk factor. *Haemophilus influenzae* used to be a common cause in children, but is uncommon now since the introduction of widespread vaccination. *Listeria monocytogenes* is an important cause in pregnant women, elderly patients, and patients with heavy alcohol use or immunosuppression. Coxsackievirus is an enterovirus that can cause aseptic meningitis.

18. **D: Dipyridamole-thallium scan (Ischemic heart disease).** This patient's history is concerning for ischemic heart disease. A stress test would be helpful to diagnose this. All stress tests consist of a stressor (e. g., exercise, dipyridamole, dobutamine) and some imaging modality (e.g., ECG, thallium, echocardiography, sestamibi). Because of the patient's severe osteoarthritis, she is unlikely to be able to perform exercise stress testing. An echocardiogram without a stressor is less useful for diagnosing ischemic heart disease. A dipyridamole-thallium scan would not require exercise, and the thallium scan can be interpreted despite the presence of a left bundle branch block on ECG (in contrast to a stress test using ECG as the imaging modality).

19. **A: Subdiaphragmatic "free" air (How to read an abdominal film).** The patient's presentation of severe abdominal pain with hemodynamic instability and peritoneal findings on exam, coupled with his

history of alcohol and aspirin use, is concerning for a perforated gastric or duodenal ulcer. "Free air" under the diaphragm is consistent with a GI perforation (leakage of air into the peritoneal space). Pancreatic calcifications are diagnostic for chronic pancreatitis. Dilated loops of bowel suggest bowel obstruction. Air in the bowel wall is a concerning finding for necrotic bowel.

20. **D: Paracentesis (Basic procedures).** The appropriate initial test for evaluating the cause of ascites is paracentesis with ascites fluid analysis. The SAAG (serum albumin level minus the ascites albumin level) can distinguish between ascites resulting from portal hypertension (e.g., cirrhosis, CHF—SAAG ≥ 1.1) and non–portal hypertension–related ascites (e.g., peritoneal carcinomatosis, peritoneal TB—SAAG <1.1). The other tests may be useful in confirming the presence of related conditions (e.g., pelvic ultrasound might detect ovarian cancer; abdominal ultrasound might confirm a cirrhotic liver and presence of ascites), but ascites fluid analysis is indispensable.

21. **C: AFP (Abnormal laboratory tests).** AFP is a tumor marker used to screen individuals with cirrhosis (or HBV without cirrhosis) for hepatocellular carcinoma. β-HCG and AFP are markers for germ cell tumors (e.g., certain testicular and ovarian cancers). CA-125 is a marker for ovarian cancer. BRCA1 is a genetic test; mutations in the BRCA1 gene are associated with high rates of breast, ovarian, and other cancers. In general, tumor markers do not have the specificity to diagnose or screen patients for their associated cancers. They are often used to follow patients with known cancer for response to treatment or recurrence or to aid in the diagnosis of nonspecific findings (e.g., abdominal mass on CT).

22. **D: Ceftazidime (Antibiotics).** Antibiotic options for *Pseudomonas aeruginosa* are limited; ceftazidime and cefoperazone are the only third-generation cephalosporins with significant activity against *Pseudomonas*. Other options include antipseudomonal penicillins (e.g., piperacillin), cefepime (fourth-generation cephalosporin), aminoglycosides, imipenem, ciprofloxacin, and aztreonam. None of the other answer choices has good activity against *Pseudomonas*. Ideally, you should put this patient on two antibiotics with pseudomonal activity.

23. **A: Mesenteric duplex (Abdominal pain).** Mesenteric angiography evaluates for bowel ischemia in this patient with risk factors for atherosclerosis (high cholesterol) and thrombus (atrial fibrillation), although mesenteric duplex is more common now. Further evidence is acute maroon stools from bowel wall infarct and sloughing. A key exam finding is the soft abdominal exam disproportionate to the patient's level of pain. Acidosis occurs with infarction of bowel tissue.

24. **D: Hypersegmented neutrophils (Anemia).** This patient has a macrocytic anemia as a result of chronic alcohol use. Deficiencies of folate

and vitamin B_{12} are often associated with heavy alcohol use and can cause macrocytosis. All of these conditions can cause a megaloblastic process (cells getting "stuck" in the middle of cell division because of impaired DNA synthesis); hypersegmented neutrophils are suggestive of this process. Teardrop cells also can be associated with megaloblastosis to a lesser extent. They also are associated with myelophthisic anemia (e.g., bone marrow replacement by cancer, fibrosis) and thalassemia. Schistocytes (fragmented RBC) suggest hemolysis. Döhle's bodies (light blue spots in periphery of neutrophils) are most commonly seen in patients with infection. Spherocytes (RBC with loss of central pallor) are seen with hereditary spherocytosis and autoimmune hemolytic anemia.

25. **E: Omeprazole (Cough).** The most common causes of chronic cough in a nonsmoker are postnasal drip, asthma, and GERD. Weight gain, large meals, supine position, and alcohol all can exacerbate GERD symptoms. PPI (e.g., omeprazole) can be used to treat the cough associated with GERD. Antibiotics are unlikely to be useful in chronic cough. Diphenhydramine and nasal steroids can be used to treat postnasal drip. Albuterol can be used to treat asthma (including cough-variant asthma).

26. **B: Irritable bowel syndrome (Diarrhea).** This patient's history is classic for IBS, a common disorder characterized by alternating constipation and diarrhea, plus crampy abdominal pain relieved by defecation. Lactose intolerance can cause many of these symptoms (although usually not constipation), but is related to dairy intake. Chronic giardiasis typically causes foul-smelling and fatty stools. Nighttime symptoms or bloody stools would be concerning for a more serious cause of diarrhea, but these symptoms are absent in this patient. IBD might manifest with weight loss and bloody stools. Celiac sprue is a malabsorptive disorder that may be associated with weight loss, iron deficiency anemia, and vitamin D deficiency.

27. **A: Benign positional vertigo (Dizziness).** BPV manifests with brief (often <1 minute) episodes of vertigo associated with positional changes, but without other neurologic symptoms. Rotary nystagmus on Hallpike-Dix is consistent with BPV. Acute labyrinthitis causes a constant vertigo that lasts for days to weeks and is often associated with a viral illness. Meniere's syndrome and acoustic neuroma are associated with tinnitus and hearing loss. Vertigo with Meniere's syndrome typically lasts for hours, whereas vertigo with acoustic neuroma is generally very mild. Brainstem ischemia is usually associated with other cranial nerve findings (e.g., diplopia, dysarthria, facial weakness or numbness).

28. **C: Esophageal spasm (Chest pain).** Esophageal spasm may appear very similar to cardiogenic chest pain, with substernal pain, diaphoresis, and nausea and response to nitroglycerin, which relaxes the muscle. MI should have altered vital signs and an abnormal ECG during pain. PE usually has associated tachycardia, and any chest pain

would not be relieved with nitroglycerin. Aortic dissection would have tachycardia, and similar to pericarditis, pain would not be relieved with nitroglycerin.

29. **E: Peptic ulcer disease (Dyspepsia).** *Helicobacter pylori* has a causative role in PUD, which responds to *H. pylori* eradication. GERD may be worsened by *H. pylori* treatment; IBS, gastroparesis, and pancreatitis are unaffected.

30. **A: Symptoms relieved by sleep (Fatigue).** With physical causes of fatigue, such as cancer, most patients feel rested when they awaken in the morning, but worsen as the day progresses. In contrast, psychogenic fatigue is present from awakening, improves throughout the day, and worsens with increased stress or grief. Longer duration without diagnosis favors a psychogenic cause.

31. **D: Nadolol (GI bleed/liver disease).** Beta blockers such as nadolol have been shown to reduce rates of variceal bleeding recurrence. Omeprazole, ACEI, perphenazine, and metoclopramide do not change the rate.

32. **A: ANA (Rheumatology).** ANA serves as one more finding in a list of conditions and lab tests suggestive of SLE. This patient has small joint swelling characteristic of RA and SLE. Anemia may occur with both chronic inflammatory conditions. Spontaneous abortions are particularly seen with SLE. The renal findings of elevated creatinine and probably nephritis are consistent with SLE, not RA. cANCA occurs with Wegener's granulomatosis, which may affect the kidneys, but not with a nephritic picture. Complement CH50 may be decreased, but is nonspecific and would not aid in diagnosis.

33. **C: Total cholesterol (Healthy patient).** Cholesterol screening guidelines vary, but generally agree that men ≥35 years old should be screened. Prostate cancer screening with PSA is controversial and should not start until age 50 if performed. Annual fecal occult blood testing or flexible sigmoidoscopy or both every 3-5 years (*or* colonoscopy alone every 10 years) are recommended for colorectal cancer screening, but not until age 50 for patients with average risk. There is no recommendation for *Helicobacter pylori* screening in asymptomatic individuals.

34. **A: New onset marked constipation (Low back pain).** Bowel and bladder dysfunction or saddle anesthesia or both in low back pain are concerning for cauda equina syndrome (acute compression of the lumbosacral nerve roots in the distal spinal canal). This condition can cause permanent loss of function and requires emergent imaging and surgical consultation when suspected. Failure to improve with anti-inflammatories is concerning, but less so than new constipation. Evidence supporting chiropractic intervention for relief of back pain is limited. Pain limited to the low back with straight leg raise is nonspecific. Even if the test was truly positive (symptoms radiating down the leg in a radicular pattern), the

most likely cause is disc herniation, which would still be managed conservatively. Prolonged bed rest seems to worsen back pain; patients should be encouraged to return to normal activities as soon as tolerated.

35. **E: Efavirenz + zidovudine + lamivudine (HIV).** This patient has a CD4$^+$ count <200, so he should receive therapy. All patients who receive antiretroviral therapy should be treated with three antiretroviral drugs. There is no role in the treatment of HIV disease for one-drug or two-drug therapy.

36. **D: Candidal esophagitis: (HIV).** This patient has AIDS with a CD4$^+$ count of 100. In patients with HIV who have esophageal symptoms, if they have thrush on exam, almost 100% have candidal esophagitis as the cause of their esophageal symptoms. This patient should be treated for candidal esophagitis and have endoscopy only if there is no improvement with antifungal therapy.

37. **A: UA (UTI).** UA is an adequate test in this low-risk patient to evaluate for UTI, the most likely diagnosis. Urine culture is indicated when a patient is having recurrent episodes or lack of response to treatment. *Chlamydia* screening is indicated in women with multiple partners in the past year and one baseline *Chlamydia* screening once sexually active. Gonorrhea is usually symptomatic with discharge, but should be tested for in this patient if the genitourinary symptoms do not resolve with UTI treatment.

38. **C: *Mycobacterium tuberculosis* (TB and HIV).** This patient has AIDS with a low CD4$^+$ count of 80. He has a febrile illness with weight loss and cough. The presence of hilar and paratracheal lymphadenopathy strongly suggests TB. In patients with HIV disease and a low CD4$^+$ count, TB is manifested by hilar, paratracheal, and mediastinal lymphadenopathy. More than half of HIV patients with TB and CD4$^+$ counts <200 also have extrapulmonary TB. This patient has axillary and cervical adenopathy, which is consistent with extrapulmonary TB. *Pneumocystis carinii* pneumonia does not cause adenopathy. Endocarditis in an IDU would likely cause patchy pulmonary infiltrates as opposed to adenopathy. Sarcoid is possible, but not more likely in an HIV patient. Persistent generalized lymphadenopathy would not explain the weight loss or fevers.

39. **D: cANCA (Rheumatology/vasculitis).** This patient's sinus disease, abnormal lung findings, and evidence of glomerular disease are consistent with Wegener's granulomatosis. cANCA would be helpful for the diagnosis. ANA can be used to evaluate for SLE, but is less useful in the absence of other findings of SLE. SLE can cause glomerular disease, but sinus disease and pulmonary nodules would not be typical. Anticardiolipin antibody is a test for antiphospholipid syndrome, which is generally characterized by arterial and venous thromboses and pregnancy loss. ESR is a nonspecific marker for inflammation. CEA is a tumor marker typically associated with colon cancer.

40. **D:** *Mycoplasma pneumoniae* **(Pneumonia).** The myalgias, nonproductive cough, mild fever, and near-normal WBC all suggest *Mycoplasma pneumoniae*, rather than *Haemophilus influenzae* or *Streptococcus pneumoniae*. The CXR is subsegmental, which can be seen in mycoplasmal pneumonia; a viral etiology usually results in more diffuse x-ray changes. Anaerobes are unlikely because she has no risk for aspiration.

41. **E: ERCP (Biliary disease).** With ascending cholangitis (fever, jaundice, and elevated WBC), the physical blockage must be removed to decompress the bile duct. The gallbladder itself is not inflamed; there is no wall thickening or pericholic fluid. Intravenous antibiotics are warranted, but are secondary to the procedure.

42. **A: Two sets of blood cultures (Endocarditis).** This patient has fever, murmur, and endocarditis risk with injection drug use. An echocardiogram does not always identify a vegetation, so a normal echocardiogram does not exclude endocarditis. The patchy infiltrates seen on CXR are most likely due to bacterial seeding from a right-sided heart valve lesion. Further testing for TB by sputum Gram stain and culture, given the relative high likelihood in this patient, and CT may be indicated to evaluate for cavitary lesions from bacterial seeding to the lung. At this point, however, the key issue is blood culture to nail down the diagnosis of endocarditis and to identify organism and antibiotic sensitivity. Two cultures are indicated; a single culture may be misconstrued as a skin contaminant.

43. **D: Menorrhagia, increased CPK, increased cholesterol, carpal tunnel syndrome (Thyroid disease).** Patients with hypothyroidism can develop macroglossia, menorrhagia, increased cholesterol, muscle aches with increased CPK, infiltration of the carpal tunnel causing carpal tunnel syndrome, and bradycardia. Menorrhagia is caused by decreased estrogen metabolism, leading to increased endometrial proliferation and heavier periods. Hyperthyroidism is associated with increased estrogen metabolism and amenorrhea.

44. **B: Metformin (DM).** Metformin has numerous desirable properties in this patient: It promotes weight loss rather than weight gain, it does not cause hypoglycemia, and it's relatively inexpensive. Insulin and sulfonylureas promote weight gain. Rosiglitazone and pioglitazone are available, but would not be the first choice in this patient because of their substantial cost and concerns for increased cardiac mortality in patients on rosiglitazone.

45. **C: Begin ACEI (DM).** The JNC VII recommends a goal BP of <130/80 mm Hg in patients with DM. Her proteinuria makes an ACEI the initial antihypertensive of choice; it can reduce progression of diabetic nephropathy. The other three treatment options all might be reasonable second-line agents if she needs further BP reduction.

46. **E: Mitral stenosis (Valvular heart disease).** Mitral stenosis causes a diastolic murmur, and as atrial pressure increases, it can result in

increased pulmonary pressure and occasionally hemoptysis. Pregnancy increases total blood volume and accelerates this process. The likely cause of her mitral stenosis is rheumatic fever as a child in Cambodia. Primary pulmonary hypertension does not cause a murmur. Although AR would cause a diastolic murmur, it should be heard best at the right upper sternal border, not the apex. There is no fever to indicate pneumonia. AS would cause a systolic murmur.

47. **B: Contrast head CT (Meningitis).** This patient has a $CD4^+$ count <100, fever, and headache. He is at risk for CNS mass lesions secondary to toxoplasmosis. He should have a contrast CT scan first. If CT scan is negative, he would need LP. He should have diagnostic tests instead of empiric treatments, such as acyclovir or amphotericin.

48. **D: IIB NHL.** Fever and night sweats indicate B symptoms, and disease that is in multiple sites but above the diaphragm is staged as II; this is IIB.

49. **E: Diabetic peripheral neuropathy (Lower extremity).** The nocturnal worsening, decreased vibration and proprioception, and progressive symmetry all support diabetic neuropathy. Normal ABI rules out significant peripheral vascular disease—no edema or plethora to argue for venous obstruction. Nocturnal cramps would be episodic and unilateral. Multiple myeloma may have attendant paraneoplastic neurologic changes, but given his underlying DM and the characteristic pattern, diabetic peripheral neuropathy is the correct answer.

50. **D: Nephrotic syndrome (Lower extremity).** Nephrotic syndrome is a common end pathway for many renal diseases. High protein loss into the urine results in compensatory hepatic production of proteins, including clotting factors. Consequently, venous thromboses are more likely. Laparoscopic cholecystectomy does not result in patient immobility to a significant extent. Prednisone therapy, MI, and asthma do not increase thrombosis risk.

51. **E: Normal chest x-ray (Pulmonary embolism).** This patient presents with dyspnea, pleuritic chest pain, and an elevated JVP suggesting right heart failure after a long plane flight back from Europe. He also has risk factors for coronary heart disease. The top two items in the differential diagnosis should be pulmonary embolism and ischemic heart disease, both of which most often have a normal CXR.

52. **C: 45-year-old with fever and normal neurologic exam (How to perform basic procedures).** Head CT is obtained before LP when a CNS mass lesion is a possibility, as is the case of a 43-year-old woman with a history of breast cancer, an HIV patient with a low $CD4^+$ count (could have toxoplasmosis or CNS lymphoma), or a patient with a seizure who is febrile (CNS abscess). A CT scan also is reasonable in a patient with depressed mental status in whom a full neurologic exam is compromised.

53. **A: Ruptured aneurysm (Informed consent—how to perform basic procedures).** Implied consent is possible only with immediately life-threatening situations. Otherwise, surrogate decision makers must be contacted.

54. **E: Biopsy (Lymphadenopathy).** This patient has a large firm neck mass. He is a smoker, so the possibility of a mouth or pharyngeal cancer is high. He also could have a lymphoma. The best choice would be removal of the mass for diagnosis. An ENT surgeon also would do a careful exam to look for a primary tumor.

55. **C: Admission and pacing (Cardiac arrhythmias).** The patient's history of a syncopal episode is concerning for arrhythmia. His rhythm strip shows complete dissociation between the atrial rhythm (P waves) and ventricular rhythm (QRS complexes). This is third-degree heart block, which requires treatment with a permanent pacemaker.

56. **E: Iron saturation (Heart failure).** Clinically, the patient seems to have heart failure, as seen in his elevated JVP and basilar crackles; this is the likely cause of his dyspnea. Clues to the etiology of his heart failure appear in the form of his hyperglycemia, small testes, hepatomegaly, and diffuse "tan" including areas without sun exposure. All of these together point to hemochromatosis as the most likely underlying problem and iron saturation as the most valuable test.

57. **B: Autosomal recessive (CHF).** Hereditary hemochromatosis (the most common cause of hemochromatosis) is usually the result of a mutation in the *HFE* gene on chromosome 6, with autosomal recessive inheritance. In a U.S. sample, 83% of patients had the same C282Y missense mutation, making genetic testing for hemochromatosis possible.

58. **D: Admission (Ischemic heart disease).** This patient has known CAD and presents with stuttering anginal pain at rest—unstable angina. Unstable angina is a high-risk situation and requires admission for management and possible intervention depending on the patient's preferences and clinical course.

59. **D: Metoprolol (Ischemic heart disease).** Beta blockers have been shown to be of proven mortality benefit after MI. The other medications listed may have symptomatic benefits (amlodipine) or reduce rates of recurrent MI (clopidogrel, warfarin), but the evidence for mortality benefit isn't as strong.

60. **C: Urine metanephrines (Adrenal disorders).** Urine metanephrines are elevated in pheochromocytoma. This is suggested by the labile hypertension, occasional palpitations and sweating, and notable postural hypotension. These all suggest pheochromocytoma. Thyroid, ACTH, and aldosterone aberrations may increase BP, but the BP readings are generally consistent rather than labile. Low potassium can suggest either Cushing's syndrome or hyperaldosteronism, but Cushing's syndrome has exam findings (striae, hirsutism), and both cause consistent, not episodic, hypertension.

61. **B: Cosyntropin stimulation test (Adrenal disorders).** This patient has a clinical presentation consistent with glucocorticoid withdrawal syndrome. The cosyntropin stimulation test would be positive because her adrenals would be atrophic after long courses of exogenous steroids and would be unable to respond appropriately to cosyntropin, a synthetic ACTH analogue.

62. **D: ACTH (Adrenal disorders).** This patient presents with history, physical, and lab findings suggestive of adrenal insufficiency. The hyperpigmentation is helpful because it results from the common precursor of ACTH and MSH, suggesting high ACTH levels and primary adrenal insufficiency. Her history of pernicious anemia and hypothyroidism is suspicious for an autoimmune etiology.

63. **D: Insulin peaking when he is not eating (DM).** This patient is using NPH insulin, which peaks 6–10 hours after it is injected. If patients taking NPH insulin miss meals or their meals are late, the insulin peaks, and they can have hypoglycemic events. Dinnertime NPH peaks hours after eating dinner. If patients eat a lighter than expected dinner, it increases the chance of hypoglycemia.

64. **A: Switch NPH to glargine (DM).** The best way to avoid hypoglycemia owing to insulin peaks is to use a long-acting insulin that doesn't peak. Insulin glargine does not peak, so this would be a good choice. Decreasing his short-acting insulin given with his meals would not solve the problem. Switching to an insulin pump could help the problem, but would not be done before trying a long-acting, nonpeaking insulin such as glargine.

65. **D: Diet, exercise, and statin (Hyperlipidemia).** This patient has two risk factors—hypertension and low high-density lipoprotein cholesterol. The overall 10-year risk for developing CHD is >20%. The most recent NCEP guidelines recommend a target low-density lipoprotein of <100 in patients with 10-year risk >20. Treatment with diet is recommended at any low-density lipoprotein >100 with this 10-year risk, and drug therapy should be used if the low-density lipoprotein cholesterol is >130. A statin would be the best option to lower his low-density lipoprotein from its high level (175).

66. **B: Atorvastatin (Hyperlipidemia).** All of the options offered would likely improve this patient's lipid profile. Statins have been shown to be of benefit in diabetics regardless of their baseline cholesterol, however. Those data, combined with the low-density lipoprotein target of <100 because of her DM, make a statin the best choice.

67. **D: RBC casts (Acute renal failure).** Accompanying hepatitis C infection may be a glomerulonephritis, with resultant RBC casts. Pigmented casts suggest ATN. WBC casts occur with interstitial nephritis. Oxalate and uric acid crystals are not indicators of glomerular disease.

68. **C: Carotid duplex (Neurology).** All of the choices offered are possible options in the evaluation of a patient with an acute stroke. In this

patient with risk factors for atherosclerosis and carotid bruit on exam, the most appropriate place to look first is at her carotids.

69. **B: Amyotrophic lateral sclerosis (Neurology).** The constellation of symptoms in this patient is highly suggestive of amyotrophic lateral sclerosis. Amyotrophic lateral sclerosis is an upper motor neuron disease that results in secondary denervation of skeletal muscles. The relatively denervated motor units are prone to fasciculations, and the loss of upper motor neurons results in hyperreflexia, seen in this patient's up-going toe. Guillain-Barré syndrome and lumbar radiculopathy are isolated to lower motor neurons and should not produce hyperreflexia. Stroke is an upper motor neuron disease, but would be limited to a contiguous distribution in the brain; this patient has swallowing and extremity symptoms, so stroke is unlikely. Multiple sclerosis could present in this way, in theory; however, usually patients with multiple sclerosis have more than just motor involvement, making amyotrophic lateral sclerosis more likely.

70. **A: Start heparin and order CT angiogram (Hypercoagulable states).** This patient has a history that is strongly suggestive of an underlying hypercoagulable state: The presence of SLE, prior spontaneous abortions, and a prior DVT all are suspicious. Her presentation is notable for acute dyspnea, tachycardia, and hypoxemia; her pretest probability of pulmonary embolism is intermediate to high. The appropriate next step is to begin heparin therapy while finalizing the diagnosis. CT pulmonary angiogram is less invasive and more easily obtained than catheter angiography. Thrombolytic therapy is indicated only in patients who are hemodynamically unstable, and inferior vena caval filters should be reserved for patients who cannot be anticoagulated (e.g., trauma with risk of bleeding). A D-dimer would likely be positive, and even if it were negative, it wouldn't be sufficient to exclude PE in this high-risk patient.

71. **C: S1Q3T3 (Pulmonary embolism).** Although pulmonary embolism can cause many "classic" findings, such as right bundle branch block and the "S1Q3T3" right ventricular strain pattern, the most common finding is sinus tachycardia.

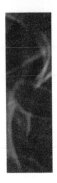

APPENDIX A

Important Drug Side Effects

Symptom	Associated Medications
Constipation	Antihistamines
	Calcium
	Calcium channel blockers (nondihydropyridines > dihydropyridines*)
	Iron
	Narcotics
	TCA
Diarrhea	Antibiotics
	Beta blockers
	Colchicine
	Digoxin
	Magnesium-containing antacids
	Metformin
	Milk of magnesia
	SSRI
Edema	Calcium channel blockers, dihydropyridines
	Estrogen
	NSAID
	Pioglitazone
	Progesterone
	Proton pump inhibitors
	Rosiglitazone
	Testosterone
Urinary retention	Calcium channel blockers
	Sedating antihistamines (diphenhydramine, chlorpheniramine)
	TCA
Confusion	Antidepressants
	Benzodiazepines

(Continued)

H$_2$ blockers
Narcotics
NSAID (rare)
Quinolones
Oxybutinin
Sedating antihistamines
(diphenhydramine,
chlorpheniramine)

*Nondihydropyridines = diltiazem, verapamil. Dihydropyridines = amlodipine, felodipine, nifedipine

Common Drug-related Changes in Electrolytes and Glucose

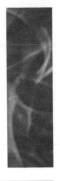

Bicarbonate	
Decreased	NRTI
	Metformin
	Topiramate
Increased	Corticosteroids
	Diuretics (especially thiazides)
Calcium	
Increased	Thiazide diuretics
Glucose	
Increased	Niacin, protease inhibitors, corticosteroids, megestrol
Magnesium	
Decreased	Diuretics, amphotericin B, cisplatin
Potassium	
Decreased	Diuretics—thiazide and loop
	Carboplatin/cisplatin
	Corticosteroids, especially fludrocortisone
	Gentamicin, tobramycin
Increased	ACEI
	Cyclosporine
	NSAID
	Potassium-sparing diuretics
	TMP-SMX
Sodium	
Decreased	ACEI
	Antidepressants (SSRI > TCA)
	Carbamazepine, valproic acid
	Chlorpropamide
	Cyclophosphamide
	Neuroleptics
	Thiazide diuretics
Increased	Lithium (via nephrogenic diabetes insipidus)

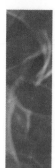

APPENDIX C

Frequently Used Medical Equations

Fractional Excretion of Sodium

$$\text{FeNa} = \text{Cr}^S \times \text{Na}^U / \text{Cr}^U \times \text{Na}^S \times 100$$

Creatinine Clearance

$$\text{CrCl} = (140 - \text{age} \times \text{ideal weight (kg)}/72 \times \text{(serum creatinine)}$$

Osmolal Gap

$$\text{Osm gap} = \text{(measured serum Osm)} - \text{(calculated Osm)}$$

Osmolality

$$\text{Osm} = 2(\text{sodium}) + \text{BUN}/2.8 + \text{glucose}/18$$

Free Water Deficit

$$\text{Free water deficit} = [(\text{serum sodium}/140) - 1] \times 0.6 \times \text{weight(kg)}$$

Alveolar Oxygen Concentration (P_{AO_2})

$$P_{AO_2} = F_{IO_2}(PB - 47) - P_{CO_2}/0.8$$

= approximately 100 at sea level with normal
Where: PB = atmospheric pressure = 760 mm Hg at sea level
F_{IO_2} = fraction of inspired oxygen = 0.21 at sea level
P_{AO_2} = arterial oxygen concentration = blood gas P_{O_2}
P_{CO_2} = arterial carbon dioxide concentration

Alveolar-Arterial Oxygen Gradient (A-a gradient)

$$\text{A-a gradient} = P_{AO_2} - P_{aO_2}$$

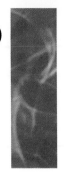

Common Normal Laboratory Test Values

Laboratory Test	Normal Value*
Albumin	3.5-5.2 g/dL
Alkaline phosphatase	38-172 U/L
ALT (SGOT)	10-44 U/L
Amylase	27-144 U/L
Arterial P_{CO_2}	33-48 mm Hg
Arterial pH	7.35-7.45
Arterial P_{O_2}	70-100 mm Hg
AST (SGPT)	11-39 U/L
Bicarbonate (HCO_3^-)	24-31 mEq/L
Bilirubin—direct (conjugated)	0.0-0.3 mg/dL
Bilirubin—indirect (unconjugated)	0.1-0.7 mg/dL
Bilirubin—total	0.1-1 mg/dL
BUN	8-21 mg/dL
Calcium (Ca)	8.9-10.2 mg/dL
Chloride (Cl)	98-108 mEq/L
CPK	30-285 U/L
Creatine (Cr)	0.3-1.2 mg/dL
ESR	0-15 mm/h
Glucose (Glu)	62-125 mg/dL
HCT	36%-45% female, 38%-50% male
LDH	0-190 U/L
Lipase	7-51 U/L
MCV	81-98 fL
Osmolality	280-300 mOsm/kg
Platelets	150,000-400,000/µL
Potassium (K)	3.7-5.2 mEq/L
Sodium (Na)	136-145 mEq/L
Uric acid	2.4-5.7 mg/dL female, 3.4-7 mg/dL male
WBC	4300-10,000/µL

*Normal values for the University of Washington Medical Center Laboratory.

Index

Page numbers followed by an *f*, *t*, or *b* indicate figures, tables and boxed material, respectively.